Medical Radiology

# Diagnostic Imaging

The book series *Medical Radiology – Diagnostic Imaging* provides accurate and up-to-date overviews about the latest advances in the rapidly evolving field of diagnostic imaging and interventional radiology. Each volume is conceived as a practical and clinically useful reference book and is developed under the direction of an experienced editor, who is a world-renowned specialist in the field. Book chapters are written by expert authors in the field and are richly illustrated with high quality figures, tables and graphs. Editors and authors are committed to provide detailed and coherent information in a readily accessible and easy-to-understand format, directly applicable to daily practice.

*Medical Radiology – Diagnostic Imaging* covers all organ systems and addresses all modern imaging techniques and image-guided treatment modalities, as well as hot topics in management, workflow, and quality and safety issues in radiology and imaging. The judicious choice of relevant topics, the careful selection of expert editors and authors, and the emphasis on providing practically useful information, contribute to the wide appeal and ongoing success of the series. The series is indexed in Scopus.

Mariano Scaglione • Cem Çalli
Mario Muto • Stefan Wirth
Editors

# Emergency Radiology of the Head and Spine

Springer

*Editors*
Mariano Scaglione
Department of Medical, Surgical and Experimental Sciences
University of Sassari
Sassari
Italy

Department of Radiology
Pineta Grande Hospital
Castel Volturno
Italy

Department of Radiology
James Cook University Hospital/
Teesside University
Middlesbrough
UK

Mario Muto
Neuroradiology Department
Cardarelli Hospital
Naples
Italy

Cem Çalli
Department of Radiology
Ege University Medical School
Izmir
Turkey

Stefan Wirth
Department of Radiology and Nuclear Medicine
Schwarzwald-Baar Hospital
Villingen-Schwenningen
Germany

ISSN 0942-5373 ISSN 2197-4187 (electronic)
Medical Radiology
ISSN 2731-4677 ISSN 2731-4685 (electronic)
Diagnostic Imaging

ISBN 978-3-030-91046-4 ISBN 978-3-030-91047-1 (eBook)
https://doi.org/10.1007/978-3-030-91047-1



This Springer imprint is published by the registered company Springer Nature Switzerland AG
The registered company address is: Gewerbestrasse 11, 6330 Cham, Switzerland

**Mariano Scaglione:**
*This book is dedicated to my sons Peter and Ruben and my love Teresa!*

**Cem Çalli:**
*I dedicate my work to my beloved wife Basak and my lovely daughters Ece and Cemre.*

**Mario Muto:**
*This book is dedicated to my wife Olga and my sons Alessandra and Gianluca for their daily support to my work!*

# Preface

Emergency Radiology of the Head and Spine is a complex topic involving not only specialists and experts in neuroscience but quite often involving radiologists in the front line in peripheral hospitals, without support by neuro-specialists.

More and more MR units are going to be installed worldwide considering the importance of this diagnostic technology not only for elected patients but very often in emergency too.

This book, which is the last book of trilogy (*Emergency Radiology of the Abdomen, Emergency Radiology of the Chest and Cardiovascular System*), has the ambition to become the first-line support for all colleagues in neuroscience departments and for those in peripheral hospitals needing suggestions for diagnostic decisions, important to manage acute clinical condition and to decide about the best treatment for our patients.

We want to thank all the co-authors for their support and book chapters authors; they all did a fantastic work making this book a great support for our daily work!


Sassari, IT — Mariano Scaglione
Izmir, TR — Cem Çalli
Naples, IT — Mario Muto
Villingen-Schwenningen, DE — Stefan Wirth

# Contents

# Part I

# Brain: Traumatic Emergent Injuries (M. Muto, IT – P Vilela, Portugal – S. Wirth, DE)

# Imaging of Cranial and Facial Fractures

Mehmet Ruhi Onur, Ilkay Idilman, and Erhan Akpinar

## Contents



M. R. Onur (✉) · I. Idilman · E. Akpinar
Faculty of Medicine, Department of Radiology,
Hacettepe University, Ankara, Turkey



M. Scaglione et al. (eds.), *Emergency Radiology of the Head and Spine*,
Medical Radiology Diagnostic Imaging, https://doi.org/10.1007/978-3-030-91047-1_1

**Abstract**

Craniofacial fractures represent one of the most frequent encountered emergency settings after motor vehicle accidents, assaults, fall, or other trauma types. Appropriate management of patients with craniofacial fractures depends on a comprehensive assessment of imaging findings including fracture sites, patterns, and associated injuries. Computed tomography is the mainstay imaging technique in craniofacial fractures with its superiorities including thin-section image acquisition and multiplanar and three-dimensional image generation capability. Decision of treatment method and preoperative planning necessitates assessment of imaging features according to current classifications of maxillofacial fractures. Cranial fractures should be evaluated with accompanying intracranial injuries. Maxillofacial fractures manifest with imaging features that usually represent injury mechanism and disruption of facial buttresses. Management of patients with craniofacial fractures can be accomplished by multidisciplinary approach including assessment of imaging features and decision of treatment method to prevent further complications.

## 1 Introduction

Craniofacial skeleton is formed by multiple articulating bones, which encase critical anatomical structures including the brain and sensorineural organs such as eye, ear, and olfactory system. Craniofacial fractures may result from blunt or penetrating traumas including motor vehicle and pedestrian accidents, work, and sport-related accidents, falls, and assaults. Primary imaging technique in craniofacial trauma is computed tomography (CT) due to its capability of fast imaging, thin-section (submillimeter) acquisition, easy patient positioning and multiplanar reconstruction (MPR), and three-dimensional (3D) reconstruction facilities. 3D post-processing techniques including surface-shaded display (SSD) and volume rendering (VR) have been widely used in craniofacial fractures. Cinematic rendering (CR) is a novel 3D post-processing CT technique that enables to generate more photo-realistic representations of the human body by using different lightmaps from CT or magnetic resonance imaging (MRI) datasets (Fig. 1) (Dappa et al. 2016). Awareness of imaging findings, anatomical key points, and classifications of fractures is necessary for comprehensive assessment of craniofacial fractures. Appropriate management of craniofacial fractures necessitates assessment of fracture patterns, classifications, and implications for preoperative planning.

## 2 Cranium

The cranium is a bony structure formed by calvarium (dome-like superior portion of the cranium) and skull base (floor of the cranium). Cranial bones are separated from each other by cranial sutures. The frontal and occipital bones are also included in the calvarial bones and contribute to the skull base skeleton with their horizontally oriented portions. In this section, cranial fractures including squamous part of frontal bone and parietal and occipital bones are presented. Frontal sinus fractures are mentioned in maxillofacial skeleton section since frontal sinus fractures are usually encountered with the fractures of facial skeleton.

### 2.1 Calvarium

The calvarium is formed by the squamous (superior) portion of the frontal bone anteriorly, parietal bones laterally, and the occipital bone posteriorly. Frontal bone is a smooth, broad, and a bowl-shaped bone that surrounds the anterior cranial fossa. Frontal bone is divided into vertical (squamous) and horizontal (orbital) parts. Squamous part of the frontal bone forms the skeletal part of forehead, while orbital part forms the thin roofs of the orbits. Frontal bones articulate with two parietal bones via the coronal suture and

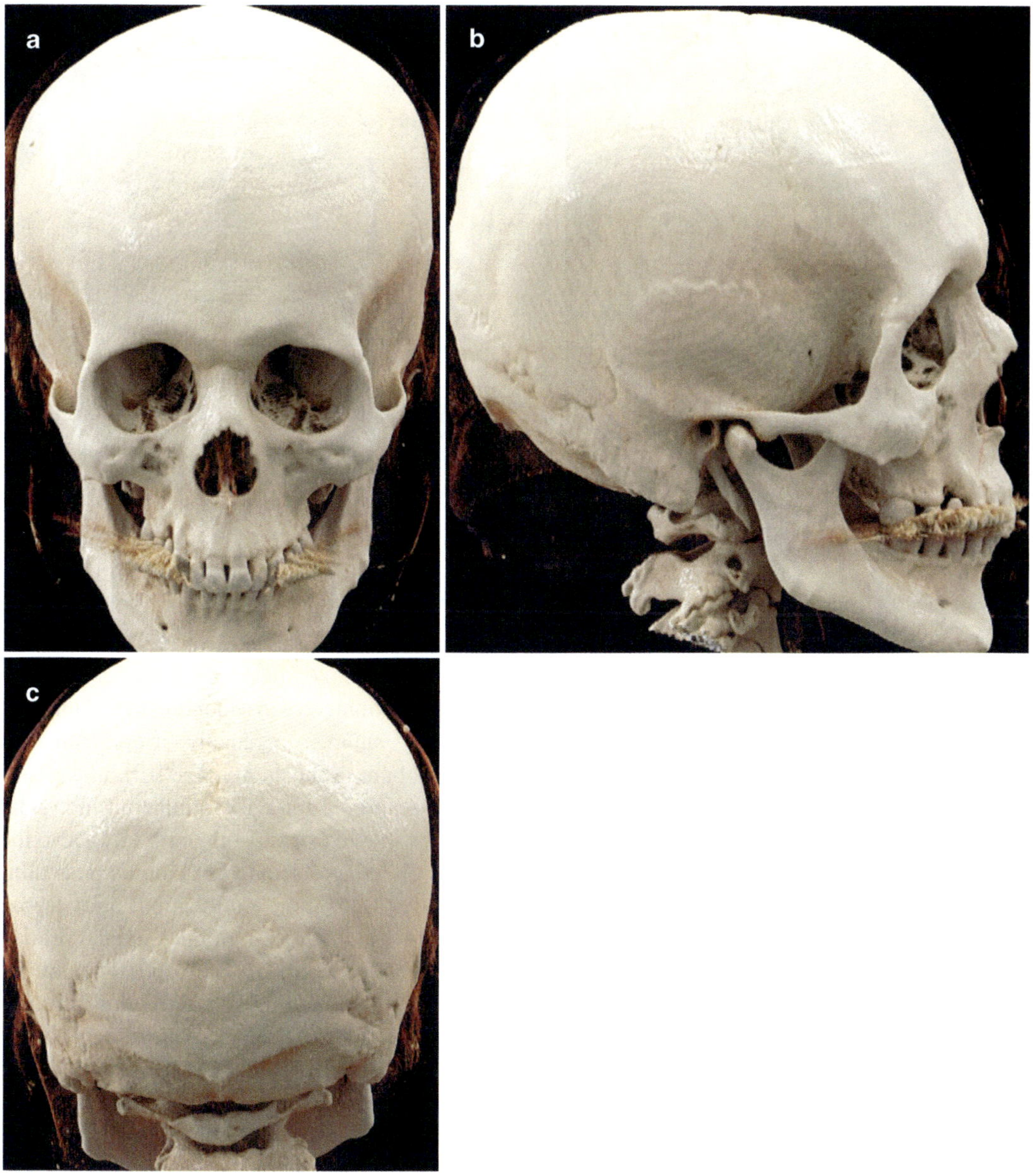


**Fig. 1** CR images of cranium. Anterior (**a**), lateral (**b**), and posterior (**c**) view of cranium on CR images

with nasal bones at the frontonasal suture. Zygomatic, lacrimal, ethmoid, and sphenoid bones constitute other cranial bones, which articulate with the frontal bone. In infants, the halves of the frontal squama are divided by the metopic suture, which is not visible after the age of 6. A remnant of the metopic suture may be visible in 8% of adults and mimic fracture on radiographs (Fig. 2) (Zdilla et al. 2018).

Parietal bones are smooth convex bones, which form superior and lateral aspect of the calvarium. Two parietal bones join in the midline via the sagittal suture. Lambdoid suture is located between parietal bones and occipital bone. Other bony structures that articulate with parietal bones are temporal bones and greater wings of the sphenoid bone. An accessory suture named as intraparietal or sub-sagittal suture in the parietal bone

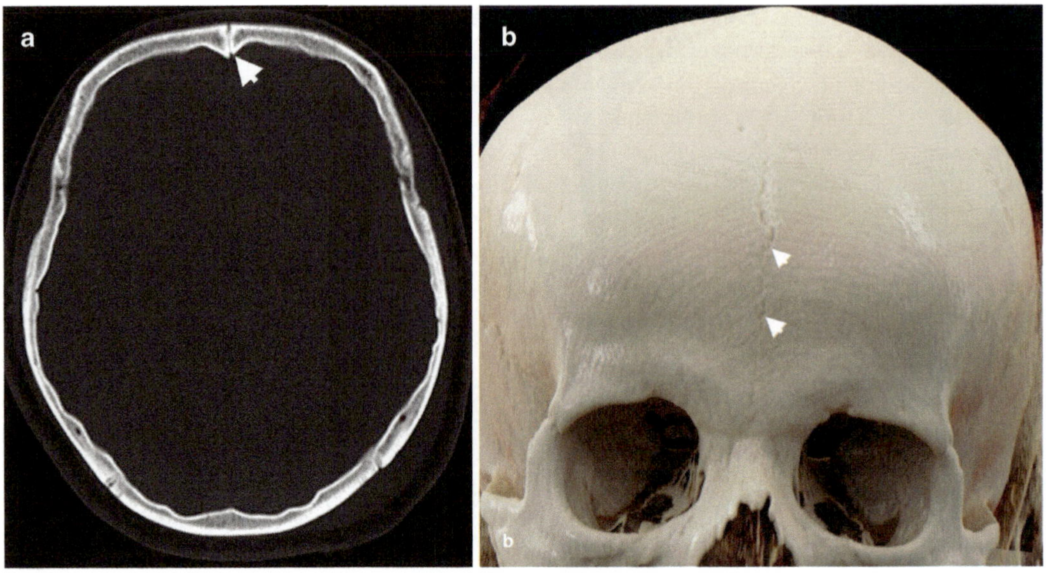


**Fig. 2** Metopic suture. Axial CT (**a**) and CR (**b**) images of a 54-year-old woman demonstrate a metopic suture (arrowheads) in the midline extending from bregma to the nasion

may mimic a linear fracture on radiographs (Sanchez et al. 2010).

Occipital bone forms the posterior and inferior parts of the calvarium. Occipital bones articulate with first cervical vertebrae via occipital condyles. Persistent occipital suture that extends from the dorsal aspect of the foramen magnum may mimic occipital fracture. This accessory suture has been shown not to extend more than 2 cm from the edge of the foramen magnum (Sanchez et al. 2010). A longer fissure in the same location represents a fracture.

## 2.2 Imaging Techniques

Primary imaging modality in the diagnosis of craniofacial fractures is CT. Although plain film radiography is not primarily used in craniofacial fractures, familiarity with radiographic imaging features of craniofacial fractures may be helpful in emergency settings. Skull fractures can be evaluated on radiographs obtained at anteroposterior (A-P) and lateral views of the skull. Occipital fractures can be depicted at the Towne view. The assessment of cranial fractures on radiographs can be difficult in children due to the presence of numerous synchondroses and unusual accessory sutures, especially in parietal and occipital bones (Sanchez et al. 2010).

The scan area for CT examination in cranial fractures should extend from the skull base to the vertex. CT images should be acquired with thin-section ($\leq$1.25 mm) collimation and reconstructed with at least 2-mm-thick axial, coronal, and sagittal images. CT images should be reviewed at bone and soft-tissue window settings. Bone window setting enhances the margins of the bony cortex and provides the ability to depict localization and extension of cranial fractures, while scalp injuries and intracranial injuries such as extra-axial and intracranial hemorrhages and parenchymal injuries can be detected at soft-tissue window setting.

## 2.3 Cranial Fractures and Imaging Features

Cranial fractures may be caused by blunt or penetrating trauma. Blunt trauma usually occurs as motor vehicle accidents (MVA), falls, and assaults, whereas penetrating trauma consists of gunshot injury, stabbing, and impalement

(Hijaz et al. 2011). Frontal bone fractures, being the most frequent calvarial bone fracture, occur in 37% of all cranial fractures (Pappachan and Alexander 2006). Blow effects of trauma in parietal and occipital bones are usually minimized secondary to the distribution of impact force through the convexity of these bones. Cranial fractures can manifest as linear (nondisplaced and most frequent form), depressed, diastatic, and comminuted (fragmentation into multiple parts) forms. Linear fractures are characterized by separation of bone edges without displacement. Depressed fracture is defined as displacement of fracture segment deeper than the uninvolved skull. Comminuted fracture is defined as fragmentation of involved calvarial bone into multiple parts and radiation of multiple linear fractures from the point of impact through areas of weakness.

Cranial fractures manifest on radiographs as radiolucent line or depressed osseous fragments (Fig. 3). CT images at bone window setting reveal linear fracture as separation of bone portions with non-sclerotic edges (Fig. 4). Depressed fractures present as displacement of fracture fragment from the uninvolved skull (Fig. 5). Diastatic fracture refers to fracture type that follows a cranial suture and causes widening of the suture (Fig. 6). Comminuted cranial fractures are characterized by multiple fracture fragments with more significant fracture displacement (Fig. 7). In infants and children, cranial fractures more commonly present as diastatic fractures that may also manifest as growing fractures secondary to herniation of cerebrospinal fluid (CSF) or brain parenchyma into the subcutaneous tissue through the relevant dural tear (Mulroy et al. 2012). In children, plain film radiographs demonstrate growing fractures as persistent diastatic fracture enlarging on follow-up imaging. Cross-sectional imaging techniques can demonstrate extension of intracranial tissue or a leptomeningeal cyst between the edges of the growing fracture (Fig. 8) (Carter and Anslow 2009). Differentiation between cranial sutures

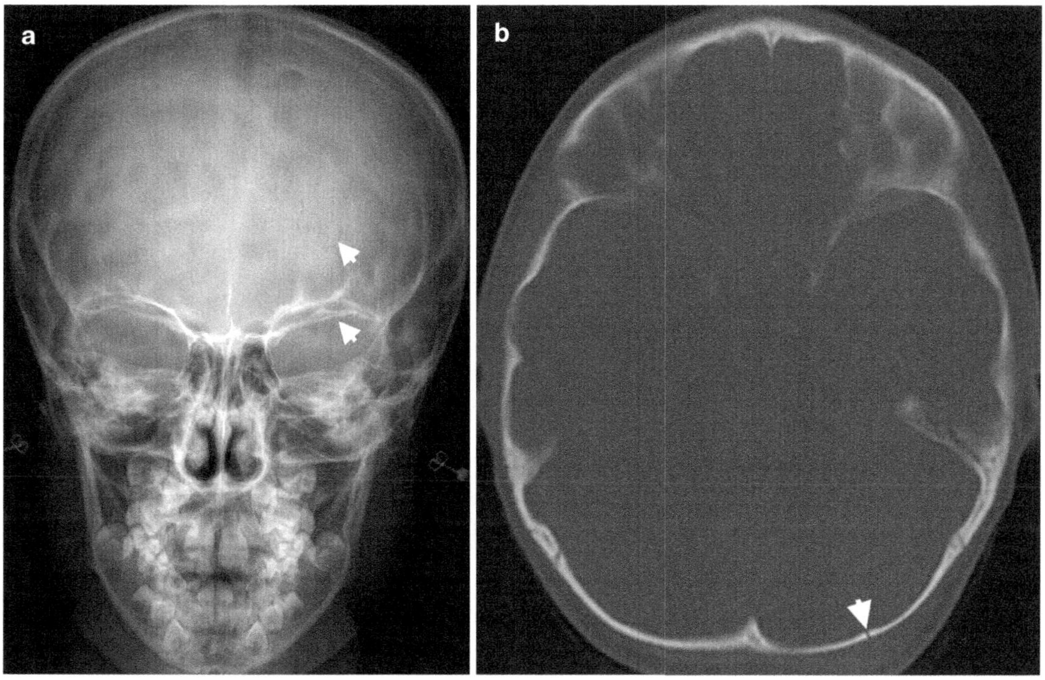


**Fig. 3** Linear fracture in occipital bone. (**a**) A-P view of skull radiograph of a 6-year-old female patient presented to emergency department after fall reveals a unilateral linear vertically extending radiolucency (arrowheads) in left side of occipital bone. (**b**) Axial CT image confirms the presence of linear fracture (arrowhead) in the occipital bone

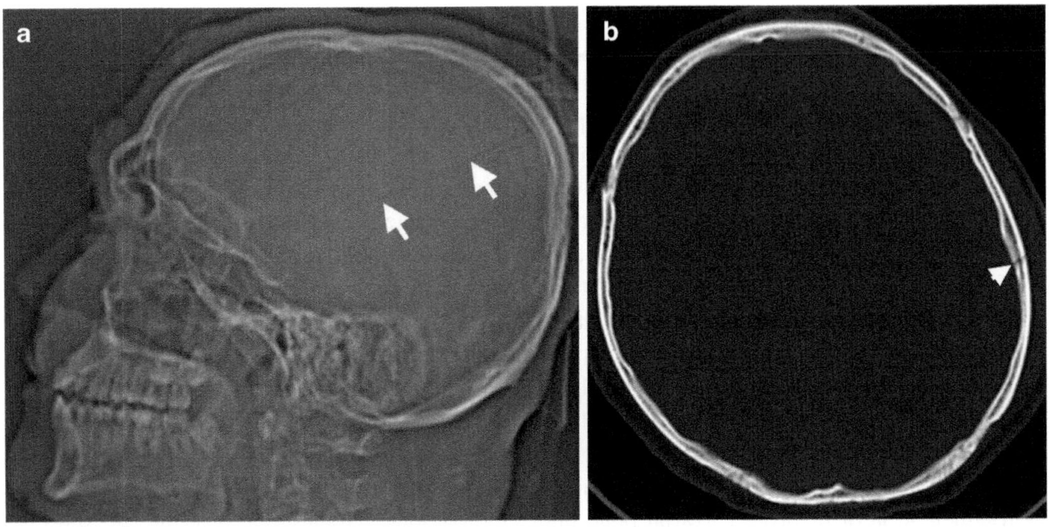


**Fig. 4** Linear fracture in parietal bone. (**a**) Scenogram image reveals fracture as radiolucent line extending through temporal and parietal bones (short arrows). (**b**) Axial CT image of the same patient demonstrates linear fracture (arrowhead) in parietal bone

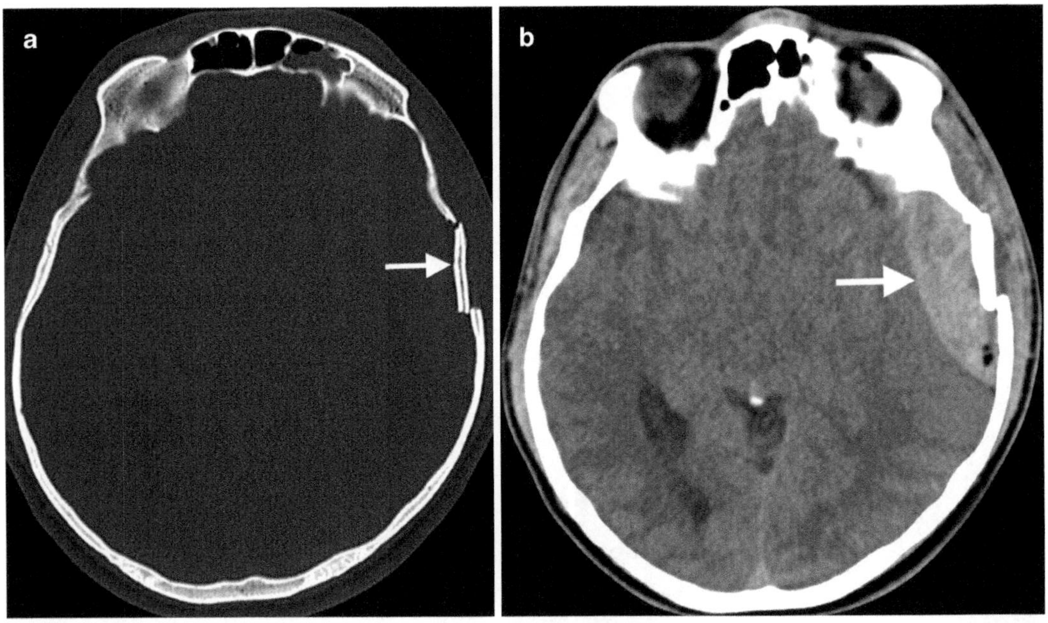


**Fig. 5** Depressed fracture in temporal bone. (**a**) Axial CT image on bone window shows a depressed temporal bone fracture characterized by displacement of fracture fragment (arrow) from the uninvolved temporal bone part. (**b**) Axial CT image on soft-tissue window demonstrates accompanying epidural hemorrhage (arrow) resulting from depressed fracture

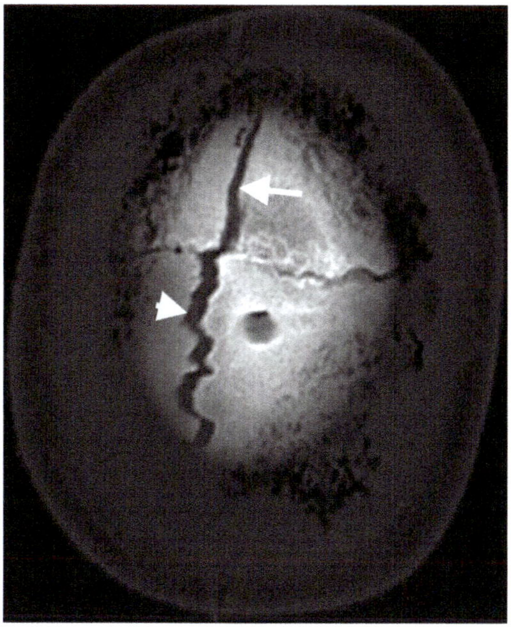

**Fig. 6** Cranial fracture with diastasis of neighboring suture. Axial CT image shows linear fracture (arrow) in the vertex that extends from the frontal bone and results in diastasis of the sagittal suture (arrowhead)

and fractures on plain radiographs and CT is crucial for avoiding misdiagnosis (Table 1). Non-depressed fractures in cranial bones appear as sharp lucencies with non-sclerotic edges, while accessory sutures present as radiolucent lines with irregular interdigitations, also known as zigzag pattern, and sclerotic borders (Fig. 9). Cranial fractures usually manifest with adjacent soft-tissue swelling indicating a scalp hemorrhage or edema. Widening of fracture line as it extends to the suture or synchondrosis is another helpful feature in depicting fracture. Cranial fractures resulting from high-impact trauma can cross suture lines in contrast to accessory sutures, which join with the major suture (Sanchez et al. 2010). Accessory sutures often present bilaterally and fairly symmetric in appearance, especially in the parietal bones (Weir et al. 2006). Skull fractures caused by high-energy trauma may also occur bilaterally; however, bilateral skull fractures almost always appear as comminuted and depressed fractures with marked asymmetry due

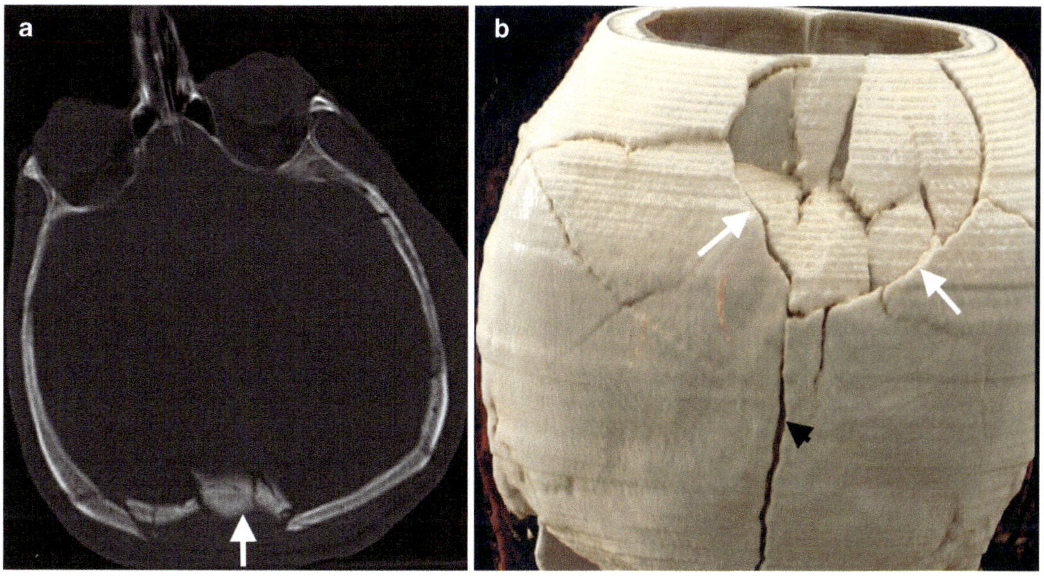


**Fig. 7** Comminuted fracture in cranium. (**a**) Axial CT image of a 58-year-old male patient reveals comminuted fracture (arrow) of occipital bone, and (**b**) CR image shows comminuted fracture (arrows) in the occipitoparietal bone. A linear fracture (black arrowhead) is radiating from the comminuted fracture extending through the occipital bone

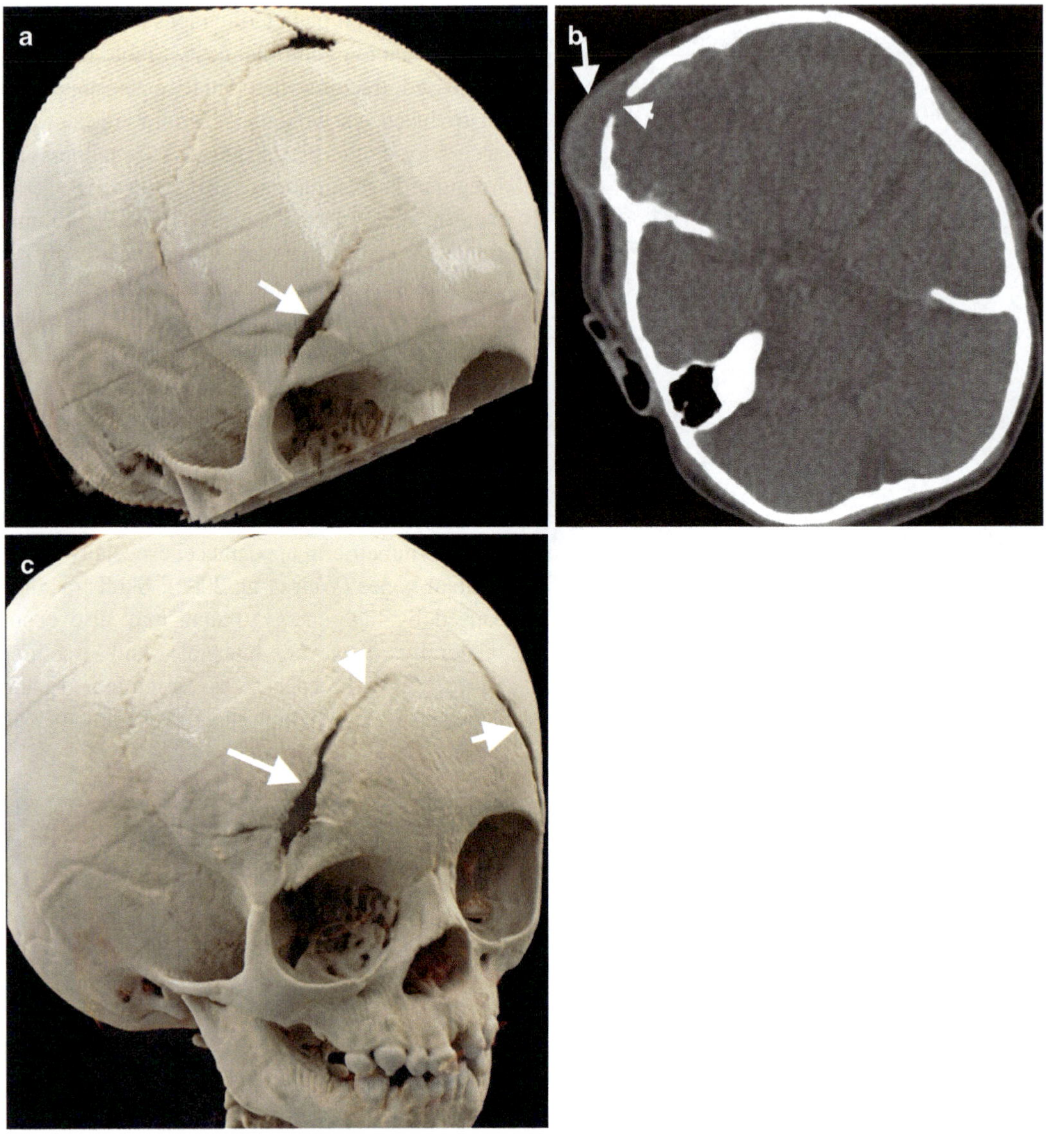


**Fig. 8** Growing fracture. (**a**) CR image of a 1-year-old child shows a fracture in right frontal bone with separated bony edges (arrow). (**b**) Axial image of follow-up CT performed 1-month after initial CT demonstrates a low attenuated fluid collection (arrow) representing leptomeningeal cyst herniating from the scalp through fracture defect (arrowhead). (**c**) CR image of follow-up CT reveals increased distance between the bony edges of right frontal fracture (long arrow and arrowhead) with accompanying left frontal fracture (short arrow)

to the underlying high-energy impact (Sanchez et al. 2010). Vascular or peripheral nerve grooves should also be distinguished from linear fractures. Well-corticated margins, decreased sharpness, and asymmetric extension of the grooves created by neurovascular structures may be helpful to distinguish vascular grooves in cranial bones from linear fractures.

Linear, depressed, and comminuted fractures of cranium can cause extra-axial hemorrhage when they cross vessel grooves such as those encompassing the middle meningeal artery or dural venous sinuses. Venous injuries may also result in thrombosis of the veins leading to venous infarction. Parietal bone fractures may cause injuries in the parietal branch of middle

**Table 1** Imaging features for differentiation between cranial fracture and suture (Sanchez et al. 2010)

| Cranial fracture | Cranial suture |
|---|---|
| Linear radiolucency with sharp edges | Extends with zigzag pattern |
| Non-sclerotic edges | Sclerotic edges |
| Often associated with diastasis of suture | No associated diastasis |
| Widens as approaching to suture | Joins adjacent suture |
| May cross adjacent suture lines | No crossing suture lines |
| Usually unilateral, asymmetric if bilateral | Often bilateral, fairly symmetric (accessory sutures) |
| Soft-tissue swelling (subgaleal hematoma, scalp hematoma) | No soft-tissue swelling |

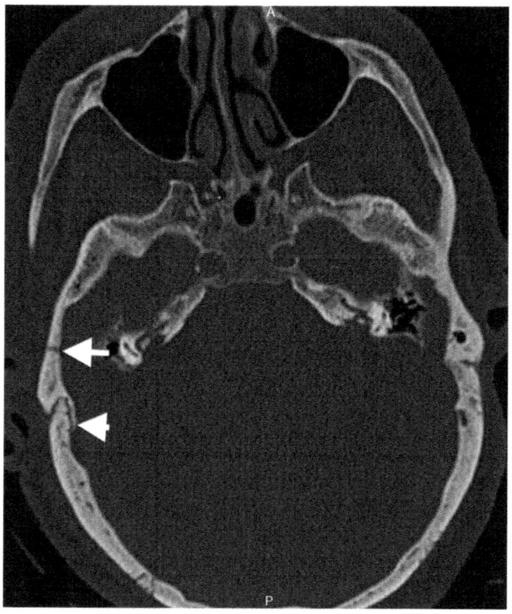


**Fig. 9** Cranial fracture and suture. Axial CT image at bone window shows a linear fracture in right temporal bone with sharp and non-sclerotic edges (arrow) nearby occipitomastoid suture, which manifests with interdigitating appearance and sclerotic edges (arrowhead)

meningeal artery and veins. Frontal branch of the middle meningeal artery may also be injured since this vessel traverses the underlying anterior part of the parietal bone superior to the pterion where four cranial bones (frontal, parietal, sphenoid, and temporal bones) articulate. Parietal bone fractures may damage the parietal branch of superficial temporal artery and posterior auricular artery in the scalp. Occipital bone fractures may cause injury to the transverse sinus, confluence of sinuses, and caudal portion of superior sagittal sinus (Fig. 10).

Dural tears and arachnoid tears may occur as an immediate consequence of calvarial fractures. Dural tears can result in subdural hygroma and CSF leakage, which may present as rhinorrhea or otorrhea depending on the location of the dural tear. Arachnoid tears may also cause subdural hygroma formation (Hijaz et al. 2011).

## 3 Temporal Bone

### 3.1 Anatomy

Temporal bone forms inferolateral aspect of lateral calvarial vault and contributes to the skull base skeleton. Temporal bone articulates with occipital bone posteriorly, parietal bone superiorly, and greater wing of the sphenoid bone anteriorly. Temporal bone contains five distinct portions as squamous, mastoid, petrous, tympanic part, and styloid process. Squamous part of the temporal bone is the thinnest and weakest part of calvarial bones that contains the posterior zygomatic process and anterior part of the mandibular fossa. Mastoid portion includes mastoid air cells and connects to epitympanum via aditus ad antrum. Skull base part of temporal bone constitutes petrous and mastoid portions. Tympanic part divides into epitympanum, mesotympanum, and hypotympanum. Mesotympanum encloses ossicles named as malleus, incus, and stapes, which articulate with each other via incudomalleal and incudostapedial joints. Tympanic portion is separated from external auditory canal (EAC) by tympanic membrane. The boundaries of middle ear consist of tympanic membrane laterally, inner ear medially, tegmen tympani superiorly,

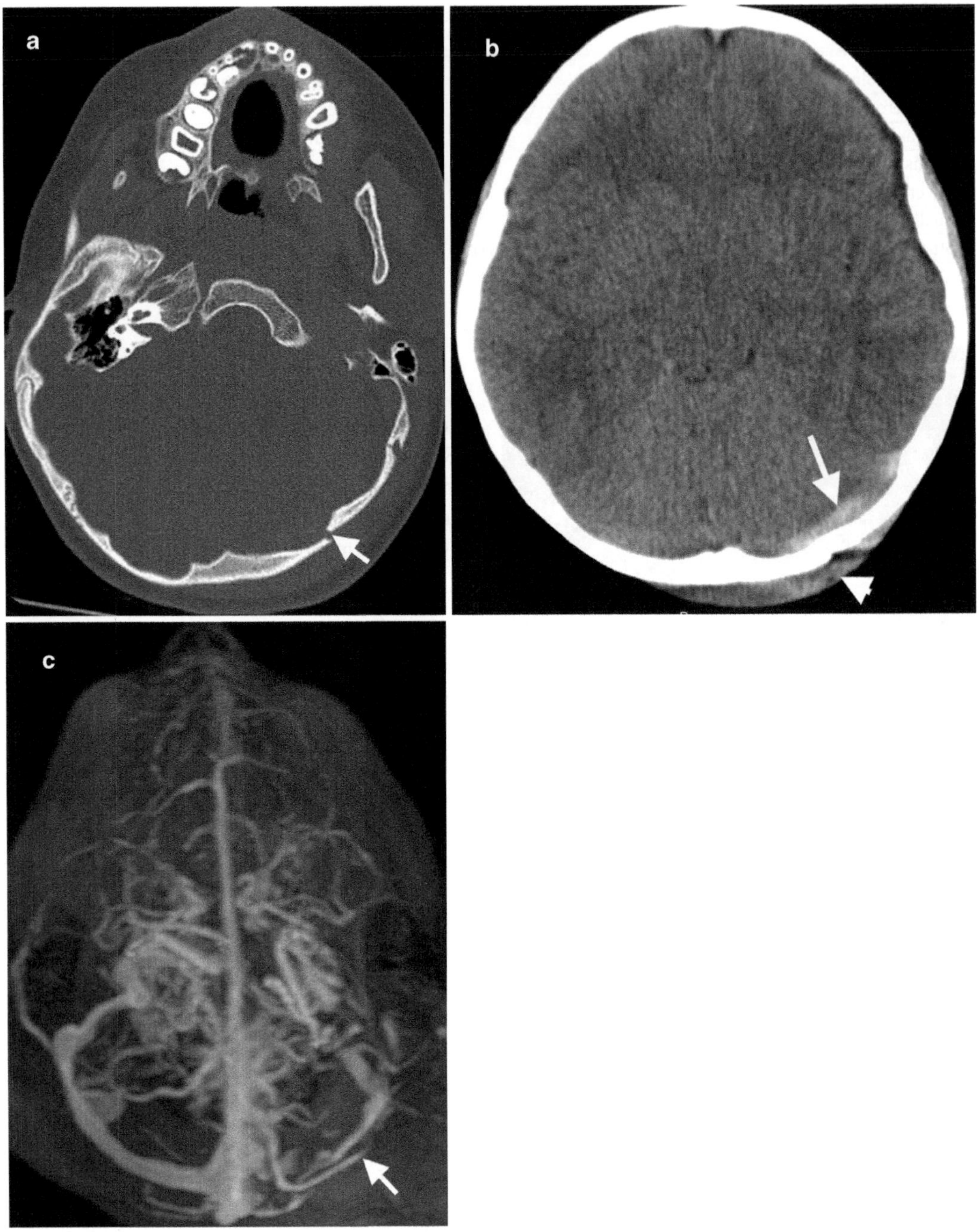

**Fig. 10** Cranial fracture resulting in venous sinus thrombosis. (**a**) Axial CT image of a 5-year-old boy demonstrates a depressed fracture (arrow) in left occiput. (**b**) Axial CT image at soft-tissue window shows increased density in left transverse sinus trajectory (arrow) suggestive of sinus thrombosis. A scalp hematoma (arrowhead) can be seen as an accompanying imaging feature at the fracture site. (**c**) MR venography reveals thrombosis of the left transverse sinus with loss of blood flow signal in the sinus (arrow)

and jugular wall inferiorly. Petrous portion of the temporal bone contains inner ear that is comprised of cochlea, vestibule, and semicircular canals within the osseous labyrinth. Osseous labyrinth is surrounded by the otic capsule, which is the densest part of the temporal bone. Carotid

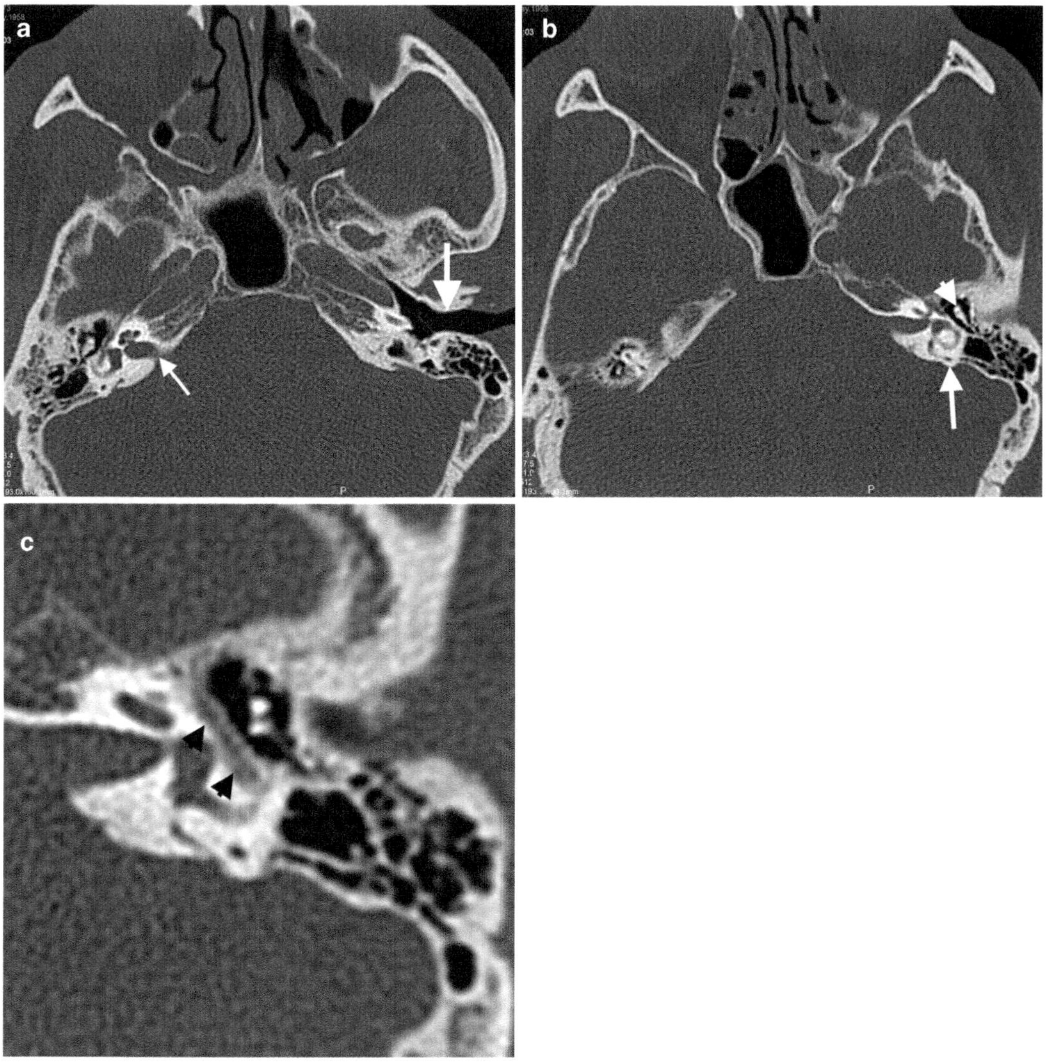


**Fig. 11** Temporal bone anatomy. (**a**) Axial CT image at bone window demonstrates left EAC (thick arrow) and right inner ear (thin arrow). (**b**) Ice cream appearance of incudomalleal complex (arrowhead) in tympanic portion and otic capsule (arrow) in the left temporal bone. Ice cream scoop and cone represent malleolar head and short process of the incus, respectively. (**c**) Axial CT image shows tympanic segment of facial canal (black arrowheads) coursing medial to the left middle air

canal is located posteriorly to the petrous ridge of temporal bone.

Facial nerve traverses the temporal bone from its inferolateral portion to the superomedial portion. Integrity of facial nerve can be assessed on CT by visualizing the facial canal. Facial nerve has different portions in the temporal bone called according to temporal bone portions as labyrinthine, mastoid, and tympanic segments (Fig. 11) (Juliano et al. 2013).

## 3.2 Fractures

Temporal bone fractures constitute 18–22% of skull fractures occurred secondary to major head traumas (Cannon and Jahrsdoerfer 1983). A substantial force (at least 1875 lb) is required for fracture of the temporal bone that indicates high probability of concomitant cranial bone fractures (Tress et al. 2014). Clinical signs and symptoms of temporal bone fractures include hemorrhagic

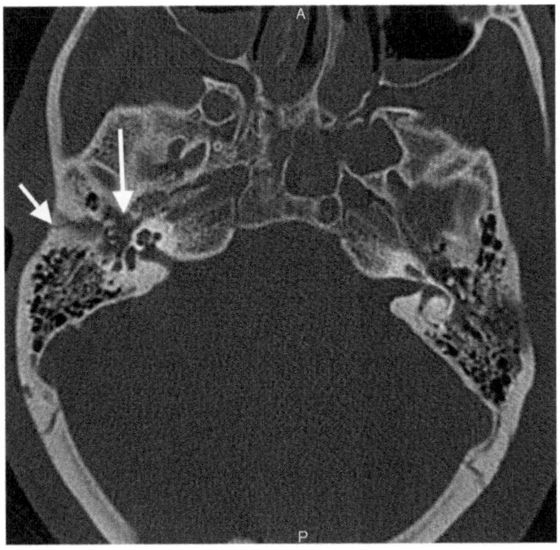


**Fig. 12** Hemotympanum. Axial head CT image demonstrates a linear fracture (short arrow) in the right temporal bone with hemotympanum (long arrow)

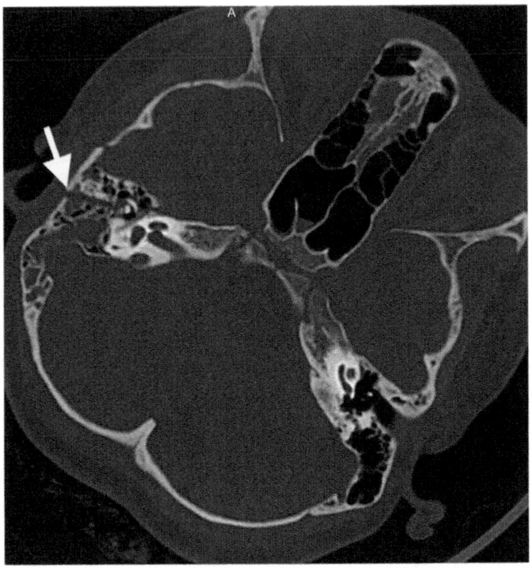


**Fig. 13** Longitudinal temporal bone fracture. Axial CT image of a 10-year-old girl after MVA reveals a longitudinal fracture (arrow) extending parallel to the orientation of petrous ridge of right temporal bone with separated fracture fragments

otorrhea, tympanic membrane perforation, vertigo, hearing loss, and facial nerve palsy (Juliano et al. 2013). Fractures traversing the mastoid portion can result in "Battle sign" (postauricular ecchymosis) due to traumatic rupture of the mastoid emissary vein (Watanabe and Kida 2012). CT examination in temporal bone fractures should be performed with slice thickness ≤1 mm and field of view (FOV) <10 cm. Additional evaluation with MPR images including coronal plane, Stenvers view (oblique coronal orientation parallel to the petrous ridge), and Pöschl view (oblique coronal orientation perpendicular to the petrous ridge) may be helpful for acquisition of CT images parallel to orientation of ossicles and facial nerve. As head trauma is often assessed with head CT, it may be helpful to know imaging findings of temporal bone fractures on head CT. Head CT findings that may be associated with temporal bone fractures include EAC, tympanic cavity and mastoid air cell opacification, air within the temporomandibular joint, intracranial air adjacent to the temporal bone, and pneumolabyrinth (Fig. 12) (Kennedy et al. 2014).

Temporal bone fractures are traditionally classified as longitudinal, transverse, or mixed according to their orientation relative to the long axis of the petrous pyramid. Mixed fractures refer to fracture types occurring in both transverse and longitudinal planes. Longitudinal fractures constitute 50–80% of temporal bone fractures and extend parallel to the long axis of the petrous pyramid (Fig. 13) (Little and Kesser 2006; Nosan et al. 1997; Ishman and Friedland 2004). This fracture type usually begins from squamosal portion of temporal bone, extends along the posterosuperior border of the EAC bony margin, and exits in middle cranial fossa anterior to the labyrinth (Juliano et al. 2013). Longitudinal fractures may also extend into jugular fossa, carotid canal, and facial canal. Ossicular injuries and tympanic membrane perforation are usually associated with longitudinal fractures. Ossicular dislocation and hemotympanum occur in 32% and 90% of patients, respectively (Meriot et al. 1997). Transverse fractures are oriented perpendicular to the axis of the petrous pyramid and traverse the temporal bone in superoinferior orientation. Transverse fractures usually result from fronto-occipital impacts and may occur laterally through the cochlea or vestibule or medially through the internal acoustic canal (IAC) and petrous pyramid (Collins et al. 2012). Although transverse fractures occur at a frequency of one third to one fifth to that of longitudinal fractures, the probability of facial nerve injury, which can occur in 7% of patients in this type of injury, increases its clinical importance (Brodie and Thompson 1997). Cochlear nerve injury can also occur secondary to transverse fractures that involve the IAC apex. Oblique fractures that refer to coexistence of both longitudinal and transverse fractures are found approximately 10–75% of patients in previous studies (Dahiya et al. 1999; Ghorayeb and Yeakley 1992; Juliano et al. 2013; Little and Kesser 2006; Nosan et al. 1997; Ishman and Friedland 2004).

Although traditional classification depending on fracture orientation in temporal bone as longitudinal, transverse, or mixed type is widely used, it was shown that there is no satisfying correlation between this classification system with clinical outcomes and further complications. Thereby, several investigators recommended different classification systems that classify temporal bone fractures according to the involved portions of temporal bone such as petrous and non-petrous types or otic capsule-spared or violated type. Petrous fractures involve the petrous apex and otic capsule, while non-petrous fractures involve the middle ear and mastoid portion (Ishman and Friedland 2004). Complications of petrous fracture group include facial nerve injury, CSF leak, and sensorineural hearing loss. Involvement of ossicular chain in non-petrous group causes increased incidence of conductive hearing loss (CHL). Temporal bone fracture classification regarding involvement of otic capsule is mainly focused on clinical outcome. The most common injury type according to this classification system is otic capsule-sparing form that occurs in 94–97% of patients resulting from temporoparietal blow. This form causes CHL due to ossicular injury. The other form, otic capsule-violating fracture, occurs in 3–6% of cases and usually results from occipital blow. This type has a high association with facial nerve injury (30–50%), sensorineural hearing loss, and CSF fistula (Juliano et al. 2013). High spatial resolution CT examinations with MPR images can demonstrate the involvement of vestibule, vestibular aqueduct, semicircular canals, cochlea, and/or facial canal in otic capsule-violating fractures (Juliano et al. 2013).

Temporal bone fractures may cause various complications including tympanic membrane perforation, ossicular chain derangement, injury of vestibulocochlear apparatus, facial nerve and vessels, CSF leakage, and meningitis. Traumatic CHL, being the most common complication with an occurrence rate of 24–81% following temporal bone trauma, can result from massive hemorrhage in EAC, tympanic membrane perforation, hemotympanum, and derangement of the ossicular chain (Kennedy et al. 2014; Dahiya et al. 1999; Brodie and Thompson 1997; Nosan et al. 1997; Rafferty et al. 2006). Ossicular injuries include fractures of the malleus, incus, or stapes, dislocation or subluxation of incudomalleolar, incudostapedial, and/or stapediovestibular joint, and disruption of the suspensory ligaments of the ossicles (Meriot et al. 1997; Yetiser et al. 2008). Ossicular injuries may be caused by direct traumatic forces or associated with simultaneous contraction of the stapedius and tensor tympani muscles after trauma (Basson and van Lierop 2009; Swartz 2001). Longitudinal fractures that extend into the middle ear more often cause ossicular injury compared to transverse fractures (Kennedy et al. 2014). The most frequently injured ossicle in the middle ear is incus, which has the weakest ligamentous support in the tympanic cavity. Mild separation of ossicles in ossicular joints is named as subluxation, while frank separation is called as dislocation. Total incus dislocation may also occur and presents on CT as absence of incus in its normal position and displacement within the incuidal fossa or not found at all (Swartz 2001). Incudomalleolar joint normally appears as an ice cream configuration on axial CT sections. In this configuration, the ice cream scoop and cone represent malleolar head and short process of incus, respectively (Fig. 11b). Any widening of incudomalleolar joint space or any offset of the malleus head relative to the incus indicate incudomalleolar subluxation since interface between these ossicles should be very thin (Fig. 14) (Collins et al. 2012). Incudomalleolar dislocation is characterized by

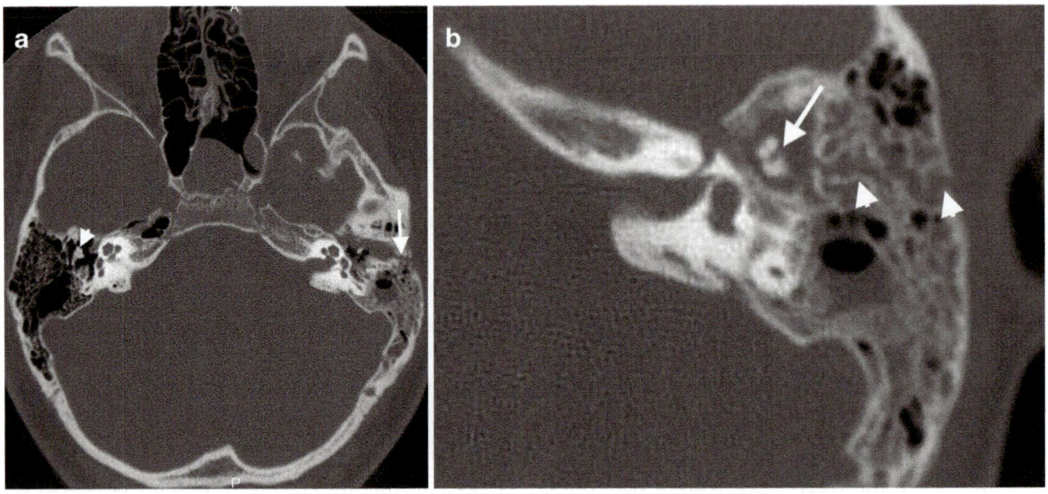

**Fig. 14** Incudomalleolar subluxation in a 17-year-old man after MVA. (**a**) Axial CT image shows a longitudinal fracture (arrow) in the left temporal bone. Normal ice cream cone appearance (arrowhead) is shown on the right temporal bone. (**b**) Axial CT image of the same patient demonstrates longitudinal fracture (arrowheads) associated with widening of incudomalleolar joint space (arrow)

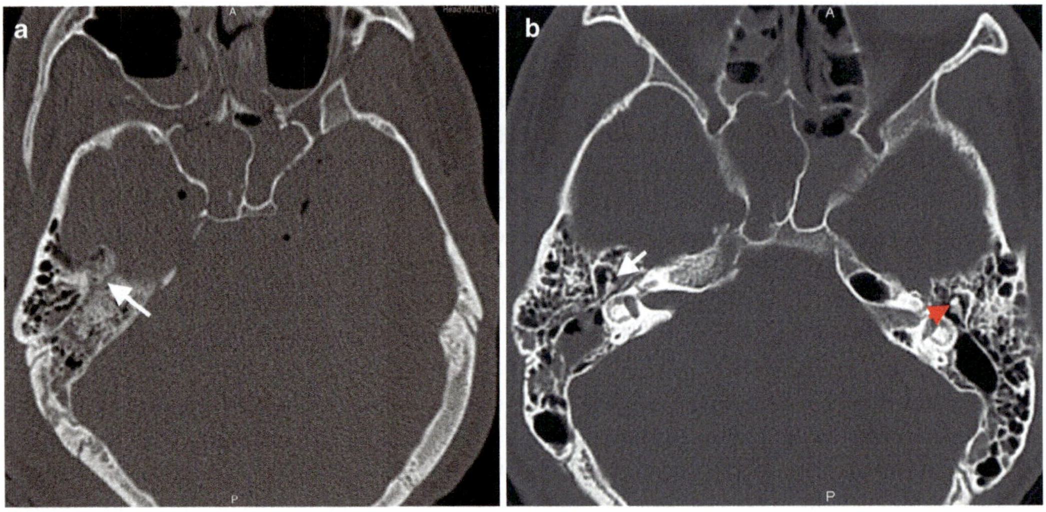

**Fig. 15** Incudomalleolar dislocation. (**a**) Axial CT image demonstrates right temporal bone fracture (arrow) with oblique orientation. (**b**) Ice cream cone appearance (red arrowhead) represents normal incudomalleolar joint alignment in the left temporal bone. Incudomalleolar dislocation presents with displacement of head of the malleus (scoop of ice cream) from the body and short process of the incus (cone) (arrow)

falling off ice cream scoop from cone (Fig. 15). The presence of both incus and malleus in the same image on a coronal scan is abnormal and suggestive of incudomalleolar dislocation (Lourenco et al. 1995). Stapediovestibular joint disruption rarely occurs and is being reported in 3% of cases due to the strong attachment of annular ligament of this joint (Meriot et al. 1997). Incudostapedial joint injury may be difficult to assess on CT compared to incudomalleolar joint in the setting of hemotympanum. It is important to define the joint injuries as mild or severe on imaging studies since minor ossicular derangements can be managed conservatively, while frank dislocations require surgical management to prevent CHL.

Fractures of ossicles may be encountered in 2–11% of patients with temporal bone trauma (Nosan et al. 1997; Meriot et al. 1997). Ossicular fractures appear as a lucent line through the ossicles and/or displaced bone fragment within the tympanic cavity on axial CT images. Vertical position of the manubrium and long process of the incus make the fractures of these incus components more easily detectable on coronal CT images. The fractures of the stapes footplate may be associated with perilymphatic fistula (PLF) (Kennedy et al. 2014).

Sensorineural hearing loss (SNHL) may result from injuries of otic capsule or cochlear nerve. The imaging findings of SNHL and vertigo include injury of the bony labyrinth, injury of the IAC, brainstem/nerve root zone, and pneumolabyrinth. Isolated intralabyrinthine hemorrhage in the absence of fracture may also cause SNHL. Although transverse fractures were reported to be more commonly associated with SNHL, new classification schemes regarding involvement of petrous bone or otic capsule were found to be more correlated with occurrence of SNHL. Otic capsule-violating fractures occur in 2–6% of temporal bone fractures, and SNHL invariably occurs in these fractures (Dahiya et al. 1999; Brodie and Thompson 1997; Little and Kesser 2006). Temporal bone fractures traversing cochlea, vestibule, or semicircular canal on CT strongly suggest otic capsule injury (Fig. 16). In the absence of fracture, hemorrhage within the otic capsule that may not be shown on CT can be depicted on MRI with high signal intensity on T1-weighted images.

Another potential complication of temporal bone fracture is vertigo, which may be caused by violation of vestibule, semicircular canals, vestibular aqueduct, or vestibular nerve. Vertigo may also be caused by labyrinthine concussion, shearing of nerve root entry zone, or brainstem injury (Kennedy et al. 2014). Cochlear concussion refers to injury or disruption of membranous labyrinth due to the traumatic force (Collins et al. 2012). CT images reformatted in the Stenvers and Pöschl views are most beneficial to demonstrate superior and posterior semicircular canals due to the compatibility of orientation of these views with alignment of semicircular canals.

PLF refers to abnormal connection between perilymph and middle ear cavity and should be suspected when CT shows fracture/dislocation of the stapes footplate oval window and the fracture traverses the round or oval window. Secondary signs of PLF include unexplained middle ear fluid and pneumolabyrinth on CT.

CSF leak may be encountered in 13–45% of patients with temporal bone fractures, which increases the risk of meningitis (Brodie and Thompson 1997; Dahiya et al. 1999; Nosan et al. 1997; Rafferty et al. 2006). CSF leaks after temporal bone fractures may present as otorrhea and otorhinorrhea in the setting of tympanic membrane disruption and intact tympanic membrane with Eustachian tube drainage, respectively (Prosser et al. 2011). The determination of CSF leak site on CT or MRI is crucial in surgical management of these patients (Fig. 16). The assessment of CSF leaks on CT necessitates scrutinizing the integrity and position of the tegmen tympani on coronal and sagittal images in terms of bone defects, fracture fragments, and associated encephalocele (Fig. 17). The sensitivity of CT was reported as 92% for detection of the site of bone defect, which may cause dural tear and CSF leak (Lloyd et al. 2008). CSF leak and accompanying multiple osseous defects may necessitate cisternography, which may be performed with CT and MRI to determine the source of active leak. CT cisternography technique should begin with precontrast thin-section CT images to determine the baseline density in sinuses formed by blood or high protein content. This should be followed by a scan performed after introducing intrathecal iodinated contrast agent via lumbar puncture in head-down position with provocative maneuvers. Post-contrast images should be obtained in both prone coronal and supine axial positions. CSF leaks appear as increased density and pooling of contrast in the sinuses and mastoids (Baugnon and Hudgins 2014). MR cisternography technique includes heavily T2-weighted, fat-saturated spin-echo,

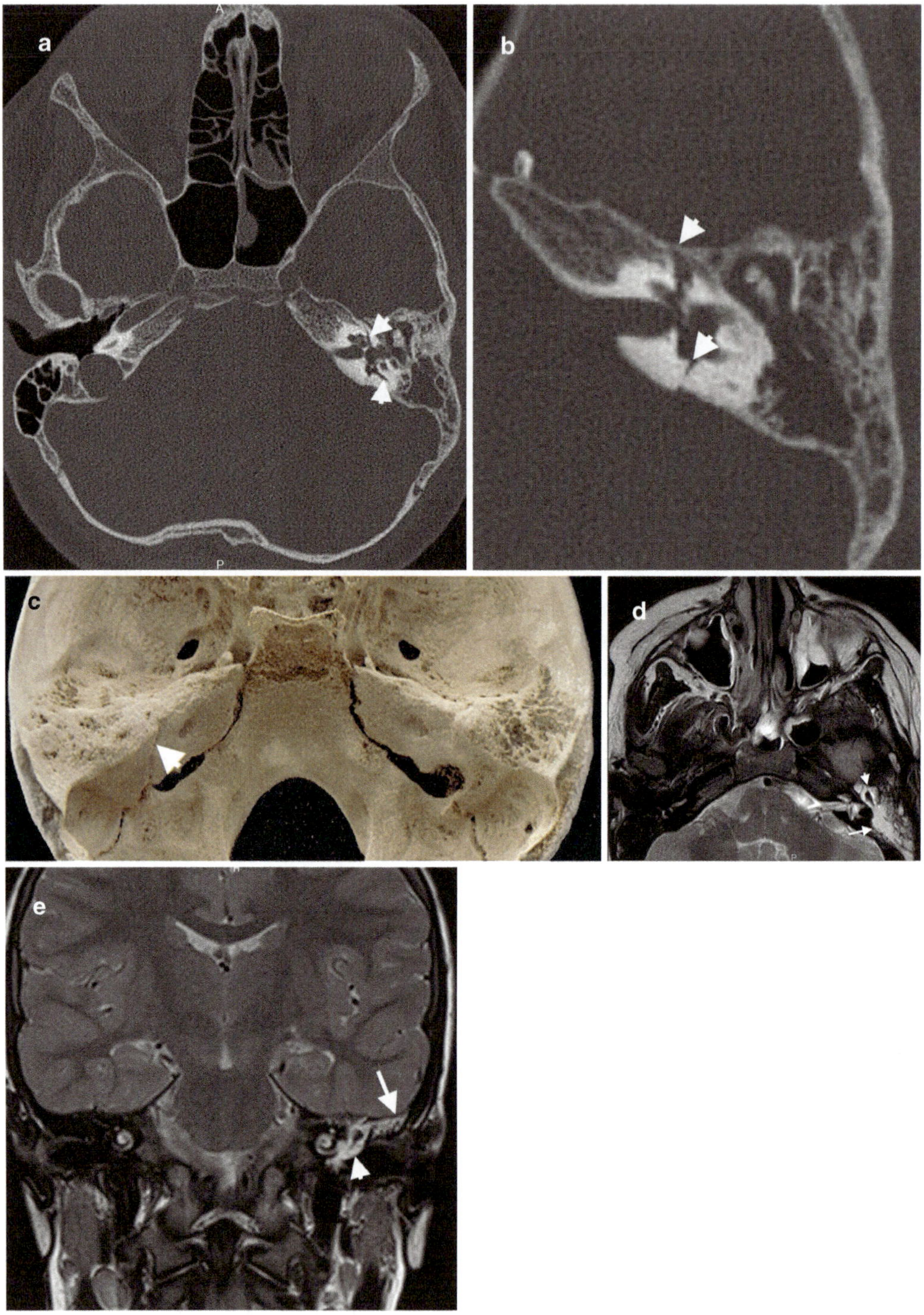

**Fig. 16** Otic capsule-violating temporal bone fracture in an 8-year-old male patient with a history of MVA. (**a**) Axial CT image demonstrates a horizontally oriented fracture violating otic capsule (arrowheads) in the left temporal bone. (**b**) Enlarged axial view shows hemotympanum and hemomastoideum with horizontal fracture (arrowheads) traversing petrous portion of the temporal bone with anteroposterior orientation. (**c**) CR image demonstrates the horizontal fracture as a subtle linear fracture line (arrowhead) traversing petrous portion of left temporal bone. Axial (**d**) and coronal (**e**) T2-weighted MR images obtained 15 days after trauma reveal hyperintense fluid in the left mastoid cells (arrows) and tympanic cavity (arrowheads) consistent with CSF leakage

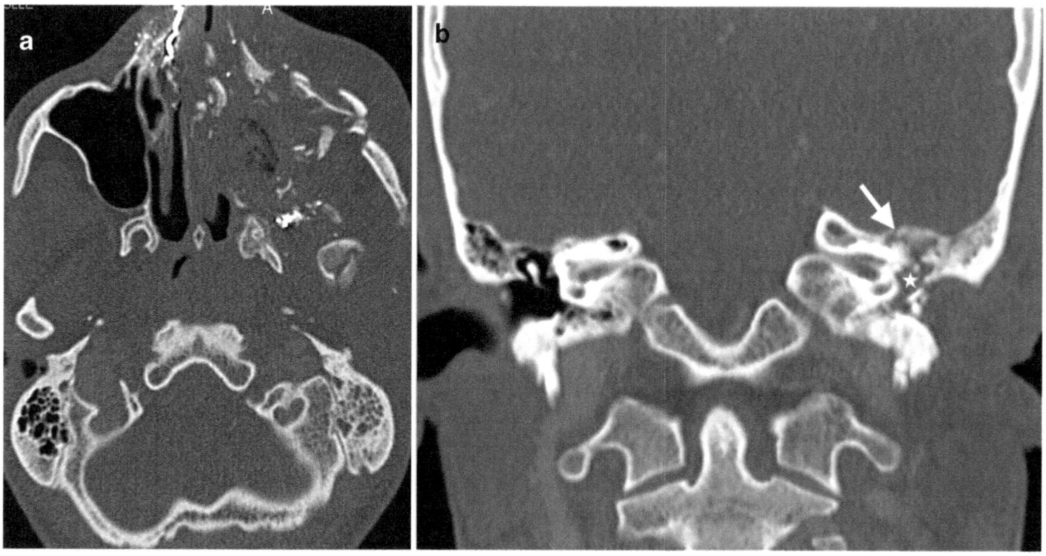


**Fig. 17** Tegmen tympani fracture. (**a**) Axial CT image of a 24-year-old man with a history of gunshot injury reveals multiple maxillofacial bone fractures in right side of the face. (**b**) Coronal CT image demonstrates displaced tegmen tympani fracture (arrow) and hemotympanum (*)

high-resolution 3D GRE sequences in addition to precontrast and post-contrast T1-weighted images. CSF leaks present as continuous column of T2 hyperintense material extending from the subarachnoid space. Localization and size of encephaloceles may be better evaluated on T2-weighted MR images. Dural enhancement adjacent to suspected fracture site may indicate dural tear and subsequent CSF leak.

Facial nerve injury may be encountered in 5–10% of patients with temporal bone fractures (Brodie and Thompson 1997; Yetiser et al. 2008). This injury occurs in 48% of otic capsule-violating and 6% of otic capsule-sparing fractures (Brodie and Thompson 1997). Displacement or violation of facial canal boundaries in temporal bone on CT is suggestive of facial nerve injury (Fig. 18). Most common injury site of facial nerve is geniculate ganglion, followed by the second genu of the nerve, and the tympanic and the mastoid portions. Distal facial nerve injury may also occur in styloid process fractures (Collins et al. 2012). Signs and symptoms of facial nerve injury may exist even in the absence of facial canal injury. In this setting, MRI may be helpful, which can demonstrate T1 hyperintensity in the facial canal suggestive of perineural hematoma. Enhancement of cisternal, canalicular, or labyrinthine segments of facial nerve is always pathologic, while geniculate ganglion and tympanic and mastoid segments may enhance normally after intravenous gadolinium administration (Collins et al. 2012).

Vascular complications of temporal bone fracture include injury to the internal carotid artery (ICA) and jugular vein. As ICA passes through the petrous portion of the temporal bone, the risk of ICA injury increases in temporal bone fractures, especially traversing the petrous portion (Fig. 19). ICA complications after temporal bone fractures include dissection, transection, pseudoaneurysm formation, occlusion, and arteriovenous fistula. The distal transverse and sigmoid sinuses may also be injured in fractures extending into the jugular foramen. Temporal bone CT examinations should be reviewed with soft-tissue algorithms for the depiction of venous sinus thrombosis that appears as hyperdense clot or air within the vein lumen. CT and MR venography can be preferred to assess venous injury more comprehensively (Kennedy et al. 2014) (Fig. 18).

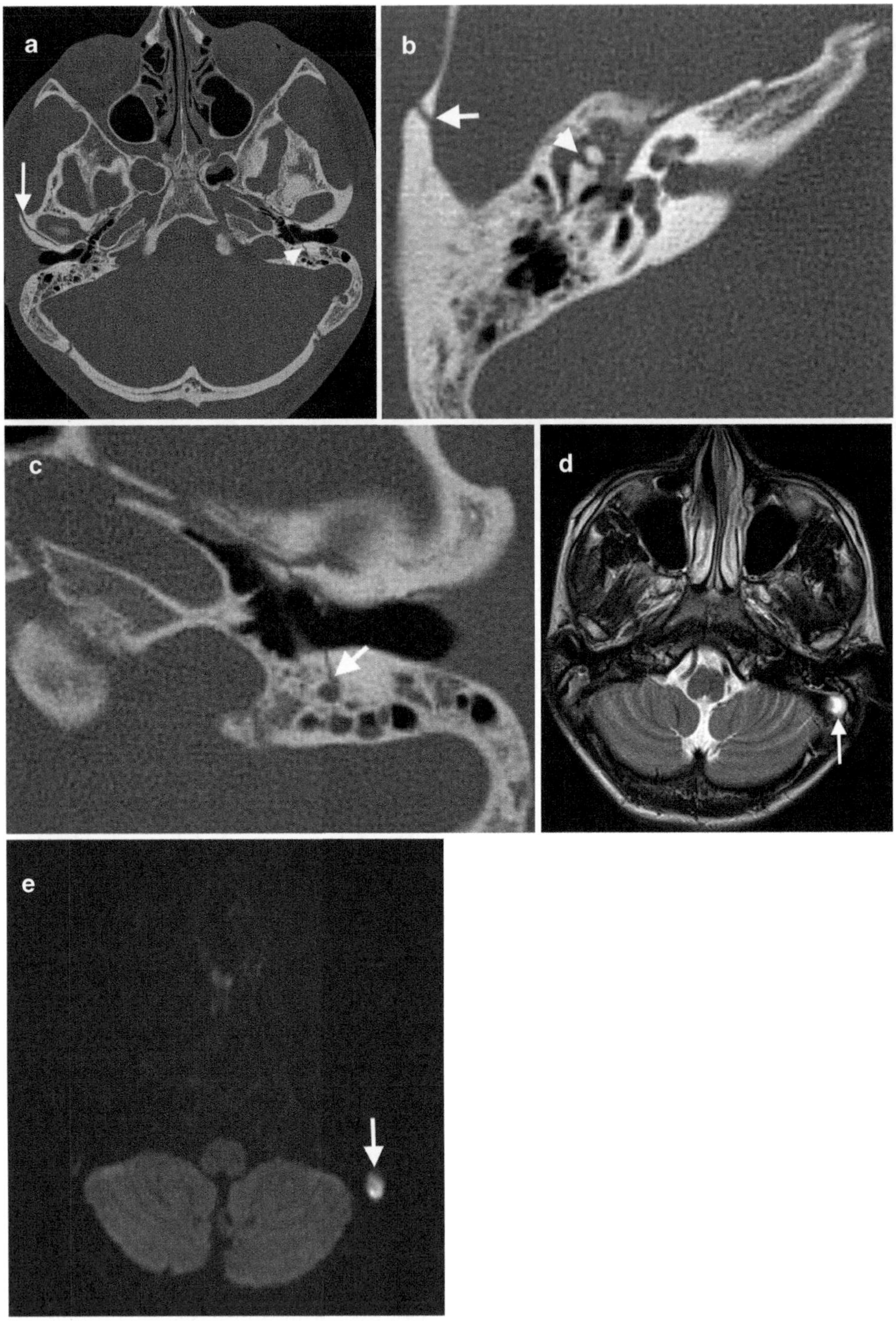


**Fig. 18** Bilateral temporal bone fractures in a 16-year-old man with a history of a wall fell on him 10 days ago. (**a**) Axial CT image demonstrates a linear fracture (arrow) oriented longitudinally through anterior wall of the right EAC and horizontally oriented fracture extending through left otic capsule (arrowhead). (**b**) Enlarged view of axial CT image of the same patient reveals fracture in the squamous part of the right temporal bone and dislocation of the incudomalleolar joint (arrowhead). (**c**) Enlarged view of left temporal bone axial CT image depicts extension of fracture through the anterior wall of left facial canal (arrow). (**d**) Axial T2-weighted MR image shows loss of signal void (arrow) in left sigmoid sinus adjacent to the left temporal bone suggestive of sigmoid sinus thrombosis. (**e**) Axial DWI reveals increased signal intensity due to thrombosis of sigmoid sinus

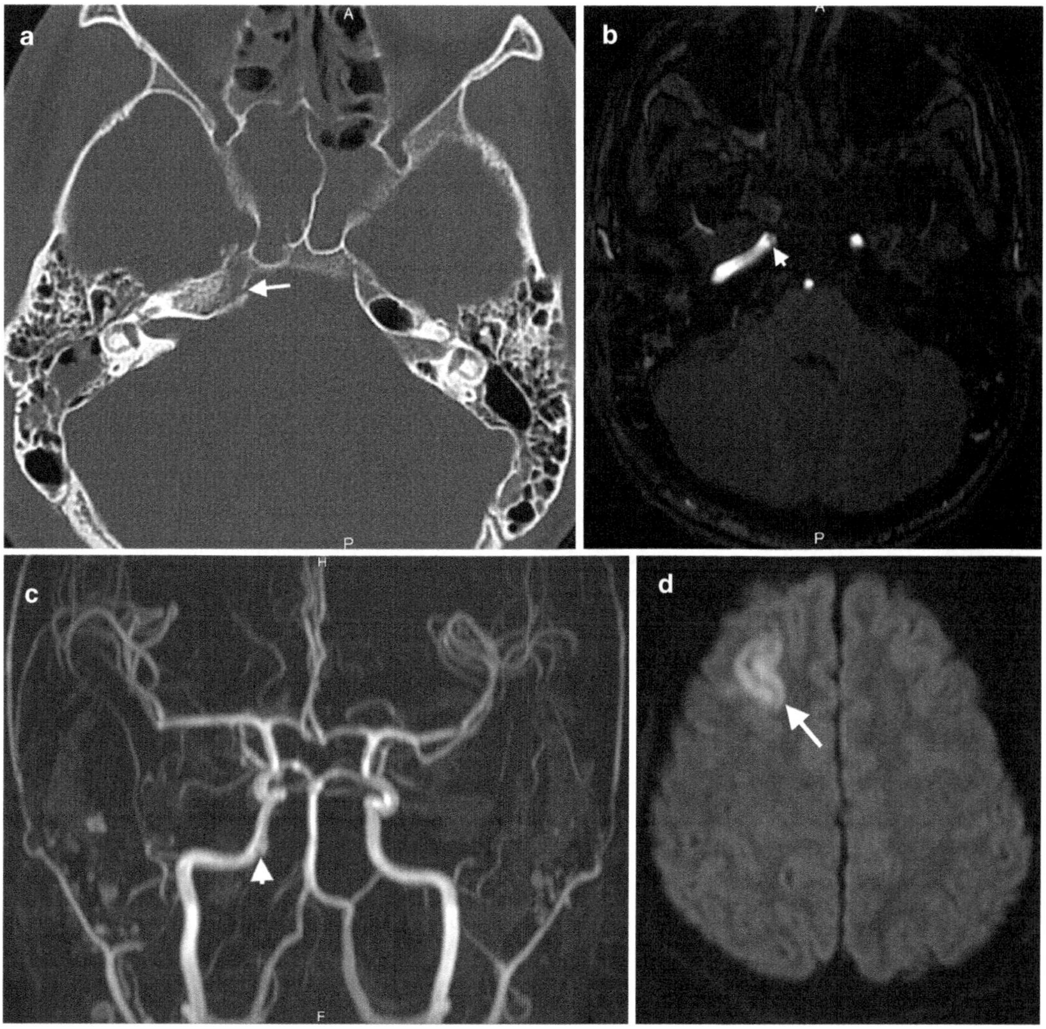


**Fig. 19** Temporal bone fracture with carotid artery injury in a 17-year-old man with a history of fall. (**a**) Axial CT image reveals right petrosal ridge fracture (arrow) involving right carotid artery. Axial 2D (**b**) and 3D (**c**) TOF MR angiography images show linear hypointense filling defect (arrowheads) representing dissection at the junction of petrous and cavernous segments of the right ICA. (**d**) DWI of the same patient demonstrates increased signal intensity (arrow) secondary to acute ischemia in the right frontal lobe

## 4 Skull Base

### 4.1 Anatomy

The skull base forms the floor of the intracranial compartment and separates intracranial and extracranial compartments. Skull base is constituted from three components including anterior skull base (ASB), middle skull base (MSB), and posterior skull base (PSB) and made up of seven bones as paired frontal and temporal bones with the unpaired ethmoid, sphenoid, and occipital bones. ASB, MSB, and PSB form the floor of the anterior cranial fossa, middle cranial fossa, and posterior cranial fossa, respectively (Fig. 20). ASB is formed by orbital plates of frontal bone and posterior table of frontal sinus and separates anterior fossa structures from the orbits and sinonasal cavity. Cribriform plate (CP) and roof of the ethmoid sinuses form the floor of ASB. ASB

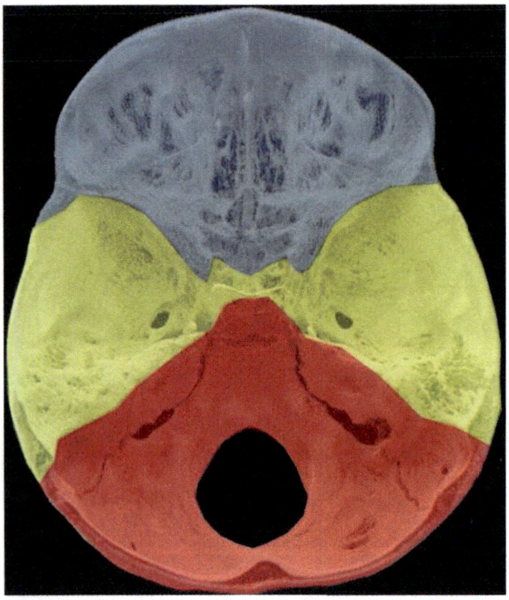

**Fig. 20** Skull base anatomy. Colored axial CR image of SB demonstrates ASB with blue, MSB with yellow, and PSB with red colors

is separated from MSB by the lesser wing of sphenoid bone. Bilateral fovea ethmoidalis as medial extensions of orbital plates is located in the inferomedial wall of the ASB superolaterally to CP. Connection between CP and fovea ethmoidalis is maintained by lateral lamellae (Fig. 21a) (Manson et al. 2009; Madhusudan et al. 2006). MSB is a critical anatomic structure as it contains several foramina that transmit vessels and nerves between intracranial and extracranial compartments. MSB is mainly constituted from sphenoid bone and temporal bone portion anterior to the petrous ridge (Figs. 20 and 21b). Sphenoid bone is a bat-like bone composed of a central body, greater and lesser wings laterally, and pterygoid processes inferiorly. MSB is formed by central skull base (CSB) and lateral skull base. CSB is composed of sphenoid bone and anteromedial aspect of the petrous part of temporal bone (Baugnon and Hudgins 2014). PSB is formed by the occipital bone and posterior aspect of the petrous part of the temporal bone. Occipital condyles and mastoid portion of the temporal bone form the inferior boundaries of PSB (Figs. 20 and 21c). In the midline, basis of the PSB is formed by clivus, which is constituted from basisphenoid and basioccipitus in sphenoid and occipital bones, respectively. Major anatomical landmarks in PSB are foramen magnum as the largest SB foramen, IAC, jugular foramen, and hypoglossal canal.

## 4.2 Fracture

Skull base fractures occur due to high-velocity blunt trauma, motorcycle collisions, pedestrian injuries, sport accidents, falls, or assault (Yilmazlar et al. 2006). These fractures are encountered in 7–16% of non-penetrating head injuries (Baugnon and Hudgins 2014). Ten percent of skull base fractures are caused by penetrating injuries most commonly from gunshot wounds (Samii and Tatagiba 2002). Clinical signs suggestive of SB fracture include Battle's sign, unilateral periorbital ecchymosis, bloody otorrhea, and acute cranial nerve deficits. Radiologists should be aware of the normal variant lucencies in pediatric SB to prevent false-positive diagnosis of SB fractures. The assessment of CT with MPR images on bone and soft-tissue windows is mandatory for comprehensive management of patients. It is important to detect SB fractures and displacement of bone fragments since dural tears are usually caused by fracture fragments.

Skull base fractures are frequently associated with complex facial fractures and might lead to important complications such as CSF leak, injury of cranial nerves and vessels, and meningitis. These fractures appear on CT as a non-corticated, non-interdigitating lucencies, with or without adjacent pneumocephalus, sinus or middle ear/mastoid opacification, or intraorbital emphysema (Fig. 22) (Baugnon and Hudgins 2014). Widening and diastasis of suture lines may also be encountered on CT.

Severe trauma to the midface or frontal region may result in ASB fracture. ASB fractures may involve posterior frontal sinus, roof of ethmoid, CP, and orbita (Figs. 23 and 24) (Kienstra and Van Loveren 2005; Manson et al. 2009). This fracture type carries a risk of CSF leak, which

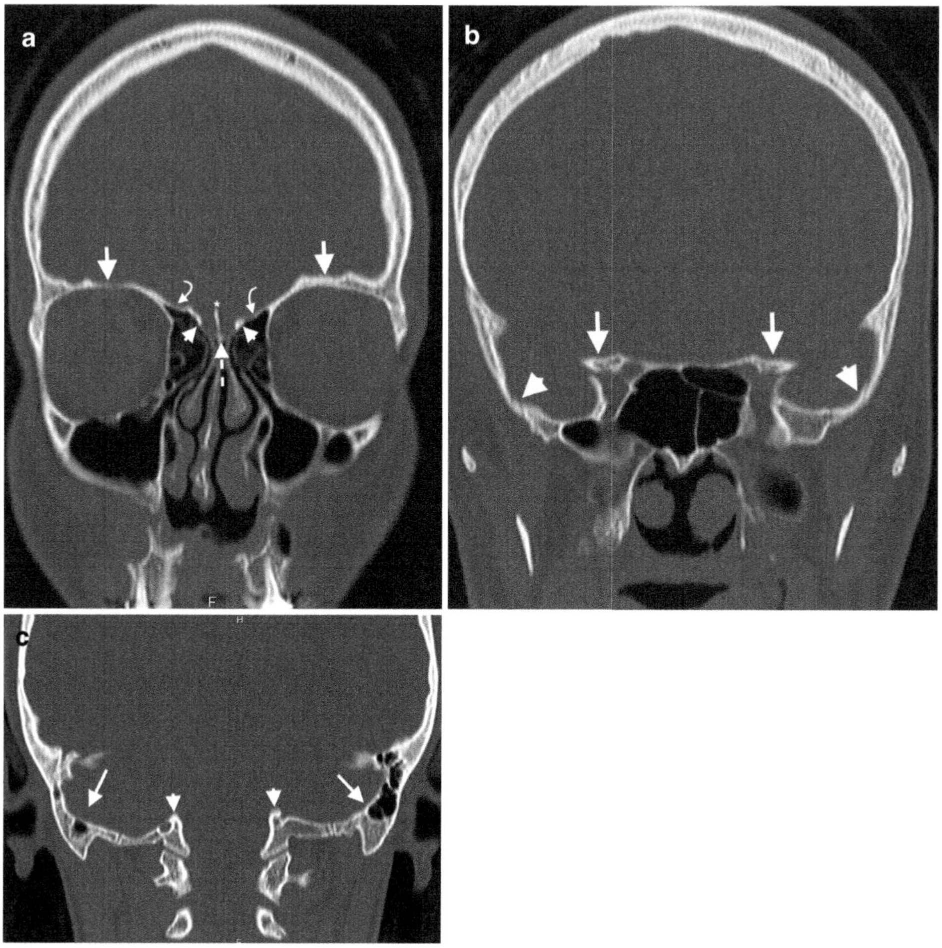


**Fig. 21** Coronal CT images revealing anatomic structures in ASB, MSB, and PSB. (**a**)ASB. Coronal CT image of ASB reveals bilateral orbital roofs (arrows), fovea ethmoidalis (curved arrows), lateral lamellae (arrowheads), CP (dashed arrow), and crista galli (*). (**b**) MSB. Coronal CT image shows MSB formed by sphenoid bone (arrows) and petrous parts of the temporal bones (arrowheads). (**c**) PSB. Coronal CT image shows posterior part of the mastoid portion of the temporal bones (arrows) and occipital condyles (arrowheads)

usually presents with unilateral rhinorrhea 1 week after the trauma (Policeni and Smoker 2015). Frontobasal fractures included in ASB fractures are classified according to the localization and severity as type I, type II, and type III fractures (Table 2). CSF leak is associated with frontobasal fractures in 25% of cases (Madhusudan et al. 2006). ASB fractures may cause other complications including intraorbital injury, meningoencephalocele, and anosmia due to cranial nerve (CN) I injury (Baugnon and Hudgins 2014). Anterior and posterior ethmoidal artery grooves located in ASB may mimic fractures. Characteristic location and corticated and tapering nature of margins of these artery boundaries can be helpful in distinguishing grooves from the fracture. Supraorbital canal and sphenofrontal suture may also mimic ASB fractures (Connor et al. 2005).

MSB fractures are most frequently encountered as oblique or sagittal fractures (Bobinski et al. 2016). Transverse fractures of MSB usually result from direct blow to the lateral skull and zygoma. All CSB fractures involve sphenoid sinus (Fig. 25). Cranial nerves traversing neural foramina, fissures, or canals may be injured due

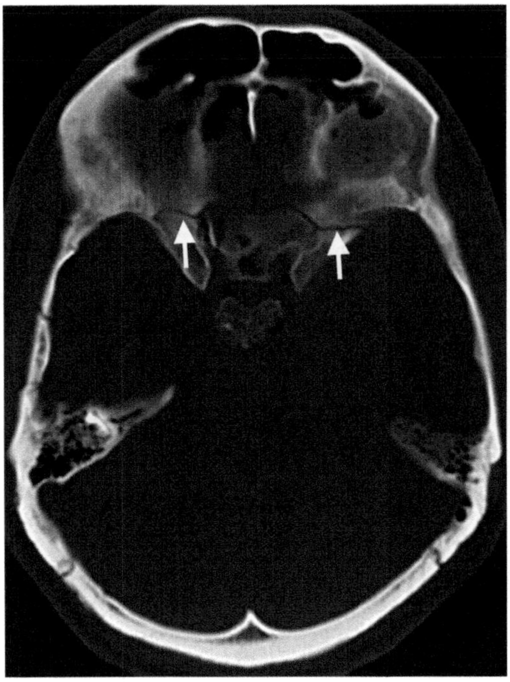

**Fig. 22** Axial CT image of a 31-year-old man with MVA reveals a linear fracture (arrows) traversing bilateral lesser sphenoid wings and posterior orbital plate of the frontal bone

to laceration, stretching, or transection, especially in coronally oriented CSB fractures (Feiz-Erfan et al. 2007; Mundinger et al. 2013). Carotid artery injury should be suspected in the setting of intracanalicular air after MSB fracture, especially extending to the clivus (Baugnon and Hudgins 2014). CTA or MRA should be performed in this setting in order to assess carotid artery injury. Involvement of ICA in this fracture type may result in transection, dissection, aneurysm/pseudoaneurysm, carotid-cavernous fistula, and vascular entrapment (Fig. 19) (Feiz-Erfan et al. 2007; Mundinger et al. 2013; Liang et al. 2007). Carotid dissection or occlusion presents on MRI as loss of flow voids and increased T1 and T2 signal around the periphery of the carotid arteries in crescentic shape (Baugnon and Hudgins 2014). Transverse fractures in the sphenoid sinus anteriorly or posteriorly can propagate laterally through the greater sphenoid wing and squamosal temporal bones. Greater sphenoid wing fracture may result in anterior middle cranial fossa epidural hematomas due to associated sphenoparietal venous sinus injury. Palatovaginal canal that extends from pterygopalatine fossa to the roof of pharynx may mimic CSB fracture on axial CT images (Connor et al. 2005). Spheno-occipital synchondrosis, a transverse clival cleft in children between basisphenoid and basiocciput, and petro-occipital fissure between the clivus and the petrous apex comprise other mimickers of CSB fractures (Fig. 26) (Koch 2014).

PSB fractures include fractures of clivus, basilar part of the occipital bone, and condyles (Figs. 27 and 28). Clivus fractures are very uncommon, but cranial nerve defects involving cranial nerves II, III, IV, V, VI, VII, or VIII almost invariably accompany these fractures (Menku et al. 2004). Brainstem may also be injured in clival fractures, especially in those oriented longitudinally (Bobinski et al. 2016). Longitudinal fractures of clivus may cause vertebrobasilar artery and brainstem injury, while transverse fractures may present with carotid artery injury (Menku et al. 2004). PSB fractures most commonly cause epidural hematoma in posterior fossa due to injury to the transverse or sigmoid dural sinuses or jugular bulb (Lui et al. 1993; Karasu et al. 2008). Occipital condylar fractures are classified into three types as type I, comminuted impaction fracture of occipital condyle caused by axial loading; type II, skull base linear fracture extending into occipital condyle; and type III, avulsion fracture at the attachment site of alar ligament (Bobinski et al. 2016). PSB fractures can be mimicked by emissary vein foramens, occipitomastoid, tympanomastoid, tympanosquamous, and petrosquamous sutures.

## 5 Orbita

### 5.1 Anatomy

Bony orbit is pyramidal in shape with a roof, floor, medial wall, lateral wall, orbital opening directed anterolaterally, and an apex directed posteromedially. Orbital roof is mainly formed by orbital plate of frontal bone with contribution of the lesser wing of sphenoid bone. Medial

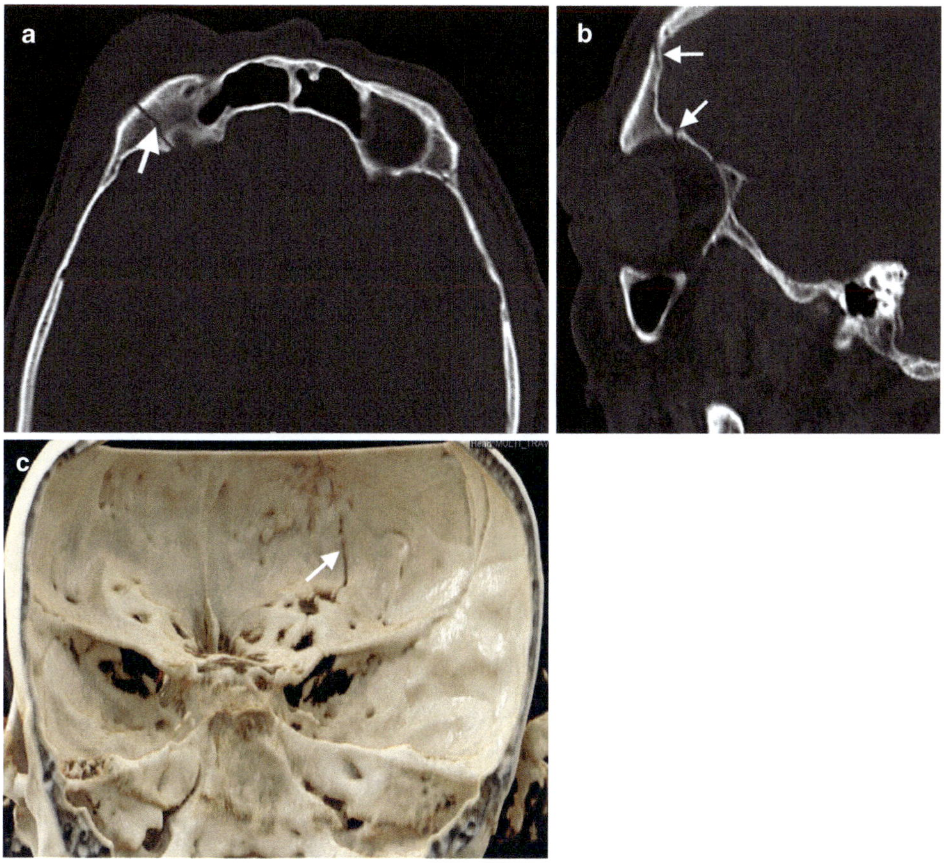


**Fig. 23** Linear fracture of ASB. Axial (**a**) and coronal (**b**) CT images present a nondisplaced linear fracture (arrows) of orbital part of the frontal bone (right orbital roof) (**c**) CR image with posteroanterior view reveals that the fracture (arrow) extends from squamosal part of the frontal bone to the right orbita roof

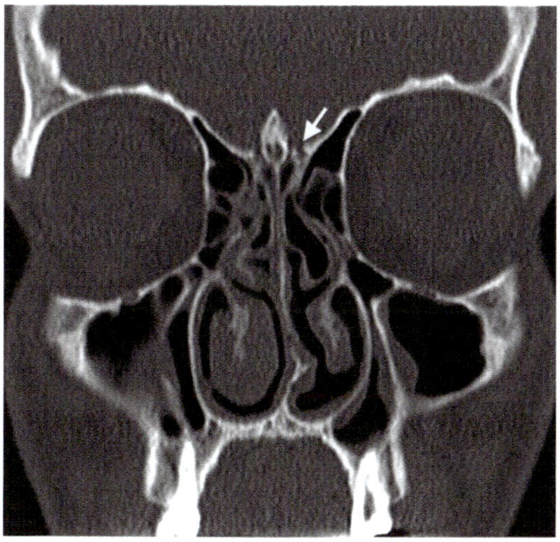

**Fig. 24** ASB fracture. Coronal CT image of a 18-year-old man with a history of assault demonstrates a fracture (arrow) involving left lateral lamella

**Table 2** Classification of frontobasal fractures (Manson et al. 2009)

| Fracture type | Features |
|---|---|
| Type I | Isolated linear fractures of the cranial base involving the medial third of the supraorbital rim and extending posteriorly along the sella |
| Type II | Vertical linear fractures involving the lateral two-thirds of the supraorbital rim, orbital roof, and the lateral orbital wall |
| Type III | Comminuted fractures combining central and lateral frontobasilar fractures involving frontal bone and orbital roof |

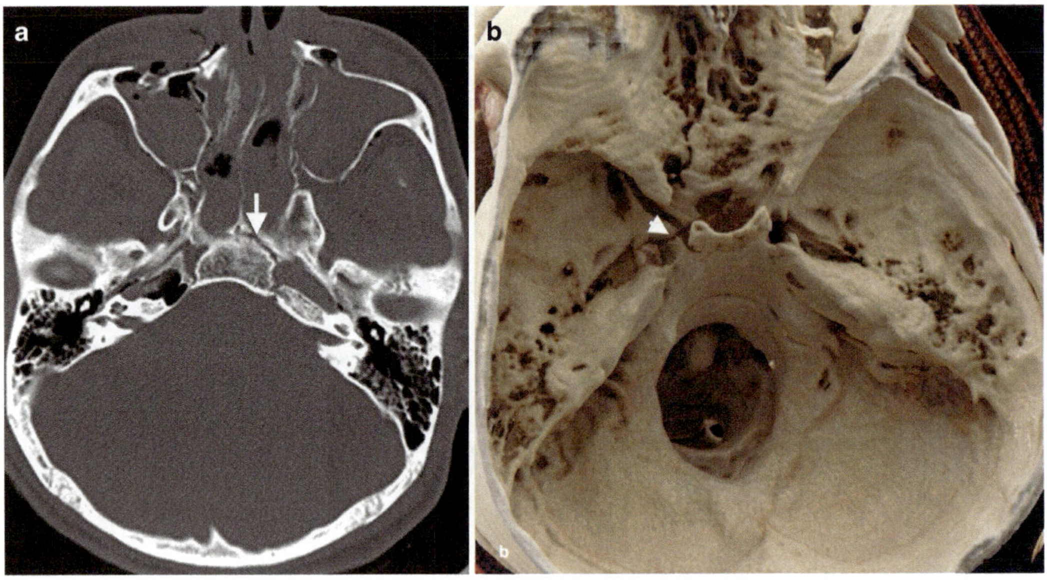

**Fig. 25** MSB fracture involving left lateral wall of the sphenoid sinus. (**a**) Axial CT image reveals an obliquely oriented fracture (arrow) through left anterolateral wall of the sella. (**b**) CR image demonstrates fracture (arrowhead) of the left lateral wall of the sphenoid sinus

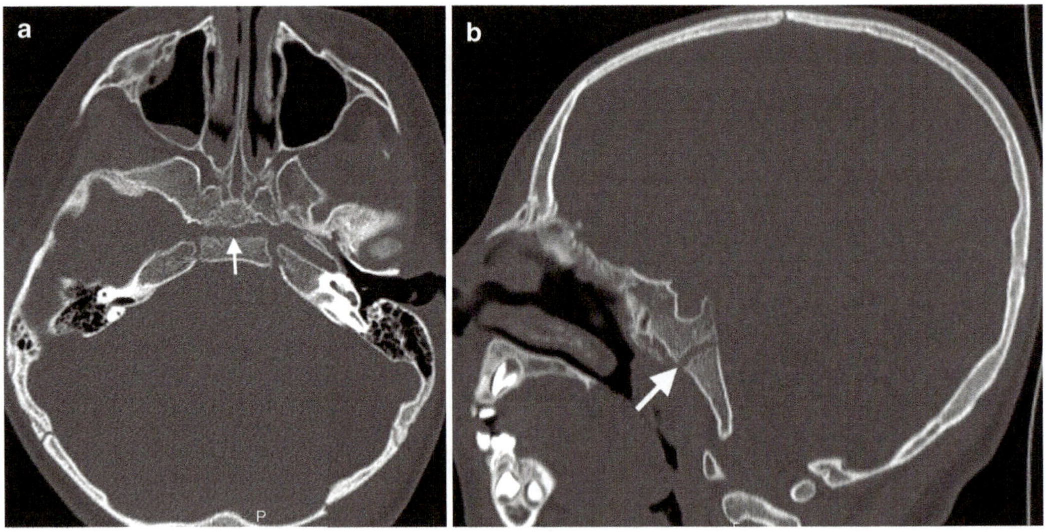

**Fig. 26** Sphenooccipital synchondrosis. Axial (**a**) and sagittal (**b**) CT images reveal sphenooccipital synchondrosis (arrows) mimicking clivus fracture

orbital wall consists of ethmoid bone, lacrimal bone, frontal process of maxilla, and body of the sphenoid. Orbital floor is formed by the orbital part of the maxilla, and orbital processes of palatine and zygomatic bones. Lateral wall is comprised of frontal process of zygomatic bone in

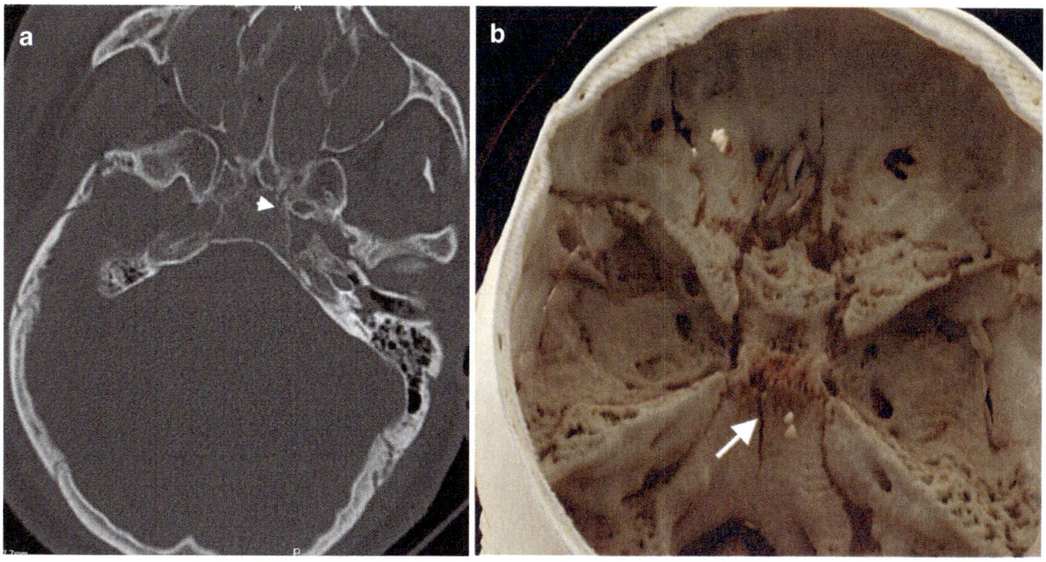

**Fig. 27** Linear fracture in clivus. (**a**) Axial CT image on bone window demonstrates a subtle linear fracture (arrowhead) in clivus. (**b**) CR image demonstrates longitudinally oriented linear fracture (arrow) at the cranial aspect of the clivus

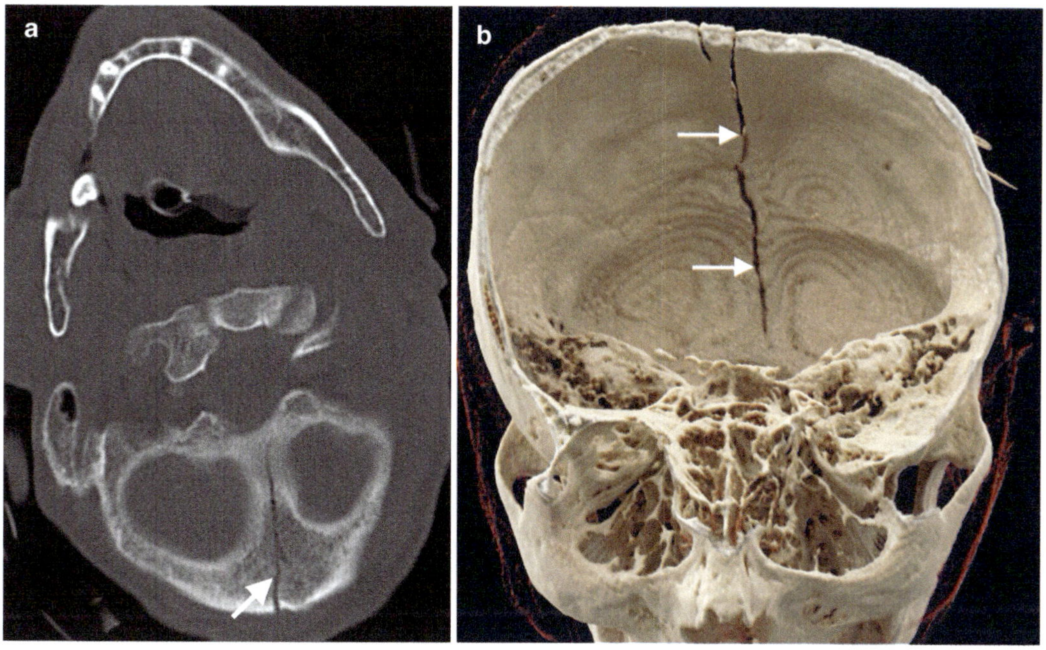

**Fig. 28** Occipital bone fracture involving PSB. (**a**) Axial CT image demonstrates a linear fracture (arrow) extending from squamosal part of occipital bone through basilar part. (**b**) Superoinferior view of CR image shows fracture (arrows) involving squamous and basilar parts of occipital bone

front and greater wing of sphenoid in behind. Optic canal and superior orbital fissure form orbital apex. Lateral wall is the thickest orbital wall, whereas medial wall formed by the lamina papyracea is the thinnest wall followed by orbital floor.

## 5.2 Fracture

Orbital fractures maintain 10–30% of facial fractures (Ellis 2012; Roth et al. 2010). Injury of bony orbit may be seen as isolated fractures such as fracture of the orbital floor, medial wall, lateral wall, and roof or occurs as a part of combined fracture such as zygomaticomaxillary complex (ZMC), naso-orbitoethmoid (NOE), and Le Fort fractures. Although outer rim of the orbits is composed of thick bones, inner orbit bones are susceptible to fractures due to their thin structures.

Orbital fractures should be assessed with MPR CT images. Coronal CT images have the greatest utility to depict the fracture, size of the orbital wall defect, and the change in orbital shape and volume (Roth et al. 2010; Rothman et al. 1998). Posterior extent of orbital floor defects may be depicted on sagittal images, while axial images can show posterior extent of medial wall fractures (Dreizin et al. 2018). Soft-tissue content of orbita including extraocular muscles, globe, and fibrofatty tissue should be assessed by reviewing MPR CT images on soft-tissue window. Majority of orbital fractures is comprised of blow-out and blow-in fractures. Blow-out fractures result from a direct blunt force to the orbit and increased intraorbital pressure. This fracture type mainly affects the medial wall and orbital floor as weakest parts of the bony orbit results in displacement of bone fragments into the ethmoid cells/nasal cavity or maxillary sinus and herniation of orbital fat content with extraocular muscles to these regions (Winegar et al. 2013). An accurate diagnosis of blow-out fracture can be accomplished by reviewing sagittal and coronal CT images to evaluate the size of the wall defect and possible herniation of soft tissues or extraocular muscles. Immobilization of the herniated muscle in the fracture site (entrapment) is a potential complication of blow-out fractures (Fig. 29). Medial rectus and inferior rectus muscles should appear flattened on axial and coronal CT images, respectively (Lo Casto et al. 2012). Entrapment of extraocular muscles manifests on CT and MR images as an abrupt kink or rounding of the muscle characterized by a 1:1 height-to-width ratio with protrusion into the adjacent ethmoidal or maxillary sinus (Fig. 30) (Lo Casto et al. 2012). Only fat content herniation may also cause entrapment of muscles due to the retractile effect of fibrous septations between herniated fat and extraocular muscles. Orbital emphysema may be encountered on CT in blow-out fractures secondary to wall defect between orbita and maxillary sinus; however, it should be kept in mind that increased intranasal pressure can also cause air passage from nasal cavity to the orbita. In pediatric population, orbital floor fracture may present as trapdoor fracture in which the flexible bone fracture fragment returns to the orbital floor with inferior rectus muscle persisting in the maxillary sinus. This fracture occurs secondary to relatively deficient mineralization of the orbital floor (Koch 2014). Trapdoor fractures may present with silent clinical features with absence of swelling and ecchymosis and are called as "white-eyed blow-out fracture" (Jordan et al. 1998). Coronal CT images demonstrate inferior rectus muscle below orbital floor with or without fracture fragment of the orbital floor (Fig. 31) (Winegar et al. 2013; Grant 3rd et al. 2002). Trapdoor fracture may cause ischemia and necrosis of the entrapped muscle leading to fibrosis, scarring, and persistent diplopia (Koch 2014). Clinically important late enophthalmos can be predicted by the following the initial CT criteria: defect's surface area greater than 2 $cm^2$, more than 25–50% orbital floor or medial wall involvement, collapse of the junctional bulge and internal orbital buttress, and soft-tissue herniation with volume displacement greater than 1.5 mL (Ellis 3rd 2012; Roth et al. 2010; Burm et al. 1999). It should be noted that small fractures affecting medial wall may manifest just as an opacification of ethmoid cells or herniation of intraorbital fat with no displaced bone fragment. Developmental dehiscence of the lamina papyracea can mimic orbital blow-out fractures with the appearance of bowed medial orbital wall toward the ethmoid complex and herniated medial extraconal fat through the defect (Fig. 32). Orbital blow-out fractures may present with intraorbital hemorrhage, globe injury, and injury of the infraorbital nerve in the setting of orbital floor fracture (Figs. 33, 34 and 35) (Winegar et al. 2013).

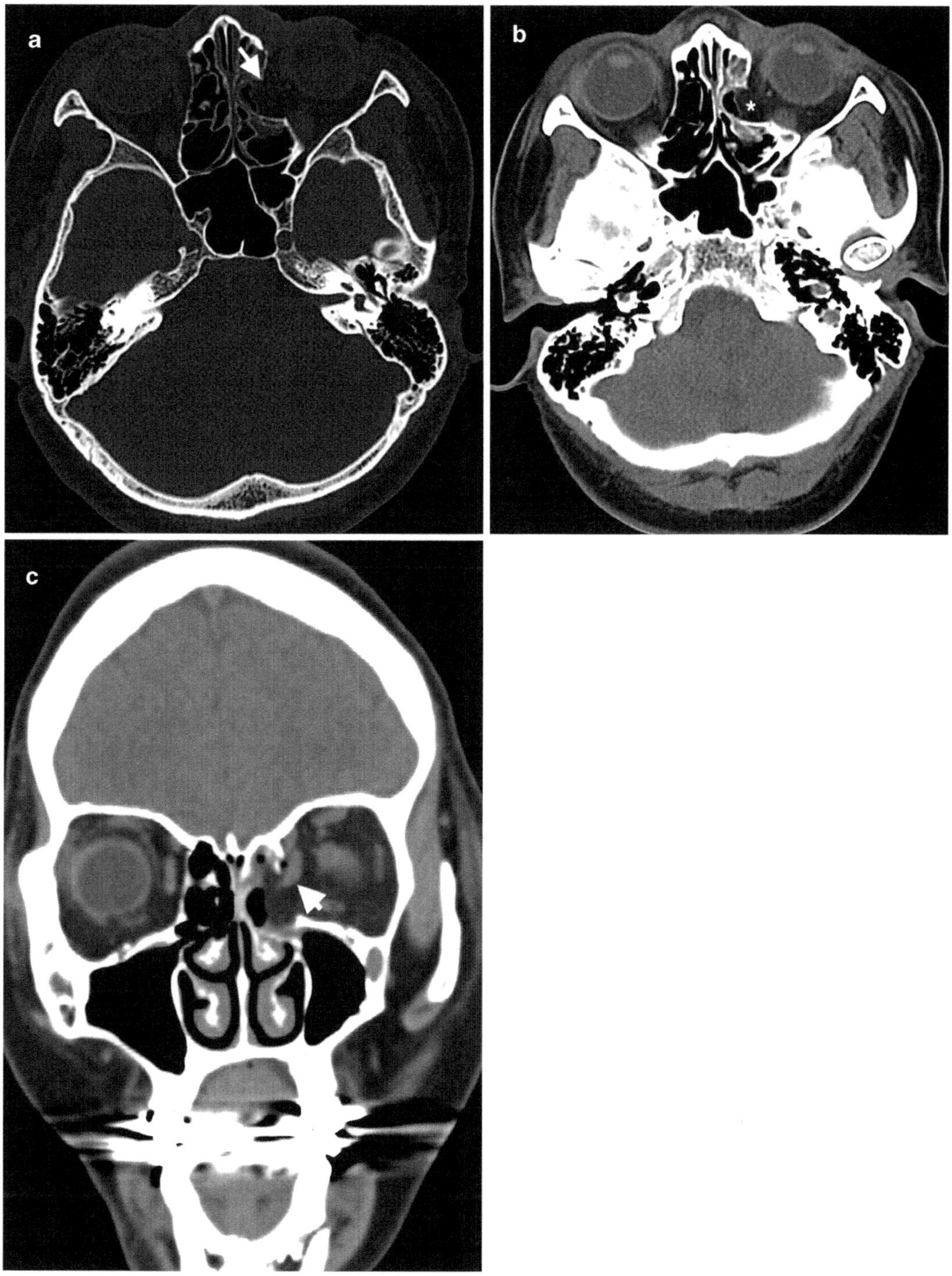


**Fig. 29** Blow-out fracture. (**a**) Axial CT image of a 39-year-old woman with a history of fall demonstrates a medial orbital wall defect (arrow). (**b**) Axial CT image on soft-tissue window reveals herniation of extraconal fat (*) through the medial wall defect. (**c**) Coronal CT image on soft-tissue window shows kinking and entrapment of left medial rectus muscle (arrowhead) herniating through the medial orbital wall defect into the ethmoidal cells

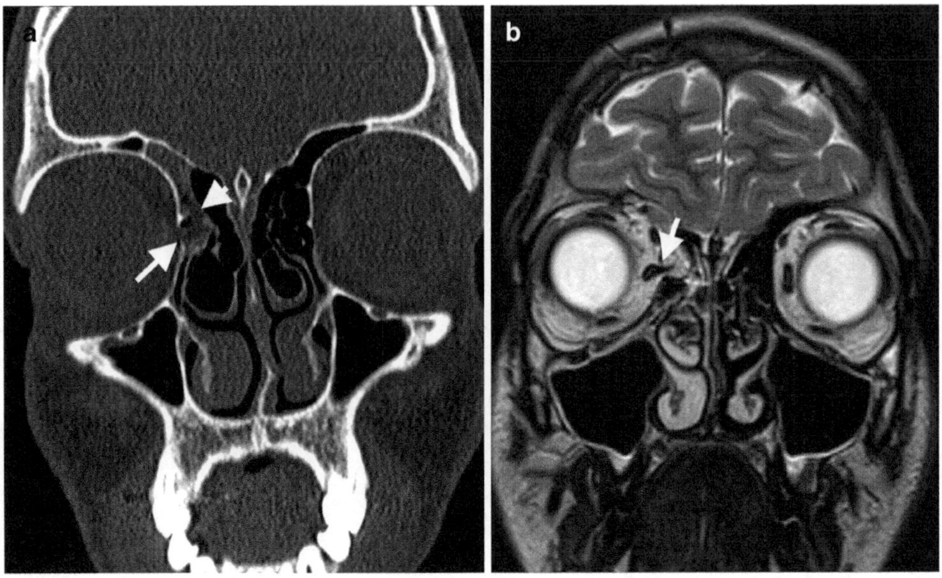


**Fig. 30** Blow-out fracture with entrapment of medial rectus muscle in a 14-year-old man with a history of assault. (**a**) Coronal CT image reveals a defect (arrow) in right medial orbital wall with fat herniation to the adjacent ethmoidal sinuses (arrowhead). (**b**) Coronal T2-weighted MR image demonstrates entrapment of right medial rectus muscle (arrow)

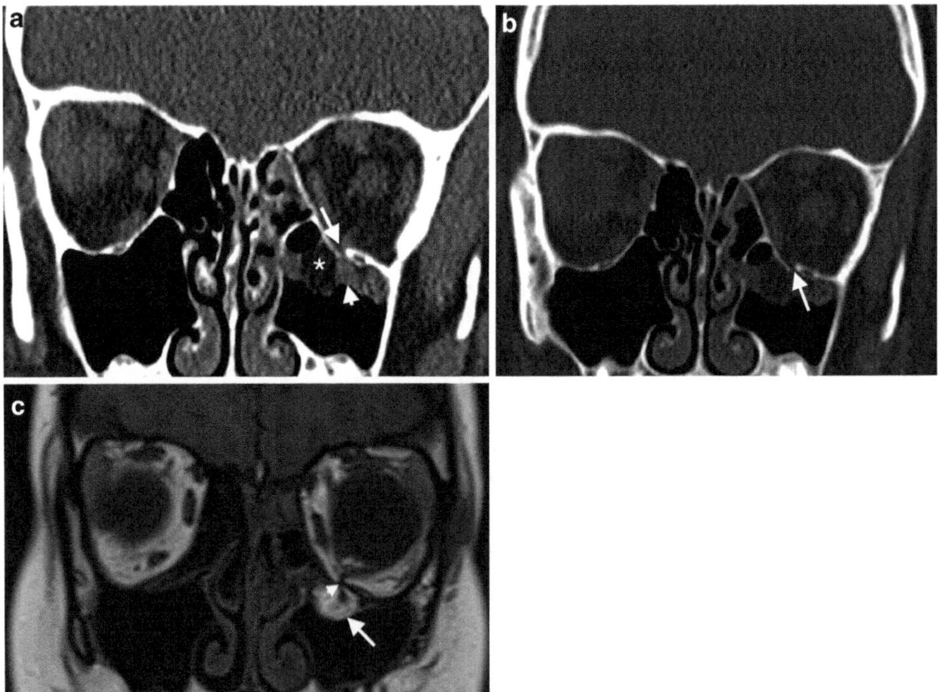


**Fig. 31** Trapdoor fracture in a 11-year-old woman with a history of MVA. Coronal CT images on soft (**a**) and bone (**b**) window images reveal left inferior orbital wall fracture (arrows) with fat (*) herniation into the left maxillary sinus. (**c**) Coronal T1-weighted MR image reveals herniation of left orbital extraconal fat (arrow) into the left maxillary sinus. Although fracture defect is almost closed, inferior rectus muscle is entrapped in the left maxillary sinus below the left orbital floor (arrowhead) consistent with trapdoor fracture

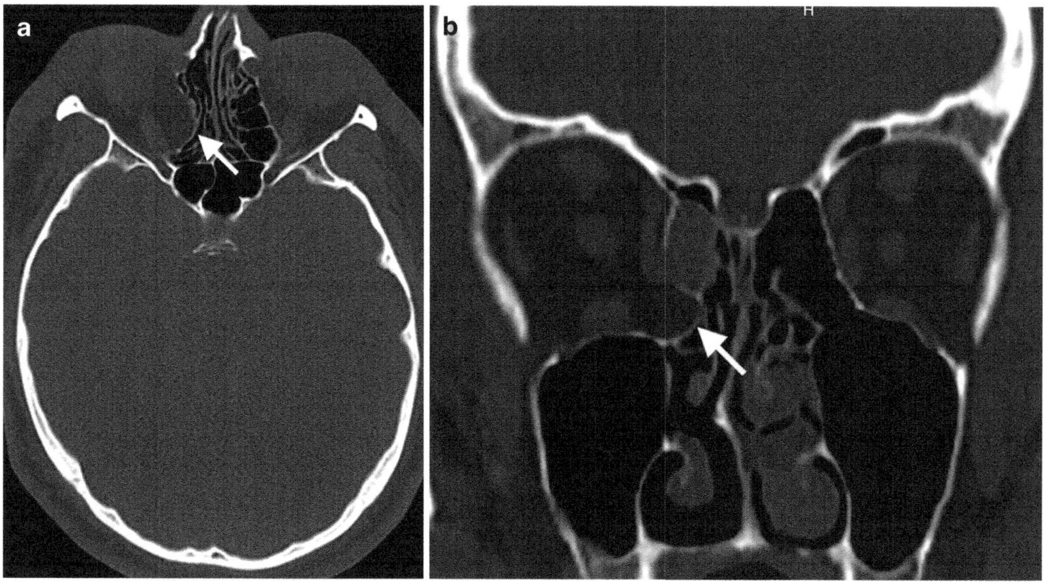


**Fig. 32** Axial (**a**) and coronal (**b**) CT images of a patient reveal dehiscence of the right lamina papyracea (arrows) that mimic blow-out fracture of right orbita. No medial wall defect exists as well as accompanying orbital soft-tissue injury suggestive of blow-out fracture

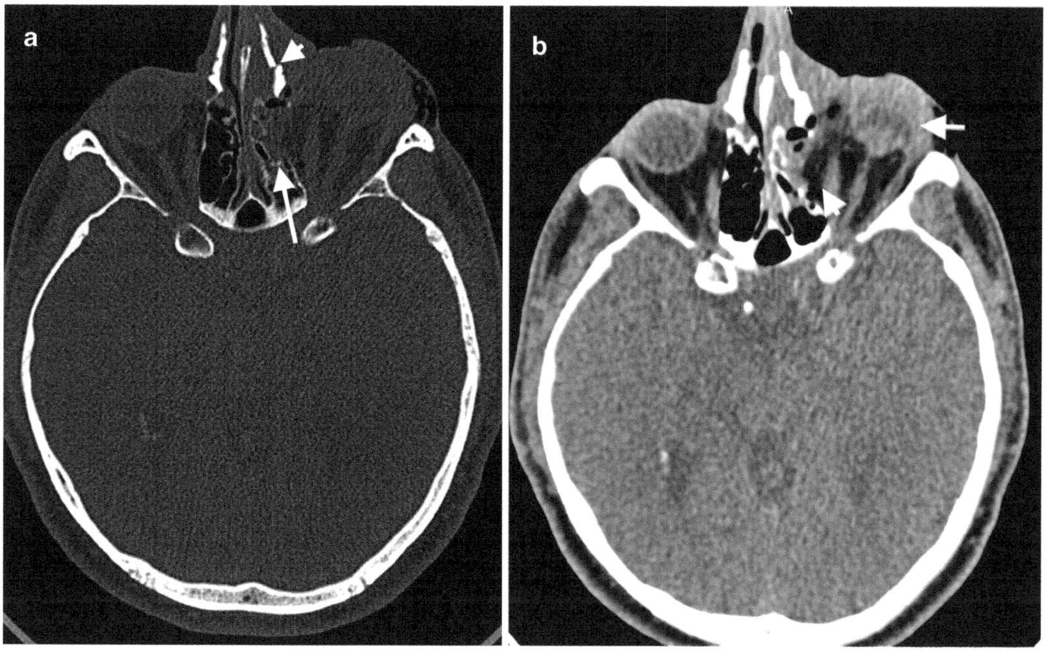


**Fig. 33** Blow-out fracture with globe perforation in a 46-year-old man with a history of assault. (**a**) Axial CT image on bone window shows blow-out fracture of left orbital wall (arrow) and left nasal bone fracture (arrowhead). (**b**) Axial CT image on soft-tissue window reveals perforation of left globe with volume loss and intraocular hemorrhage (arrow)

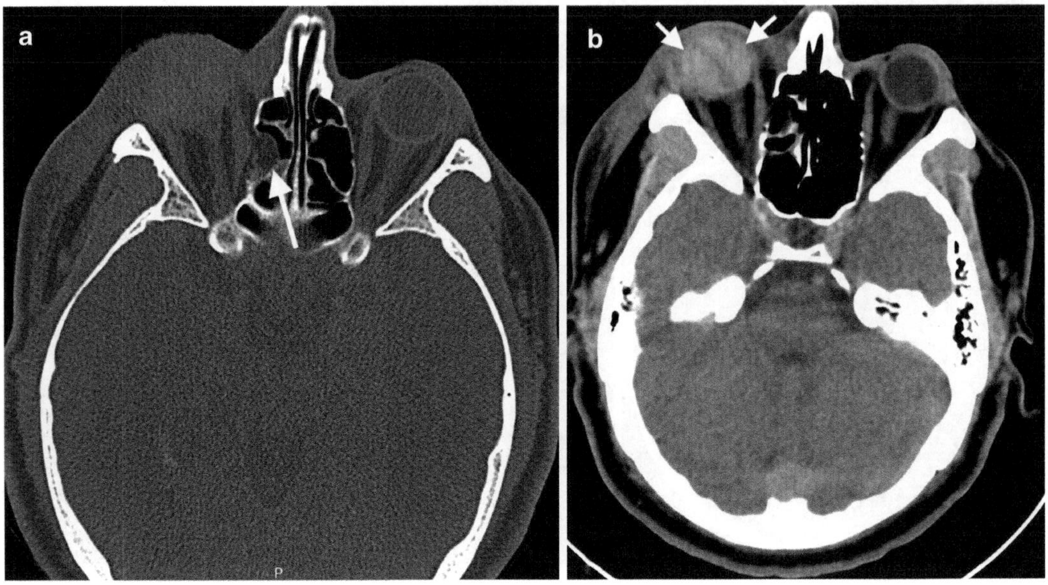


**Fig. 34** Blow-out fracture with globe hemorrhage in a 42-year-old man with a history of MVA. (**a**) Axial CT image on bone window shows blow-out fracture of right orbital wall (arrow). (**b**) Axial CT image on soft-tissue window reveals hyperdense hemorrhage within the right globe (arrow)

Penetrating injuries may also cause orbital wall fractures (Fig. 36).

Blow-in fractures are characterized by displacement of bony fragments of frontal bone into the intraorbital soft tissues through the orbital roof. This fracture type occurs due to direct impact to the supraorbital rim or frontal bone with the transmitting force directed toward the orbital roof (Fig. 37) (Uzelac and Gean 2014). Free bone fragments may cause orbital muscle or globe laceration. Orbital roof fractures are more common in pediatric population (Koch 2014). Posterior extension of the orbital roof fractures should also be evaluated for a possible orbital apex injury that has a potential for optic nerve and oculomotor nerve injury. The presence of orbital apex fractures necessitates exclusion of retrobulbar hematoma and bony impingement on the optic nerve (Koch 2014). Orbital roof fractures may be associated with CSF leak, pneumocephalus, and intracranial complications.

Orbital rim fractures occur due to high-energy trauma and may involve superior, lateral, and inferior orbital rims. Superior orbital rim fracture, being the most common, may result in inferior and anterior displacement of the globe. Subperiosteal hematoma may accompany orbital rim fractures. Extension of orbital floor fractures to the superior orbital fissure may cause superior orbital fissure syndrome, which occurs due to injury of cranial nerve III, IV, VI, and ophthalmic branch of the V nerve (Winegar et al. 2013). Extension of fracture through orbita apex may result in orbital apex syndrome, which is characterized by optic nerve impingement resulting in decreased vision clinically. Fractures of lateral orbital wall are usually associated with ZMC fractures (Fig. 38) (Dreizin et al. 2018). Inferior orbital rim fractures may involve inferior orbital foramen, thereby inferior orbital nerve resulting in anesthesia of cheek and upper lip. Orbital rim fractures may be complicated with other ocular injuries including globe rupture, retrobulbar hematoma, optic nerve injury, and lens dislocation. The assessment of globe in the setting of orbita fracture may be crucial.

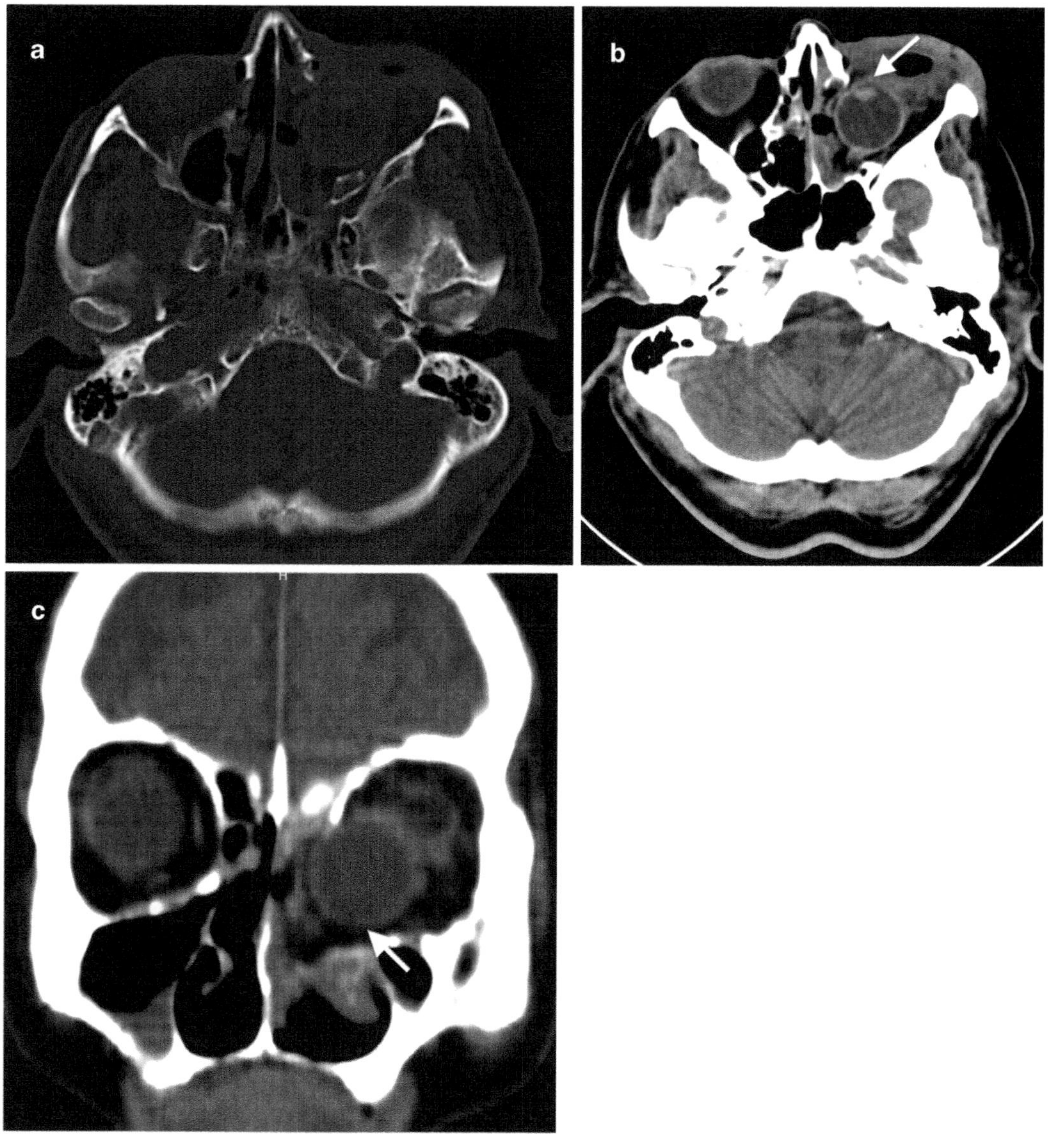


**Fig. 35** Internal globe herniation secondary to blow-out fracture in a 75-year-old man. (**a**) A blow-out fracture with a large defect of left orbital wall is seen at bone window axial CT image. Axial (**b**) and coronal (**c**) CT images at soft-tissue window demonstrate inferomedial herniation of the left globe (arrows) into the ethmoidal cells through the inferomedial wall defect

Anterior chamber of globe can be evaluated by volume change. Volume decrease in anterior chamber may indicate corneal laceration or anterior displacement of the lens. Increase in the anterior chamber volume may indicate posterior chamber rupture (Uzelac and Gean 2014). Lens should be assessed in terms of dislocation. Posterior chamber should be interrogated in terms of globe rupture, retinal detachment, and hemorrhage.

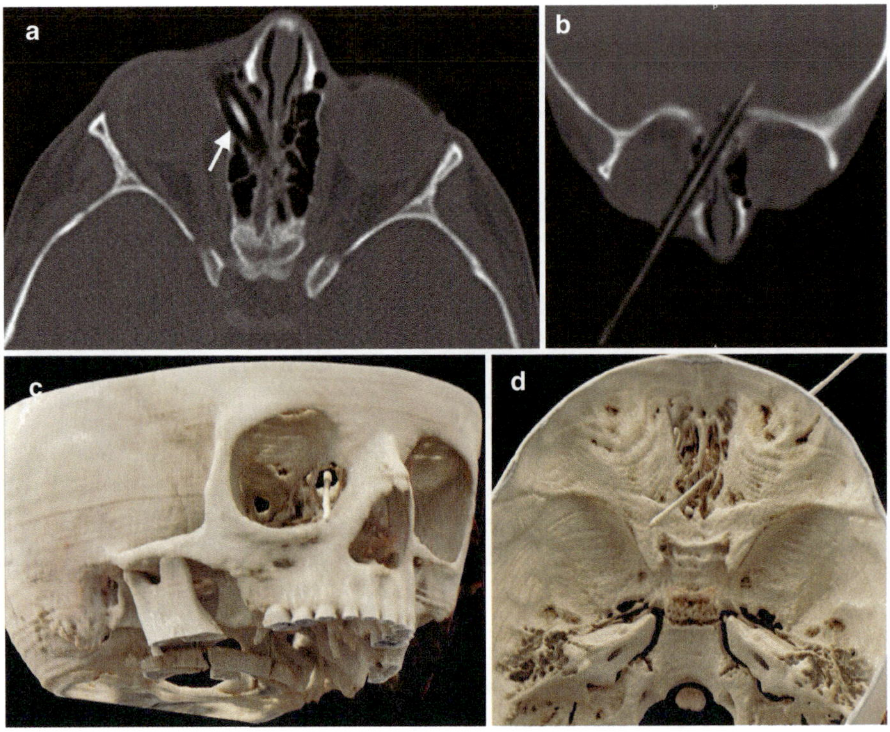


**Fig. 36** Penetrating trauma of orbital wall in a 4-year-old man with a history of pencil stuck. Axial bone window CT (**a**), coronal MPR image (**b**), and CR (**c**, **d**) images demonstrate a penetrating pencil passing through right medial orbital wall and stucking into the frontal lobe crossing the CP

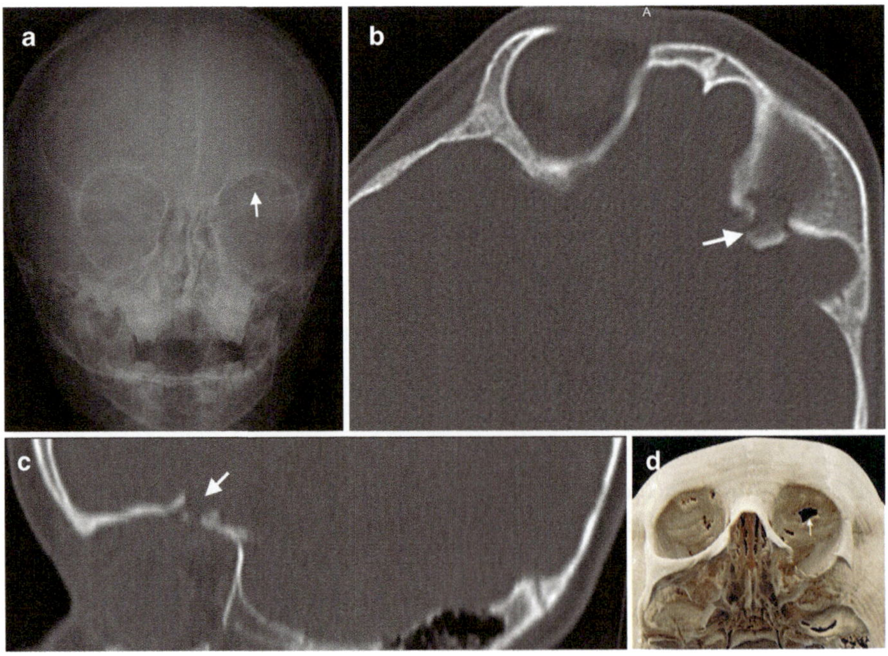


**Fig. 37** Orbital roof fracture. (**a**) Skull radiograph in A-P position demonstrates an oval shape radiolucency (arrow) representing a defect in the left orbital roof. Axial (**b**) and sagittal (**c**) bone window CT images demonstrate the fracture (arrows) in the left orbital roof. (**d**) CR image shows the bone defect (arrow) in the orbital roof

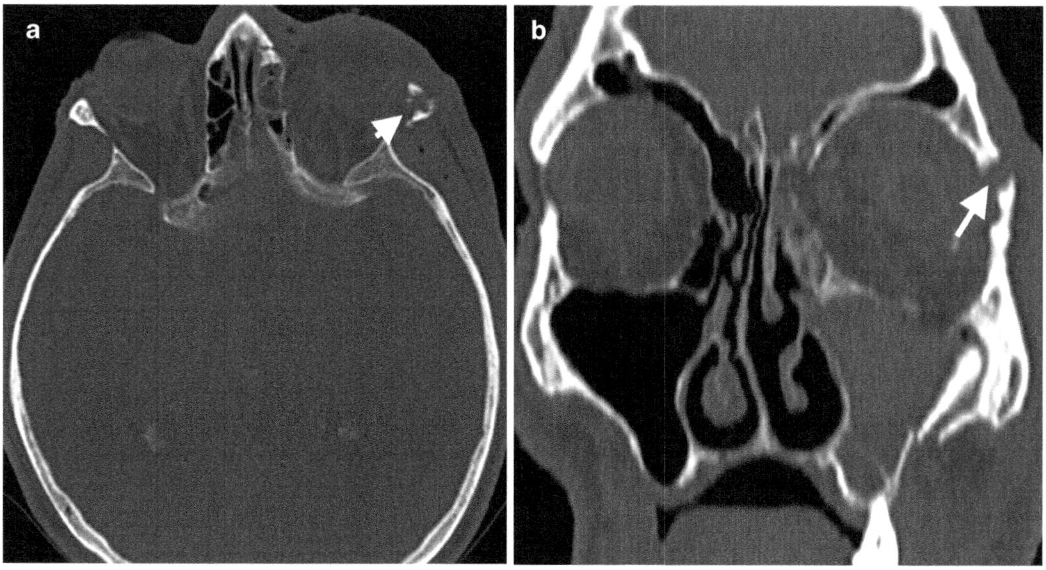


**Fig. 38** Lateral wall fracture of the orbita. Axial (**a**) and coronal (**b**) CT images of a 52-year-old male patient with MVA show lateral wall fracture (arrows) of left orbita

## 6 Maxillofacial Bones

### 6.1 General Information

Maxillofacial skeleton is composed of zygomatic, maxillary, nasal, lacrimal, palatine, and mandible bones. Facial skeleton is considered as a network of horizontally and vertically aligned bony buttresses, which refer to bony structures of substantial thickness and lines of osseous thickening formed by articulating facial bones. Facial buttresses increase the resistance of facial skeleton to trauma and provide a rigid framework for orbital contents, sinuses, teeth, and nasal cavity (Winegar et al. 2013). Maxillofacial buttress network distributes mechanical energy resulting in propagation of fractures through facial bones. Importance of facial buttresses is based on the fact that disruption of these buttresses results in change in facial dimensions. Horizontal buttresses of facial skeleton are comprised of superior orbital rim, upper transverse maxillary, lower transverse maxillary, upper transverse mandibular, and lower transverse mandibular buttresses. Vertical buttresses of facial skeleton consist of medial maxillary (nasomaxillary), lateral maxillary (zygomaticomaxillary), posterior maxillary (pterygomaxillary), and posterior vertical mandibular (mandibular) buttresses (Table 3 and Fig. 39).

Maxillofacial fracture patterns may differ in children due to flexible suture lines, greater flexibility of osseous structures of the face, and a thicker subcutaneous fat as a protective layer that makes facial skeleton of children more resistant to fractures (Zimmermann et al. 2005; Alcala-Galiano et al. 2008). Incomplete development of paranasal sinuses in children increases the stability and decreases the incidence of midface fractures (Koch 2014).

### 6.2 Imaging Techniques

#### 6.2.1 Radiography

Plain film radiography has a very limited role in evaluation of facial skeleton fractures due to overlap of maxillofacial bones on 2D imaging. Patient positioning for radiography may be difficult and potentially dangerous in the setting of trauma. Caldwell (P-A) or axial view radiographies may be helpful for delineation of the zygomatic arch. Occipitomental or Waters view can delineate inferior and lateral orbital walls and the

**Table 3** Vertical and horizontal facial buttresses network (Fig. 39) (Winegar et al. 2013; Lo Casto et al. 2012)

| Vertical buttress system | Localization |
|---|---|
| Medial maxillary buttress (nasomaxillary) | Extends from the nasofrontal suture inferiorly along the lateral margin of the pyriform aperture to the maxillary alveolar process |
| Lateral maxillary buttress (zygomaticomaxillary) | Extends from zygomaticofrontal suture inferomedially along the lateral orbital rim across the zygomaticomaxillary suture to terminate in the maxillary alveolar process |
| Posterior maxillary buttress (pterygomaxillary) | Between the posterior maxillary alveolus and pterygoid processes of the sphenoid bone |
| Posterior mandibular buttress (mandibular) | Portions of angle, ramus, and condyle, along the posterior border of the mandible |
| *Horizontal buttress system* | |
| Superior orbital rim | Includes orbital roofs, CP, and fovea ethmoidalis |
| Upper transverse maxillary buttress (inferior orbital rim) | Extends inferiorly from the level of the nasofrontal suture, proceeds along the inferior edge of the orbit, and ends in zygomaticotemporal suture |
| Lower transverse maxillary buttress (maxillary alveolar rim) | Oriented horizontally along the maxillary alveolar process. Extends posteriorly to include the hard palate |
| Upper transverse mandibular buttress (mandibular alveolar rim) | Encompasses the mandibular alveolar process |
| Lower transverse mandibular buttress (inferior mandible border) | Inferior margin of the mandible |

zygomatico-alveolar arch. Craniofacial fractures may manifest on radiographs as interruption in bony continuity, abnormal bony overlap with double density of bone appearance and abnormal linear densities secondary to rotated fracture fragments, and air density in adjacent soft tissues.

### 6.2.2 CT

Maxillofacial CT scanning area should extend from the top of the frontal sinus to the bottom of the hyoid bone to include the entire maxillofacial skeleton. Axial CT images should be acquired at submillimeter thickness (<1 mm) or 1.25 mm thickness with overlap to acquire high spatial resolution images with 3D images. CT images may be reviewed at 1.5–2-mm-thick reformatted images in the axial, coronal, and sagittal planes on soft tissue and bone window settings. Complex fractures involving multiple planes should be assessed with 3D images. 3D imaging is also preferred by surgeons owing to 360° rotation facility to simulate facial alignment for preoperative planning (Lo Casto et al. 2012). 3D imaging has limitations due to relevant artifacts during the reformation process, which may result in decreased ability to visualize nondisplaced fractures (Saigal et al. 2005). Additional oblique or curved reformations may be helpful to delineate the fracture.

MR imaging, thanks to high soft-tissue contrast, can be used to demonstrate soft-tissue injury and cranial nerve deficits associated with facial skeleton injury. MRI cannot be used in evaluation of craniofacial fractures due to signal loss in cortical bones.

## 6.3 Frontal Sinus

### 6.3.1 Anatomy

Frontal sinus is located inferiorly to the squamous part of the frontal bone and represents superior portion of the facial skeleton. Frontal sinus consists of air between a thick anterior and thin and relatively delicate posterior walls (Mehta et al. 2012). The dura and frontal lobes lie just behind the posterior wall of frontal sinus. Drainage of the frontal sinus is maintained by nasofrontal duct, also known as frontal recess, located at the inferomedial aspect of frontal sinus and extends into the middle meatus of nasal cavity (Fig. 40) (Mehta et al. 2012).

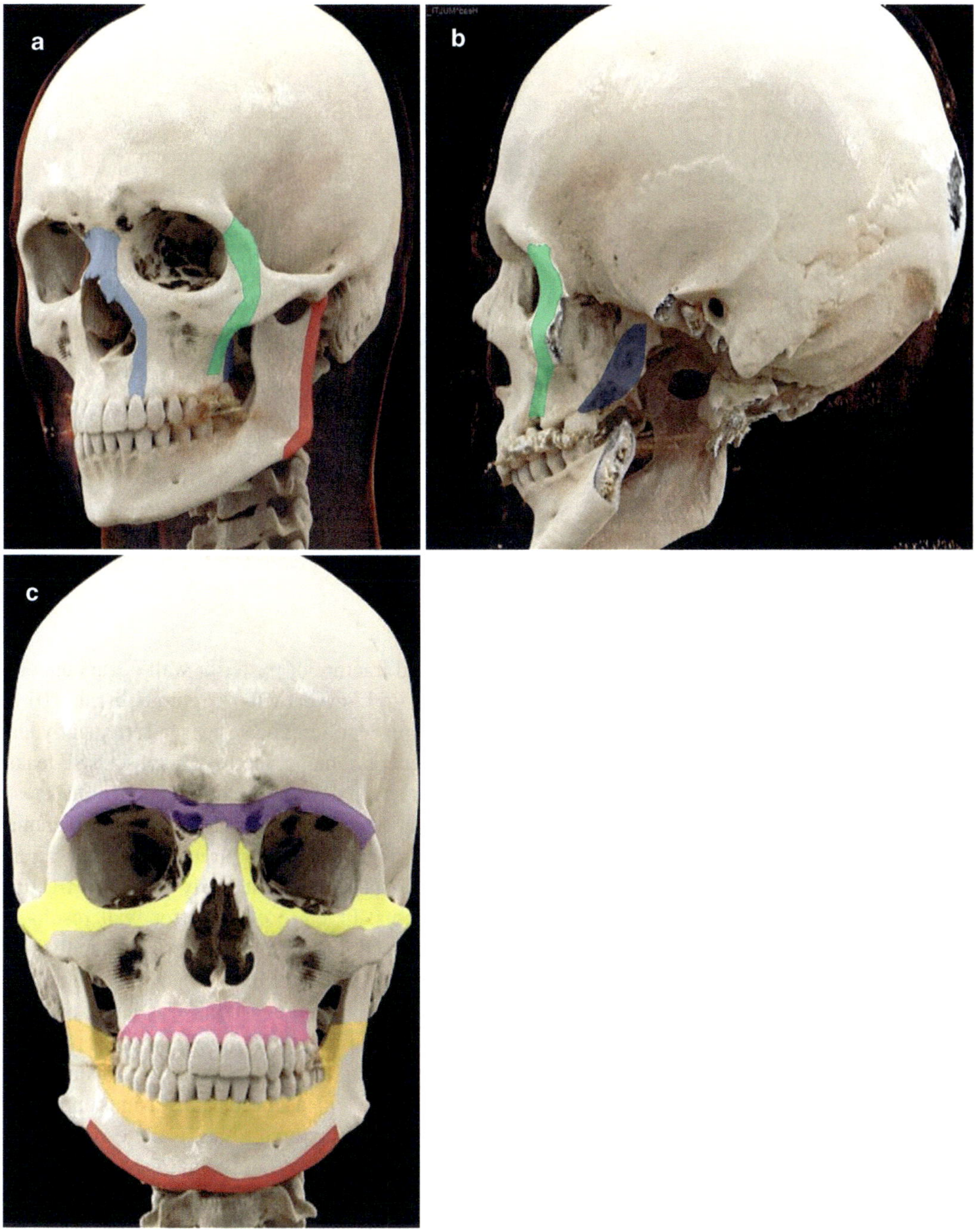


**Fig. 39** Facial buttresses are shown as colored regions on CR images. Left oblique (**a**) and lateral (**b**) views reveal vertical facial buttresses. Medial maxillary buttress (blue), lateral maxillary buttress (green), posterior maxillary buttress (dark blue), and posterior mandibular buttress (red). (**c**) Horizontal facial buttresses. Superior orbital rim (purple), upper transverse maxillary buttress (yellow), lower transverse maxillary buttress (pink), upper transverse mandibular buttress (orange), and lower transverse mandibular buttress (red)

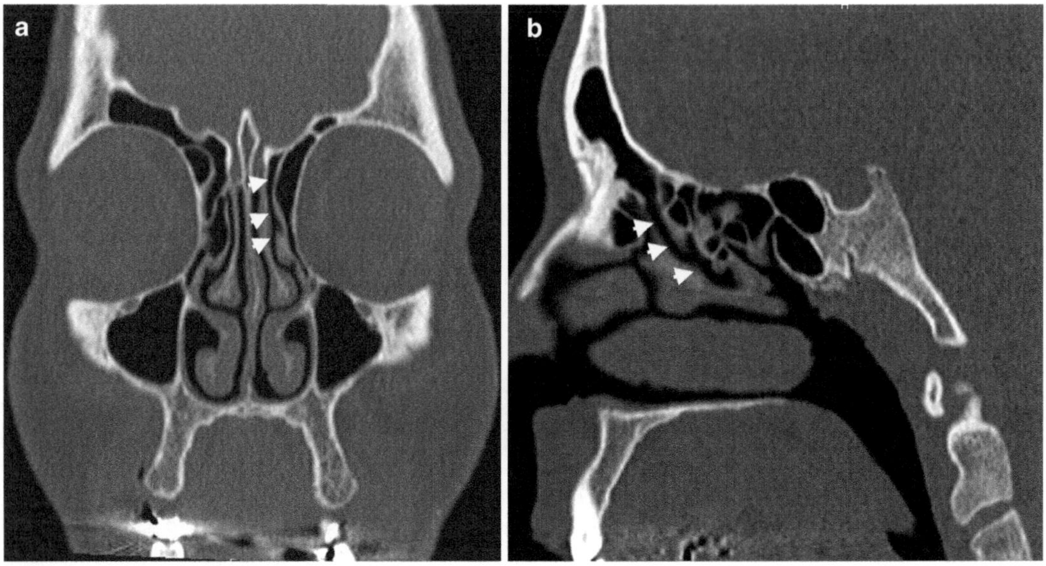


**Fig. 40** Coronal (**a**) and sagittal (**b**) CT images demonstrate nasofrontal duct (arrowheads) extending from frontal sinus to the middle meatus

### 6.3.2 Fracture

Frontal sinus fractures may occur in patients with direct trauma to the sinus part or extension of a calvarial bone fracture into the sinus (Metzinger et al. 2005). Considerable force is required to cause frontal sinus fractures, which were found to be accompanied by another facial fracture in 83% of patients and intracranial injury in 54% of patients (McRae et al. 2008).

Axial CT images have the greatest utility in assessment of frontal sinus. Opacification of frontal sinus with air–fluid level highly indicates traumatic hemorrhage in the frontal sinus.

Involvement of anterior and/or posterior frontal sinus walls and presence or absence of displacement constitute the mainstay issues to be mentioned in assessment of frontal sinus fractures. Displaced frontal sinus fracture refers to displacement of involved bone segment higher than 2 mm or thicker than the width of the sinus wall. Two-thirds of cases with frontal sinus fracture present with involvement of only anterior wall (Fig. 41). Internal mucosal lining is invariably teared after anterior wall fractures, which present almost always with hemorrhage in the sinus. In these patients, cosmetic treatment is only needed if a displaced fracture is observed. Isolated fracture of posterior wall occurs uncommonly (5% of patients) (Schmitt et al. 2014). Fractures involving posterior wall frequently tear adjacent dura mater and may result in CSF leaks, pneumocephalus, meningitis, encephalitis, posttraumatic encephalocele, and abscess. Intracranial hemorrhage and direct traumatic brain injury may be caused by posteriorly projected fracture fragments. Fracture of posterior wall results in communication with the anterior cranial fossa and necessitates to interrogate intracranial air (pneumocephalus) and bone fragments on bone window CT images (Fig. 42). Another potential complication of frontal sinus fracture is intracranial spread of a pre-existing sinus infection through the fractured sinus wall. Frontal sinus fractures also may rarely cause orbital emphysema and CSF leakage into the orbit. Comminuted fractures present with multiple fracture fragments (Fig. 43).

Association of frontal sinus fractures with NOE injuries is not infrequent (Kienstra and Van Loveren 2005). Involvement of the base of frontal sinus, anterior ethmoids, or both in the setting of frontal sinus fracture may cause nasofrontal duct injury. Imaging findings suggestive of nasofrontal duct injury include fracture

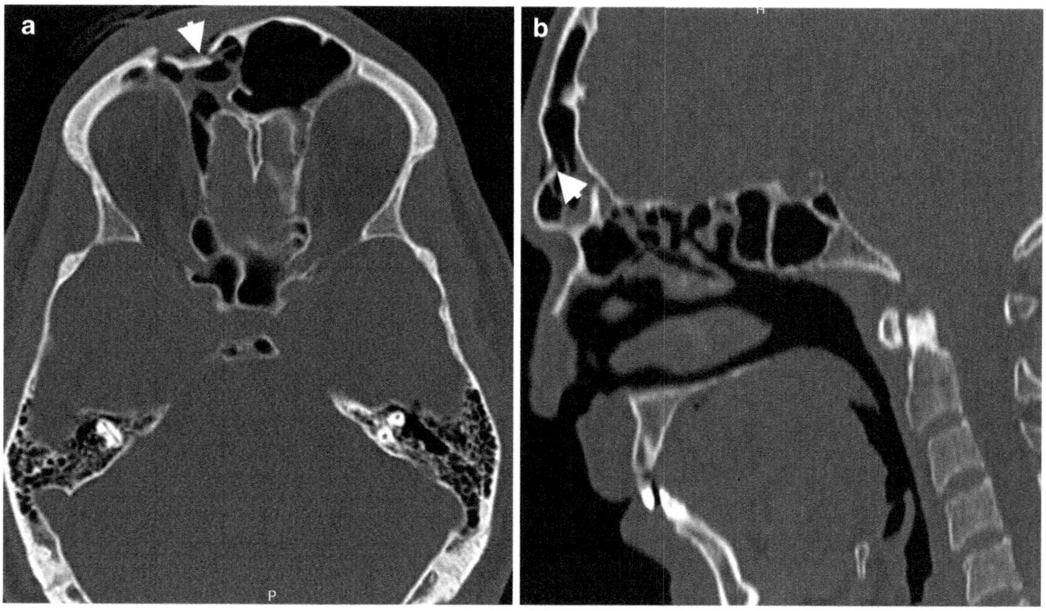

**Fig. 41** Anterior frontal sinus wall fracture. Axial (**a**) and sagittal (**b**) CT images reveal depressed fracture (arrowheads) of the anterior wall of the frontal sinus

fragments within the nasofrontal outflow tract and frontal sinus floor fracture oriented anteromedially (Rodriguez et al. 2008). Nasofrontal duct injury in frontal sinus fractures may be complicated with formation of mucocele, mucopyocele, osteomyelitis, and abscess secondary to impaired frontal sinus drainage (Fig. 44) (Patel et al. 2012). Medial wall fracture of frontal sinus may result in propagation of the fracture through CP and the roof of ethmoidal cells leading to dural tear (Schmitt et al. 2014). Fractures through the lateral aspect of frontal sinus can extend to the orbital roof depending on lateral extent of frontal sinus pneumatization (Schmitt et al. 2014).

Key imaging findings that influence surgical management of frontal sinus fractures include involvement of frontal sinus walls, presence of displacement, involvement of nasofrontal duct, and presence of a dural tear. Anterior wall fractures of frontal sinus can be managed observed if nondisplaced. Displaced fractures may necessitate surgical repair in terms of cosmetic considerations. Posterior wall fractures, if nondisplaced, can be treated conservatively with close imaging follow-up. Displaced posterior wall fractures with pneumocephalus need to be repaired by surgery.

## 6.4 Nasal Bone

### 6.4.1 Anatomy

The nasal skeleton, also called as bony nasal pyramid, is comprised of two nasal bones that articulate with each other in the midline forming the nasal bridge. Nasal bones articulate with nasal process of frontal bone superiorly at the frontonasal suture and the frontal process of maxilla laterally at the nasomaxillary sutures (Dreizin et al. 2018). Nasal septum is formed by vomer inferiorly and perpendicular plate of the ethmoid superiorly, nasal crest of maxilla, and nasal crest of palatine bone posteriorly. The upper portion of nasal bone is the thicker and more resistant to fractures than the lower and thinner portion.

### 6.4.2 Fracture

Nasal bone fractures are encountered in approximately 50% of all facial fractures and are usually caused by blunt forces applied from anterior and lateral directions

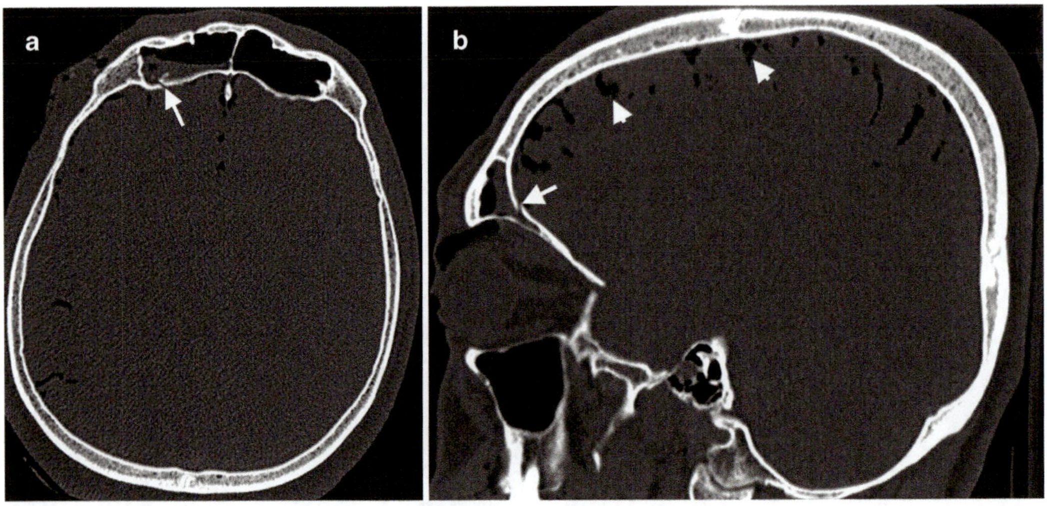


**Fig. 42** Posterior frontal sinus wall fracture. Axial (**a**) and sagittal (**b**) CT images demonstrate depressed fracture of posterior wall of the frontal sinus (arrows) and resultant pneumocephalus (arrowheads)

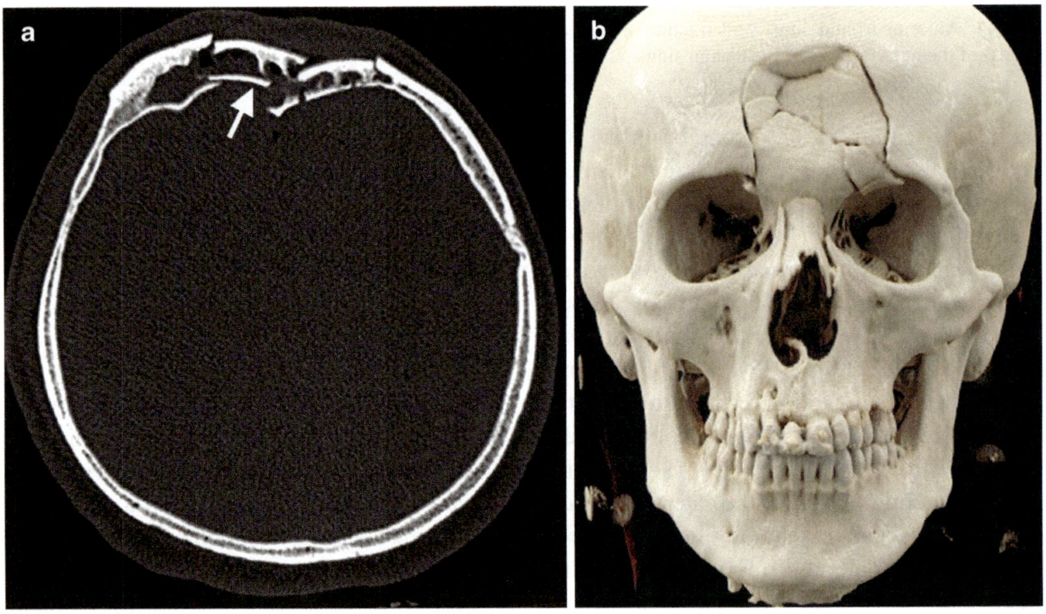


**Fig. 43** Comminuted fracture of frontal sinus. Axial CT (**a**) and (**b**) CR image demonstrate comminuted fracture of frontal sinus with multiple fracture fragments (arrow)

(Mehta et al. 2012). Most of the nasal bone fractures occur in transverse plane, and fractures can be differentiated from nasociliary groove and sutures by the midline crossing nature of fracture (Koch 2014). Nasal bone fractures can be classified as simple, comminuted, and complex fractures. Complex nasal fracture is characterized by involvement of nasal bone with associated nasal septal hematoma or open nasal laceration (Table 4) (Rohrich and Adams Jr. 2000). Most nasal fractures are managed by closed reduction, while nasal bone fractures with septal fracture or dislocation with severe soft-tissue injury may necessitate

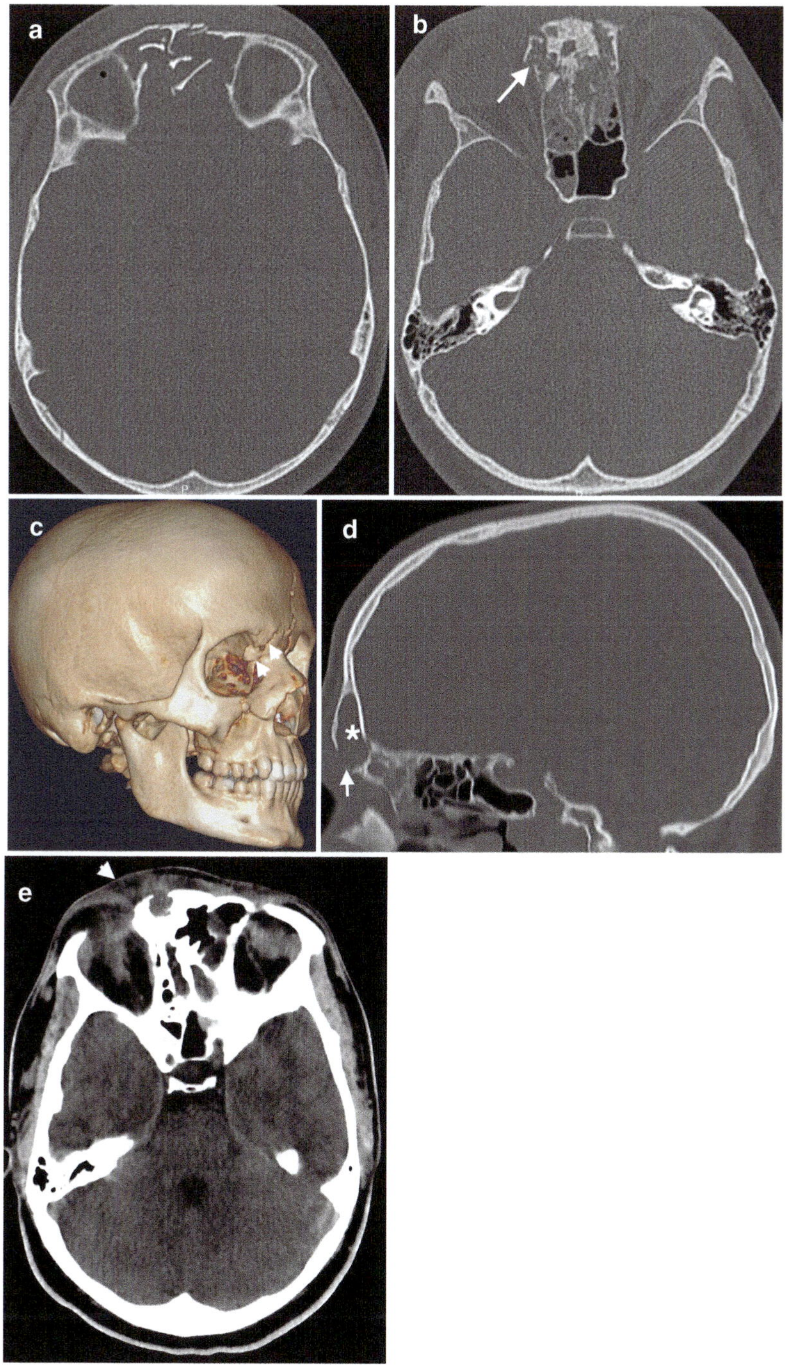


**Fig. 44** Mucopyocele formation secondary to nasofrontal duct injury. (**a**) Axial CT image reveals comminuted fracture of frontal sinus. (**b**) CT image at the level of nasofrontal recess reveals extension of fracture (arrow) along anterior and middle ethmoid air cells and nasofrontal duct region. (**c**) VR image demonstrates fracture (arrowheads) involving inferomedial part of the right frontal sinus. (**d**) Sagittal image of follow-up CT examination obtained 1 month after the trauma shows defect in the anterior wall of frontal sinus (arrow). Expansion of frontal sinus with high-density content is consistent with mucocele/mucopyocele (*) formation. (**e**) Axial CT image on soft-tissue window reveals propagation of inflammation to the subcutaneous tissue (arrowhead) through wall defect that indicates mucopyocele formation

**Table 4** Classification of nasal fractures (Rohrich and Adams Jr. 2000)

| Type | Category | Characteristics |
|---|---|---|
| I | Simple | Unilateral |
| II | Simple | Bilateral |
| III | Comminuted | Unilateral<br>Bilateral |
| IV | Complex | Associated with septal hematoma<br>Associated with open nasal laceration |
| V | | Associated with NOE fracture/midface fracture |

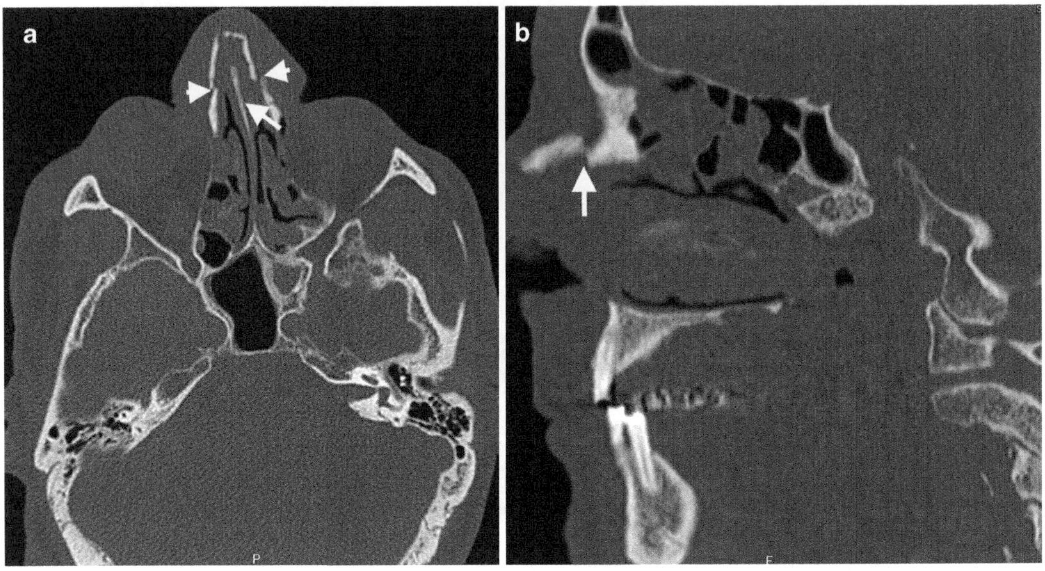


**Fig. 45** Simple nasal fracture in a 60-year-old man with a history of assault. (**a**) Axial CT image demonstrates bilateral nasal bone fractures (arrowheads). The nasal septum is spared (arrow). (**b**) Sagittal CT image reveals displacement of fracture fragment (arrow)

open repair (Ondik et al. 2009). Radiographic position preferred in nasal bone fracture is lateral nasal view. However, the sensitivity of lateral view radiography in nasal bone fracture ranges between 53% and 90% (Lo Casto et al. 2012). Nasal bone and septum injuries should be assessed with MPR CT images since 25% of nasal pyramid fractures may be missed on axial CT images, while sagittal reformatted images can demonstrate these fractures with a sensitivity of 85–99% (Figs. 45 and 46) (Kim et al. 2010). Missed nasal fractures may result in bony malunion, and further osteotomy can be required to reduce fracture fragments. Axial CT images are especially helpful to demonstrate telescoping and/or comminution of nasal bone and septum. Bowing of the bony nasal septum should also be assessed on coronal CT images. Septal fractures and dislocations may cause deforming forces on fractured nasal bones during healing by exerting force on upper lateral cartilages. This may result in malunion of nasal bones after rhinoplasty (Dreizin et al. 2018). Anterior nasal spine fractures may be detected on axial and sagittal CT images (Fig. 47). Nasal fractures usually extend in transverse orientation and can cross the midline in contrast to sutures and nasociliary grooves in nasal region, which are vertically oriented and cannot cross the midline (Schmitt et al. 2014).

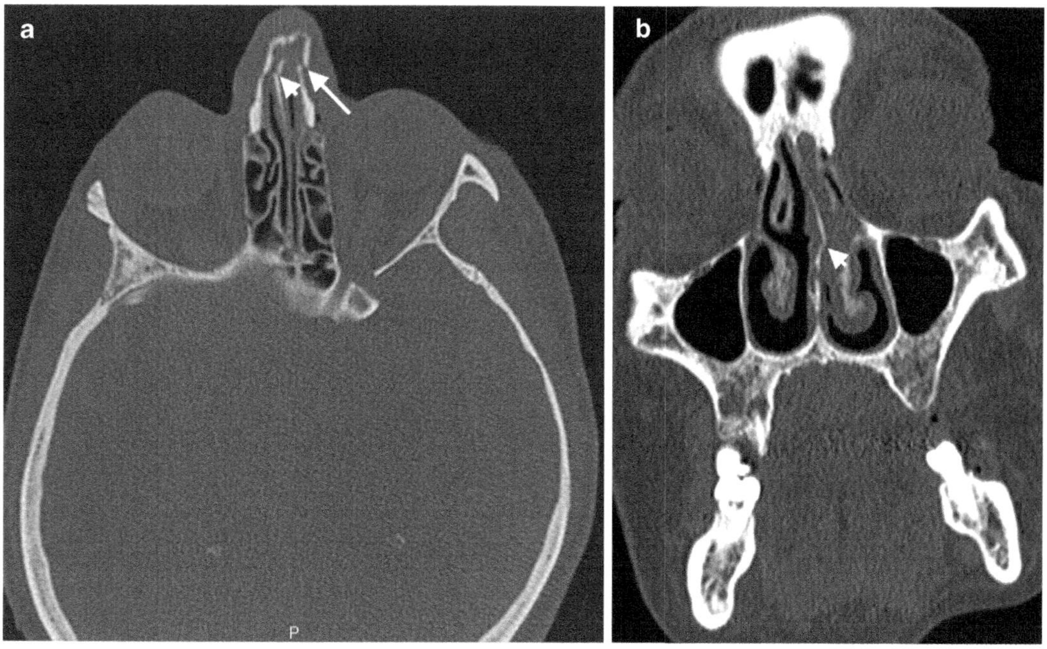


**Fig. 46** Nasal bone and septum fracture in a 50-year-old woman with a history of assault. Axial (**a**) and coronal (**b**) CT images demonstrate fracture of nasal bone (arrow) and nasal septum (arrowheads)

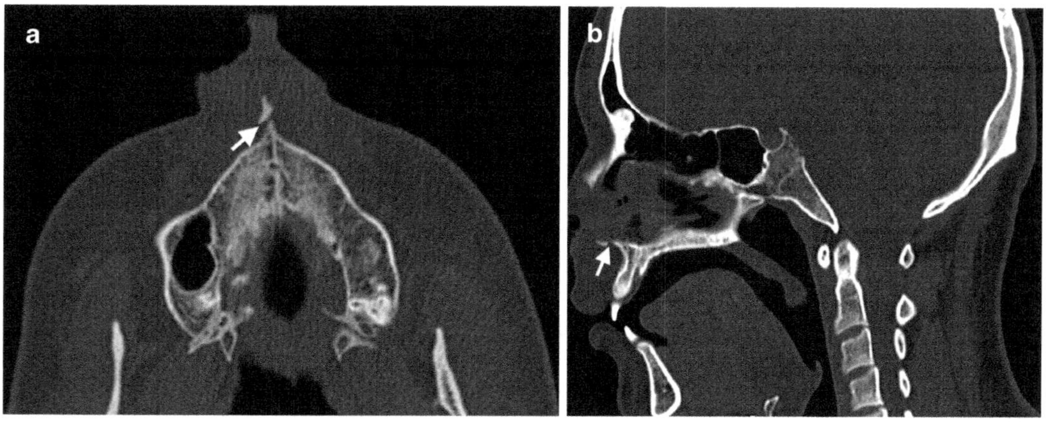


**Fig. 47** Anterior nasal spine fracture in a 21-year-old woman after MVA. Axial (**a**) and sagittal (**b**) CT images demonstrate anterior nasal spine fracture (arrows)

Injury of the nasal cartilage may result in disruption of the perichondrium and formation of septal hematoma, abscess, and necrosis leading to perforation and collapse of nasal septum (Fig. 48) (Rohrich and Adams Jr. 2000). Early and prompt diagnosis of nasal bone fracture is crucial for avoiding clinical complications and cosmetic deformities such as saddle nose.

Radiation exposure and high cost of CT increase the controversies about the utility of CT for isolated nasal bone fractures since isolated bones may be detected and even reducted with manual palpation. Cone-beam tomography has been introduced as an alternative technique as an alternative with the advantages of lower radiation dose and submillimetric resolution (Bremke et al. 2009).

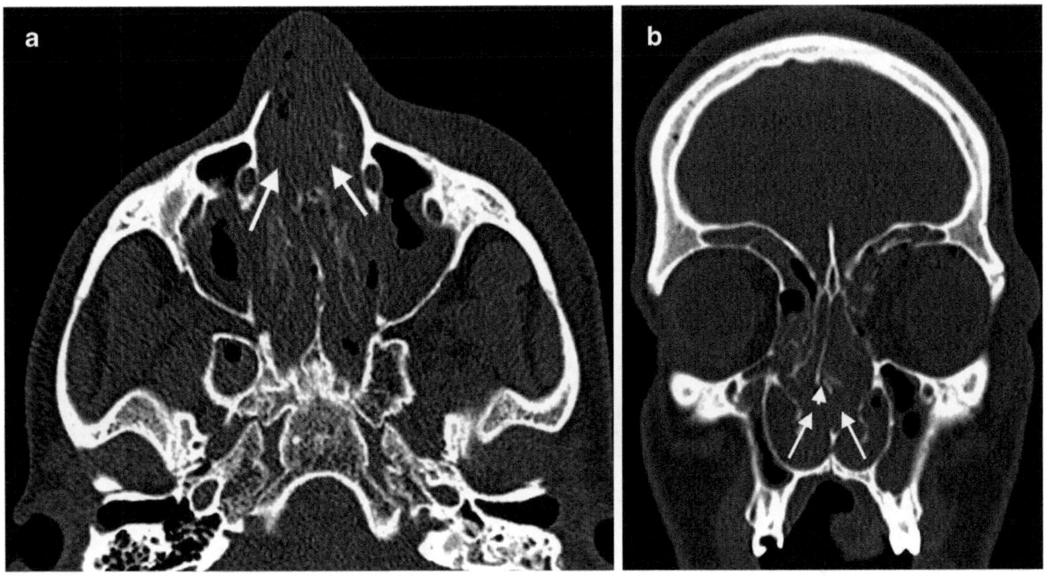


**Fig. 48** Septal hematoma in a 21-year-old man after MVA. Axial (**a**) and coronal (**b**) CT images reveal abundant hemorrhage (arrows) resulted from nasal fracture

## 6.5 Naso-Orbital-Ethmoid Fractures

### 6.5.1 Anatomy

Naso-orbitoethmoid (NOE) region is the junction point where nose, orbita, maxilla, and ethmoid bones meet. This area is bordered superiorly by CP, laterally by thin medial orbital walls, anteriorly by bony pillar (proximal part of nasal bone, nasal process of frontal bone, and frontal process of maxilla) and posteriorly by sphenoid sinus. NOE region contains important anatomical structures including olfactory nerves, lacrimal sac, frontonasal and nasolacrimal duct, medial canthal tendon (MCT), and ethmoidal vessels (Mehta et al. 2012). MCT inserts on the lacrimal crest bordering lacrimal fossa (Ellis 3rd 2012; Elbarbary and Ali 2014). MCT supports canthus (palpebral commissures), approaches eyelid to bulbus, and maintains drainage of the lacrimal sac.

### 6.5.2 Fracture

Fracture of NOE complex results from high-impact force applied anteriorly to the nose. NOE fractures disrupt the confluence of medial maxillary buttress and upper transverse maxillary buttress with involvement of ethmoid bone, nasal bone, medial orbital wall, frontal process of maxilla, and inferior orbital rim (Sargent 2007; Koch 2014). Telescoping of involved bones that is characterized by posterior displacement of anterior nasal structures into the medial orbital rim, nasal septum, nasofrontal junction, and ethmoid sinuses may occur in NOE fractures (Avery et al. 2011). Diagnosis of NOE fracture is difficult compared to other midface fractures due to camouflaging effect of facial swelling in NOE area during physical examination. NOE fractures are classified according to the Markowitz and Manson classification system that is based on a central bone fragment in medial orbital rim that contains attachment of MCT (Markowitz et al. 1991). Type I NOE fracture refers to a single large segment fracture fragment of the medial orbital rim without comminution and MCT injury. In type II fractures, there is a comminuted fracture with small pieces of bones in medial orbital rim and MCT is attached to the single bone fragment. Type III NOE fracture is characterized by comminution of central fragment and disruption or avulsion of MCT from the bone (Fig. 49) (Markowitz et al. 1991). CT assessment of NOE fractures should include the type of

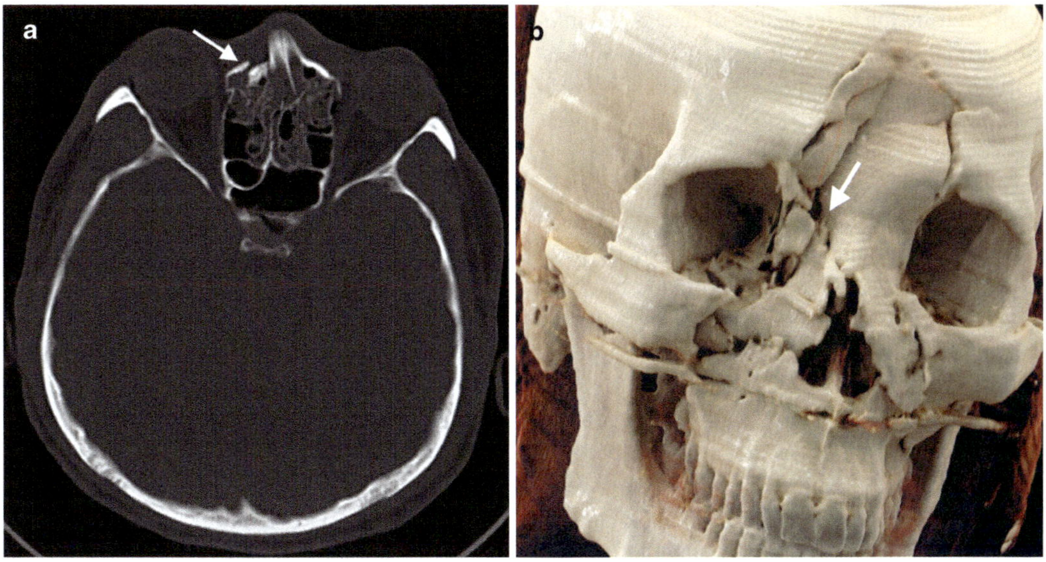


**Fig. 49** Type III NOE fracture in a 19-year-old man with a history of MVA. (**a**) Axial CT image reveals right NOE fracture involving nasolacrimal duct (arrow). (**b**) CR image demonstrates type III NOE fracture (arrow) with multiple bone fragments

injury, degree of comminution and displacement, associated fractures, and soft-tissue injury. In addition to MPR images, NOE fractures necessitate assessment with 3D VR or CR images to visualize multiple curving planes of NOE region (Dreizin et al. 2018).

Injuries of NOE region are usually anteriorly directed and affect the thick nasal bone portions known as nasal bridge. Fracture of nasal bones usually presents with ethmoidal air cell fractures since ethmoidal air cells have low resistance to the impacting force compared to the nasal bone. Injury or occlusion of frontonasal duct should be suspected when axial CT images demonstrate intrusion of nasal dorsum into the anterior ethmoid complex (Potter et al. 2006; Jain et al. 2010). NOE fractures may cause impaction of nasal saddle and buckling of nasal septum resulting in the appearance of nose pushed back between the eyes. Complications of NOE fractures include CSF rhinorrhea secondary to fracture of CP, obstruction of the lacrimal system, telecanthus (increased intercanthal and interpupillary distance) due to MCT injury, facial deformity, and exophthalmos caused by decreased orbital volume (Winegar et al. 2013).

Since fractures of NOE are encountered following high-energy traumas, isolated NOE fractures uncommonly occur and Le Fort 2 and Le Fort 3 fractures usually accompany the NOE fractures (Ellis 3rd 2012). Involvement of CP should be interrogated on CT in NOE fractures due to potential complications including olfactory nerve disruption, CSF leak, pneumocephalus, or tension pneumocephalus resulting from resuscitation efforts through airways (Mehta et al. 2012).

## 6.6 Zygomatic Bone

### 6.6.1 Anatomy

Zygomatic bone, also called malar bone, contributes to the anterolateral aspect of superior face and inferior orbital rim. Zygomatic bone is an integral part of facial buttress system by articulating with frontal, maxillary bones, arch of the temporal bone, and greater wing of the sphenoid bone with the following sutures as zygomaticofrontal, zygomaticomaxillary, zygomaticotemporal, and zygomaticosphenoid suture. Zygomatic bone provides support to the orbital soft tissue with contribution to formation of lateral and inferior orbital walls (Schmitt et al. 2014). Weakest portion of zygomatic bone is zygomaticosphenoid joint.

### 6.6.2 Fracture

Zygomatic bone has a tendency to fracture in maxillofacial trauma due to its superficial position and convex alignment. Zygomatic fractures occur most frequently in the form of zygomaticomaxillary complex (ZMC) fractures that result from anterolateral impact to the cheek and are characterized by separation of the zygomatic bone along its sutural attachments with spectrum of fractures with varying displacements (Mehta et al. 2012). ZMC fractures are defined as quadripod fractures since four surrounding sutures across the zygomatic bone are involved in these fractures. The four breakpoints involved in ZMC fractures are zygomaticomaxillary buttress in the inferior orbital rim, zygomaticosphenoid suture along the lateral orbital wall, zygomaticofrontal suture of the lateral orbital rim, and zygomaticotemporal suture (Sung et al. 2012).

ZMC fractures are classified with Zingg classification. Zingg type A ZMC fracture is isolated incomplete fracture involving only one limb of the zygoma (Fig. 50); type B fracture refers to classic tetrapod fracture characterized by liberated zygomatic mono-fragment (Fig. 51); and type C fracture is defined as comminuted fracture. Zingg type A fractures are subdivided into three subtypes as type A1 involving zygomatic arch, type A2 involving lateral orbital rim or wall, and type A3 involving inferior orbital rim (Dreizin et al. 2018; Zingg et al. 1992).

Zygomatic bone fractures may present on axial CT images as malar retrusion, rotation of zygomaticosphenoid suture and zygomaticomaxillary buttress, and depressed or comminuted zygomatic arch. MPR images can reveal overall ZMC malalignment and orbital volume changes (Ellis 3rd 2012; Marinho and Freire-Maia 2013). Depressed ZMC fractures usually result from rotational forces applied by masseter muscle on zygomatic bone. Severe depression or impingement of depressed zygoma fracture fragments on the coronoid process of mandible and/or temporalis muscle may cause inclosure of the jaw and trismus (Marinho and Freire-Maia 2013; Dreizin et al. 2018). ZMC fractures involving lateral orbital wall may cause enophthalmos due to increased orbital volume. Frank zygomatic arch fractures may present as zygomaticotemporal suture diastasis.

Nondisplaced fractures of zygomatic bones do not require surgical treatment; however, in the setting of comminuted fractures, displacement of bone fragments and comminution degree determine the surgery planning.

## 6.7 Maxilla Fractures

### 6.7.1 Anatomy

Maxillary bones form the skeleton of face between the mouth and eye as being the projectory of midface in anteroposterior plane. Each maxillary bone consists of body, containing maxillary sinus, zygomatic, frontal, palatine, and alveolar processes. Two maxillary bones unite in the midline with intermaxillary suture and form the entire upper jaw. Maxillary bones contribute to the facial buttress system, lateral wall of the nasal cavity, orbital floor, and anterior wall of the infratemporal fossa.

### 6.7.2 Fracture

Fractures of maxillary bones are usually associated with the injury to the midface bony structures. Classification of maxillary fractures was made by René Le Fort in 1901 as Le Fort I, II, and III fractures. Le Fort classification mainly depends on the level of fracture line in posterior maxilla. Common imaging feature of Le Fort fractures is pterygoid plate fracture. Le Fort fractures usually present asymmetrically, and different combinations of Le Fort fractures may coexist in the same side. Le Fort I, II, and III fractures represent palatofacial dysjunction, midfacial separation, and craniofacial separation, respectively.

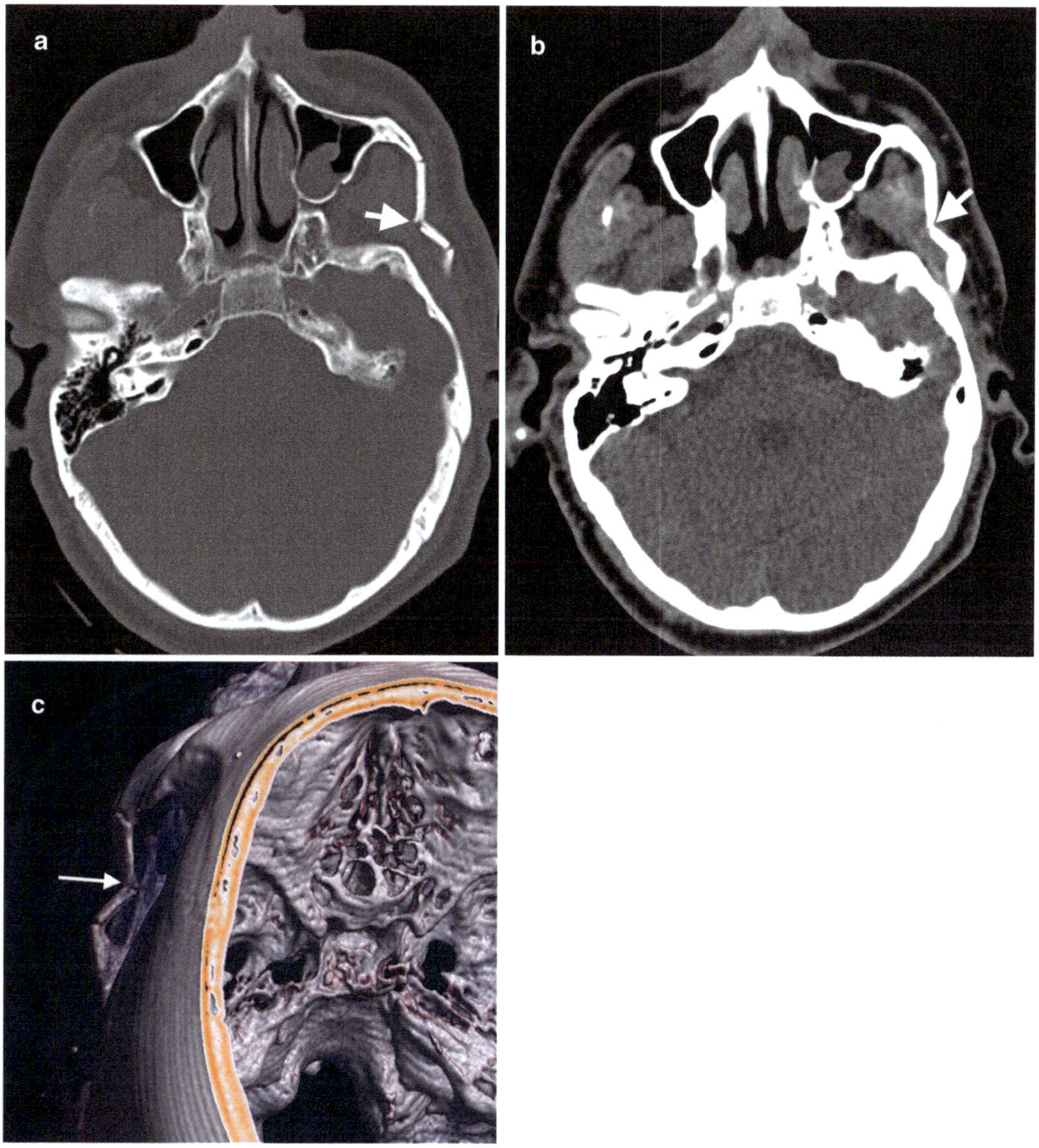


**Fig. 50** Zygomatic arch fracture in a 51-year-old man presented to emergency service with malar pain and malocclusion after MVA. (**a**) Axial CT image on bone window shows depressed fracture of left zygomatic bone (arrow) with medial angulation. (**b**) Axial CT image on soft-tissue window reveals impingement of the left temporalis muscle (arrow). (**c**) VR image demonstrates depressed fracture (arrow) of left zygomatic bone

Le Fort I fracture results from horizontal impact to the upper jaw and is characterized by a transverse fracture immediately superior to the maxillary alveolar process. This fracture type crosses the floor of the maxillary sinus and lower nasal septum, anterior, medial, and lateral maxillary walls, and inferior margin of pyriform aperture and extends posteriorly into the pterygoid plates (Fig. 52). Le Fort I fracture results in separation of maxillary alveolus and/or hard palate from upper face creating malocclusion with a free-floating alveolus and hard palate

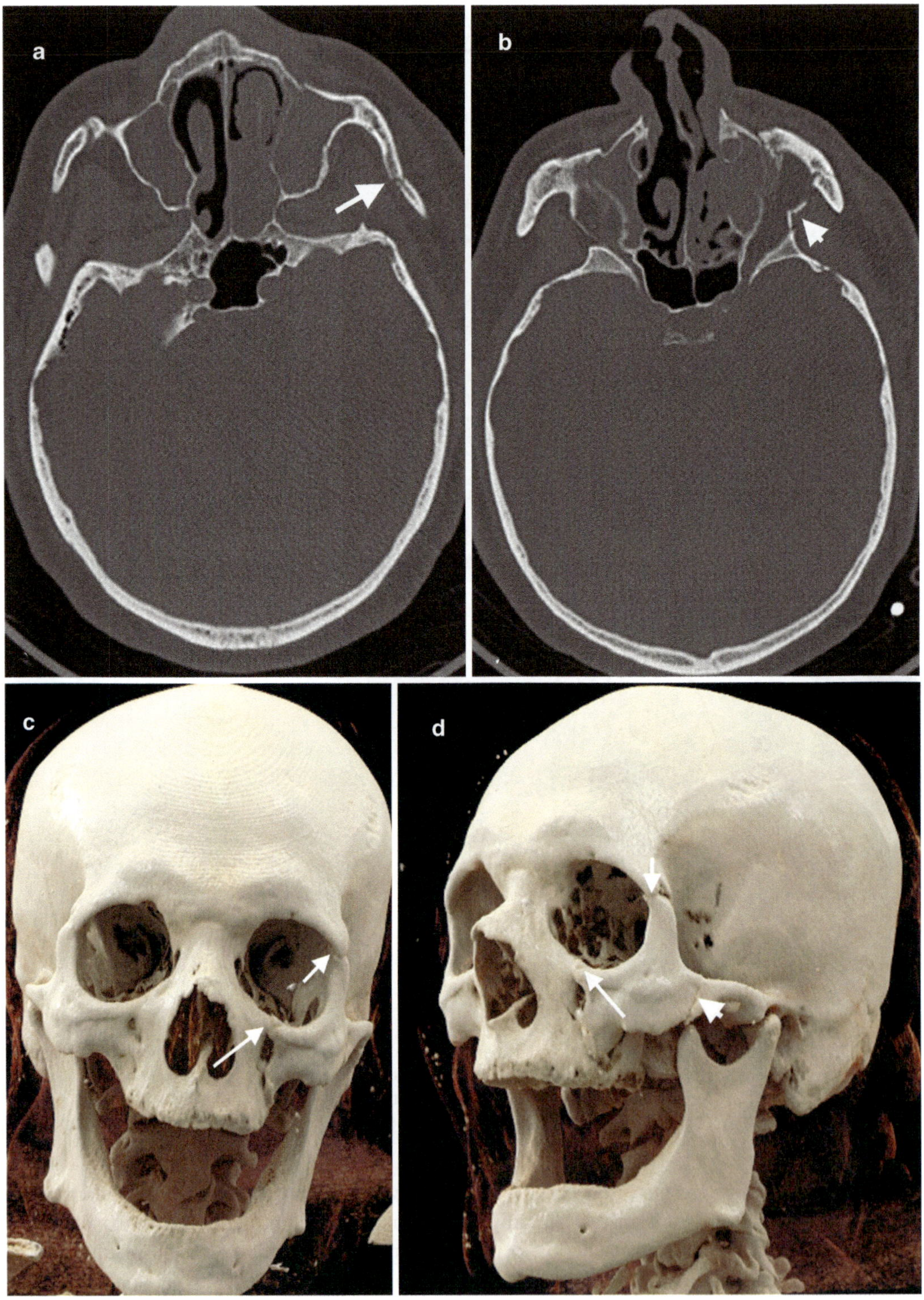


**Fig. 51** Fracture of ZMC complex in a 56-year-old man after MVA. (**a**) Axial CT image shows left zygomatic arch (arrow) fracture. (**b**) Axial CT image of the same patient reveals a fracture (arrowhead) involving zygomaticosphenoid suture. CR images with AP (**c**) and left oblique (**d**) views reveal ZMC fracture with involvement of zygomaticomaxillary suture (long arrows) and zygomaticofrontal sutures (short arrows) consistent with quadripod fracture

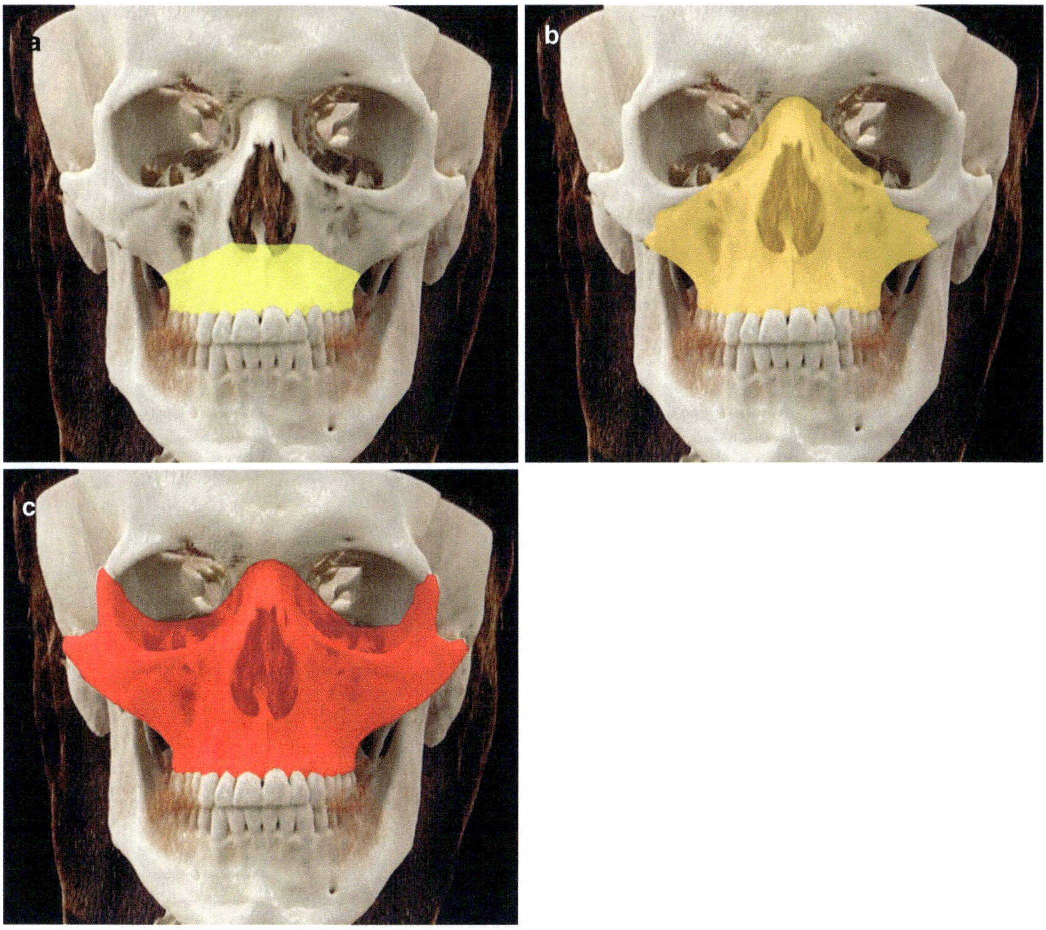


**Fig. 52** Involvement areas of Le Fort fractures. (**a**) Le Fort I fracture area (yellow). (**b**) Le Fort II fracture area (orange). (**c**) Le Fort III fracture area (red)

(Mehta et al. 2012; Lo Casto et al. 2012). Infraorbital rims are spared in Le Fort I fracture. Le Fort I fractures can be best depicted on coronal and 3D CT images due to anteroposterior orientation of these fractures (Fig. 53) (Winegar et al. 2013). Fracture of pterygoid plates can be best assessed on axial CT images.

Le Fort II fracture, also called as pyramidal shape fracture, is defined as a fracture involving frontonasal suture, bilateral zygomaticomaxillary sutures, inferior orbital rim and floor, maxillary sinuses, medial orbital walls, and posteriorly pterygoid plates (Fig. 52) (Dreizin et al. 2018). Nasal bridge may be involved or spared. Le Fort II fracture creates a pyramid-shaped maxillary fragment and separates the nasal region from the cranium. This fracture type is conceptualized as a floating maxilla. Characteristic finding of the Le Fort II fractures includes involvement of inferior orbital rim and floor. Zygomatic bone is spared in Le Fort II fractures although zygomaticomaxillary suture may be involved. Superior parts of medial maxillary, inferior part of lateral maxillary, upper transverse maxillary, and posterior maxillary buttresses are involved in Le Fort II fractures (Fig. 54).

Le Fort III fracture refers to complete craniofacial dissociation caused by suprazygomatic fracture extending horizontally from the frontonasal suture to the frontozygomatic sutures and

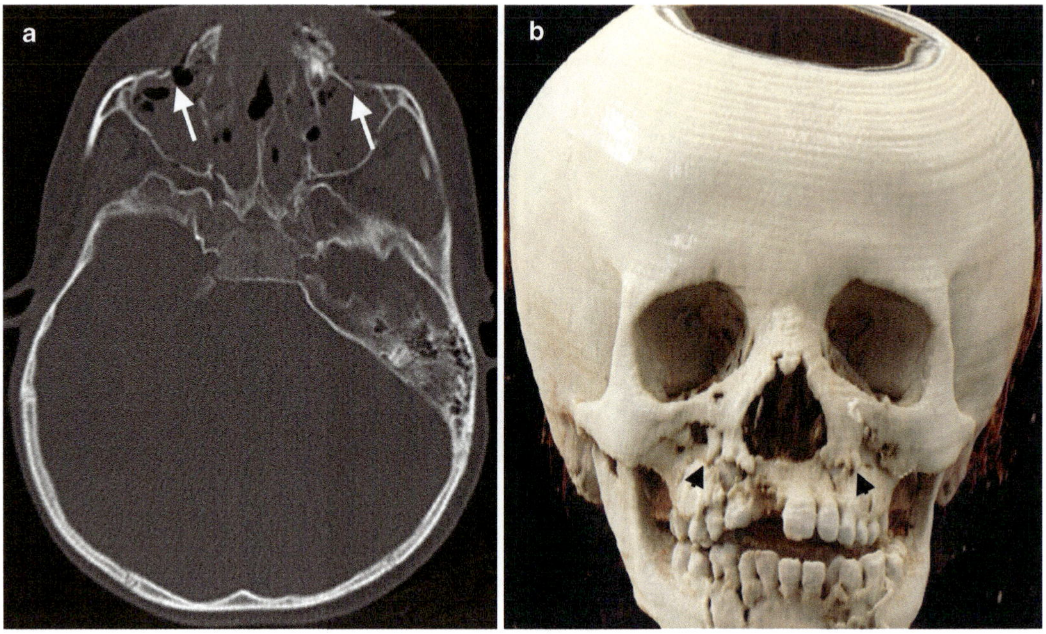


**Fig. 53** Le Fort I fracture. (**a**) Axial CT image shows bilateral anterior maxillary sinus wall fractures (arrow). (**b**) CR image demonstrates Le Fort I fracture (black arrowheads) extending through superior to the maxillary alveolar process

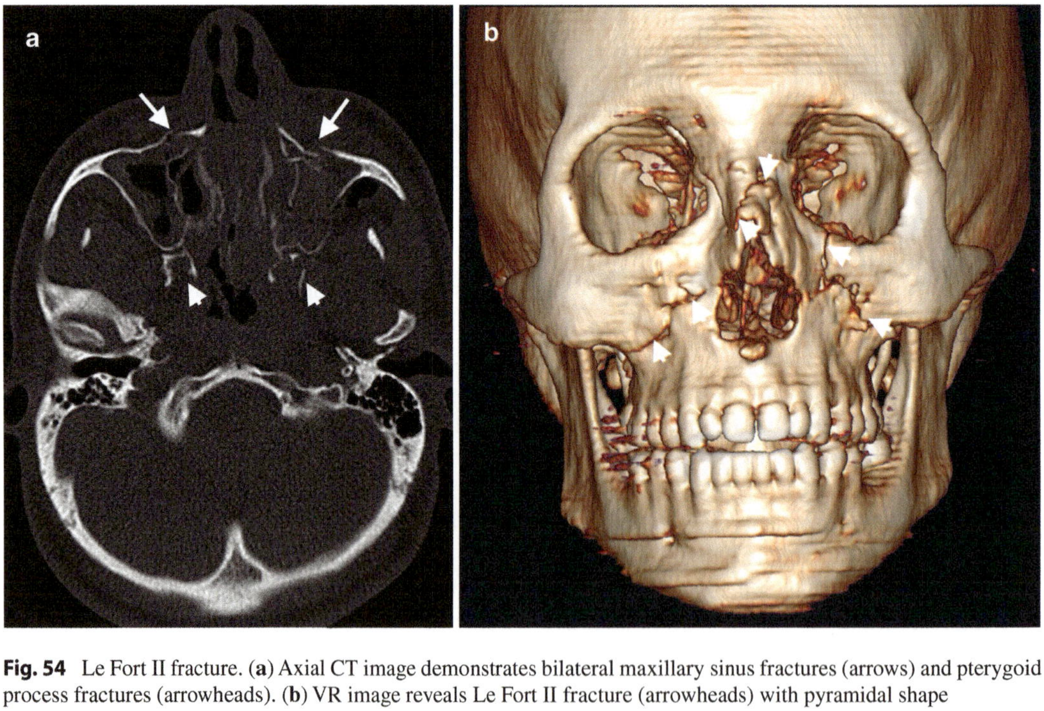


**Fig. 54** Le Fort II fracture. (**a**) Axial CT image demonstrates bilateral maxillary sinus fractures (arrows) and pterygoid process fractures (arrowheads). (**b**) VR image reveals Le Fort II fracture (arrowheads) with pyramidal shape

zygomatic arches in the line traversing medial and lateral orbital walls. This fracture type separates the zygomaticofrontal sutures and zygomatic arches and terminates through the pterygoid plates resulting in separation of face from the skull base (Fig. 55) (Mehta et al. 2012). Le Fort III fractures present frequently as combinations of ZMC and NOE fractures (Dreizin et al. 2018). Superior portions of the medial maxillary and lateral maxillary, upper transverse maxillary, and posterior maxillary buttresses are involved in Le Fort III fractures (Winegar et al. 2013). Unique imaging finding of Le Fort III fracture is involvement of lateral orbital rim and zygomatic arch.

There are distinguishing imaging key points that can be used in differentiation of Le Fort fractures. Anterolateral margin of the nasal fossa is involved in only Le Fort I fracture. Le Fort II fracture differs from others by involvement of the inferior orbital rim. Le Fort III fracture is characterized as the only type that involves the zygomatic arch (Sung et al. 2012). Although nasofrontal suture and medial orbital wall are involved in Le Fort II and III fractures, these two fracture types can be distinguished by involvement of lateral orbital wall and zygomatic arch in Le Fort III fracture (Fig. 56) (Winegar et al. 2013). Le Fort fractures may cause significant functional and cosmetic problems and complications such as rhinorrhea, otorrhea, pneumocephalus, and intracranial complications with potential extension to carotid canal and orbital apex (Bellamy et al. 2013).

Isolated alveolar process fracture in maxillary bone involves lower transverse maxillary buttress and results from direct force applied to the alveolar process or indirect force transmitted from the underlying teeth via the base of dental crown (Winegar et al. 2013). Alveolar process fracture may cause dental root avulsion, crown or root fracture, dental intrusion or extrusion, and malocclusion (Fig. 57) (Lieger et al. 2009).

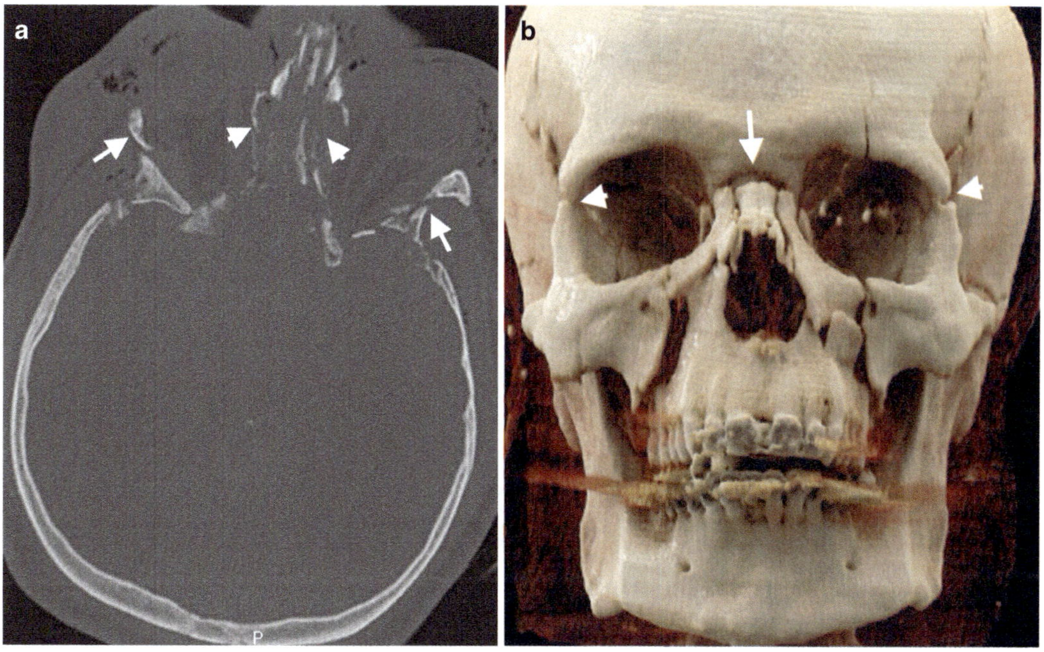


**Fig. 55** Le Fort III fracture. (**a**) Axial CT image demonstrates medial (arrowheads) and lateral walls (arrows) fractures of bilateral orbita. (**b**) CR image shows Le fort III fracture extending through bilateral zygomaticofrontal suture (arrowheads) and nasal bridge (arrow). CR image also reveals bilateral Le Fort II fracture with involvement of bilateral maxillary bones extending into inferior orbital rims

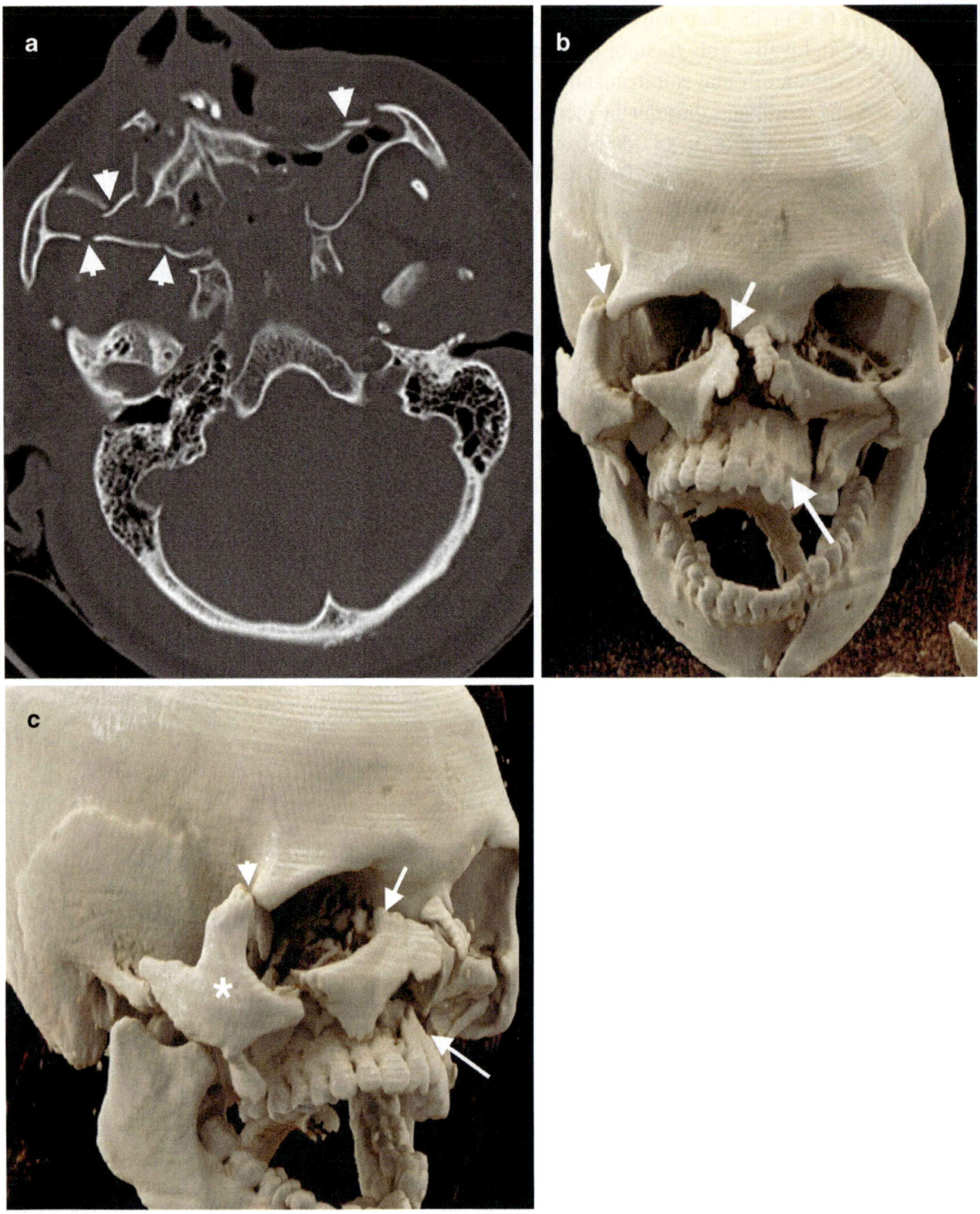

**Fig. 56** Concurrent Le Fort I, II, and III fracture. (**a**) Axial CT image demonstrates multiple maxillofacial fractures (arrowheads) with telescoping. CR images at AP (**b**) and right oblique (**c**) views demonstrate Le Fort I fracture as floating palate (long arrows), Le Fort II fracture (short arrow), and Le Fort III fracture with right ZMC fracture (arrowheads). Zygomatic bone is seen as a liberated fragment (*) secondary to quadripod fracture

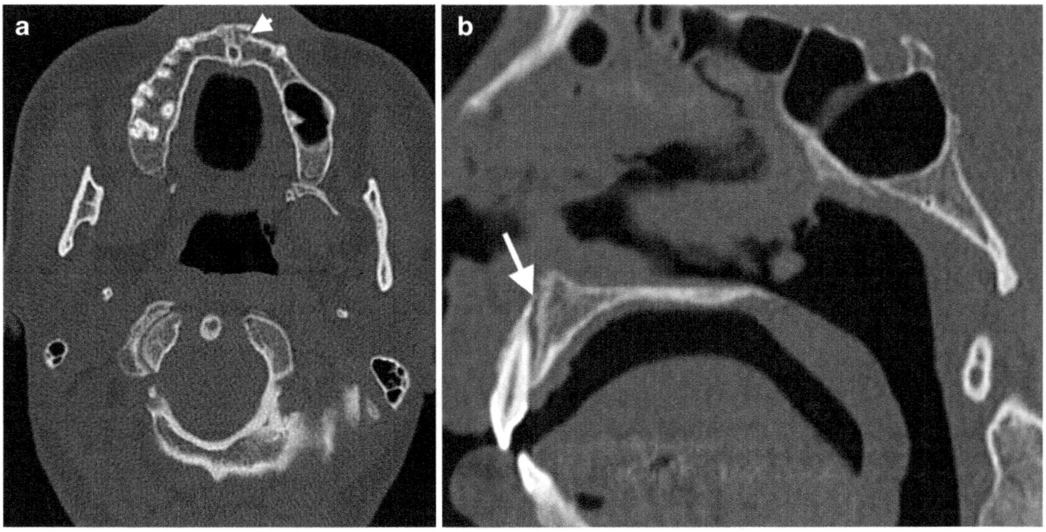


**Fig. 57** Alveolar process fracture. (**a**) Axial CT image reveals a fracture (arrowhead) of left first incisive root. (**b**) Sagittal CT image demonstrates fracture (arrow) oriented in oblique position involving tooth root

## 6.8 Palatine Bone

### 6.8.1 Anatomy

The palatine bone is an L-shaped, paired bone located between the maxilla and sphenoid bone. Palatine bone is formed by a horizontal and perpendicular plate and the pyramidal process. Horizontal plate forms the posterior 1/3 portion of the hard palate, while perpendicular plate contributes to the lateral wall of the nasal cavity neighboring the pterygoid process of sphenoid bone.

### 6.8.2 Fracture

Palatal fractures are encountered in up to one-half of Le Fort fractures (Chen et al. 2008). These fractures should be assessed on MPR CT images. Palatal fractures separate maxilla into left and right symmetric or asymmetric pairs (Avery et al. 2011). Classification of palatal fractures is based on direction of fractures. Type 1 palatal fractures account for 90% of fractures and oriented sagittally beginning at the maxillary alveolus and propagating to paramedian or para-alveolar locations (Fig. 58). Type 2 fractures extend horizontally dividing the hard palate in the coronal plane. Type 3 fractures refer to complex and comminuted fractures (Chen et al. 2008).

## 6.9 Mandibular Fractures

### 6.9.1 Anatomy

The mandible is the only mobile bone in face with attachment to the skull base via two temporomandibular joints. It has a central anterior unit containing symphyseal and parasymphyseal region with bilateral horizontal body, angle, and vertical units as ramus containing condylar neck, head, subcondylar region, coronoid process, and finally alveolar process (Dreizin et al. 2016; Morrow et al. 2014). The upper border of mandibular body is the alveolar part, and the lower part is the base of the mandible. A vertical line drawn from the lower canine tooth separates parasymphysis and mandibular body,

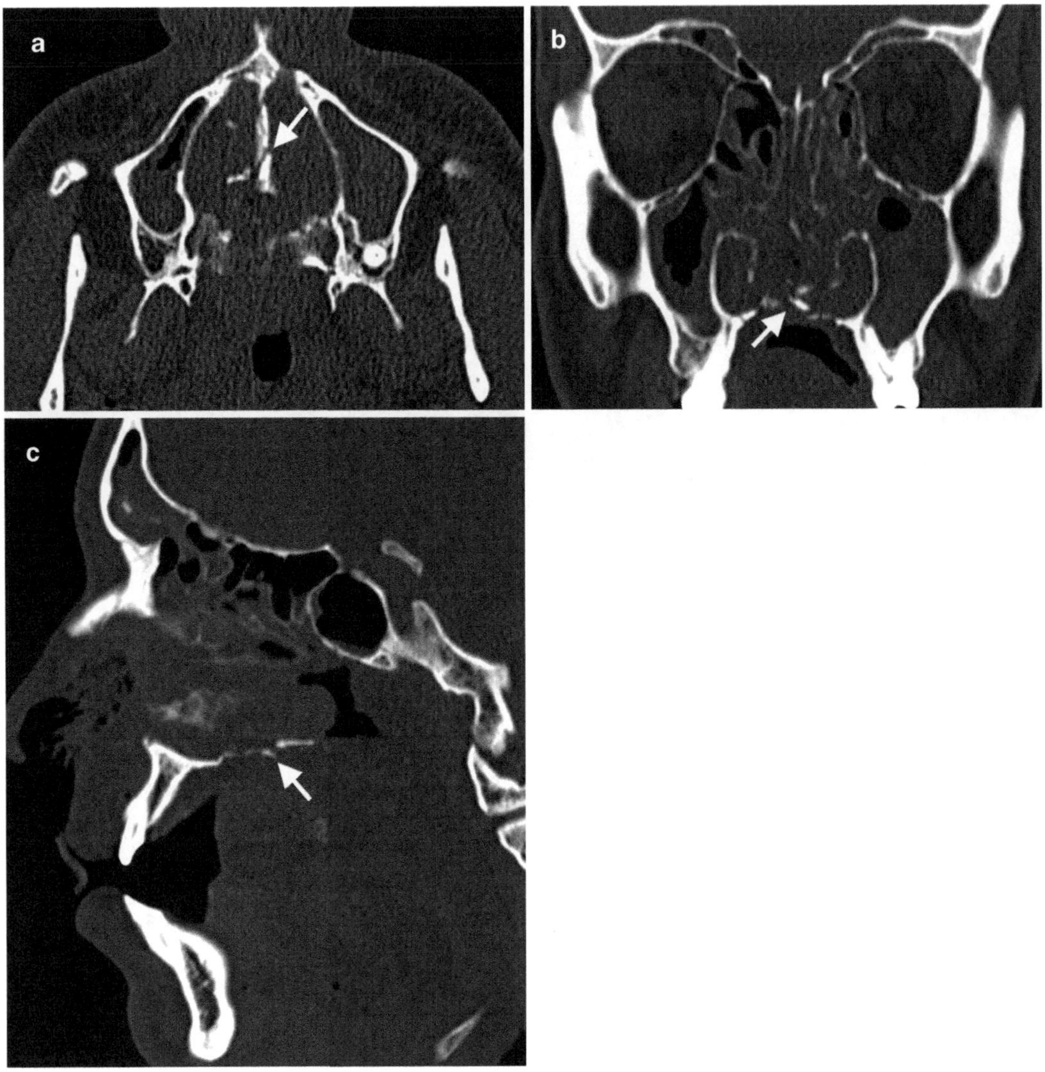


**Fig. 58** Palatine bone fracture. Axial (**a**), coronal (**b**), and sagittal (**c**) CT images demonstrate displaced fracture (arrows) of the hard palate

whereas a vertical line drawn from third molar tooth socket superiorly and masseter muscle insertion inferiorly separates angle from the body. Condyle and glenoid fossa form the synovial temporomandibular joint (Dreizin et al. 2016; Avery et al. 2011).

### 6.9.2 Fracture

Mandibular fractures are the second most common facial fractures with high complication rates. Motor vehicle collisions, falls, and assaults are the leading causes of mandibular fractures. Mandibular fractures tend to involve multiple places due to curved or ring-like shape of the bone. Unifocal fractures occur in 30–40% of cases, and unilateral fractures are more likely in childhood than their adult counterparts (Koch 2014; Escott and Branstetter 2008). Mandibular fractures can be classified according to the localization of fracture, which depends on the type of

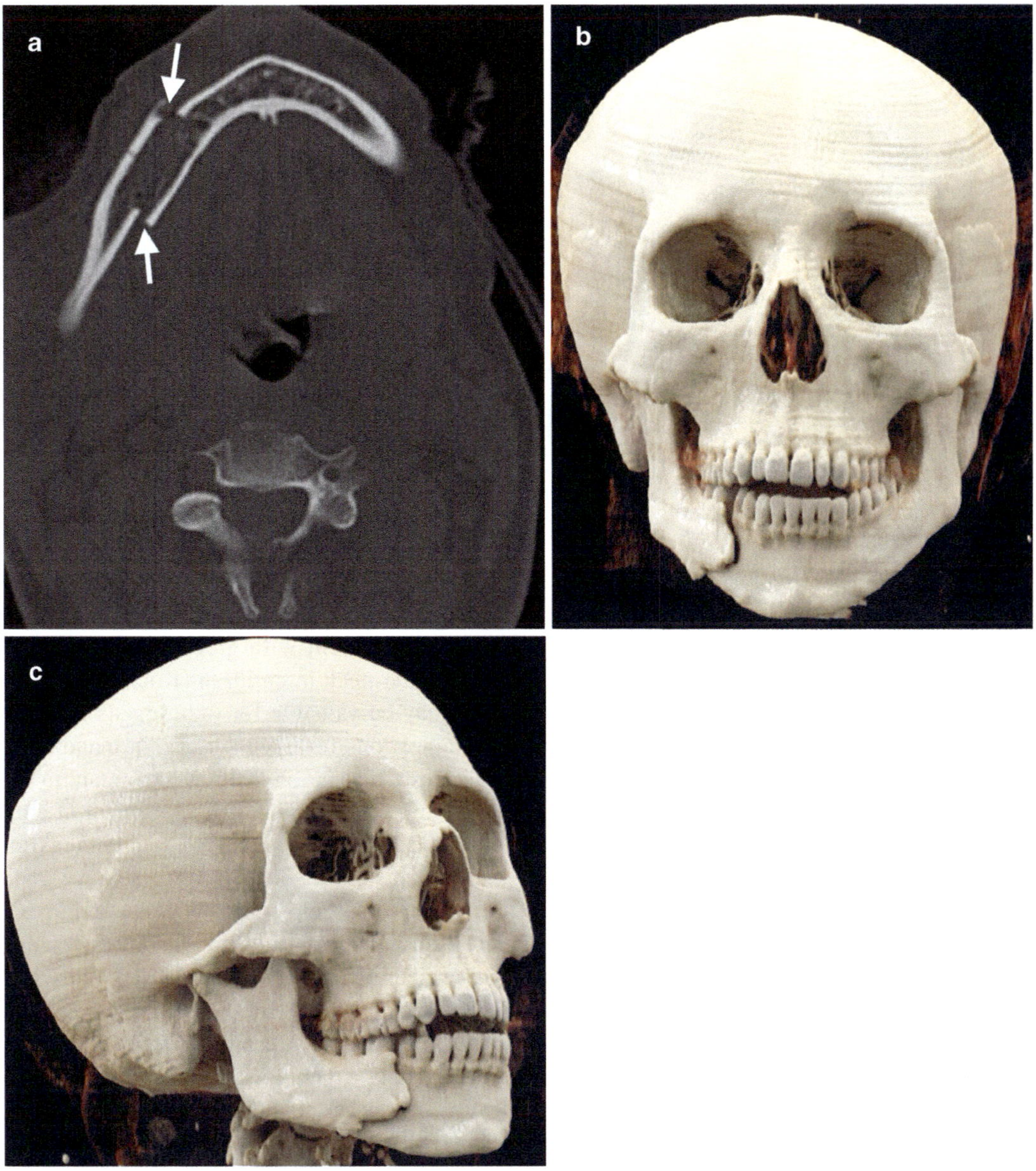


**Fig. 59** Mandible body fracture. (**a**) Axial CT image reveals displaced fracture (arrows) involving right side of the body. CR images with AP (**b**) and right oblique view (**c**) reveal body fracture with superoinferior course

impact, the degree of comminution, and the presence of displaced fragments (Winegar et al. 2013). An anterior impact causes symphyseal, parasymphyseal, or condylar fractures, whereas a lateral impact ends up with an angle or body fracture (King et al. 2004).

The most common mandibular fracture region is mandibular condyle and body followed by the mandibular angle and parasymphyseal region (Patel et al. 2012). Both body and angle fractures are unfavorable fractures since masseter, temporalis, and medial pterygoid muscles may distract the proximal segment of the fractured bone superomedially (Figs. 59 and 60) (Alimohammadi 2018). Complex fracture of the mandible is observed

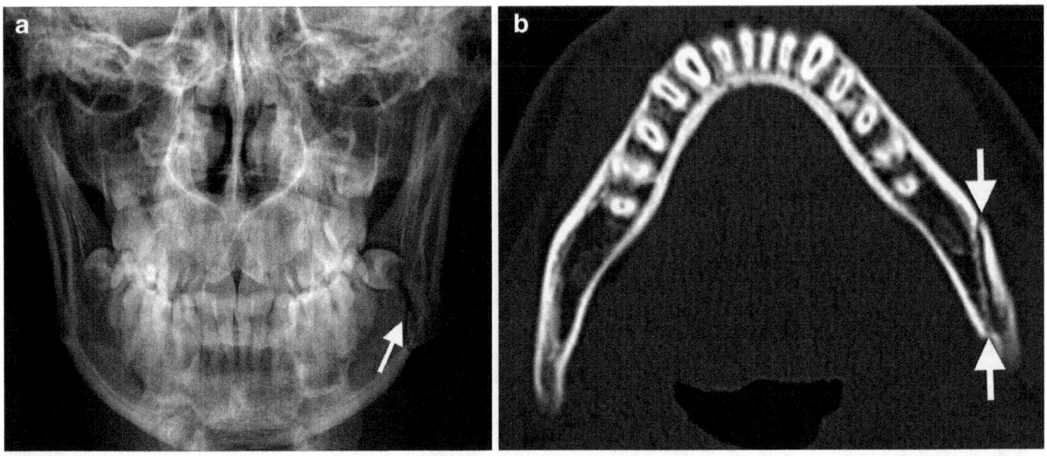


**Fig. 60** Mandible angle fracture. (**a**) AP skull radiograph reveals radiolucent line (arrow) representing fracture across the left mandible angle. (**b**) Axial CT image demonstrates linear fracture (arrows) in the left mandible angle

approximately in 50% of cases, meaning that a second fracture should always be searched in a patient with mandible fracture, which is generally located contralateral side of the mandible (Fig. 61) (Alimohammadi 2018). Flail mandible is characterized by floating mandibular segment resulted from multiple fracture sites such as bilateral angle, bilateral body, or parasymphyseal and bicondylar fractures (Fig. 62). Mandible fractures with associated soft-tissue injuries may cause airway compromise and have a greater risk of malocclusion. Mandible fractures may extend to the tooth socket resulting in tooth avulsions or luxations, which is common in symphysis, body, and angle fractures. Radiologists should evaluate the airway for a possible tooth aspiration in the case of a radiolucent socket, which indicates acute tooth loss or a fragmented tooth (Raval and Rashiduddin 2011). Involvement of teeth roots in mandibular fractures should be scrutinized in radiology reports due to increased risk of subsequent osteomyelitis (Dreizin et al. 2016). Fractures involving mandibular canal by traversing the mandibular ramus, angle, and body may cause inferior alveolar nerve injury. A high association rate was also reported with mandibular fractures and cervical spine injury, which necessitates performing CT of the cervical spine in the setting of mandible fractures after high-speed trauma (Roccia et al. 2007). Subcondylar fractures may present with greenstick fracture of mandibular neck in children (Koch 2014).

It may be valuable for radiologists to know the indications for open surgery in mandibular fractures. Classic indications of mandibular condyle fractures include displacement of condyle into the middle cranial fossa, lateral extracapsular displacement, failure to achieve good reduction and occlusion with closed reduction techniques, bilateral subcondylar fractures, and intraarticular foreign body (Zide and Kent 1983; Montazem and Anastassov 2009). Fractures limited to condylar head, defined as intracapsular fractures, are treated conservatively or with maxillomandibular fixation. However, condylar neck fractures are defined as extracapsular fractures and generally need open surgical treatment.

Temporomandibular joint (TMJ) dislocation usually accompanies mandible fractures due to its ring-like shape. CT images demonstrate empty glenoid fossa secondary to the force of traction by lateral pterygoid muscle on condylar fracture fragments toward medially and anteriorly (Koch 2014). Fractures of mandible involving temporomandibular joint may present with otorrhea or otorrhagia secondary to the injury of EAC (Avrahami et al. 1994).

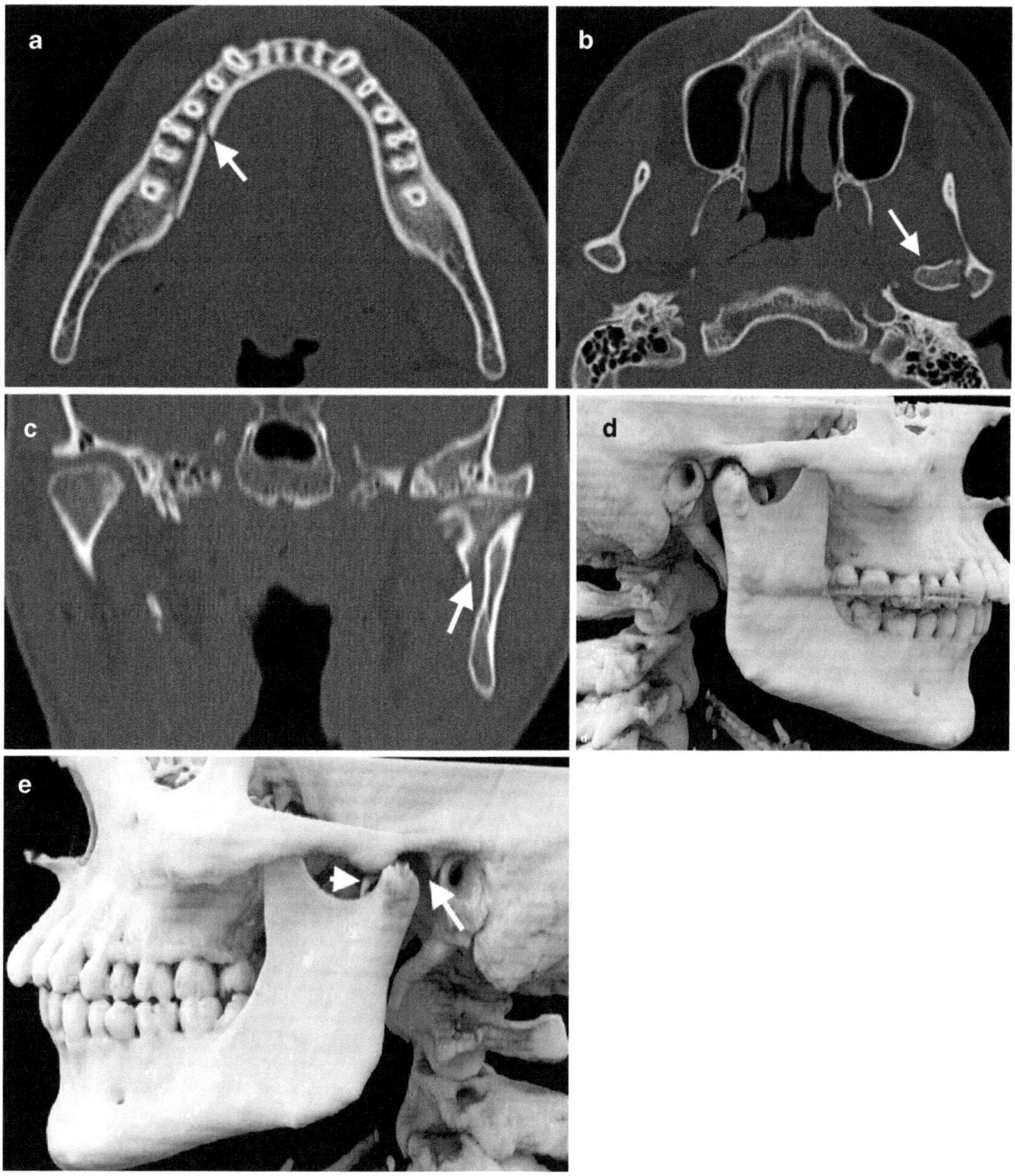


**Fig. 61** Complex mandible fracture. (**a**) Axial CT image reveals a linear right mandible corpus fracture (arrow). Axial (**b**) and coronal (**c**) CT image of the same patient demonstrates left condylar fracture (arrows). (**d**) CR image demonstrates normal appearance of right mandible condyle and temporomandibular joint. (**e**) CR image reveals condylar fracture (arrow) with liberated condyle from the temporomandibular joint (arrowhead)

Dental fractures may be encountered in mandible fractures. Dental root fractures after trauma are usually horizontal and involve the single-rooted teeth. The majority of these fractures are encountered at the level of the midheight of the root (Alimohammadi 2018).

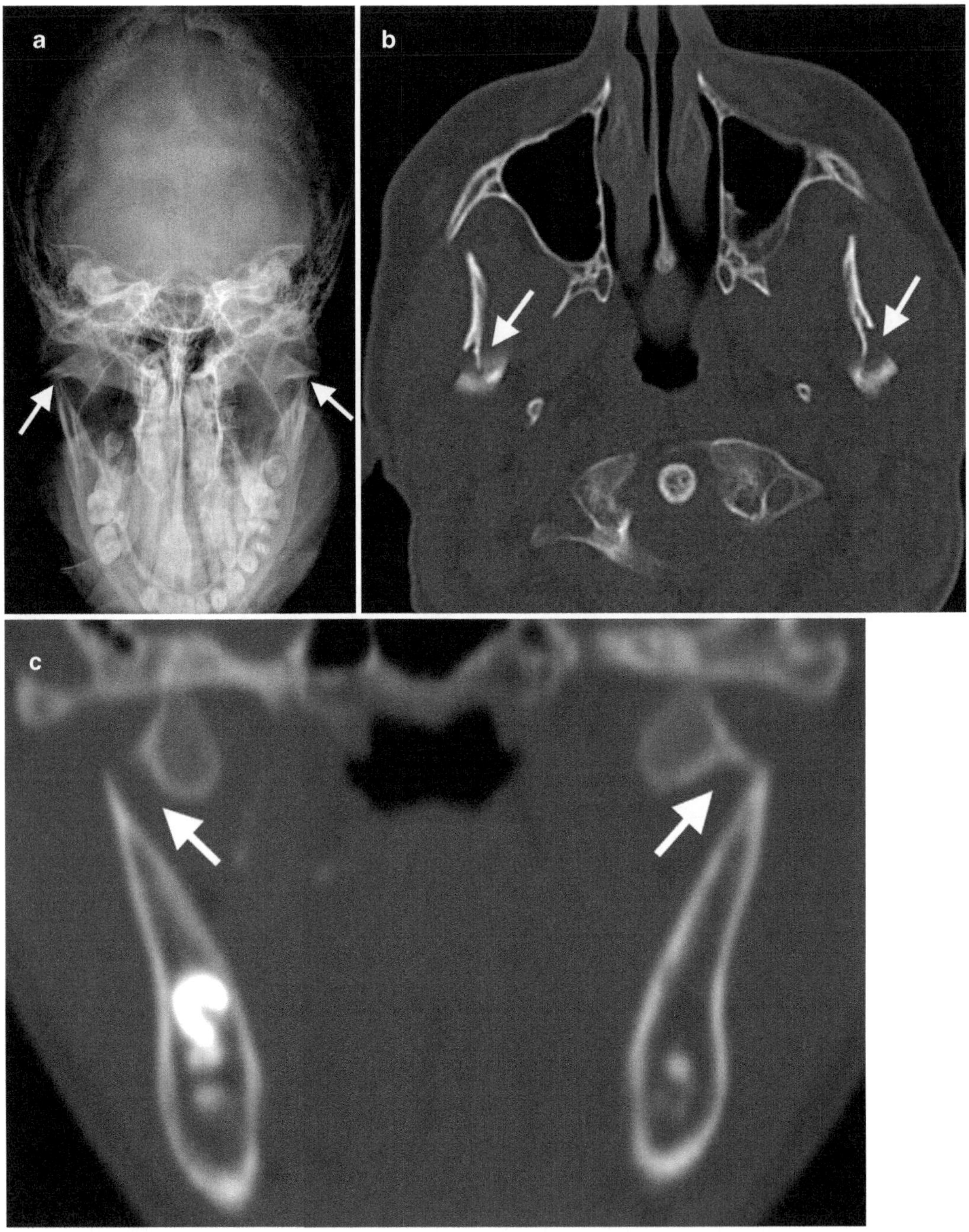


**Fig. 62** Bicondylar fracture. (**a**) Towne radiography reveals bilateral condylar fractures (arrows). Axial (**b**) and coronal (**c**) CT images show bilateral condylar fractures (arrows)

## 7 Conclusion

Craniofacial fractures may present with simple or complex imaging findings in emergency service. A comprehensive approach with thorough knowledge of anatomy and mechanisms of traumatic craniofacial injury are necessary for comprehensive imaging assessment and management of patients. CT is a mainstay imaging technique in craniofacial fractures, which demonstrates the

**Table 5** Complications of maxillofacial fractures

| Fracture type | Complication |
|---|---|
| Cranium | Extra-axial hemorrhage<br>Parenchymal injuries<br>Sinus thrombosis<br>Dural tears |
| Temporal Bone | CHL<br>SNHL<br>Facial and cochlear nerve injury<br>CSF leak<br>PLF<br>Vascular injury |
| Skull base | CSF leak<br>CN injury<br>Vascular injury<br>Meningitis<br>Brainstem injury (PSB) |
| Orbita | Entrapment of extraocular muscles<br>CN injury<br>CSF leak<br>Glob hemorrhage, perforation<br>Lens dislocation |
| Frontal sinus | CSF leakage<br>Intracranial infection<br>Mucocele, mucopyocele |
| Nasal bone | Saddle nose |
| Naso-orbitoethmoid complex fracture | MCT injury, telecanthus<br>CSF rhinorrhea<br>Obstruction of the lacrimal system<br>Facial deformity and exophthalmos |
| ZMC | Enophthalmos<br>Trismus |
| Maxilla (Le Fort fractures) | Rhinorrhea<br>Otorrhea<br>Pneumocephalus<br>Intracranial infection |
| Mandibular | Flail mandibular<br>Tooth avulsions<br>TMJ dislocation<br>Otorrhea or otorrhagia |

presence, localization, and pattern of fractures with highlighting further complications (Table 5). Multiplanar and 3D images are mandatory for delineating for complex fractures and for preoperative planning. Craniofacial fractures may present with different patterns in children due to the incomplete skeletal development. Imaging assessment of maxillofacial fractures might be more helpful for clinicians whether fractures are classified according to well-known classification schemes. Management of patients with craniofacial fractures mainly depends on imaging findings depicted on CT.

## References


Alcala-Galiano A, Arribas-Garcia IJ, Martin-Perez MA, Romance A, Montalvo-Moreno JJ, Juncos JM (2008) Pediatric facial fractures: children are not just small adults. Radiographics 28(2):441–461.; quiz 618. https://doi.org/10.1148/rg.282075060

Alimohammadi R (2018) Imaging of dentoalveolar and jaw trauma. Radiol Clin N Am 56(1):105–124. https://doi.org/10.1016/j.rcl.2017.08.008

Avery LL, Susarla SM, Novelline RA (2011) Multidetector and three-dimensional CT evaluation of the patient with maxillofacial injury. Radiol Clin N Am 49(1):183–203. https://doi.org/10.1016/j.rcl.2010.07.014

Avrahami E, Frishman E, Katz R (1994) CT evaluation of otorrhagia associated with condylar fractures. Clin Radiol 49(12):877–878

Basson OJ, van Lierop AC (2009) Conductive hearing loss after head trauma: review of ossicular pathology, management and outcomes. J Laryngol Otol 123(2):177–181. https://doi.org/10.1017/S0022215108002454

Baugnon KL, Hudgins PA (2014) Skull base fractures and their complications. Neuroimaging Clin N Am 24(3):439–465., vii-viii. https://doi.org/10.1016/j.nic.2014.03.001

Bellamy JL, Mundinger GS, Reddy SK, Flores JM, Rodriguez ED, Dorafshar AH (2013) Le Fort II fractures are associated with death: a comparison of simple and complex midface fractures. J Oral Maxillofac Surg 71(9):1556–1562. https://doi.org/10.1016/j.joms.2013.04.007

Bobinski M, Shen PY, Dublin AB (2016) Basic imaging of skull base trauma. J Neurol Surg B Skull Base 77(5):381–387. https://doi.org/10.1055/s-0036-1583540

Bremke M, Wiegand S, Sesterhenn AM, Eken M, Bien S, Werner JA (2009) Digital volume tomography in the diagnosis of nasal bone fractures. Rhinology 47(2):126–131

Brodie HA, Thompson TC (1997) Management of complications from 820 temporal bone fractures. Am J Otol 18(2):188–197

Burm JS, Chung CH, Oh SJ (1999) Pure orbital blowout fracture: new concepts and importance of medial orbital blowout fracture. Plast Reconstr Surg 103(7):1839–1849

Cannon CR, Jahrsdoerfer RA (1983) Temporal bone fractures. Review of 90 cases. Arch Otolaryngol 109(5):285–288

Carter R, Anslow P (2009) Imaging of the calvarium. Semin Ultrasound CT MR 30(6):465–491

Chen CH, Wang TY, Tsay PK, Lai JB, Chen CT, Liao HT, Lin CH, Chen YR (2008) A 162-case review of palatal fracture: management strategy from a 10-year experience. Plast Reconstr Surg 121(6):2065–2073. https://doi.org/10.1097/PRS.0b013e3181706edc

Collins JM, Krishnamoorthy AK, Kubal WS, Johnson MH, Poon CS (2012) Multidetector CT of temporal

bone fractures. Semin Ultrasound CT MR 33(5):418–431. https://doi.org/10.1053/j.sult.2012.06.006
Connor SE, Tan G, Fernando R, Chaudhury N (2005) Computed tomography pseudofractures of the mid face and skull base. Clin Radiol 60(12):1268–1279. https://doi.org/10.1016/j.crad.2005.05.016
Dahiya R, Keller JD, Litofsky NS, Bankey PE, Bonassar LJ, Megerian CA (1999) Temporal bone fractures: otic capsule sparing versus otic capsule violating clinical and radiographic considerations. J Trauma 47(6):1079–1083
Dappa E, Higashigaito K, Fornaro J, Leschka S, Wildermuth S, Alkadhi H (2016) Cinematic rendering - an alternative to volume rendering for 3D computed tomography imaging. Insights Imaging 7(6):849–856. https://doi.org/10.1007/s13244-016-0518-1
Dreizin D, Nam AJ, Tirada N, Levin MD, Stein DM, Bodanapally UK, Mirvis SE, Munera F (2016) Multidetector CT of mandibular fractures, reductions, and complications: a clinically relevant primer for the radiologist. Radiographics 36(5):1539–1564. https://doi.org/10.1148/rg.2016150218
Dreizin D, Nam AJ, Diaconu SC, Bernstein MP, Bodanapally UK, Munera F (2018) Multidetector CT of midfacial fractures: classification systems, principles of reduction, and common complications. Radiographics 38(1):248–274. https://doi.org/10.1148/rg.2018170074
Elbarbary AS, Ali A (2014) Medial canthopexy of old unrepaired naso-orbito-ethmoidal (noe) traumatic telecanthus. J Craniomaxillofac Surg 42(2):106–112. https://doi.org/10.1016/j.jcms.2013.03.003
Ellis E 3rd (2012) Orbital trauma. Oral Maxillofac Surg Clin North Am 24(4):629–648. https://doi.org/10.1016/j.coms.2012.07.006
Escott EJ, Branstetter BF (2008) Incidence and characterization of unifocal mandible fractures on CT. AJNR Am J Neuroradiol 29(5):890–894. https://doi.org/10.3174/ajnr.A0973
Feiz-Erfan I, Horn EM, Theodore N, Zabramski JM, Klopfenstein JD, Lekovic GP, Albuquerque FC, Partovi S, Goslar PW, Petersen SR (2007) Incidence and pattern of direct blunt neurovascular injury associated with trauma to the skull base. J Neurosurg 107(2):364–369. https://doi.org/10.3171/JNS-07/08/0364
Ghorayeb BY, Yeakley JW (1992) Temporal bone fractures: longitudinal or oblique? The case for oblique temporal bone fractures. Laryngoscope 102(2):129–134. https://doi.org/10.1288/00005537-199202000-00005
Grant JH 3rd, Patrinely JR, Weiss AH, Kierney PC, Gruss JS (2002) Trapdoor fracture of the orbit in a pediatric population. Plast Reconstr Surg 109(2):482–489. discussion 490-485
Hijaz TA, Cento EA, Walker MT (2011) Imaging of head trauma. Radiol Clin N Am 49(1):81–103. https://doi.org/10.1016/j.rcl.2010.07.012
Ishman SL, Friedland DR (2004) Temporal bone fractures: traditional classification and clinical relevance. Laryngoscope 114(10):1734–1741. https://doi.org/10.1097/00005537-200410000-00011
Jain SA, Manchio JV, Weinzweig J (2010) Role of the sagittal view of computed tomography in evaluation of the nasofrontal ducts in frontal sinus fractures. J Craniofac Surg 21(6):1670–1673. https://doi.org/10.1097/SCS.0b013e3181f3c5f1
Jordan DR, Allen LH, White J, Harvey J, Pashby R, Esmaeli B (1998) Intervention within days for some orbital floor fractures: the white-eyed blowout. Ophthalmic Plast Reconstr Surg 14(6):379–390
Juliano AF, Ginat DT, Moonis G (2013) Imaging review of the temporal bone: part I. anatomy and inflammatory and neoplastic processes. Radiology 269(1):16–32. https://doi.org/10.1148/radiol.13120733
Karasu A, Sabanci PA, Izgi N, Imer M, Sencer A, Cansever T, Canbolat A (2008) Traumatic epidural hematomas of the posterior cranial fossa. Surg Neurol 69(3):247–251.; discussion 251-242. https://doi.org/10.1016/j.surneu.2007.02.024
Kennedy TA, Avey GD, Gentry LR (2014) Imaging of Temporal Bone Trauma. Neuroimag Clin N Am 24(3):467–486. https://doi.org/10.1016/j.nic.2014.03.003
Kienstra MA, Van Loveren H (2005) Anterior skull base fractures. Facial Plast Surg 21(3):180–186. https://doi.org/10.1055/s-2005-922857
Kim BH, Seo HS, Kim AY, Lee YS, Lee YH, Suh SI, Lee DH (2010) The diagnostic value of the sagittal multiplanar reconstruction CT images for nasal bone fractures. Clin Radiol 65(4):308–314. https://doi.org/10.1016/j.crad.2009.12.006
King RE, Scianna JM, Petruzzelli GJ (2004) Mandible fracture patterns: a suburban trauma center experience. Am J Otolaryngol 25(5):301–307
Koch BL (2014) Pediatric considerations in craniofacial trauma. Neuroimaging Clin N Am 24(3):513–529., viii. https://doi.org/10.1016/j.nic.2014.03.002
Liang W, Xiaofeng Y, Weiguo L, Wusi Q, Gang S, Xuesheng Z (2007) Traumatic carotid cavernous fistula accompanying basilar skull fracture: a study on the incidence of traumatic carotid cavernous fistula in the patients with basilar skull fracture and the prognostic analysis about traumatic carotid cavernous fistula. J Trauma 63(5):1014–1020.; discussion 1020. https://doi.org/10.1097/TA.0b013e318154c9fb
Lieger O, Zix J, Kruse A, Iizuka T (2009) Dental injuries in association with facial fractures. J Oral Maxillofac Surg 67(8):1680–1684. https://doi.org/10.1016/j.joms.2009.03.052
Little SC, Kesser BW (2006) Radiographic classification of temporal bone fractures - clinical predictability using a new system. Arch Otolaryngol Head Neck Surg 132(12):1300–1304. https://doi.org/10.1001/archotol.132.12.1300
Lloyd KM, DelGaudio JM, Hudgins PA (2008) Imaging of skull base cerebrospinal fluid leaks in adults. Radiology 248(3):725–736. https://doi.org/10.1148/radiol.2483070362
Lo Casto A, Priolo GD, Garufi A, Purpura P, Salerno S, La Tona G, Coppolino F (2012) Imaging evaluation of facial complex strut fractures. Semin Ultrasound

CT MR 33(5):396–409. https://doi.org/10.1053/j.sult.2012.06.003
Lourenco MT, Yeakley JW, Ghorayeb BY (1995) The "Y" sign of lateral dislocation of the incus. Am J Otol 16(3):387–392
Lui TN, Lee ST, Chang CN, Cheng WC (1993) Epidural hematomas in the posterior cranial fossa. J Trauma 34(2):211–215
Madhusudan G, Sharma RK, Khandelwal N, Tewari MK (2006) Nomenclature of frontobasal trauma: a new clinicoradiographic classification. Plast Reconstr Surg 117(7):2382–2388. https://doi.org/10.1097/01.prs.0000218794.28670.07
Manson PN, Stanwix MG, Yaremchuk MJ, Nam AJ, Hui-Chou H, Rodriguez ED (2009) Frontobasal fractures: anatomical classification and clinical significance. Plast Reconstr Surg 124(6):2096–2106. https://doi.org/10.1097/PRS.0b013e3181bf8394
Marinho RO, Freire-Maia B (2013) Management of fractures of the zygomaticomaxillary complex. Oral Maxillofac Surg Clin North Am 25(4):617–636. https://doi.org/10.1016/j.coms.2013.07.011
Markowitz BL, Manson PN, Sargent L, Vander Kolk CA, Yaremchuk M, Glassman D, Crawley WA (1991) Management of the medial canthal tendon in nasoethmoid orbital fractures: the importance of the central fragment in classification and treatment. Plast Reconstr Surg 87(5):843–853
McRae M, Momeni R, Narayan D (2008) Frontal sinus fractures: a review of trends, diagnosis, treatment, and outcomes at a level 1 trauma center in Connecticut. Conn Med 72(3):133–138
Mehta N, Butala P, Bernstein MP (2012) The imaging of maxillofacial trauma and its pertinence to surgical intervention. Radiol Clin N Am 50(1):43–57. https://doi.org/10.1016/j.rcl.2011.08.005
Menku A, Koc RK, Tucer B, Durak AC, Akdemir H (2004) Clivus fractures: clinical presentations and courses. Neurosurg Rev 27(3):194–198. https://doi.org/10.1007/s10143-004-0320-2
Meriot P, Veillon F, Garcia JF, Nonent M, Jezequel J, Bourjat P, Bellet M (1997) CT appearances of ossicular injuries. Radiographics 17(6):1445–1454. https://doi.org/10.1148/radiographics.17.6.9397457
Metzinger SE, Guerra AB, Garcia RE (2005) Frontal sinus fractures: management guidelines. Facial Plast Surg 21(3):199–206. https://doi.org/10.1055/s-2005-922860
Montazem AH, Anastassov G (2009) Management of condylar fractures. Atlas Oral Maxillofac Surg Clin North Am 17(1):55–69. https://doi.org/10.1016/j.cxom.2008.11.002
Morrow BT, Samson TD, Schubert W, Mackay DR (2014) Evidence-based medicine: mandible fractures. Plast Reconstr Surg 134(6):1381–1390. https://doi.org/10.1097/PRS.0000000000000717
Mulroy MH, Loyd AM, Frush DP, Verla TG, Myers BS, Bass CR (2012) Evaluation of pediatric skull fracture imaging techniques. Forensic Sci Int 214(1–3):167–172. https://doi.org/10.1016/j.forsciint.2011.07.050
Mundinger GS, Dorafshar AH, Gilson MM, Mithani SK, Manson PN, Rodriguez ED (2013) Blunt-mechanism facial fracture patterns associated with internal carotid artery injuries: recommendations for additional screening criteria based on analysis of 4,398 patients. J Oral Maxillofac Surg 71(12):2092–2100. https://doi.org/10.1016/j.joms.2013.07.005
Nosan DK, Benecke JE Jr, Murr AH (1997) Current perspective on temporal bone trauma. Otolaryngol Head Neck Surg 117(1):67–71. https://doi.org/10.1016/S0194-59989770209-2
Ondik MP, Lipinski L, Dezfoli S, Fedok FG (2009) The treatment of nasal fractures: a changing paradigm. Arch Facial Plast Surg 11(5):296–302. https://doi.org/10.1001/archfacial.2009.65
Pappachan B, Alexander M (2006) Correlating facial fractures and cranial injuries. J Oral Maxillofac Surg 64(7):1023–1029. https://doi.org/10.1016/j.joms.2006.03.021
Patel R, Reid RR, Poon CS (2012) Multidetector computed tomography of maxillofacial fractures: the key to high-impact radiological reporting. Semin Ultrasound CT MR 33(5):410–417. https://doi.org/10.1053/j.sult.2012.06.005
Policeni BA, Smoker WR (2015) Imaging of the skull base: anatomy and pathology. Radiol Clin N Am 53(1):1–14. https://doi.org/10.1016/j.rcl.2014.09.005
Potter JK, Muzaffar AR, Ellis E, Rohrich RJ, Hackney FL (2006) Aesthetic management of the nasal component of naso-orbital ethmoid fractures. Plast Reconstr Surg 117(1):10e–18e
Prosser JD, Vender JR, Solares CA (2011) Traumatic cerebrospinal fluid leaks. Otolaryngol Clin N Am 44(4):857–873., vii. https://doi.org/10.1016/j.otc.2011.06.007
Rafferty MA, Mc Conn Walsh R, Walsh MA (2006) A comparison of temporal bone fracture classification systems. Clin Otolaryngol 31(4):287–291. https://doi.org/10.1111/j.1749-4486.2006.01267.x
Raval CB, Rashiduddin M (2011) Airway management in patients with maxillofacial trauma - A retrospective study of 177 cases. Saudi J Anaesth 5(1):9–14. https://doi.org/10.4103/1658-354X.76476
Roccia F, Cassarino E, Boccaletti R, Stura G (2007) Cervical spine fractures associated with maxillofacial trauma: an 11-year review. J Craniofac Surg 18(6):1259–1263. https://doi.org/10.1097/scs.0b013e31814e0581
Rodriguez ED, Stanwix MG, Nam AJ, St Hilaire H, Simmons OP, Christy MR, Grant MP, Manson PN (2008) Twenty-six-year experience treating frontal sinus fractures: a novel algorithm based on anatomical fracture pattern and failure of conventional techniques. Plast Reconstr Surg 122(6):1850–1866. https://doi.org/10.1097/PRS.0b013e31818d58ba
Rohrich RJ, Adams WP Jr (2000) Nasal fracture management: minimizing secondary nasal deformities. Plast Reconstr Surg 106(2):266–273
Roth FS, Koshy JC, Goldberg JS, Soparkar CN (2010) Pearls of orbital trauma management.

Semin Plast Surg 24(4):398–410. https://doi.org/10.1055/s-0030-1269769
Rothman MI, Simon EM, Zoarski GH, Zagardo MT (1998) Superior blowout fracture of the orbit: the blowup fracture. AJNR Am J Neuroradiol 19(8):1448–1449
Saigal K, Winokur RS, Finden S, Taub D, Pribitkin E (2005) Use of three-dimensional computerized tomography reconstruction in complex facial trauma. Facial Plast Surg 21(3):214–220. https://doi.org/10.1055/s-2005-922862
Samii M, Tatagiba M (2002) Skull base trauma: diagnosis and management. Neurol Res 24(2):147–156. https://doi.org/10.1179/016164102101199693
Sanchez T, Stewart D, Walvick M, Swischuk L (2010) Skull fracture vs. accessory sutures: how can we tell the difference? Emerg Radiol 17(5):413–418. https://doi.org/10.1007/s10140-010-0877-8
Sargent LA (2007) Nasoethmoid orbital fractures: diagnosis and treatment. Plast Reconstr Surg 120(7 Suppl 2):16S–31S. https://doi.org/10.1097/01.prs.0000260731.01178.18
Schmitt PJ, Barrett DM, Christophel JJ, Leiva-Salinas C, Mukherjee S, Shaffrey ME (2014) Surgical perspectives in craniofacial trauma. Neuroimaging Clin N Am 24(3):531–552., viii-ix. https://doi.org/10.1016/j.nic.2014.03.007
Sung EK, Nadgir RN, Sakai O (2012) Computed tomographic imaging in head and neck trauma: what the radiologist needs to know. Semin Roentgenol 47(4):320–329. https://doi.org/10.1053/j.ro.2012.05.002
Swartz JD (2001) Temporal bone trauma. Semin Ultrasound CT MR 22(3):219–228
Tress EE, Clark RS, Foley LM, Alexander H, Hickey RW, Drabek T, Kochanek PM, Manole MD (2014) Blood brain barrier is impermeable to solutes and permeable to water after experimental pediatric cardiac arrest. Neurosci Lett 578:17–21. https://doi.org/10.1016/j.neulet.2014.06.020
Uzelac A, Gean AD (2014) Orbital and facial fractures. Neuroimaging Clin N Am 24(3):407–424., vii. https://doi.org/10.1016/j.nic.2014.03.008
Watanabe K, Kida W (2012) Images in clinical medicine. Battle's sign. N Engl J Med 367(12):1135. https://doi.org/10.1056/NEJMicm1100820
Weir P, Suttner NJ, Flynn P, McAuley D (2006) Lesson of the week - Normal skull suture variant mimicking intentional injury. Brit Med J 332(7548):1020–1021. https://doi.org/10.1136/bmj.332.7548.1020
Winegar BA, Murillo H, Tantiwongkosi B (2013) Spectrum of critical imaging findings in complex facial skeletal trauma. Radiographics 33(1):3–19. https://doi.org/10.1148/rg.331125080
Yetiser S, Hidir Y, Gonul E (2008) Facial nerve problems and hearing loss in patients with temporal bone fractures: demographic data. J Trauma 65(6):1314–1320. https://doi.org/10.1097/TA.0b013e3180eead57
Yilmazlar S, Arslan E, Kocaeli H, Dogan S, Aksoy K, Korfali E, Doygun M (2006) Cerebrospinal fluid leakage complicating skull base fractures: analysis of 81 cases. Neurosurg Rev 29(1):64–71. https://doi.org/10.1007/s10143-005-0396-3
Zdilla MJ, Russell ML, Koons AW, Bliss KN, Mangus KR (2018) Metopism: a Study of the Persistent Metopic Suture. J Craniofac Surg 29(1):204–208. https://doi.org/10.1097/SCS.0000000000004030
Zide MF, Kent JN (1983) Indications for open reduction of mandibular condyle fractures. J Oral Maxillofac Surg 41(2):89–98
Zimmermann CE, Troulis MJ, Kaban LB (2005) Pediatric facial fractures: recent advances in prevention, diagnosis and management. Int J Oral Maxillofac Surg 34(8):823–833. https://doi.org/10.1016/j.ijom.2005.06.015
Zingg M, Laedrach K, Chen J, Chowdhury K, Vuillemin T, Sutter F, Raveh J (1992) Classification and treatment of zygomatic fractures: a review of 1,025 cases. J Oral Maxillofac Surg 50(8):778–790

# Traumatic Haemorrhage

Leonora Schmidt, Andrea Irma Diettrich,
Francesca Iacobellis, and Stefan Wirth

## Contents



**Abstract**

Computed tomography (CT) is the key tool to diagnose intracranial haemorrhage following craniocerebral trauma. MRI provides additional information in cases when this seems appropriate such as a more detailed clarification of traumatic neurological disabilities, differentiation between oedema and ischaemia or imaging of shear damage to the neuronal fibre pathways.

Most common is subarachnoid haemorrhage (SAH), followed by subdural (SDH) and epidural haemorrhage (EDH). Besides trauma, SAH may also emerge spontaneously due to rupture of an aneurysm, most likely at

L. Schmidt
Department of Radiology, Helios Clinic, Munich West, Germany

A. I. Diettrich
Radiology Division, SS Annunziata, Naples, Italy

F. Iacobellis
Radiology Department, Cardarelli Hospital, Naples, Italy

S. Wirth (✉)
Department of Radiology and Nuclear Medicine, Schwarzwald-Baar Hospital, Villingen-Schwenningen, Germany
e-mail: Stefan.Wirth@sbk-vs.de



M. Scaglione et al. (eds.), *Emergency Radiology of the Head and Spine*, Medical Radiology Diagnostic Imaging, https://doi.org/10.1007/978-3-030-91047-1_2

the Willis circle. In contrast to spontaneous subarachnoidal bleeding, traumatic SAH does not normally occur at the Sylvian fissure or the basal cisterns, but rather at the cortical, surface sulci and in the interhemispheric gap. As a consequence, the distribution pattern may cause clarification by CT angiography. Subdural haematomas are common concomitant injuries of craniocerebral trauma, especially within elderly patients. They impress computer tomographically as falciform hyperdense bleeding, which can spread along the interhemispheric gap or the falx cerebri and are, therefore, able to cross the adhesion points of the dura and calotte, in contrast to epidural haematomas. Because of their mostly venous origin, neurologic symptoms are commonly subacute. Despite the very early stage of SDH up to 1 h, SDH loses density with time but may show several bleeding events, making it variable in density, especially in CT follow-ups. Epidural haematomas are rather rare, but often dramatic consequences of craniocerebral trauma are associated with skull fractures in up to 90% of cases. They emerge especially temporally at the coup site and are mostly of arterial origin with subsequent secondary complications, such as mass effects. In acute diagnostics, the CT shows a biconvex and hyperdense bleeding, which does not cross the sutures. EDHs with surgical decompression in time have a good outcome, which is why quick and correct diagnosis is of extraordinary importance. A clinically symptom-free interval between the time of injury and the start of mass effects can aggravate diagnosis.

Contusions are one of the most common complications of SHT and occur when the gyri collide with the cranial calotte or dura mater. They manifest themselves as multiple hyperdense lesions with perifocal oedema, preferably at the frontobase and in the temporal lobe, and are often associated with other intracranial haemorrhages, especially SAB. Their peculiarity is that they tend to haemorrhagic progression in up to 50% of cases. Contrast extravasation can predict this. According to this background, control CTs play an important role and can be prognostically decisive. An intravenous administration of KM should be weighed up accordingly in follow-up examinations.

Diffuse axonal damage occurs primarily on the basis of high-speed trauma with associated rapid head rotation. The axonal integrity is destroyed. Since a haemorrhagic component is often absent or can be extremely discreet, the detection with CT is often not possible, and instead, MRI is the imaging method of choice. DAI lesions are most frequently found in descending order at the medullary cortex border, the corpus callosum and in the brainstem. DAI is associated with a very unfavourable prognosis, especially in severe SHT, and is a frequent cause of persistent disabilities up to maximum forms such as apallic syndrome.

At present, however, there is still no clear evidence of an increase in risk of patients under anticoagulation after mild craniocerebral trauma, especially for the endpoint of compulsory therapy, if the data situation is unsatisfactory. For a final evaluation, a significantly more mature study situation on patients under anticoagulation with mild SHT is required. This should only be possible with very large numbers of patients in a multicentre approach.

In order to be able to cope with the presumably increasing incidence of SHT with increasing age in the future, a continuous reduction in the radiation exposure of the CT and a better availability of the MRT will be necessary. Further positive effects may arise from the establishment of dual-energy CT in SHT diagnostics. It is possible that the virtual native representation will help in the assessment of the course after KM administration. In addition, it may even be possible to identify active bleeding components in haematomas.

## Abbreviations

| | |
|---|---|
| A | Arteria |
| ASS | Acetylsalicylic acid |
| CCT | Cranial computed tomography |

| | |
|---|---|
| CCTHR | Canadian CT head rule |
| CHIP | CT in Head Injury Patients Prediction Rule |
| CI | Confidence interval |
| CT | Computed tomography |
| DAI | Diffuse axonal injury |
| EDH | Epidural haematoma |
| EFNS | European Federation of Neurological Societies Guideline |
| GCS | Glasgow Coma Scale |
| ICB | Intracranial bleeding |
| INR | International normalized ratio |
| ISS | Injury Severity Score |
| LDGN | Guideline of the German Society of Neurosurgery |
| LOC | Loss of consciousness |
| MRT | Magnetic resonance scanner |
| NEXUS II | National Emergency X-Ray Utilization Study II |
| NI | Neurosurgical intervention |
| NICE | National Institute for Health and Care Excellence (Guidelines) |
| NMH | Low molecular weight heparin |
| NOAK | New oral anticoagulants |
| NOC | New Orleans criteria |
| OR | Odds ratio |
| SAH | Subarachnoid haemorrhage |
| SDH | Subdural haemorrhage |
| SHT | Craniocerebral trauma |
| PACS | Picture archiving and communicating system |
| UFH | Unfractionated heparin |

## 1 Extra-Axial Traumatic Haemorrhage

### 1.1 Epidemiology

Craniocerebral trauma can lead to various primary intracranial forms of bleeding, which are classified as extra- or intra-axial haemorrhage by their relation to the cerebral parenchyma or, respectively, the pia mater. Therefore, extra-axial bleeding is located outside the cerebral parenchyma (e.g. subarachnoidal, subdural and epidural bleeding) and intra-axial bleeding is located inside the cerebral parenchyma (e.g. contusion bleeding and diffusely axonal damage).

The most common form of extra-axial bleeding is subarachnoidal bleeding, with a rate of 32–45% (Brown et al. 2004; Sarkar et al. 2014a, b; Servadei et al. 2002; Steyerberg et al. 2008; Wong et al. 2011a, b). In the case of mild craniocerebral trauma, isolated subarachnoidal bleeding is mostly found; however, this only sometimes shows haemorrhagic progression (Borczuk et al. 2013a, b; Phelan et al. 2014a, b). In a retrospective study by Phalen et al. 15% of all intracranial bleeding after craniocerebral trauma was isolated subarachnoidal bleeding (Phelan et al. 2014a, b).

The second most common form is subdural bleeding, with a rate of 28–44% (Brown et al. 2004; Sarkar et al. 2014a, b). Leitgeb et al. reported a 49% incidence of subdural haematomas after severe craniocerebral trauma with a mortality of 47% (Leitgeb et al. 2012a, b). Mortality in hospital settings generally ranges from 12 to 16% (Kalanithi et al. 2011a, b; Ryan et al. 2012a, b). Adult patients suffer a subdural haematoma more often than children. The main factors for a bad outcome measured by the so-called Glasgow Coma Scale are age, neurologic status and severity of the craniocerebral trauma (Leitgeb et al. 2012a, b).

The least common form is epidural bleeding, with a rate of 10–13% (Brown et al. 2004; Sarkar et al. 2014a, b; Steyerberg et al. 2008), which occurs significantly more frequently in children and is the second most common of all extra-axial bleeding in children (Sarkar et al. 2014a, b). In the case of mild craniocerebral trauma, patients require neurological surgery most often (18%) (Sweeney et al. 2015a, b).

### 1.2 Biomechanics

Extra-axial bleeding in the case of craniocerebral trauma is caused by the deformation resulting from collision forces and acceleration of the cerebral mass and its partly immobile vessels. One distinguishes between the site of direct force impact, the coup focus and the contralateral contrecoup focus. The latter is mostly severer, because the cerebrum hits the calvaria without decelerating. The impact on the coup focus, on the other hand, is reduced by the calvaria itself and by the cervical muscles. Severe clinical symptoms of the injury are set by the site of the bleeding and the secondary consequences, such as elevated cerebral pressure and herniation.

Epidural haematomas often evolve after low-energy craniocerebral trauma. They are associated with calvaria fracture in 75–90% of cases (Heinzelmann et al. 1996; Paiva et al. 2013a, b) and are more likely to occur isolated rather than in combination with other intracranial injuries. If these occur, then they are mostly combined with contusion (Heinzelmann et al. 1996; Paiva et al. 2013a, b). The associated fractures play the main role in pathogenesis: if the fracture line crosses a vascular meatus, structures beneath—preferably the arteria meningea media (Crooks 1991)—are injured. Subsequently, the bleeding dissolves the dura mater from the calvarial periosteum and an unphysiological epidural space evolves (Fig. 1). Because the dura mater sticks very strongly to the periosteal layer of the sutures, epidural bleeding normally respects the sutures and does not cross them. In contrast to subdural haematomas, epidural bleeding can cross the median or the tentorium cerebelli, because the duplicates of the dura do not touch the epidural space. The area of the temporal lobe is most commonly affected, followed by temporal–frontal and frontal areas (Crooks 1991; Heinzelmann et al. 1996; Paiva et al. 2013a, b). The posterior cranial fossa or the clivus is rare locations of epidural haematomas, and epidural haematomas close to the vertex can also be overseen easily. Bilateral epidural haematomas have a lower incidence of up to 2% and are probably caused by a simultaneous laceration of the left and right arteria meningea media (Paiva et al. 2013a, b).

Subdural haematomas, however, evolve between the dura mater and the arachnoidea. An unphysiological space emerges through displacement by the haematomas. The cause of the bleeding is most commonly of venous origin on the grounds of disruption of bridging veins (Fig. 2). An acute subdural haematoma in the context of craniocerebral trauma firstly reflects a massive force impact, for example, by deceleration trauma. Because of the viscid elastic features of the bridging veins and the loose attachment to the arachnoidea, they are the predilection sites of rupture in the case of sudden acceleration (Crooks 1991). The immobile parasagittal bridging veins

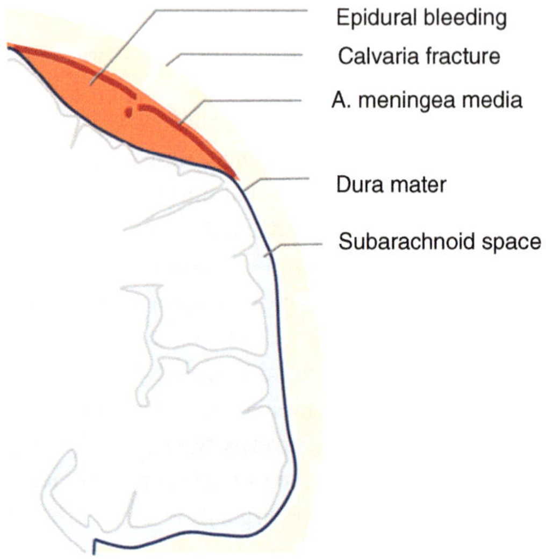


**Fig. 1** Epidural bleeding. Typical spreading between the dura mater and calvaria. The main predilection site is the arteria meningea media shown. The shape is caused by the limiting adhesion between the dura mater and the calvaria at the sutures

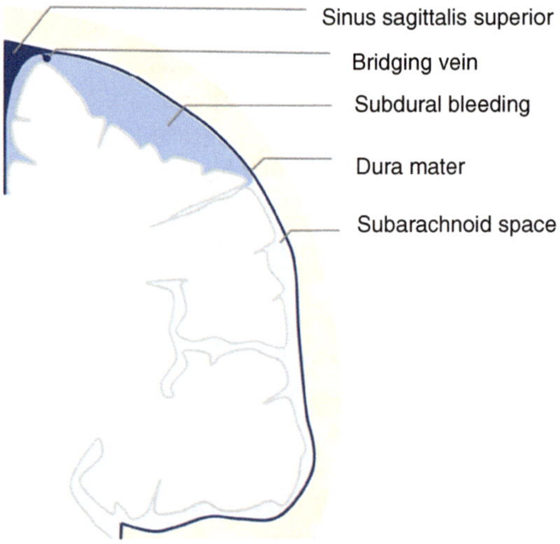


**Fig. 2** Subdural bleeding. The leading cause is venous bleeding of disrupted bridging veins. They spread into the subdural space emerging between the dura mater and arachnoidea

are especially affected by acceleration with a position change in the posterior–anterior direction (Tsutsumi et al. 2017). That is why it is suspected that an impact on both the frontal and occipital regions is a risk factor for the development of a subdural haematoma (Post et al. 2015a, b). Subdural haematomas preferably evolve supratentorially and parietotemporally, and, less commonly, frontally.

In contrast to the epidural haematoma, osseous sutures are crossed according to the anatomical situation. The haematoma is limited in its expansion only by the falx cerebri and the tentorium cerebelli and, therefore, spreads preferably over the whole hemisphere. As a result, subdural haematomas are often more extensive than epidural haematomas. They can occur on the site of coup and contrecoup, the latter more frequently (Kim and Gean 2011). An age-specific feature lies within the bigger subdural space in older people (Sigurdsson et al. 2012). This is caused, on the one hand, by involution of the cerebral mass, i.e. physiological atrophy, and, on the other hand, in the context of neurodegenerative diseases. This explains the higher incidence of subdural haematomas within the elderly population (Yokobori et al. 2016a, b).

Subarachnoidal bleeding evolves in the subarachnoidal space, located between the arachnoidea and pia mater (Fig. 3). Unchecked movements of the head and blunt trauma including the neck are the most common circumstances of accident, especially concerning the contrecoup site (Kim and Gean 2011). Subarachnoidal bleeding can present both with localized and diffuse injury patterns (Andriessen et al. 2010). It can be of venous or arterial origin. There are different theories regarding the possible injury mechanisms (Modi et al. 2016). On the one hand, small intracranial cortical vessels migrating through the subarachnoidal space can disrupt through hyperextension by trauma. Following that, an isolated traumatic subarachnoidal bleeding can be caused by a disrupted basilar arteria (Salvatori et al. 2012; van Gijn and Rinkel 2001). On the other hand, a subarachnoidal bleeding can occur as an extension of an intraparenchymal bleeding and contusion, for example, through diffusion (Modi et al. 2016) or through a shifting of an intraventricular haemorrhage (Kim and Gean 2011). Traumatic subarachnoidal bleeding in combination with other intracranial bleeding is found preferably on the site of direct force impact, for example the superficial sulci in direct proximity to a bordering focus of contusion. Yuh et al. suspect a similar injury mechanism for both subarachnoidal bleeding and contusions because of the strong connotation (Yuh et al. 2013).

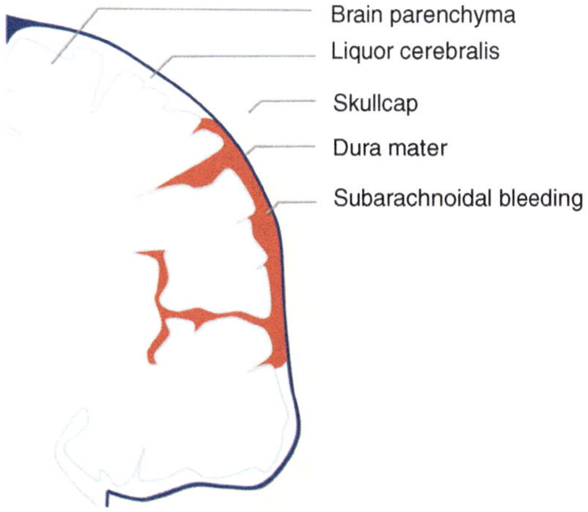


**Fig. 3** Subarachnoidal bleeding. Bleeding spreads in the subarachnoidal space following the sulci after the rupture of smaller cortical vessels or diffusion of intraparenchymal haemorrhages. Venous bleeding next to the calvaria or arterial bleeding of disrupted aneurysms of the cranial base is typical

## 1.3 Types of Injury

### 1.3.1 Epidural Bleeding

The epidural haematoma classically presents as hyperdense biconvexity at the site of the coup in immediate proximity to the calvaria. Cranial fractures are associated in 90% of the cases, which is why searches for interrupted contours and eventual dislocations of calvaria fractures must be made. Impact injuries of soft parts of the scalp are seen as an expression of direct force. Arterial bleeding is the cause in about 90% of cases (Currie et al. 2016a, b); venous epidural haematomas occur predominantly at the posterior cranial fossa and are caused by a disruption of the sinus. Epidural haematomas on the frontal part of the intermediate cranial fossa are based most likely on an injury of the sphenoidal sinus and should be classified as benign (Gean et al. 2010a, b). The arrangement of the haematoma displays with different grades of density as a clue to active bleeding. The so-called swirl sign, i.e. a swirl caused by hypodense layers, is seen as a sign of active bleeding and a resulting expansion of the haematoma (Selariu et al. 2012a, b). Guo et al. showed that the swirl sign in patients with epidural haematoma is accompanied significantly by a worse outcome (death: OR 4.61, 95%, CI 1.34–15.82, $p < 0.05$) (Guo et al. 2017a, b). In the case of post-traumatic bilateral haematomas, the epidural haematoma is the most common entity and shows a preferred association with intraparenchymal haematoma (Fig. 4), respectively, contusions followed by epidural haematoma and subarachnoidal bleeding (Pandey et al. 2017).

As described above, epidural haematomas do not usually cross the sutures. By contrast, Huisman et al. found a crossing of the sutures in 11% of epidural haematomas in children. Possible factors according to the authors are, on the one hand, post-traumatic diastasis of the sutures or, on the other hand, the fracture line crossing the sutures (Huisman and Tschirch 2009). Epidural haematomas frequently show a delayed bleeding progress. This explains that there is a symptom-free interval in about half of the cases. This is represented by the sequence between the time of injury and blurring again at the time of mass effects, such as cerebral compression with a shift of the median line and consecutive herniation. Because this requires rapid surgical decompression, the damage caused by pressure and destroyed cerebral tissue is mostly reversible (Steyerberg et al. 2008). At the same time, in 6% of the cases, a delayed epidural haematoma can occur after decompressive hemicraniectomia following craniocerebral trauma—mostly after subdural bleeding. A skull fracture, found in pre-surgical

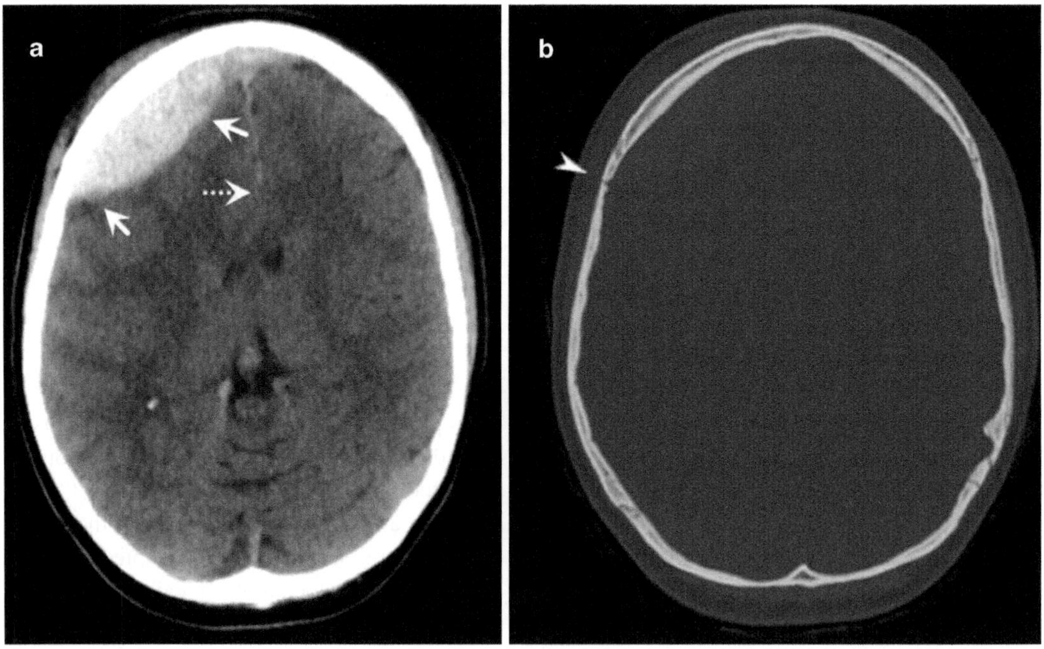


**Fig. 4** Characteristics of epidural bleeding (21-year-old patient after craniocerebral trauma). (**a**) Bleeding presents as a hyperdense convex structure on the front right in the immediate proximity to the calvaria (arrows). Spreading is limited by the dura sticking to the sutures, which causes the biconvex shape. In addition, there is a shift of the median line to the left with a possible subfalcine herniation (dotted arrow; also see Fig. 12). (**b**) Bone window: an important criterion is a skull fracture, which is frequently associated (arrowhead)

computed tomography (CT), was identified as a highly sensitive marker for this complication (Talbott et al. 2014a, b).

Special forms of post-traumatic epidural haematomas affect the localization at the clivus, in the posterior fossa and at the vertex. Clivar epidural haematomas presumably evolve because of an occipitoatlantoaxial ligamental instability. In a third of the cases, they are associated with bilateral paralysis of cranial nerves (Malik et al. 2007a, b). Bleeding in the posterior fossa accounts for 3% of all epidural haematomas and is accompanied by occipital fractures in about 85% of the cases (Malik et al. 2007a, b). A fracture line of the posterior fossa can be a hint of delayed epidural bleeding (Kircelli et al. 2016a, b). Rather rare epidural haematoma close to the vertex may be suspected in the CT after a direct impact on the vertex and in the case of signs of increased intracerebral pressure. In this case, coronary reconstruction should be used for diagnosis, to prevent misinterpreting the epidural haematoma for an artefact (Ramesh et al. 2017a, b). There is no difference between a chronic and acute traumatic epidural haematoma in terms of the localization of the haematoma, whereas the temporal lobe is the most frequent (Kach et al. 1992a, b).

The development of a pseudoaneurysm of the arteria meningea media after craniocerebral trauma, which is susceptibly caused by a lacerating vascular wall, is rare but not irrelevant. This can show a small acute epidural haematoma (de Andrade et al. 2008). This laceration of the vascular wall is probably closed by a clot and forms a pseudo-lumen after recanalization. As reported by De Andrade et al., the incidence of a pseudoaneurysm within an acute epidural haematoma and a fracture line crossing the arteria meningea media occurs in up to 30% of cases (de Andrade et al. 2008). The problem with a pseudoaneurysm is that it can grow in the course of time and disrupt secondarily (de Andrade et al. 2008). Subsequently, it can lead to a new epidural haematoma. There are also reports of subdural and intraparenchymal bleeding. Computed tomography angiography is an appropriate non-invasive method for spotting a post-traumatic aneurysm (Paiva et al. 2014). The Brain Trauma Foundation views CT criteria, such as a volume of more than 30 $cm^3$, a diameter of 15 mm or a shift of the median line of more than 5 mm, as indications for a surgical intervention (Soon et al. 2016).

Basically, CT evidence of an epidural haematoma after craniocerebral trauma is prognostically advantageous in comparison with the other forms of intracranial bleeding (Steyerberg et al. 2008).

### 1.3.2 Subdural Bleeding

The subdural haematoma in acute settings can be seen in CT as a homogenous, mostly hyperdense semilunar structure in proximity to the calvaria. Accurate examination of the falx cerebri and tentorium cerebelli is needed, because small subdural haematomas here are mostly very subtle. Again, coronary visualization and thinner layers can help. The subdural haematoma in an acute post-traumatic form presents typically with hyperdense density values (Lee et al. 1997a, b). With very early imaging (e.g. in the first hour after trauma), a subdural haematoma can initially present in an isodense form and become hyperdense with density values of >50–60 HU stepwise through the bleeding. Subsequently, the density declines after this maximum and the subdural haematoma can become subacute (mostly isodense) or chronic (hypodense or with mixed density) (Scotti et al. 1977a, b). An acute subdural haematoma, on the other hand, can lose density in the CT if the patient is or becomes anaemic (haemoglobin < 8–10 g/dl) (Grelat et al. 2016). Furthermore, a disruption in the arachnoidea and the subsequent flow of liquor can dilute the bleeding (Kim and Gean 2011). If the bleeding appears inhomogeneous, it may be a sign of active bleeding or a coagulopathy (Grelat et al. 2016). Regarding the latter, a so-called haematocrit fluid level can also evolve, because no sufficient clot can be formed quickly (Sharma and Gaillard 2018a, b).

Subdural haematomas can lead to significant mass effects, which present predominantly as a shift of the median line or herniation. Occult isodense subdural haematomas can catch one's eye indirectly through mass effects occurring.

However, if haematomas are on both sides, they may balance pressure and aggravate detection in CT (Provenzale 2007). However, they can usually be identified through application of a contrast agent or magnetic resonance imaging (MRT), but these methods are usually unnecessary (Fig. 5).

Measurement of the maximum width should be performed carefully, because the decision to evacuate surgically is also based on the spreading of the haematoma. Bullock et al. advised decompression at a width of over 10 mm or a shift of the median line over 5 mm (Bullock et al. 2006). Lentiform subdural haematomas are special cases, which are similar to epidural haematomas and can, therefore, lead to mistakes. Causes can be subdural adhesions, for example, after previous surgery (Su et al. 2010). Computed tomographically, the haematoma is a distinctive feature, especially when enhancing the ratio of the dura line (Su et al. 2010). Further hints for distinction are falciform extensions of the haematoma or an obtuse angle of the inner haematoma line and the skull (see Fig. 6) (Su et al. 2010). In addition, it was observed that haematomas in a peripheral direction increasingly adopt their semilunar structure (Su et al. 2010).

There are reports of subdural haematomas dissolving spontaneously within a few hours (Inamasu et al. 2002a, b; Kapsalaki et al. 2007a, b). Reasons can be the dilution through an arachnoidal disruption and the following flow of liquor mentioned above (Inamasu et al. 2002a, b; Kapsalaki et al. 2007a, b). Another possibility is the reallocation of the subdural haematoma in other compartments caused by increased pressure through cerebral swelling, compressing the haematoma (Kapsalaki et al. 2007a, b). A hypodense cushion between the haematoma and the inner wall of the skull bone was identified by Fujimoto et al. and Vital et al. as a predictive factor for a spontaneous dissolution (Fujimoto et al. 2014a, b; Vital et al. 2016a, b). As with many other types of bleeding, an active extravasation of the contrast agent can be a hint of active bleeding and its fast progression. Romero et al. identified a significantly higher risk of expansion of haematoma (OR 4.5, 95% CI 2.0–10.1, $p = 0.0001$) and found increased hospital mortality (OR 7.6; 95% CI 2.6–22.3, $p = 0.0004$) or patients with acute subdural haematomas (Romero et al. 2013a, b).

In addition, subdural hygroma can evolve post-traumatically. These are accumulations of liquor in the subdural space, which presumably follow a disruption of the arachnoidea (Kazam and Tsiouris 2015). Subdural hygroma mostly occurs days to weeks after trauma, but there are also reports of acute hygroma (Kamezaki et al.

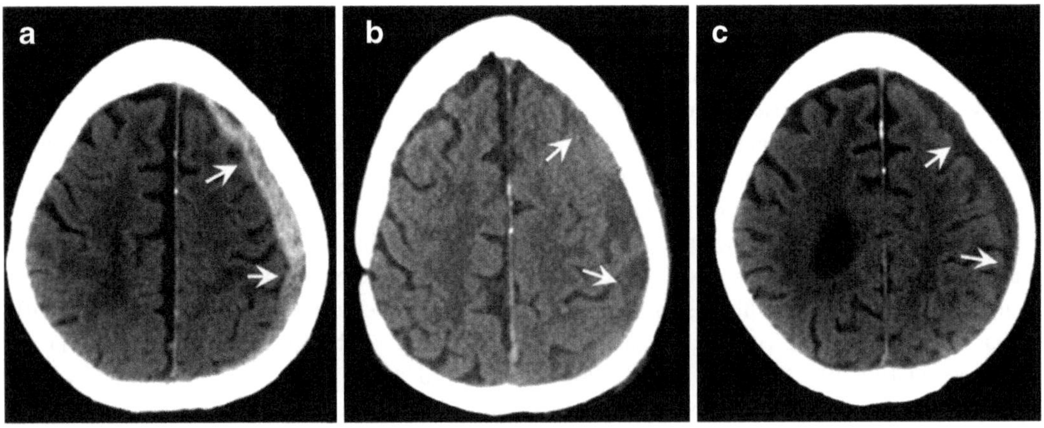


**Fig. 5** Subdural bleeding in the course of time. (**a**) Acute hyperdense subdural bleeding in the form of a hyperdense falciform consolidation (arrows) is shown, which spreads over almost the whole hemisphere. (**b**) After 10 days, the density of the same bleeding has lowered and is now partly isodense to the cerebral parenchyma (arrows). (**c**) After 19 days, chronic subdural bleeding is now hypodense compared to the cerebral parenchyma (arrows)

2004a, b). Differentiation from the beginning of cerebral involution may be difficult. Here, the CT so-called cortical vein sign may be helpful: in cerebral involution, veins cross the subarachnoidal space; in an acute accumulation of liquids, these shift to the inner side (Kazam and Tsiouris 2015). Most significant information is delivered by MRT, which can differentiate between subdural hygroma, (chronic) subdural bleeding or cerebral involution.

### 1.3.3 Subarachnoidal Bleeding

Subarachnoidal bleeding shows in CT as hyperdense bleeding in the subarachnoidal space and can spread over the whole area filled with liquor. It is mostly found at the contrecoup site and can occur locally or diffusedly, especially in severe craniocerebral trauma (Heit et al. 2017). Differentiating between traumatic subarachnoidal bleeding and a primary aneurysm disruption can sometimes be difficult, because the latter can also lead to a craniocerebral trauma through triggered neurological deficiencies. Basically, the relation between both entities has not yet been explained in detail (Song et al. 2016a, b). The main distinctive feature is the localization of appearance, and other features of traumatic and spontaneous subarachnoidal bleeding are mostly identical. Traumatic subarachnoidal bleeding occurs predominantly at the cortical superficial sulci and in the interhemispheric gap (Heit et al. 2017; Rinkel et al. 1993; Song et al. 2016a, b; Wong et al. 2011a, b; Wu et al. 2010a, b) (Fig. 7).

By contrast, spontaneous subarachnoidal bleeding is found primarily in the centre at the Sylvian fissure and basal cisterns, which explains why these localizations are a highly predictive factor (OR 4.78, 95% CI 1.33–17.1) for a disrupted aneurysm after trauma (Balinger et al. 2015a, b; Cummings et al. 2000a, b). Basically, the ratio of aneurysms being the cause of traumatic subarachnoidal bleeding is estimated as low (Cummings et al. 2000a, b). In this context, further diagnostic is performed with CT angiography usually excessively and an unnecessary radiation load is caused (Balinger et al. 2015a, b; Naraghi et al. 2015).

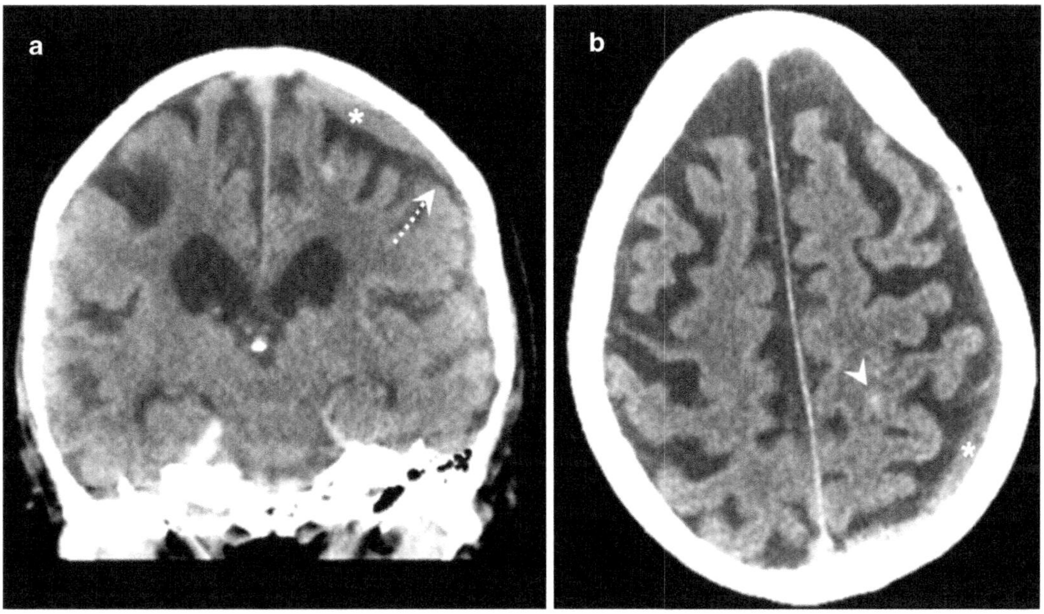


**Fig. 6** Lentiform subdural bleeding. (**a**) The subdural bleeding on the left hemisphere (star) impresses as a rather convex lesion in the coronary layer. After pointing out the obtuse angle of the inner haematoma line directed to the skull (dotted arrow), association of the bleeding with the subdural space can be made. (**b**) Subdural bleeding (star) in the axial layer. In addition, there is a little small sulcal subarachnoidal bleeding (arrowhead)

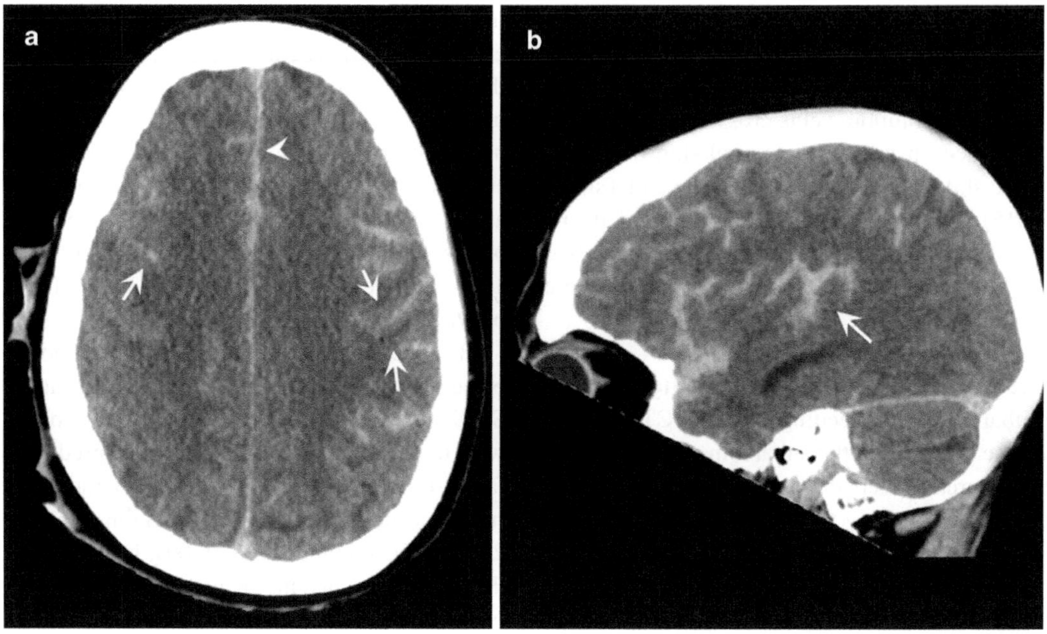


**Fig. 7** Highly developed bilateral subarachnoidal bleeding. (**a**) Traumatic subarachnoidal bleeding—in this case bilateral—appears typically at the superficial sulci (arrows) and in the interhemispheric gap (arrowhead). (**b**) Sagittal reconstruction showing the clear distribution pattern in superficial sulci (by contrast, aneurysmatic subarachnoidal bleeding develops basally and, therefore, shows another distribution pattern)

In addition, in rare cases, there is a chance of aneurysms caused by trauma. These should be considered because of the menacing secondary disruption (Nakstad et al. 2008). Nakstad et al. saw a possible association of post-traumatic aneurysm development with fractures of the skull base, particularly in young patients (Nakstad et al. 2008). Traumatic subarachnoidal bleeding is mostly accompanied by other cranial injuries, predominantly skull fractures and contusions (van Gijn and Rinkel 2001). In comparison with CT, the MRT is superior regarding the detection of smaller cases of subarachnoidal bleeding through fluid-attenuated inversion recovery sequences (FLAIR) and susceptibility sequences, such as susceptibility-weighted imaging (SWI) (Noguchi et al. 2000a, b; Verma et al. 2013). The MRT is better suited than the CT, especially in the detection of an associated intraventricular haemorrhage (Wu et al. 2010a, b). However, larger blood levels in the posterior horns of the lateral ventricles can also be detected with the CT (see Fig. 8).

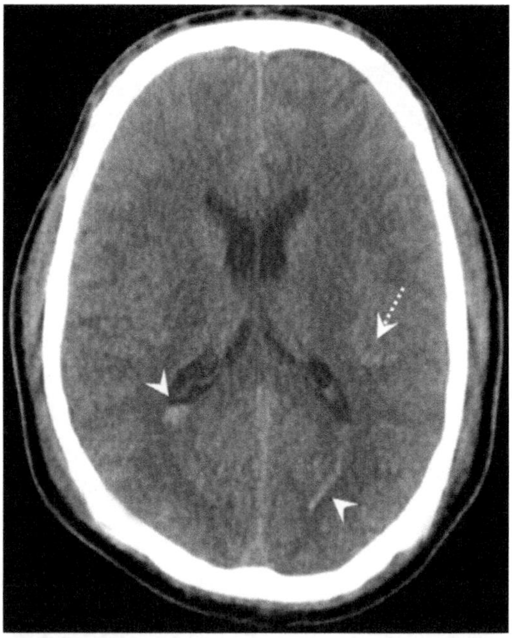

**Fig. 8** Small subarachnoidal bleeding with intraventricular blood levels. Discrete subarachnoidal bleeding on the left frontoparietal site (dotted arrow) is shown. Small blood levels are found, orthostatically lowering in both posterior horns of the lateral ventricles (arrowheads)

An independent prognostic factor of the outcome was shown within the maximum diameter of subarachnoidal bleeding in the CT, whereas the anatomical spreading of traumatic subarachnoidal bleeding had no impact (Wong et al. 2011a, b). Furthermore, pseudo-subarachnoidal bleeding should be mentioned, which can develop through a diffuse cerebral oedema. On the one hand, a focal decrease in liquor and, on the other hand, spreading of small pia vessels and the resulting increased blood flow can result in a hyperdense imitation of subarachnoidal bleeding (Given 2nd et al. 2003a, b; Provenzale 2007).

The latest studies rate isolated subarachnoidal bleeding after trauma within mild craniocerebral trauma as benign and see no necessity for routine follow-up imaging (Hayashi et al. 2016a, b; Phelan et al. 2014a, b; Quigley et al. 2013a, b). In addition, traumatic subarachnoidal bleeding very rarely needs neurosurgical intervention (Sweeney et al. 2015a, b). Quigley et al. found progression in patients with isolated subarachnoidal bleeding in less than 3%, and none of them showed neurologic deterioration, respectively, a neurosurgical intervention (Quigley et al. 2013a, b). However, the appearance of a subdural haematoma at the same time is associated with a decline in the outcome (OR 2.63, 95% CI 1.198–5.81) (Borczuk et al. 2013a, b) (Fig. 9).

Servadei et al. found a mortality rate of 43% within basal subarachnoidal bleeding, respectively, 47% within all other subarachnoidal bleeding in intermediate-to-severe craniocerebral trauma. Logistic regression analysis found a very strong association between traumatic subarachnoidal bleeding and the results (OR 2.49, 95% CI 1.74–3.55, $p < 0.001$) (Servadei et al. 2002). The authors based this on the correlation between traumatic subarachnoidal bleeding and the severity of initial mechanical damage (Servadei et al. 2002). Patients with traumatic subarachnoidal bleeding are significantly older (average of age 43 vs. 32 years), and the mortality of severe craniocerebral trauma and subarachnoidal bleeding is 18.4 vs. 9.6%, respectively, in patients without subarachnoidal bleeding ($p = 0.001$) (Servadei and Picetti 2014).

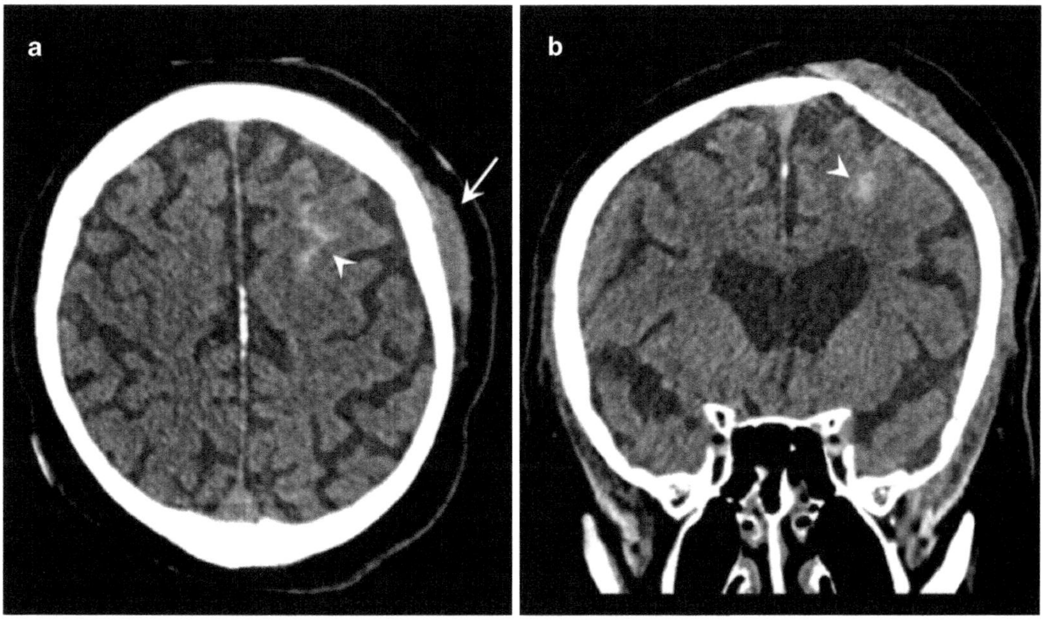


**Fig. 9** Isolated small subarachnoidal bleeding. Smaller sulcal hyperdensities are found on the left front, expressing subarachnoidal bleeding (arrowheads). (**a**) A directly neighbouring galeal haematoma (arrow) pleads for the subarachnoidal bleeding being the coup site in this case. No additional intracranial bleeding was found. (**b**) The subarachnoidal bleeding in the coronary reconstruction (arrowhead) is shown

## 2 Intra-Axial Traumatic Haemorrhage

### 2.1 Epidemiology

The group of intra-axial injuries includes all injuries within the pia mater in the brain parenchyma. In particular, a distinction can be made between intraparenchymal bleeding such as contusions and diffuse axonal damage. Contusions are a common injury pattern in craniocerebral trauma. The incidence is estimated to be up to 8.2% of all SHT cases and 13–73% of moderate and severe SHT cases (Iaccarino et al. 2014; Skandsen et al. 2010; Lobato et al. 1983). It is assumed that contusions account for slightly more than 40% of all traumatic intra-axial brain lesions (Gentry et al. 1988a). Sarkar et al. saw a more frequent occurrence of contusions (<1 cm diameter) in adults compared to children (22.4% vs. 12.4%, $p < 0.01$). Intraparenchymal hematomas (≥1 cm diameter) were detected in 30.7% of adults and 19.2% of paediatric patients ($p < 0.01$) (Sarkar et al. 2014a).

The known secondary brain damage in the form of mass effects, brain oedemas and herniation is problematic for this type of injury and determines its prognosis. This problem is exacerbated by the ability of intraparenchymal bleeding to show haemorrhagic progression. Thus, their actual extent in the first CT can easily be underestimated. So-called "talk-and-die" patients with severe contusions therefore show a normal to only slightly restricted GCS at admission and are characterized by a rapid deterioration in clinical progression (Peterson and Chesnut 2011; Davis et al. 2007).

In his retrospective review of a trauma database, Sweeney et al. found isolated contusion in mild SHT to be the intracranial injury with the least need for neurosurgical intervention (2.4% of all contusions) (Sweeney et al. 2015a).

Diffuse axonal injury (DAI), also known by synonyms such as shear injury or traumatic axonal injury, is also a common traumatic finding. It is assumed that the presence of a DAI is largely underestimated, as it often remains undetected on standard CTs. The literature reports total incidences of up to 41% (Lee et al. 2012). Occurrence in moderate SHT is found in 56%, in severe SHT even up to 72% of patients, a combination of DAI and contusion in 50% (Skandsen et al. 2010). However, DAI is not only found in cases of moderate and severe SHT, but also found in cases of mild SHT (Inglese et al. 2005). Patients with DAI are usually significantly younger, have more severe injuries, and more often the trauma is caused by a traffic accident, especially a motorcycle accident (Skandsen et al. 2010; Lee et al. 2012). DAI is one of the most frequent causes of a persistent vegetative state after trauma (Lolli et al. 2016) and is an unfavourable prognosis factor for the outcome of severe SHT (Lee et al. 2012). In their prospective cohort study, Vieira et al. found permanent disability after 6 months in 29.4% of patients with DAI, of whom 11.8% were dependent in everyday life (Vieira et al. 2016). The severity of the DAI is decisive for the outcome of the patients (Vieira et al. 2016). However, Moen et al. see only the number of cortical contusions ($p = 0.089$) instead of the DAI as more relevant to predict the outcome in patients with mean SHT (Moen et al. 2012; Moen et al. 2014). Skandsen et al. found DAI as a negative prognostic factor only if it was located in the brain stem (Skandsen et al. 2010). These intraparenchymal lesions in the brainstem account for 4% (Gentry et al. 1988a). Abu Hamdeh et al. also found a significant association with the long-term outcome for haemorrhagic bilateral brain stem lesions (OR 2.42, 95% CI 1.09–5.38, $p = 0.03$) diagnosed by SWI (Abu Hamdeh et al. 2017).

Intraventricular bleeding is a special case of intra-axial bleeding. This can occur primarily by rupture of a choroid plexus (LeRoux et al. 1992), but also secondarily by intrusion of intra-axial parenchymal haemorrhage into the ventricles. They are found in about 3% of SHT (Sarkar et al. 2014a; Brown et al. 2004).

### 2.2 Biomechanics

In intra-axial bleeding such as cerebral contusion, bruising causes injuries on the microvascular level and affect both venous and arterial vessels. They also have a coup and contrecoup injury pattern. As in the case of extra-axial bleeding, the contrecoup focal point is usually larger in terms of the severity of the injury. The pia–arachnoid complex absorbs a not negligible proportion of the force exerted by craniocerebral trauma. It consists of cerebrospinal fluid, arachnoid trabecula, pia and arachnoidea mater (Scott and Coats 2015). When accelerated, its viscoelastic properties allow it to absorb part of the force. If the force is sufficiently high, however, the brain mass at the point of impact collides with the bony inside of the skull, the falx cerebri or the tentorium cerebelli. This leads to local foci of contusion. Here, too, regional intraparenchymal areas exist, which seem to be more susceptible than others (Scott and Coats 2015). Contusions are therefore preferentially found at the frontobase (54%)—caused by the impact against the anterior skull fossa with the Crista galli—and the temporal lobe (30%), caused by the impact against the middle skull fossa and the cuneiform and petrous bone (Iaccarino et al. 2014; Bigler 2007). The remaining lesions are found in the parietal (5.9%) and occipital lobe (0.6%), the posterior fossa (5.3%) and the basal nucleus (5.2%) (Iaccarino et al. 2014). In the midbrain, bleeding occurs mainly as a result of pressure from the tentorium on the impinging brain parenchyma. Contusions of the cerebellar region, however, are relatively rare with 0.39–0.82% of all traumatic brain injuries (Sato et al. 2014), since it is comparatively immobile due to a good fixation in the posterior skull fossa during a violent impact (Sato et al. 2014; Ganpule et al. 2017). According to Sato et al., the cerebellum could have more space in the cranial fossa and be more susceptible to a resulting contusion (Sato et al. 2014) if a brain atrophy is present, e.g. in the context of a chronic alcohol abuse. In frontal trauma, a larger volume of the frontal sinus cavities appears to have a protective effect against contusions (Pajic et al. 2017).

The injury mechanism of diffuse axonal damage is still the subject of research today. What is certain is that the process of damage is dynamic and very complex and is sometimes initiated by the mechanical force at the time of trauma. If the axons are deformed by tensile stress beyond their elastic limit, microstructural injuries occur (Sullivan et al. 2015; Bigler 2016). This is mainly caused by accidents with high-speed changes such as deceleration traumas often in combination with a rotational component (Meythaler et al. 2001; Hill et al. 2016). Traffic accidents are a very frequent cause of DAI. It seems that a lateral impact of the skull more than a frontal impact increases the risk of a DAI (Post et al. 2015a; Zwahlen et al. 2007; Yoganandan et al. 2009). Since the brain parenchyma consists of heterogeneous tissues with different deformability and consistency, on which different shear forces act during a trauma (Gentry et al. 1988a), axonal damage occurs preferentially at the subcortical medullary cortex border—here especially frontotemporally bilaterally (Struffert et al. 2003), the parasagittal white matter, the corpus callosum and the brain stem (Kim and Gean 2011; Cloots et al. 2013). The basal ganglia and the capsula interna may also be affected (Forsting and Jansen 2017). The corpus callosum is particularly susceptible to axonal injury because shear forces can develop between the two mobile hemispheres, while the corpus callosum serves as a connection between them and is prevented from further movement by the falx cerebri (Hijaz et al. 2011; Chung et al. 2012). At the DAI, complex pathophysiological processes take place at the cellular level, which is currently the subject of discussion and range from biochemical changes, e.g. in the calcium balance, to mechanical disturbances of the cytoskeleton (Andriessen et al. 2010; Hill et al. 2016). In the long term, diffuse axonal damage leads to Waller's degeneration and atrophy of the white matter, the pathology of which has not yet been sufficiently clarified (Kim and Gean 2011; Johnson et al. 2013; Smith et al. 2013; Ding et al. 2008).

## 2.3 Types of Injury

### 2.3.1 Parenchymal Haemorrhage

Parenchymal haemorrhage is primarily seen as hyperdense lesions in CT. They can present as small petechiae up to confluent haematomas. In addition, perifocal oedema is very common and is expressed by a surrounding density reduction (Currie et al. 2016a). Contusions rarely appear as isolated injuries and are also present several times in a quarter of cases (Iaccarino et al. 2014). There is a predominant association with subarachnoid haemorrhages, and in Iaccarino et al., this is the case in 68.8% (Iaccarino et al. 2014). Partial volume effects should also be considered in the image morphological assessment. Thereby, hyperdense microhaemorrhages and hypodense environmental oedema can cause a contusion isodense to the surrounding brain tissue (Morales et al. 2017). Bone artefacts can overlook even small contusions near the skull.

The special feature of intraparenchymal haematomas is a dynamic injury process. The main problem is the misinterpretation in the first CT due to the progression of bleeding within the next few hours on the one hand and on the other hand due to the delayed basic occurrence. Initially, contusions cannot impress at all or only very subtly due to minimal haemorrhages or oedemas. This makes the question of serial CT examination all the more important in order to detect a mass effect requiring surgical decompression or evacuation at an early stage (Allison et al. 2017). Haemorrhagic progression is defined as the expansion of volume on the one hand and the recurrence of the lesion between the first CT and the control CT on the other. Different terminologies assume a percentage enlargement of 30% or absolute 10 ml (Iaccarino et al. 2014). This diversity also explains the different incidences of haemorrhagic progression of 30–51% (Tong et al. 2011; Iaccarino et al. 2014; Alahmadi et al. 2010; Narayan et al. 2008) (Fig. 10).

The aim of the latter studies was to identify predictors of progression. Alahmadi et al. found the initial size of the contusion ($p = 0.0212$) and the presence of subdural haematomas ($p = 0.05$) (Alahmadi et al. 2010) to be statistically significant. Depeda et al. also observed other image morphological predictors such as an initial volume of less than 5 ml (OR 2.42, $p < 0.001$), cistern compression (OR 1.95, $p < 0.001$) and the presence of multiple traumatic ICBs (OR 1.56, $p = 0.007$) (Cepeda et al. 2015). In moderate-to-severe SHT, Allison et al. identified an association of haemorrhagic progression with SAB (OR 6.33, 95% CI 1.80–22.23), SDH (OR 3.46, 95% CI 1.39–8.63) and skull fracture (OR 2.67, 95% CI 1.28–5.58) (Allison et al. 2017). In the past, special attention was paid to contrast extravasation as a possible predictor (Letourneau-Guillon et al. 2013). Huang et al. found contrast extravasation associated with bleeding progression ($p < 0.05$), clinical worsening ($p < 0.01$) and the need for subsequent surgery ($p < 0.01$) in 41% of traumatic contusions. In addition, patients with contrast extravasation had a greater volume of oedema after 24 h ($p < 0.01$) and 72 h ($p < 0.01$) (Huang et al. 2011). In Kim et al., extravasation was also an independent predictor of mortality ($p = 0.017$) and hematoma growth ($p < 0.001$) (Kim et al. 2008). Haemorrhagic progression of contusions occurs in up to 82% within the first 12–24 h, but can also manifest up to 3–4 days after trauma (Tong et al. 2011; Kurland et al. 2012). It should also be noted that the earlier the CT is performed after trauma, the greater the probability that contusions will only become visible in a subsequent scan (Kurland et al. 2012).

In the past, the pericontusional hypodense region was also examined for its character. Thus, the area similar to the penumbra in stroke is considered; i.e., the area is composed of necrotic but also vital tissue. A perfusion CT can better than a native CT define the viability of the pericontusional tissue and the delimitation of the extent of the contusion and could therefore be of importance for surgical planning (Soustiel et al. 2008). Another rather rare form of traumatic intraparenchymal bleeding is basal ganglion bleeding (Vega et al. 2015). It can also occur bilaterally and tends to be associated with a good result as long as it is not associated with damage to other cortical and subcortical structures and occurs in isolation (Pandey et al. 2014).

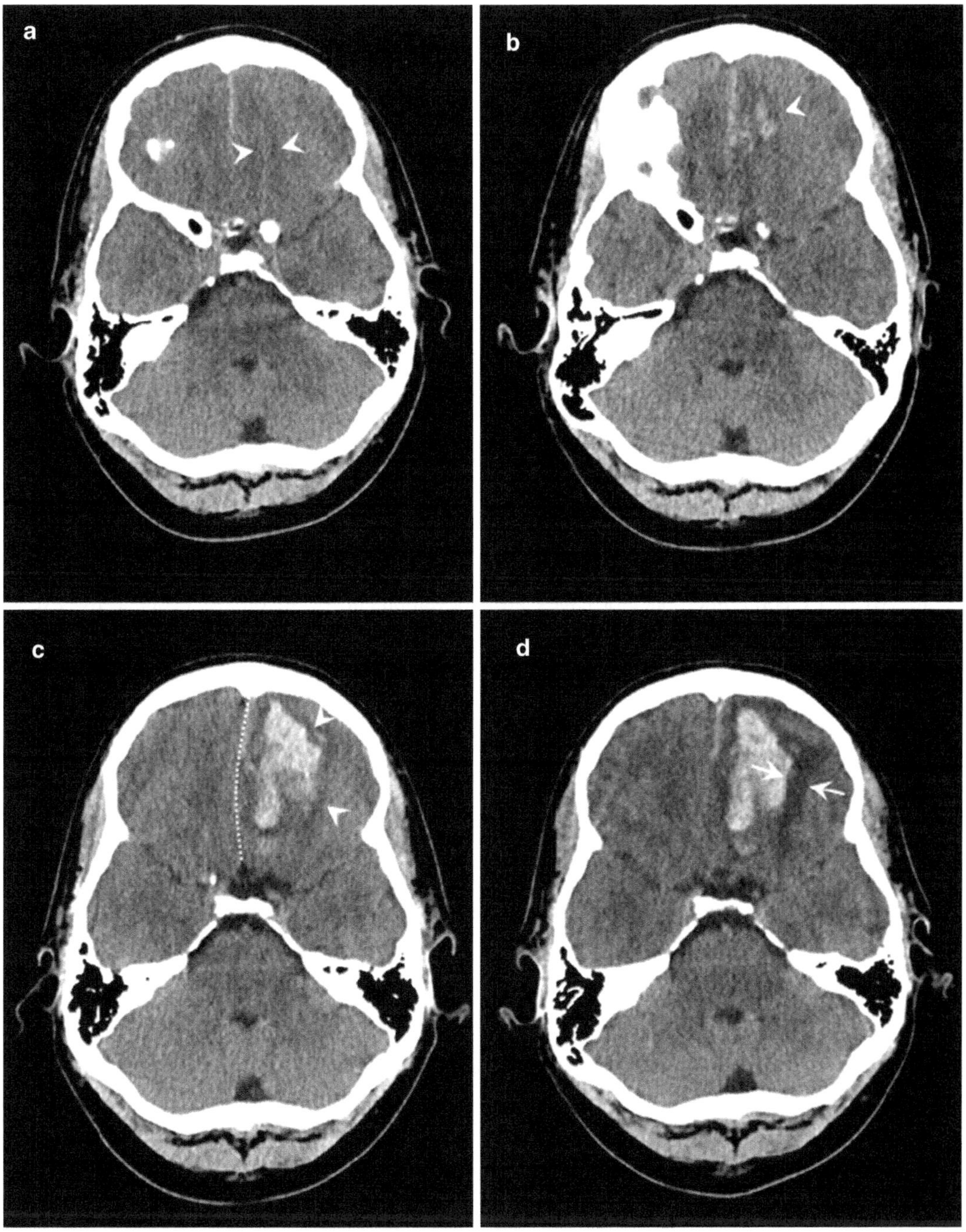


**Fig. 10** Contusion over time. (**a**) shows the first image after SHT. A side-by-side comparison shows at most a small flat hyperdense focal finding on the left frontal in loco typico (arrowheads). (**b**) In the control image after 3 h, the contusion haemorrhage slowly demarcates (arrowheads). (**c**) After a further 6 h, a clear progression (arrowheads) with perifocal oedema and space-consuming effect (dashed line) is visible. (**d**) In the course of 3 days, the still hyperdense bleeding slowly resorbs, and the perifocal oedema (arrows) has expanded further in the meantime

### 2.3.2 Diffuse Axonal Injury

The diffuse axonal damage has a special position with regard to the SHT, since it tends to be often undetectable in CT imaging. MRI is clearly superior to DAI in detection and can therefore often make a statement in cases whose neurological symptoms cannot be explained by CT (Hijaz et al. 2011). In CT, only indirect focal indications such as petechial bleeding and low blood levels in the lateral ventricle horns or the interpeduncular cisterns are visible (Struffert et al. 2003). Today, DAI is often divided into haemorrhagic and non-haemorrhagic (Forsting and Jansen 2017). Only 10–20% of DAI lesions show a sufficient haemorrhagic component to be detected on CT (Kim and Gean 2011; Hijaz et al. 2011). Mata-Mbemba et al. identified intraventricular haemorrhage as the only predictor ($p = 0.0139$) in CT for DAI in subsequent MRI (Mata-Mbemba et al. 2015). Cerebral microhaemorrhages are found in the white matter and are a radiological indication for a DAI (Greenberg et al. 2009; Scheid et al. 2007). In addition, they seem to be important for prognosis and initial neurological status (Park et al. 2009; Lawrence et al. 2017). Of the non-haemorrhagic lesions, only 19% can be detected by CT (Lolli et al. 2016). Depending on the severity of the trauma, the affected sites are found in a certain order: starting with the marrow bark border, followed in second place by the corpus callosum—here mainly in the splenium (Gentry et al. 1988b)—and then in the brainstem (Adams et al. 1977). The most common division of the DAI according to Adams et al. into three degrees (Adams et al. 1989) is also based on this order. From degree 2, the DAI of Lee et al. was strongly associated with an unfavourable result (OR 30.5, $p = 0{,}018$) (Lee et al. 2012) (Fig. 11).

MRI is clearly more sensitive for the detection of DAI. In MRI, DAI lesions often appear multiple in oval or ellipsoidal forms and are oriented to the direction of the nerve fibres (Forsting and Jansen 2017). The T1 sequence is often inconspicuous compared to the T2 sequence, and haemorrhagic lesions may be visible hyperintensively depending on the progress of blood breakdown (Struffert et al. 2003). More sensitive, however, is the T2*-weighted gradient echo imaging, the so-called 'haem sequence', which can visualize iron-containing degradation products of the blood due to their paramagnetic properties (Kim and Gean 2011). It is particularly sensitive to microhaemorrhages (Nandigam et al. 2009). A modification of gradient echo imaging is susceptibility-weighted imaging (Currie et al. 2016a). However, the FLAIR sequence can detect especially non-haemorrhagic lesions (Kim and Gean 2011). This can be done at least as sensitively with diffusion-weighted or diffusion tensor imaging. Although this is not as sensitive as the T2* sequence in the detection of haemorrhagic lesions, it can detect additional lesions—e.g. in the brainstem—that were not visible in other MRI sequences (Huisman et al. 2003; Ezaki et al. 2006; Docimo Jr. et al. 2014). This visualization—mostly hyperintensity by reduced diffusion coefficient values—seems to be based on the development of cytotoxic oedema by axonal necrosis (Lolli et al. 2016).

Moen et al. found a disappearance of non-haemorrhagic DAI lesions and lesions in the brainstem after 3 months. The haemorrhagic lesions also weakened over time, but at a much slower rate. Therefore, the authors recommend early MRI in severe SHT to improve outcome prediction and not overlook brain injury (Moen et al. 2012). The exact timing of MRI imaging needs to be further studied, but the authors recommend that this be done within the first week after trauma (Moen et al. 2012).

# 3 Secondary Complications and Impact of Anticoagulation

## 3.1 Secondary Complication

Intracranial injuries can take on devastating proportions due to secondary complications and thus become life-threatening within a short period of time. Responsible for this are processes on the microstructural level due to cytotoxic effects on the one hand, and on the macroscopic level the displacing effect when bleeding or oedema spreads on the other hand. The latter leads to an

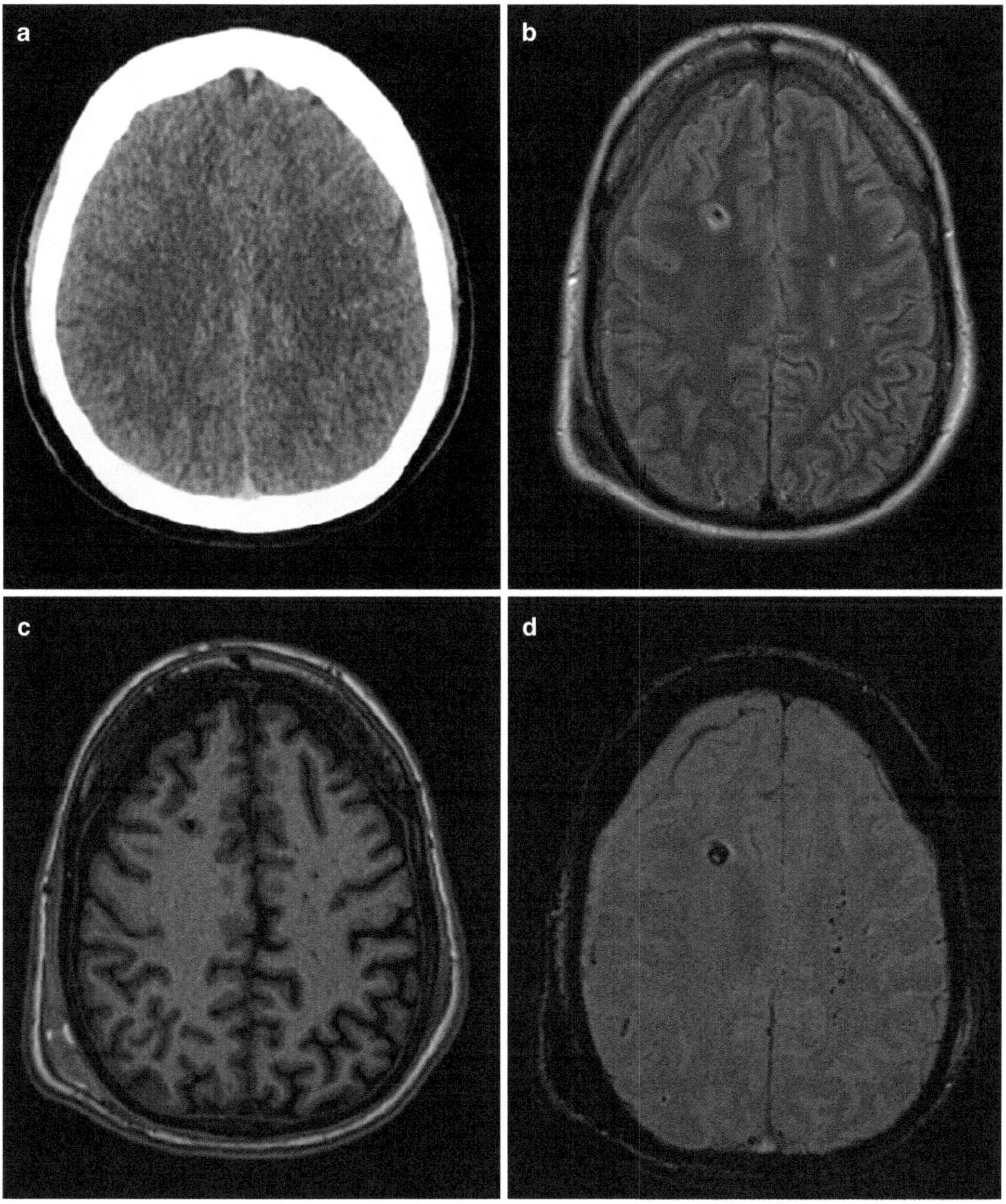


**Fig. 11** Diffuse axonal damage in cross-sectional imaging. (**a**) With CT, at most questionably small haemorrhages are visible frontoparietally at the marrow bark boundary on the left. (**b–d**) In MRI, on the other hand, the extent of the damage is more clearly shown by punctiform microbleeding, especially in the left medullary bed and partly corresponding punctiform diffusion restrictions with ADC correlation (not shown) in the left mediastromal region. In addition, a small subdural hematoma on the right frontal (*) and an intraventricular drainage (IVD, +), which has been removed, in the meantime were found. (Sequences: B T2 C FLAIR D gradient echo T2)

increase in intracranial pressure, the cardinal features of which are a midline shift and the compression of the cisterns.

Diffuse brain oedema can have various causes such as vasogenic or cytotoxic oedema. Skull–brain trauma is characterized by a mixture of both components (Hudak et al. 2014). The cerebral oedema is recognized by CT morphology by a diffuse density reduction, the loss of marrow bark differentiation with the passage of sulci and obliteration of the inner and outer CSF spaces (Ho et al. 2012).

The differentiation between density reduction due to actual brain swelling or post-traumatic hyperaemia and the resulting increased density values is often discussed. Rozsa et al. defined a density value measurement of 11–20 HU for brain swelling and 31–40 HU (Rozsa et al. 1989) for hyperaemia.

Another secondary complication, which may have been preceded by brain oedema, is herniation. Herniations can primarily manifest as subfalcine, transtentorial and tonsillary (see Fig. 12) (Kim and Gean 2011). The incarceration may also cause vessels such as the cerebral artery to be involved anteriorly or posteriorly, causing infarct patterns (Server et al. 2001). Here, too, the examination of the cerebrospinal fluid spaces and cisterns as well as the foramen magnum helps to detect the emergence of brain tissue.

Further post-traumatic complications are sometimes caused by hydrocephalus, i.e. an expansion of the internal cerebrospinal fluid spaces. This can be caused mechanically, for example, by an obstruction of drainage due to the space-consuming effect of a haematoma. The adhesion of pacchionic granulations by coagulated blood as a result of SAB can also be the cause. Post-traumatic hydrocephalus after traumatic SAB is also not a very rare event with an incidence of up to 12% (Tian et al. 2008). Increased intracranial pressure can also lead post-traumatically to haemodynamic problems with consecutive infarct patterns. Although these post-traumatic cerebral infarctions after SHT are rather rare, they have a considerable influence on mortality (Bae et al. 2014). The causes for this are manifold, e.g. secondary vasospasms after SAB or dissections.

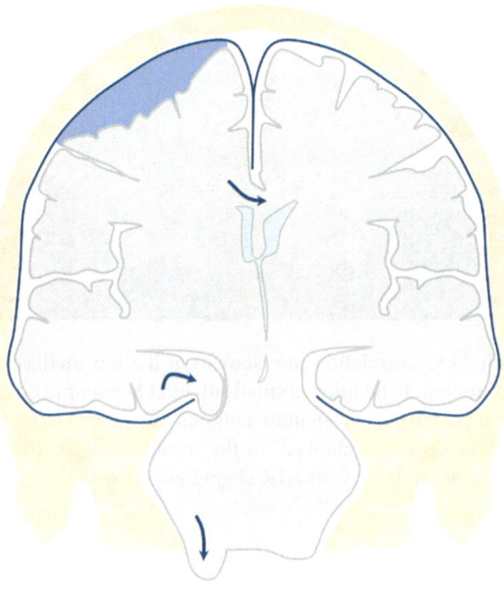

**Fig. 12** Types of herniation. Depending on the location of the intracranial post-traumatic lesion, subfalcine, uncal or transtentorial or tonsillar herniation may occur

All listed complications are decisive for the outcome, and against this background, Marshall et al. have classified them on the basis of CT morphological parameters midline shift, cisterns and the size of hyperdense or mixed hypo–/hyperdense lesions (Marshall et al. 1991) (Table 1).

Maas et al. further developed this classification to the so-called Rotterdam criteria with the following parameters: status of the basalt cisterns, intraventricular haemorrhage or subarachnoid haemorrhage and finally the presence of epidural mass lesions (Maas et al. 2005). Decompression therapy (Bor-Seng-Shu et al. 2012) is the therapeutic method of choice for increased intracranial pressure (Fig. 13).

## 3.2 Impact of Anticoagulation

Falls are the most frequent cause of SHTs, especially in the particularly affected and growing elderly patient population (Taylor et al. 2017; Giannoudis et al. 2009). The total incidence of mild SHT in patients over 65 is estimated by Feigin et al. to be 537 per 100,000 inhabitants (Feigin et al. 2013). A problem in the setting of SHT is the frequent multimorbidity of the patients, which often requires anticoagulation against the background of an underlying cardiovascular disease. The proportion of patients with such medication is growing steadily, e.g. due to

**Table 1** Mortality rates in mass effects (Marshall classification) according to (Marshall et al. 1991)

| Degree | Centre line shift | Cisterns | Hyperdense or mixed lesions ($cm^3$) | Mortality (%) |
|---|---|---|---|---|
| I | None | Delimitable | <25 | 9.6 |
| II | ≤5 mm | Delimitable | <25 | 13.5 |
| III | ≤5 mm | Compressed/ obliterated | <25 | 34 |
| IV | >5 mm | | <25 | 56.2 |
| Unloaded mass lesion | | | >25 | 53 |

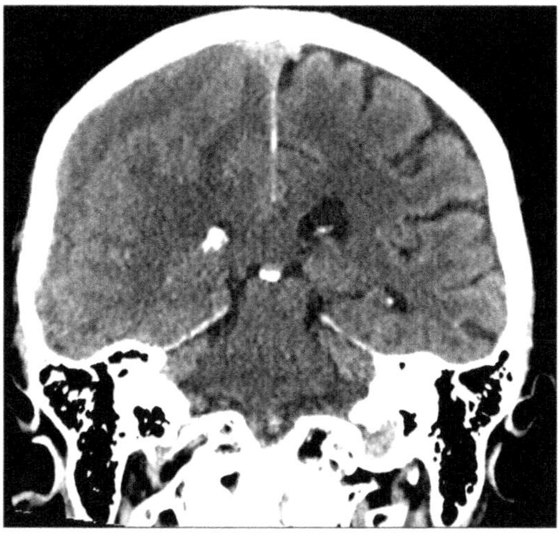

**Fig. 13** Pre-stage of a possible uncal herniation in subdural hematoma. The right hemispherical subdural hematoma leads to consecutive displacement of the ipsilateral lateral ventricle. In a lateral comparison, the beginning expansion of the brain to the right side of the tentorium is also noticeable. If a further swelling of the brain with a consecutive increase in size occurs at this point during the course of the disease, there would be an incipient uncal herniation

an increasing prevalence of atrial fibrillation (Dossett et al. 2011; Ajani et al. 2006). Classes of substances with an influence on blood coagulation are in the broadest sense vitamin K antagonists, thrombocyte aggregation inhibitors and the class of heparins. In addition, there are the new oral anticoagulants, which have only been available on the market for a few years but are still being used with increasing frequency. Here, in particular there is a pronounced lack of data to assess the risk of bleeding after trauma (Kobayashi et al. 2017).

The focus is on the question of an increase in the risk of intracranial bleeding in anticoagulated patients and the associated expansion of the indication for CCTs. In recent decades, there have been many attempts to establish evidence-based indication guidelines for each setting. Anticoagulation is an exclusion criterion for the application of the otherwise well-established Canadian head rule, which is why in such cases no statements on the CT indication can be derived from it. For the authors at that time, the cause of exclusion was too little data on anticoagulated patients with SHT (Stiell et al. 2001). The New Orleans criteria were also not evaluated for the treatment of this patient clientele due to an insufficient database (Haydel et al. 2000). The NICE criteria, on the other hand, see patients under warfarin therapy as an independent risk factor that generally indicates CCT within 8 h post-traumatic (Excellence, N.I.f.H.a.C. 2014). The current guidelines of the, on the other hand, see an indication for CCT in 'indications of a coagulation disorder (foreign anamnesis, "pass for anti-coagulant treatment", non-stilling bleeding from superficial injuries, etc.)'. (Firsching et al. 2015). Here, a recommendation level of class A (strong recommendation) is given. The EFNS guideline for mild SHT also recommends imaging for all anticoagulated patients at admission and after 24 h (Vos et al. 2002). Thus, there are no uniform and generally accepted recommendations for action for anticoagulated patients who imagine a mild SHT (GCS 13–15) without further symptoms. The subject of the discussion is the indication for CCT at presentation in the emergency room. On the other hand, even after CT has been performed, the duration of observation or the necessity of a control CT to determine delayed intracranial bleeding is controversial (Table 2).

The incidence of traumatic intracranial haemorrhage under anticoagulation varies greatly and is different for each drug subgroup. Total data

**Table 2** CCT recommendations for mild SHT with anticoagulation (Vos et al. 2012)

| Guideline | CCTHR | NICE | NOC | LDGN | EFNS | CHIP | NEXUS II |
|---|---|---|---|---|---|---|---|
| CCT recommendation | Patients with anticoagulation excluded | + | – | + | + | + | + |

*LDGN* Guideline of the German Society of Neurosurgery, *EFNS* European Federation of Neurological Societies Guideline, *CHIP* CT in Head Injury Patients Prediction Rule, *NEXUS II* National Emergency X-Ray Utilization Study II

amount to 3.5–31% (Kobayashi et al. 2017; Ganetsky et al. 2017; Li 2012; Reddy et al. 2014; Jagoda et al. 2008; Brewer et al. 2011). Garra et al. found an incidence of 0% in 39 patients (Garra et al. 1999), and in 1996, Franko et al. found an incidence of ICB in 60% of patients under warfarin anticoagulation (159 patients) (Franko et al. 2006). This diversity can be explained on one hand by the extract from trauma registers and the retrospective character of the studies, on the other hand by a small number of patients (<100 patients) or a distortion due to selection bias (Ganetsky et al. 2017; Nishijima et al. 2012). Overall, the evidence for the anticoagulants frequently used in old age as a co-factor in traumatic brain haemorrhages is poor.

## 3.3 Anticoagulation Substances

### 3.3.1 Coumarins

The coumarin class includes the two active ingredients warfarin (Coumadin®) and phenprocoumon (Marcumar®). They have an anticoagulant effect by inhibiting the synthesis of vitamin K-dependent coagulation factors II, VII, IX and X by competitively inhibiting vitamin K reductase (Karow and Lang-Roth 2017). The most frequent indications for coumarins are the prevention of systemic thromboembolism in the context of atrial fibrillation, pulmonary embolism, phlebothrombosis or mechanical heart valves. Laboratory chemistry shows a lowered quick or an increased INR value (international normalized ratio), which lies within the therapeutic target range between 2.0 and 3.0. Warfarin and phenprocoumon are both coumarin derivatives, while phenprocoumon has a half-life three to four times longer than warfarin (Beinema et al. 2008). While in the USA above all Warfarin is common, phenprocoumon is used in Germany and other European countries. Vitamin K is available as an antidote to bleeding complications.

The incidence of intracranial post-traumatic bleeding with warfarin in mild SHT is reported to be 5.1% in Nishijima et al. (37/724 patients, 95% CI 3.6–7.0%) (Nishijima et al. 2012). In the literature, higher values of 10–29% are found for SHT in some cases (Brewer et al. 2011; Major and Reed 2009; Ahmed et al. 2015).

### 3.3.2 Thrombocyte Aggregation Inhibitors

The most commonly used thrombocyte inhibitor on the current market is acetylsalicylic acid (ASS, Aspirin®). ASA is indicated for acute coronary syndrome, stent implantation and secondary prophylaxis of cerebral ischaemia and coronary heart disease. It acts by irreversibly inhibiting cyclooxygenase, thereby inhibiting thromboxane synthesis (Karow and Lang-Roth 2017). Other important representatives of platelet aggregation inhibitors are clopidogrel (Plavix®), prasugrel (Efient®) and ticagrelor (Brilique®). These ADP receptor antagonists inhibit ADP-dependent platelet activation. The field of application is very similar to that of ASS. In addition, ADP receptor antagonists can be used as a substitute for ASA or can also be given in combination with ASA as part of dual platelet inhibition after stent implantation (Karow and Lang-Roth 2017). In contrast to coumarins, the impairment of coagulation cannot be demonstrated or quantified by laboratory chemistry. In the prospective study by Fabbri et al. with 1558 participants, 35% of all patients with craniocerebral trauma received treatment with platelet aggregation inhibitors. From an age of 75, the proportion even rises to 53% (Fabbri et al. 2013).

The incidence of post-traumatic intracranial bleeding under this therapy is also subject to different data. It is indicated for clopidogrel by Nishijima et al. with 12% (33/276, 12.0%, 95% CI 8.4–16.4). Delayed haemorrhagic progression was not found in any case (0/243 patients (0%; 95% CI 0–1.5) (Nishijima et al. 2012). Ganetsky et al. find a lower incidence of 3.9% (95% CI 0.5–13.2) in combination of aspirin and clopidogrel, and a slightly higher incidence of 4.6% (95% CI 3.2–6.6) in combination of aspirin and clopidogrel (95% CI 0.5–13.2) (Ganetsky et al. 2017).

### 3.3.3 Direct Oral Anticoagulants

New oral anticoagulants (NOAK) include direct factor Xa inhibitors such as rivaroxaban (e.g. XARELTO®), apixaban (e.g. Eliquis®) and edoxaban (Lixiana®). They bind to the active site of the coagulation factor Xa and thus prevent cleavage from prothrombin to active thrombin (Samama 2011). Dabigatran (e.g. Pradaxa®) is available as a direct thrombin inhibitor. These direct oral anticoagulants have only been approved for the market since 2009 (Ganetsky et al. 2017). The indication range is similar to that of coumarins, but there is a contraindication for mechanical heart valves (Karow and Lang-Roth 2017). In comparison with coumarins, coagulation monitoring is not necessary, but an antidote has only been available for dabigatran since 2016. Additional advantages are the short half-life, the rapid onset of action and the limited interaction with food and drugs (Feeney et al. 2016). An incidence of intracranial bleeding under pre-existing therapy with NOAKs cannot be found in the current scientific literature.

### 3.3.4 Heparins

The heparins are divided into unfractionated heparin (UFH), low molecular weight heparins (NMH) such as enoxaparin (e.g. Clexane®), certoparin (e.g. Mono-Embolex®) and many more and other heparins such as fondaparinux (e.g. Arixtra), argatroban (e.g. Argatra®) or danaparoid (e.g. Orgaran®). All active ingredients bind to antithrombin III and thus enhance its anticoagulatory effect. This heparin–antithrombin III complex inactivates various coagulation factors such as thrombin, Xa, XIIa, XIa and IXa and inhibits the coagulation cascade (Karow and Lang-Roth 2017). The indication range of heparins is very broad and includes both prophylaxis and therapy of all types of phlebothromboses via pulmonary embolisms, myocardial infarctions and thrombus embolisms. The anticoagulant effect of UFH can be controlled by laboratory chemical determination of the aPTT value. In NMH, however, the anti-Xa activity can be used for monitoring. In case of need, antagonization by the administration of protamine is possible (Karow and Lang-Roth 2017). A major difference between UFH and NMH is that UFH is administered continuously by perfusor for full heparinization, whereas NMH is administered twice a day (Hirsh and Levine 1992). The other heparins are mainly reserved for the situation following heparin-induced thrombocytopenia.

Incidences of intracranial bleeding after SHT are also not yet present in heparins.

## 3.4 Risk Discussion

The discussion deals with the question to what extent patients with craniocerebral trauma under anticoagulation have an increased intracranial bleeding risk and are not covered by the common CT indication guidelines. Since for more severe SHT a further clarification with CT is already standard, it should only be considered against the background of a mild SHT, i.e. for patients with a GCS of 13–15.

As a rule, patients with older age are also subject to greater comorbidities. It can therefore be questioned whether the greater proportion of findings requiring monitoring are actually due to anticoagulation—or whether they are indirectly due to age. Although no unambiguous statement is possible, it seems at least questionable to perform CT imaging after trauma exclusively on the basis of anticoagulation. In the case of CCTHR, for example, an age above 65 represents a risk factor for its own for which CCT is indicated. This means that a large number of patients are already covered under anticoagulation. In fact, however, the proportion of anticoagulated patients under 65 is also increasing (Dossett et al. 2011). One of the most common diseases requiring anticoagulant therapy is atrial fibrillation. Schnabel et al. showed a prevalence for this disease of 4.6% in men between 55 and 64 years of age (Schnabel et al. 2012). The rate of patients with atrial fibrillation and antithrombotic therapy in this age range was 57.3%. Fabbri et al. also showed a proportion of almost 10% of the total population in Italy treated with antiplatelet agents (Fabbri et al. 2010). This reveals the relevance of a guideline for the treatment of these patients with mild SHT. One of the biggest problems in the evaluation of the current study situation is revealed by the fact that the majority of the studies only include patients above a certain age. Accordingly, many studies only consider patients aged 60/65 or older and investigate the differences between patients with and without anticoagulation. This study design therefore often excludes the respective anticoagulant as a generally valid predictive variable, since confounding is often associated with older age patients and this cannot always be completely ruled out despite all efforts. Since there is already an indication for CCT for patients over 60 or 65 years of age depending on the guideline, the question arises whether including anticoagulants as predictors can increase the age limit. Fabbri et al. have already developed a first model for this.

In fact, the number of scientific studies on this subject has increased in recent years. Many studies, however, consider the outcome of SHT patients of all GCS in order to investigate a fundamental risk increase for the respective anticoagulant—not only specifically for the mild SHT. Often the different drug groups are not diversified or only drug groups are compared with each other and not against a control group, which also leads to inconsistent results. In this case, it would be necessary to consider which endpoint creates a CT indication. While Skaga et al. basically see death as the most suitable starting point for trauma research (Skaga et al. 2008), the necessity of neurosurgical interventions as an endpoint seems even more interesting in this question. This parameter is the only one that can be indicated primarily by imaging and thus clinically influenced. The comparison of this endpoint can be used to determine how often neurosurgical intervention (indicated by CCT) can reduce mortality, assuming that neurosurgical interventions tend to reduce mortality (Shimoda et al. 2014).

### 3.4.1 Coumarins

Since coumarins, unlike all other anticoagulants, have been on the market for many decades, this is the most mature study on their risk assessment. Whereas many studies have previously found an increase in risk of intracranial haemorrhagia (Bonville et al. 2011), increased mortality (Bonville et al. 2011) and increased morbidity, more and more prospective and targeted studies are now coming to the conclusion that coumarin does not have a significant increase in risk either.

Increased mortality in trauma patients with warfarin (OR 1.72, 95% CI 1.63–1.81; $p < 0.001$) (Dossett et al. 2011) was discovered by Dossett et al. in a very large retrospective evaluation of a trauma register in 2011. Narum et al. also retrospectively investigated the 30-day mortality in 418 patients with SHT with respect to differences in warfarin ($n$ = 12.7%) and antiplatelet therapy ($n$ = 19.1%) compared to non-users. In patients without physiological impairment at ingestion (GCS 13–15, and normal respiratory rate and systolic blood pressure), warfarin was associated with increased mortality (adjusted OR 8.3; 95% CI 2.0–34.8). However, warfarin patients were significantly older than non-users (76.6 vs. 69.1 years) and also showed significantly greater comorbidity before trauma (measured by the American Society of Anesthesiologists–Physical Status Score (ASA-PS) 2.81 vs. 1.84) (Narum et al. 2016). Bonville et al. in a study with 3436 patients also showed an increased mortality for patients with SHT under warfarin (relative risk 3.2, 95% CI 1.6–6.6). However, the anticoagulant groups differed significantly in age and sex composition from those without anticoagulants (Bonville et al. 2011). Maung et al. conducted a retrospective examination of a trauma database with 3392 patients with trauma. They found a higher total trauma-related mortality among warfarin compared to a control group and a group of patients with NOAK (warfarin group (9.0%) versus NOA (2.8%) and control group (3.7%) ($p < 0.001$).) In the group of traumatic brain injuries, the warfarin group also had higher trauma-related mortality compared to NOAKs and non-anticoagulated patients (warfarin group (19.3%) compared to NOAK (16.7%) or control group (10.9%) ($p = 0.08$). However, this did not reach statistical significance (Maung et al. 2016). In 2009, McMillian identified six studies involving warfarinized head injury patients. With regard to mortality, the authors conclude that there is only a tendency towards increased mortality in older patients with warfarin (McMillian and Rogers 2009). In comparison, these studies have the largest number of patients who see an increased risk for warfarin. However, they all have in common that they have a retrospective character and at the same time age can often act as a strong confounder.

The authors investigated the occurrence of ICB in anticoagulated 982 patients who presented with mild SHT in the emergency departments of two trauma centres and four municipal hospitals. Patients with warfarin and clopidogrel use were considered, with 72.7% warfarin. No increased risk of traumatic ICB was found (relative risk 0.40, CI 0.25–0.65, in multivariable analysis 0.62, CI 0.70–5.49) (Nishijima et al. 2013).

According to that, further studies are necessary despite the already prevailing opinion that coumarin causes a risk increase due to a not clear study situation for a better risk estimate.

Based on possible risk factors, further attempts were made to stratify patients with SHT under coumarin therapy on the basis of their risk for one of the endpoints mentioned. The AHEAD study attempted to identify predictors of ICB in warfarin in a prospective design. This included a remarkable study population of 3566 patients with blunt head trauma. 81.5% had a GCS of 15. The authors identified GCS and the presence of the two neurological symptoms LOC and amnesia as significant risk factors. Increased INR (>4) was found to be a significant risk in univariate analysis. However, after exclusion of patients with GCS <15, the risk was no longer significantly increased (relative risk = 1.11, 95% CI 0.95–1.18, $p = 0.298$). The authors concluded that patients with a GCS = 15 and without evidence of symptoms had a low risk of adverse effects regardless of their INR (2.7%) (Mason et al. 2017) (see Table 3). Negative effects were defined as death, neurosurgical intervention or clinically significant CCT findings.

A problem with the risk factors LOC and amnesia as possible predictors is the fact that more than 2/3 of the patients (68.7%, $n = 2428$) did not report any neurological symptoms (amnesia, vomiting, unconsciousness or headaches). Similar to the AHEAD study, Brewer et al. showed that LOC is significantly associated with ICB in patients with mild SHT and warfarin (Brewer et al. 2011).

Nishijima et al. also tried to develop a clinical predictive rule for the use of coumarins in mild SHT in their prospective study described above, but ultimately failed to do so. They identified vomiting (adjusted odds ratio 3.68, 95% CI 1.55–8.76) and an abnormal mental status (adjusted OR 3.08, 95% CI 1.60–5.94) as additional risk factors. However, these variables were absent in more than 75% of patients with traumatic ICB. The bivariate analysis also found an increased risk of immediate ICB in headache, vomiting, drug or alcohol intoxication and abnormal mental status. Therefore, they recommend a liberal indication (Nishijima et al. 2013).

**Table 3** Outcome of coumarin therapy patients (Mason et al. 2017)

| Clinical presentation | Number total | Of which unwanted event (%) | Number |
|---|---|---|---|
| GCS = 15 + no neurological symptoms | 2243 | 2.8 | 65 |
| GCS = 15 + 1 neurological symptom | 384 | 9.0 | 38 |
| GCS = 15 + 2 neurological symptoms | 109 | 13.5 | 17 |
| GCS = 15 + 3 neurological symptoms | 15 | 26.7 | 4 |
| GCS < 15 | 358 | 20.9 | 75 |

Due to the fact that anticoagulation can or must be controlled by checking the INR value, there is the additional approach of several authors to make SHT imaging dependent on the current INR value. Gaetani et al. found a significant association of the INR value with the total mortality after SHT (Gaetani et al. 2012). In Menditto et al. with 97 patients under light SHT and warfarin therapy, a delayed bleeding after normal first CT was observed in 7 cases. Of these, 7 patients an increased INR ratio of more than 3.0 (57% vs. 5% of the comparison population) was present in 4 cases. Again, all patients were well over 65 years of age and the patient population was extremely small. For an INR ≥3, the authors determined a relative risk of 14 (95% CI 4–49) (Menditto et al. 2012). Claudia et al. also dealt with the INR as a predictive factor for ICB in patients with head trauma under coumarins. The authors found a significant association ($r = 0.37$; $p < 0.005$). As cut-off, they identified a value of 2.43. This had a sensitivity of 92%, a specificity of 66% and positive and negative predictive values of 33% and 97%, respectively (Claudia et al. 2011). On this basis, the EAST guidelines of 2012 recommend the determination of the INR value in patients with coumarins and the retention of this value for observation in patients with supratherapeutic values (recommendation level 3) (Barbosa et al. 2012).

Finally, it can be stated that the assumption of a basically increased spontaneous bleeding risk of coumarins cannot be clearly extended to patients with mild SHT. Although earlier retrospective studies also see an increase in risk, more recent research has come to different conclusions. Further research is needed to focus on patients with mild SHT who are not covered by current indication guidelines.

### 3.4.2 Thrombocyte Aggregation Inhibitor

There are also different assessments of platelet aggregation inhibitors with regard to their risk increase. The frequent problem with study designs is that no differentiation is made between the different substances. Patients under aspirin, for example, are unified with patients under clopidogrel or prasugrel, although these drug classes act via very different mechanisms. Here too, there is hardly any data on patients with mild SHT, but in most cases all grades have been included.

Aspirin was the most frequently administered anticoagulant in our study. The frequencies of the intracranial findings showed the same distribution of the entire anticoagulant group, which could not indicate a higher risk in comparison.

The prospective study mentioned above by Nishijima et al. surprisingly showed a higher risk of ICB of clopidogrel (33/276, 12.0%, 95% CI 8.4–16.4) compared to warfarin (($n$ = 37/724, 5.1%, 95% CI 3.6–7.0), relative risk 2.31, 95% CI 1.48–3.63). However, only 64% of patients with ICB had a GCS of 15. One possible reason for the increased bleeding rate is the higher severity of injury in younger patients, if it is assumed that patients under clopidogrel are usually younger than patients under coumarins. A prospective study by Farsi et al. with 1140 patients showed a proportion of patients with mild SHT of 11.8% who took aspirin or clopidogrel or 6% with dual platelet inhibition. Here, it was documented that platelet aggregation inhibitors lead to a longer hospital stay and a worse outcome (disability after 30-day follow-up). Here, too, the problem arises that comorbidities, for example, were not taken into account because the anticoagulation group was significantly older than the control group. (80.78 ± 8.76 vs. 46.33 ± 18.77 years, $p < 0.001$) (Farsi et al. 2017). Kobayashi et al. also found an increased risk of ICB in trauma patients under aspirin (478 of 1847 patients). This drug group had the highest risk of ICB compared to the other groups (35% vs. 33% clopidogrel 27% warfarin 24% NOAK) (Kobayashi et al. 2017). However, the authors see the significantly lower age and the significantly higher proportion of patients with an injury severity score ≥10 of the ASS group as possible causes. In view of this, the study's ASA patients appear to have had a larger injury mechanism. In a retrospective evaluation of 1558 patients with SHT, Fabbri et al. showed an increased risk of the progression of ICB in patients under platelet inhibitory therapy (aspirin, clopidogrel, ticlopidine, indobufen) with a relative risk of 2.09, 95% CI 1.63–2.71). However, this study included all grades of SHT. In addition, comorbidities of patients under anticoagulation were not considered (Fabbri et al. 2013).

A 2013 meta-analysis by Batchelor et al. included five studies and the effects of aspirin and clopidogrel on mortality in blunt head trauma. The authors concluded that although there was a slightly increased risk of death for both drugs, no statistical significance was achieved (Batchelor and Grayson 2013). The study by Narum et al. described above also did not show any significant change in 30-day mortality from antiplatelet therapy (Narum et al. 2016).

Cull et al. evaluated the data of 1547 trauma patients and compared the patients with platelet aggregation inhibitors (27%) with a control group. They found no significant differences in risk of ICB, neurosurgical intervention and mortality. However, patients under antiplatelet therapy and an ISS from ≥20 showed increased mortality (OR 2.34, 95% CI 1.03–5.31) (Cull et al. 2015). Spektor et al. were interested in the effect of low-dose ASA therapy before trauma and the effect on ICB, NI and death. In comparison with the control group, no significant impairment in the corresponding parameters was found prospectively for moderate-to-mild SHT (GCS 9–15) (Spektor et al. 2003). Ganetsky et al. also analysed in a prospective cohort study of 939 patients with soil fall that there were no significant differences in ICB between the group of platelet aggregation inhibitors compared to anticoagulants. Basically, the incidence of traumatic ICB in these patients was relatively low (3.5%) (Ganetsky et al. 2017). In the abovementioned study by Bonville et al., no increased mortality was observed for aspirin and clopidogrel (Bonville et al. 2011).

Fabbri et al. tried in 2010 to develop a predictive model for mild SHT (here defined as GCS 14–15) under consideration of platelet aggregation inhibitors (Fabbri et al. 2010). Aspirin and indobufen, a platelet inhibitor commonly used in Italy, were included. In contrast, clopidogrel was not included as it was not yet available on the market. 14,288 patients aged 10 years and older were examined. The risk of a clinically significant intracranial lesion was increased with platelet inhibition in univariate analysis (OR 2.6, 95% CI 2.2 to 3.1) and interacted with age in multivariate analysis (OR 2.7, CI 1.9 to 3.7); age ≥75 years (OR 1.4, CI 1.0–1.9). Using further predictors from different prediction models such as CCTHR or CHIP, the authors showed a prediction for intracranial lesions with a sensitivity of 99.7% (95% CI 98.9–99.8) and specificity of 54.0% (95% CI 53.1–54.8). These values were achieved by an increased age limit of 75 and the inclusion of platelet inhibitors as predictors. The CT rate under these conditions was 49.3%.

In fact, the present study is one of the few to include all age groups (10 years and older). Nevertheless, it should be considered that the study was evaluated retrospectively and that a selection bias can distort the results due to the unicentric trauma register. Furthermore, the study only refers to the joint predisposition of aspirin and indobufen, which are not representative for Germany or the USA.

In principle, it can therefore be stated that there are no meaningful data on an increase in the risk of antiplatelet therapy for patients with mild craniocerebral trauma after the removal of confounders in a particular age.

### 3.4.3 NOAK

Since the NOAK substance class is only used for a relatively short period of time, the study situation on traumatically caused bleeding is contemplative. Primarily, there are only studies that assess the basic bleeding risk without differentiating between spontaneous and traumatic bleeding and often compare it with coumarins (Feeney et al. 2016). The largest of these studies is the Randomized Evaluation of Long-Term Anticoagulation Therapy-RELY study, or RELY study for short. In a follow-up of 134,414 patients with 37,587 person-years follow-up, patients with dabigatran showed a lower intracranial bleeding risk with a hazard ratio of 0.34 (CI 0.26–0.46) (Graham et al. 2015; Connolly et al. 2009) compared to warfarin. Southworth et al. obtained similar results with a lower rate of intracranial bleeding events for dabigatran than for warfarin (0.3 vs. 0.8 per 100 patient-years). The authors examined the differences between warfarin and dabigatran in atrial fibrillation in a database of over 50,000 patients. The incidence of all intracranial haemorrhages was estimated at 0.8 per 100,000 patient days for dabigatran versus 2.4 for warfarin (Southworth et al. 2013). Regarding the analysis of major bleeding under rivaroxaban, 89% of bleeding is gastrointestinal and approximately 8% intracranial haemorrhages (Tamayo et al. 2015).

Despite the lower bleeding risk of NOAKs, there are isolated case reports describing the fulminant course of an ICB under dabigatran with mild SHT (Wassef et al. 2013; Garber et al. 2012). Beynon et al. investigated NOAK rivaroxaban. Here, a patient population of 70 persons with bleeding under mild SHT was divided into three groups (I: no antiplatelets, II: warfarin or thrombocyte aggregation inhibitors and finally III: rivaroxaban). Rivaroxaban showed significantly increased haemorrhagic progression and mortality. However, the significance of rivaroxaban remains very limited in a number of six patients (Beynon et al. 2015). Parra et al. (Parra et al. 2013) came to a similar conclusion. They prospectively examined patients of my SHT after a fall from the ground. The three groups were divided into dabigatran ($n = 5$), warfarin ($n = 15$) and no anticoagulants ($n = 25$). Again, there was a significantly increased haemorrhagic progression for dabigatran compared to warfarin ($p = 0.03$). However, the number of patients with 5 patients is too small to make a scientifically sound statement.

As explained above, Maung et al. performed a retrospective evaluation of trauma patients. Here, the trauma-specific mortality of patients with SHT showed a higher rate of warfarin compared to NOAKs. Nevertheless, the NOAK rate of 16.7% was higher than in the control group. However, these values were not statistically significant. In a multivariable logistic regression analysis, only warfarin (OR 2215; 95% CI 1365–3596; $p = 0.001$), but not NOAKs, was an independent predictor of mortality in all patients. Thus, NOAKs appear to have a lower risk compared to warfarin (Maung et al. 2016). Feeney et al. retrospectively compared 162 patients with traumatic ICB who took either warfarin or NOAKS with each other. NOAKs showed significantly lower mortality (4.9% vs. 20.8%; $p < 0.008$) and a lower rate of neurosurgical intervention (8.2% vs. 26.7%; $p = 0.023$) (Feeney et al. 2016). In a prospective multicentre study by Kobayashi et al. with 1847 patients, NOAKs (dabigatran, rivaroxaban or apixaban) showed a significantly lower incidence of traumatic ICB of 24% compared to older anticoagulants (warfarin, aspirin and clopidogrel) with 31% ($p = 0.04$, univariate analysis). In multivariate analysis, this was a reduced risk (incidence rate ratio 0.78, CI 0.61–1.01, $p = 0.05$) for NOAKs—but without statistical significance (Kobayashi et al. 2017). The groups did not differ in terms of bleeding progression or mortality.

In summary of the scientific results to date, there is a trend that NOAKs may have a lower incidence of traumatic bleeding compared to established anticoagulants. Against the background of the study designs, a very small number of patients who are treated with NOAKs in order to be able to make a representative statement are often problematic. Here, too, further prospective multicentre study designs are required, focusing on traumatic intracranial bleeding in SHT. Currently, there seems to be no known risk increase for this substance class.

### 3.4.4 Heparin

Current clear figures on incidences and an increased bleeding risk in SHT under pre-existing heparinization are not available. On the contrary, heparin is discussed therapeutically as a thromboprophylaxis after SHT (Matsushima et al. 2016), since especially trauma patients with brain injuries have a higher risk of venous thromboembolic events (Knudson et al. 2004). Experimental studies have shown that heparin can reduce microvascular permeability and oedema without increasing bleeding size (Li et al. 2015; Nagata et al. 2017). In this context, data on bleeding progression in SHT patients with subsequent prophylactic heparin administration have been collected. A systematic review by Chelladurai et al. from 2013 showed a mixed study situation on progression rates between patients with heparin (UFH and NMH) and a control group (Chelladurai et al. 2013). While the majority of the evaluated studies do not see any statistically significant difference, Kwiatt et al. report a significant increase in risk (progression control group vs. NMH administration: 24% vs. 42%, $p < 0.001$) (Kwiatt et al. 2012). There are also no uniform data on a significantly different bleeding risk between the two different classes of UFH and NMH (Phelan et al. 2012; Scudday et al. 2011). Only Minshall et al. saw a higher risk of bleeding for UFH than for NMH (12% vs. 5% $p < 0.05$) (Minshall et al. 2011). The overall bleeding risk of heparins is also increased by combination with NSAIDs such as aspirin (Davidson et al. 2014).

According to this study, there is no sufficient evidence on the risk assessment of a pre-existent heparin therapy for SHT.

### 3.4.5 Haemorrhagic Progression

However, the risk of haemorrhagic progression in normal primary CT does not seem to change under anticoagulation and therefore serial control CT does not seem to be necessary for all anticoagulated patients. However, very little data are available on this issue. In a prospective study in 136 patients with mild SHT under warfarin or heparin, Kaen et al. showed a progression of only 1.4% ($n = 2$). None showed neurological deterioration or the need for neurosurgical intervention. These two patients with progression were treated with warfarin and aspirin and also showed LOC after trauma. Therefore, the authors suspected these two points as predictors. However, the number of two patients is insufficient (Kaen et al. 2010). Accordingly, there does not seem to be any reliable data for an increased progression rate in anticoagulation patients, which would change management after initial imaging.

## 4 Conclusions

Epidural haematomas are rather rare, but often dramatic consequences of craniocerebral trauma and are associated with skull fractures in up to 90% of cases. They emerge especially temporally of the coup site and are mostly of arterial origin with subsequent secondary complications, such as mass effects. In acute diagnostics, the CT shows a biconvex, hyperdense bleeding, which does not cross the sutures. The swirl sign may be pointing at an acute bleeding component. Coronary reconstructions are suited to detect epidural haematomas close to the vertex. Epidural haematomas with surgical decompression in time have a good outcome, which is why quick and correct diagnosis is of extraordinary importance. A clinically symptom-free interval between the time of injury and the start of mass effects can aggravate diagnosis.

Subdural haematomas are common concomitant injuries of craniocerebral trauma, especially within elderly patients. They impress computer tomographically as falciform hyperdense bleeding, which can spread along the interhemispheric gap or the falx cerebri and are, therefore, able to cross the adhesion points of the dura and calotte, in contrast to epidural haematomas. Because of their mostly venous origin, neurologic symptoms are commonly subacute. In the course of time, the subdural haematoma loses density and may chronify. In the case of multiple events of falling down, mixed forms with fresh hyperdense and chronic parts of the bleeding can occur. Subdural haematomas can appear isodense within hyperacute bleeding with short-term imaging; however, at the same time, one should also think of a diluting liquor component or an anaemic patient. The subdural haematomas have a worse outcome than epidural haematomas, because other intracranial injuries are associated more often.

Traumatic subarachnoidal bleeding emerges most likely through the disruption of smaller, cortical vessels or because of disruptions of aneurysms. It appears as hyperdensities in the sulci and cisterns and, in contrast to spontaneous subarachnoidal bleeding, does not normally occur at the Sylvian fissure or the basal cisterns, but rather at the cortical, surface sulci and in the interhemispheric gap. A suspected aneurysm, either etiological or as a consequence, should be clarified via CT angiography.

At present, however, there is still no clear evidence of an increase in risk of patients under anticoagulation after mild craniocerebral trauma, especially for the endpoint of compulsory therapy, if the data situation is unsatisfactory. For a final evaluation, a significantly more mature study situation on patients under anticoagulation with mild SHT is required. This should only be possible with very large numbers of patients in a multicentre approach.

In order to be able to cope with the presumably increasing incidence of SHT with increasing age in the future, a continuous reduction in the radiation exposure of the CT and a better availability of the MRT will be necessary. Further positive effects may arise from the establishment of dual-energy CT in SHT diagnostics. It is possible that the virtual native representation will help in the assessment of the course after KM administration. In addition, it may even be possible to identify active bleeding components in haematomas.

**Acknowledgement** Parts of the work were created within the framework of the doctoral thesis project of L Schmidt (Schmidt 2018). Interested readers may refer to this thesis as it contains further information.

## References

Abu Hamdeh S et al (2017) Extended anatomical grading in diffuse axonal injury using MRI: hemorrhagic lesions in the substantia nigra and mesencephalic tegmentum indicate poor long-term outcome. J Neurotrauma 34(2):341–352

Adams H et al (1977) Diffuse brain damage of immediate impact type. Its relationship to 'primary brain-stem damage' in head injury. Brain 100(3):489–502

Adams JH et al (1989) Diffuse axonal injury in head injury: definition, diagnosis and grading. Histopathology 15(1):49–59

Ahmed N et al (2015) Risk associated with traumatic intracranial bleed and outcome in patients following a fall from a standing position. Eur J Trauma Emerg Surg 41(3):307–311

Ajani UA et al (2006) Aspirin use among U.S. adults: behavioral risk factor surveillance system. Am J Prev Med 30(1):74–77

Alahmadi H, Vachhrajani S, Cusimano MD (2010) The natural history of brain contusion: an analysis of radiological and clinical progression. J Neurosurg 112(5):1139–1145

Allison RZ et al (2017) Derivation of a predictive score for hemorrhagic progression of cerebral contusions in moderate and severe traumatic brain injury. Neurocrit Care 26(1):80–86

Andriessen TM, Jacobs B, Vos PE (2010) Clinical characteristics and pathophysiological mechanisms of focal and diffuse traumatic brain injury. J Cell Mol Med 14(10):2381–2392. https://doi.org/10.1111/j.1582-4934.2010.01164.x

Bae DH et al (2014) Cerebral infarction after traumatic brain injury: incidence and risk factors. Korean J Neurotrauma 10(2):35–40

Balinger KJ et al (2015a) Selective computed tomographic angiography in traumatic subarachnoid hemorrhage: a pilot study. J Surg Res 199(1):183–189

Balinger KJ, Elmously A, Hoey BA, Stehly CD, Stawicki SP, Portner ME (2015b) Selective computed tomographic angiography in traumatic subarachnoid hemorrhage: a pilot study. J Surg Res 199:183–189. https://doi.org/10.1016/j.jss.2015.04.006

Barbosa RR et al (2012) Evaluation and management of mild traumatic brain injury: an Eastern Association for the Surgery of Trauma practice management guideline. J Trauma Acute Care Surg 73(5 Suppl 4):S307–S314

Batchelor JS, Grayson A (2013) A meta-analysis to determine the effect of preinjury antiplatelet agents on mortality in patients with blunt head trauma. Br J Neurosurg 27(1):12–18

Beinema M et al (2008) Pharmacogenetic differences between warfarin, acenocoumarol and phenprocoumon. Thromb Haemost 100(6):1052–1057

Beynon C et al (2015) Rivaroxaban and intracranial haemorrhage after mild traumatic brain injury: a dangerous combination? Clin Neurol Neurosurg 136:73–78

Bigler ED (2007) Anterior and middle cranial fossa in traumatic brain injury: relevant neuroanatomy and neuropathology in the study of neuropsychological outcome. Neuropsychology 21(5):515–531

Bigler ED (2016) Systems biology, neuroimaging, neuropsychology, neuroconnectivity and traumatic brain injury. Front Syst Neurosci 10:55

Bonville DJ et al (2011) Impact of preinjury warfarin and antiplatelet agents on outcomes of trauma patients. Surgery 150(4):861–868

Borczuk P et al (2013a) Patients with traumatic subarachnoid hemorrhage are at low risk for deterioration or neurosurgical intervention. J Trauma Acute Care Surg 74(6):1504–1509

Borczuk P, Penn J, Peak D, Chang Y (2013b) Patients with traumatic subarachnoid hemorrhage are at low risk for deterioration or neurosurgical intervention. J

Trauma Acute Care Surg 74:1504–1509. https://doi.org/10.1097/TA.0b013e31829215cf
Bor-Seng-Shu E et al (2012) Decompressive craniectomy: a meta-analysis of influences on intracranial pressure and cerebral perfusion pressure in the treatment of traumatic brain injury. J Neurosurg 117(3):589–596
Brazinova A et al (2021) Epidemiology of traumatic brain injury in Europe: a living systematic review. J Neurotrauma 15(10):1411–144
Brewer ES et al (2011) Incidence and predictors of intracranial hemorrhage after minor head trauma in patients taking anticoagulant and antiplatelet medication. J Trauma 70(1):E1–E5
Brown CV et al (2004) Does routine serial computed tomography of the head influence management of traumatic brain injury? A prospective evaluation. J Trauma 57(5):939–943
Bullock MR et al (2006) Surgical management of acute subdural hematomas. Neurosurgery 58(3 Suppl):S16–S24. discussion Si-iv
Cepeda S et al (2015) Traumatic intracerebral hemorrhage: risk factors associated with progression. J Neurotrauma 32(16):1246–1253
Chelladurai Y et al (2013) Venous thromboembolism prophylaxis in patients with traumatic brain injury: a systematic review. F1000Res 2:132
Chung SW et al (2012) Locations and clinical significance of non-hemorrhagic brain lesions in diffuse axonal injuries. J Korean Neurosurg Soc 52(4):377–383
Claudia C et al (2011) Minor head injury in warfarinized patients: indicators of risk for intracranial hemorrhage. J Trauma 70(4):906–909
Cloots RJ et al (2013) Multi-scale mechanics of traumatic brain injury: predicting axonal strains from head loads. Biomech Model Mechanobiol 12(1):137–150
Connolly SJ et al (2009) Dabigatran versus warfarin in patients with atrial fibrillation. N Engl J Med 361(12):1139–1151
Crooks DA (1991) Pathogenesis and biomechanics of traumatic intracranial haemorrhages. Virchows Arch A Pathol Anat Histopathol 418(6):479–483
Cull JD et al (2015) Outcomes in traumatic brain injury for patients presenting on antiplatelet therapy. Am Surg 81(2):128–132
Cummings TJ et al (2000a) The relationship of blunt head trauma, subarachnoid hemorrhage, and rupture of pre-existing intracranial saccular aneurysms. Neurol Res 22(2):165–170
Cummings TJ, Johnson RR, Diaz FG, Michael DB (2000b) The relationship of blunt head trauma, subarachnoid hemorrhage, and rupture of pre-existing intracranial saccular aneurysms. Neurol Res 22: 165–170
Currie S et al (2016a) Imaging assessment of traumatic brain injury. Postgrad Med J 92(1083):41–50
Currie S, Saleem N, Straiton JA, Macmullen-Price J, Warren DJ, Craven IJ (2016b) Imaging assessment of traumatic brain injury. Postgrad Med J 92:41–50. https://doi.org/10.1136/postgradmedj-2014-133211
Davidson BL et al (2014) Bleeding risk of patients with acute venous thromboembolism taking nonsteroidal anti-inflammatory drugs or aspirin. JAMA Intern Med 174(6):947–953
Davis DP et al (2007) Head-injured patients who "talk and die": the San Diego perspective. J Trauma 62(2):277–281
de Andrade AF et al (2008) Intracranial vascular lesions associated with small epidural hematomas. Neurosurgery 62(2):416–420. https://doi.org/10.1227/01.neu.0000316008.11388.f2. discussion 420–1
Ding K et al (2008) Cerebral atrophy after traumatic white matter injury: correlation with acute neuroimaging and outcome. J Neurotrauma 25(12):1433–1440
Docimo S Jr, Demin A, Vinces F (2014) Patients with blunt head trauma on anticoagulation and antiplatelet medications: can they be safely discharged after a normal initial cranial computed tomography scan? Am Surg 80(6):610–613
Dossett LA et al (2011) Prevalence and implications of preinjury warfarin use: an analysis of the National Trauma Databank. Arch Surg 146(5):565–570
Excellence, N.I.f.H.a.C (2014) Head injury: assessment and early management. National Institute for Health and Care Excellence (NICE), London
Ezaki Y et al (2006) Role of diffusion-weighted magnetic resonance imaging in diffuse axonal injury. Acta Radiol 47(7):733–740
Fabbri A et al (2010) Predicting intracranial lesions by antiplatelet agents in subjects with mild head injury. J Neurol Neurosurg Psychiatry 81(11):1275–1279
Fabbri A et al (2013) Antiplatelet therapy and the outcome of subjects with intracranial injury: the Italian SIMEU study. Crit Care 17(2):R53
Farsi D et al (2017) Effects of pre-injury anti-platelet agents on short-term outcome of patients with mild traumatic brain injury: a cohort study. Bull Emerg Trauma 5(2):110–115
Feeney JM et al (2016) Compared to warfarin, direct oral anticoagulants are associated with lower mortality in patients with blunt traumatic intracranial hemorrhage: a TQIP study. J Trauma Acute Care Surg 81(5):843–848
Feigin VL et al (2013) Incidence of traumatic brain injury in New Zealand: a population-based study. Lancet Neurol 12(1):53–64
Firsching R et al (2015) Leitlinie Schädel-Hirn-Trauma im Erwachsenenalter der Deutschen Gesellschaft für Neurochirurgie. 2015 [cited 08.09.2017; Available from: http://www.awmf.org/uploads/tx_szleitlinien/008-001l_S2e_Schaedelhirntrauma_SHT_Erwachsene_2016-06.pdf
Forsting M, Jansen O (2017) Chapter 4 Head trauma. In: Forsting M, Jansen O (eds) MR Neuroimaging. Georg Thieme Verlag, Stuttgart
Franko J et al (2006) Advanced age and preinjury warfarin anticoagulation increase the risk of mortality after head trauma. J Trauma 61(1):107–110

Fujimoto K et al (2014a) Predictors of rapid spontaneous resolution of acute subdural hematoma. Clin Neurol Neurosurg 118:94–97
Fujimoto K, Otsuka T, Yoshizato K, Kuratsu J (2014b) Predictors of rapid spontaneous resolution of acute subdural hematoma. Clin Neurol Neurosurg 118:94–97. https://doi.org/10.1016/j.clineuro.2013.11.030
Gaetani P et al (2012) Traumatic brain injury in the elderly: considerations in a series of 103 patients older than 70. J Neurosurg Sci 56(3):231–237
Ganetsky M et al (2017) Risk of intracranial hemorrhage in ground-level fall with antiplatelet or anticoagulant agents. Acad Emerg Med 24(10):1258–1266
Ganpule S et al (2017) A three-dimensional computational human head model that captures live human brain dynamics. J Neurotrauma 34(13):2154–2166
Garber ST, Sivakumar W, Schmidt RH (2012) Neurosurgical complications of direct thrombin inhibitors – catastrophic hemorrhage after mild traumatic brain injury in a patient receiving dabigatran. J Neurosurg 116(5):1093–1096
Garra G, Nashed AH, Capobianco L (1999) Minor head trauma in anticoagulated patients. Acad Emerg Med 6(2):121–124
Gean AD et al (2010a) Benign anterior temporal epidural hematoma: indolent lesion with a characteristic CT imaging appearance after blunt head trauma. Radiology 257(1):212–218
Gean AD, Fischbein NJ, Purcell DD, Aiken AH, Manley GT, Stiver SI (2010b) Benign anterior temporal epidural hematoma: indolent lesion with a characteristic CT imaging appearance after blunt head trauma. Radiology 257:212–218. https://doi.org/10.1148/radiol.10092075
Gentry LR, Godersky JC, Thompson B (1988a) MR imaging of head trauma: review of the distribution and radiopathologic features of traumatic lesions. AJR Am J Roentgenol 150(3):663–672
Gentry LR, Thompson B, Godersky JC (1988b) Trauma to the corpus callosum: MR features. AJNR Am J Neuroradiol 9(6):1129–1138
Giannoudis PV et al (2009) Severe and multiple trauma in older patients; incidence and mortality. Injury 40(4):362–367
Given CA 2nd et al (2003a) Pseudo-subarachnoid hemorrhage: a potential imaging pitfall associated with diffuse cerebral edema. AJNR Am J Neuroradiol 24(2):254–256
Given CA 2nd, Burdette JH, Elster AD, Williams DW 3rd (2003b) Pseudo-subarachnoid hemorrhage: a potential imaging pitfall associated with diffuse cerebral edema. AJNR Am J Neuroradiol 24:254–256
Graham DJ et al (2015) Cardiovascular, bleeding, and mortality risks in elderly Medicare patients treated with dabigatran or warfarin for nonvalvular atrial fibrillation. Circulation 131(2):157–164
Greenberg SM et al (2009) Cerebral microbleeds: a guide to detection and interpretation. Lancet Neurol 8(2):165–174
Grelat M, Madkouri R, Bousquet O (2016) Acute isodense subdural hematoma on computed tomography scan - diagnostic and therapeutic trap: a case report. J Med Case Rep 10:43. https://doi.org/10.1186/s13256-016-0822-x
Guo C et al (2017a) Swirl sign in traumatic acute epidural hematoma: prognostic value and surgical management. Neurol Sci 38(12):2111–2116
Guo C, Liu L, Wang B, Wang Z (2017b) Swirl sign in traumatic acute epidural hematoma: prognostic value and surgical management. Neurol Sci 38:2111–2116. https://doi.org/10.1007/s10072-017-3121-4
Hayashi T et al (2016a) Delayed deterioration in isolated traumatic subarachnoid hemorrhage. World Neurosurg 86:511.e9–511.14
Hayashi T, Karibe H, Narisawa A, Kameyama M (2016b) Delayed deterioration in isolated traumatic subarachnoid hemorrhage. World Neurosurg 86(511):e519–e514. https://doi.org/10.1016/j.wneu.2015.09.108
Haydel MJ et al (2000) Indications for computed tomography in patients with minor head injury. N Engl J Med 343(2):100–105
Heinzelmann M, Platz A, Imhof HG (1996) Outcome after acute extradural haematoma, influence of additional injuries and neurological complications in the ICU. Injury 27(5):345–349. https://doi.org/10.1016/0020-1383(95)00223-5
Heit JJ, Iv M, Wintermark M (2017) Imaging of intracranial hemorrhage. J Stroke 19(1):11–27. https://doi.org/10.5853/jos.2016.00563
Hijaz TA, Cento EA, Walker MT (2011) Imaging of head trauma. Radiol Clin North Am. 49:81–103
Hill CS, Coleman MP, Menon DK (2016) Traumatic axonal injury: mechanisms and translational opportunities. Trends Neurosci 39(5):311–324
Hirsh J, Levine MN (1992) Low molecular weight heparin. Blood 79(1):1–17
Ho ML, Rojas R, Eisenberg RL (2012) Cerebral edema. AJR Am J Roentgenol 199(3):W258–W273
Huang AP et al (2011) Early parenchymal contrast extravasation predicts subsequent hemorrhage progression, clinical deterioration, and need for surgery in patients with traumatic cerebral contusion. J Trauma 71(6):1593–1599
Hudak AM et al (2014) Cytotoxic and vasogenic cerebral oedema in traumatic brain injury: assessment with FLAIR and DWI imaging. Brain Inj 28(12):1602–1609
Huisman TA, Tschirch FT (2009) Epidural hematoma in children: do cranial sutures act as a barrier? J Neuroradiol 36(2):93–97. https://doi.org/10.1016/j.neurad.2008.06.003
Huisman TA et al (2003) Diffusion-weighted imaging for the evaluation of diffuse axonal injury in closed head injury. J Comput Assist Tomogr 27(1):5–11
Iaccarino C et al (2014) Patients with brain contusions: predictors of outcome and relationship between radiological and clinical evolution. J Neurosurg 120(4):908–918

Inamasu J et al (2002a) Rapid resolution of traumatic acute subdural hematoma by redistribution. Am J Emerg Med 20(4):376–377
Inamasu J, Nakamura Y, Saito R, Kuroshima Y, Mayanagi K, Ohba S, Ichikizaki K (2002b) Rapid resolution of traumatic acute subdural hematoma by redistribution. Am J Emerg Med 20:376–377. https://doi.org/10.1053/ajem.2002.33955
Inglese M et al (2005) Diffuse axonal injury in mild traumatic brain injury: a diffusion tensor imaging study. J Neurosurg 103(2):298–303
Jagoda AS et al (2008) Clinical policy: neuroimaging and decisionmaking in adult mild traumatic brain injury in the acute setting. Ann Emerg Med 52(6):714–748
Johnson VE et al (2013) Inflammation and white matter degeneration persist for years after a single traumatic brain injury. Brain 136(Pt 1):28–42
Kach K et al (1992a) [Differences of acute and chronic epidural hematoma]. Unfallchirurg 95(9):426–430
Kach K, Imhof HG, Kunzi W, Trentz O (1992b) [Differences of acute and chronic epidural hematoma] Unfallchirurg 95:426–430
Kaen A et al (2010) The value of sequential computed tomography scanning in anticoagulated patients suffering from minor head injury. J Trauma 68(4):895–898
Kalanithi P et al (2011a) Hospital costs, incidence, and inhospital mortality rates of traumatic subdural hematoma in the United States. J Neurosurg 115(5):1013–1018
Kalanithi P, Schubert RD, Lad SP, Harris OA, Boakye M (2011b) Hospital costs, incidence, and inhospital mortality rates of traumatic subdural hematoma in the United States. J Neurosurg 115:1013–1018. https://doi.org/10.3171/2011.6.JNS101989
Kamezaki T et al (2004a) Traumatic acute subdural hygroma mimicking acute subdural hematoma. J Clin Neurosci 11(3):311–313
Kamezaki T, Yanaka K, Fujita K, Nakamura K, Nagatomo Y, Nose T (2004b) Traumatic acute subdural hygroma mimicking acute subdural hematoma. J Clin Neurosci 11:311–313. https://doi.org/10.1016/j.jocn.2003.10.013
Kapsalaki EZ et al (2007a) Spontaneous resolution of acute cranial subdural hematomas. Clin Neurol Neurosurg 109(3):287–291
Kapsalaki EZ, Machinis TG, Robinson JS 3rd, Newman B, Grigorian AA, Fountas KN (2007b) Spontaneous resolution of acute cranial subdural hematomas. Clin Neurol Neurosurg 109:287–291. https://doi.org/10.1016/j.clineuro.2006.11.005
Karow T, Lang-Roth R (2017) Allgemeine und spezielle Pharmakologie und Toxikologie: Vorlesungsorientierte Darstellung und klinischer Leitfaden für Studium und Praxis, pp 154–186
Kazam JJ, Tsiouris AJ (2015) Brain magnetic resonance imaging for traumatic brain injury: why, when, and how? Top Magn Reson Imaging 24(5):225–239. https://doi.org/10.1097/RMR.0000000000000061
Kim JJ, Gean AD (2011) Imaging for the diagnosis and management of traumatic brain injury. Neurotherapeutics 8(1):39–53. https://doi.org/10.1007/s13311-010-0003-3
Kim J et al (2008) Contrast extravasation on CT predicts mortality in primary intracerebral hemorrhage. AJNR Am J Neuroradiol 29(3):520–525
Kircelli A et al (2016a) Is the presence of linear fracture a predictor of delayed posterior fossa epidural hematoma? Ulus Travma Acil Cerrahi Derg 22(4):355–360
Kircelli A, Ozel O, Can H, Sari R, Cansever T, Elmaci I (2016b) Is the presence of linear fracture a predictor of delayed posterior fossa epidural hematoma? Ulusal Travma Acil Cerrahi Derg 22:355–360. https://doi.org/10.5505/tjtes.2015.52563
Knudson MM et al (2004) Thromboembolism after trauma: an analysis of 1602 episodes from the American College of Surgeons National Trauma Data Bank. Ann Surg 240(3):490–496. discussion 496–8
Kobayashi L et al (2017) Novel oral anticoagulants and trauma: the results of a prospective American association for the surgery of trauma multi-institutional trial. J Trauma Acute Care Surg 82(5):827–835
Kurland D et al (2012) Hemorrhagic progression of a contusion after traumatic brain injury: a review. J Neurotrauma 29(1):19–31
Kwiatt ME et al (2012) Is low-molecular-weight heparin safe for venous thromboembolism prophylaxis in patients with traumatic brain injury? A Western Trauma Association multicenter study. J Trauma Acute Care Surg 73(3):625–628
Lawrence TP et al (2017) Early detection of cerebral microbleeds following traumatic brain injury using MRI in the hyper-acute phase. Neurosci Lett 655:143–150
Lee KS et al (1997a) The computed tomographic attenuation and the age of subdural hematomas. J Korean Med Sci 12(4):353–359
Lee KS, Bae WK, Bae HG, Doh JW, Yun IG (1997b) The computed tomographic attenuation and the age of subdural hematomas. J Korean Med Sci 12:353–359. https://doi.org/10.3346/jkms.1997.12.4.353
Lee SY et al (2012) Prediction of outcome after traumatic brain injury using clinical and neuroimaging variables. J Clin Neurol 8(3):224–229
Leitgeb J et al (2012a) Outcome after severe brain trauma due to acute subdural hematoma. J Neurosurg 117(2):324–333
Leitgeb J, Mauritz W, Brazinova A, Janciak I, Majdan M, Wilbacher I, Rusnak M (2012b) Outcome after severe brain trauma due to acute subdural hematoma. J Neurosurg 117:324–333. https://doi.org/10.3171/2012.4.JNS111448
LeRoux PD et al (1992) Intraventricular hemorrhage in blunt head trauma: an analysis of 43 cases. Neurosurgery 31(4):678–684. discussion 684–5

Letourneau-Guillon L et al (2013) Traumatic intracranial hematomas: prognostic value of contrast extravasation. AJNR Am J Neuroradiol 34(4):773–779
Li J (2012) Admit all anticoagulated head-injured patients? A million dollars versus your dime. You make the call. Ann Emerg Med 59(6):457–459
Li S et al (2015) Enoxaparin ameliorates post-traumatic brain injury edema and neurologic recovery, reducing cerebral leukocyte endothelial interactions and vessel permeability in vivo. J Trauma Acute Care Surg 79(1):78–84
Lobato RD et al (1983) Outcome from severe head injury related to the type of intracranial lesion. A computerized tomography study. J Neurosurg 59(5):762–774
Lolli V et al (2016) MDCT imaging of traumatic brain injury. Br J Radiol 89(1061):20150849
Maas AI et al (2005) Prediction of outcome in traumatic brain injury with computed tomographic characteristics: a comparison between the computed tomographic classification and combinations of computed tomographic predictors. Neurosurgery 57(6):1173–1182. discussion 1173-82
Major J, Reed MJ (2009) A retrospective review of patients with head injury with coexistent anticoagulant and antiplatelet use admitted from a UK emergency department. Emerg Med J 26(12):871–876
Malik NK et al (2007a) Posterior fossa extradural hematoma: our experience and review of the literature. Surg Neurol 68(2):155–158. discussion 158
Malik NK, Makhdoomi R, Indira B, Shankar S, Sastry K (2007b) Posterior fossa extradural hematoma: our experience and review of the literature. Surg Neurol 68:155–158.; discussion 158. https://doi.org/10.1016/j.surneu.2006.10.051
Marshall LF et al (1991) A new classification of head injury based on computerized tomography. J Neurosurg 75(1s):S14–S20. Special Supplements
Mason S et al (2017) AHEAD Study: an observational study of the management of anticoagulated patients who suffer head injury. BMJ Open 7(1):e014324
Mata-Mbemba D et al (2015) Intraventricular hemorrhage on initial computed tomography as marker of diffuse axonal injury after traumatic brain injury. J Neurotrauma 32(5):359–365
Matsushima K et al (2016) Therapeutic anticoagulation in patients with traumatic brain injury. J Surg Res 205(1):186–191
Maung AA et al (2016) Trauma patients on new oral anticoagulation agents have lower mortality than those on warfarin. J Trauma Acute Care Surg 81(4):652–657
McMillian WD, Rogers FB (2009) Management of prehospital antiplatelet and anticoagulant therapy in traumatic head injury: a review. J Trauma 66(3):942–950
Menditto VG et al (2012) Management of minor head injury in patients receiving oral anticoagulant therapy: a prospective study of a 24-hour observation protocol. Ann Emerg Med 59(6):451–455
Meythaler JM et al (2001) Current concepts: diffuse axonal injury-associated traumatic brain injury. Arch Phys Med Rehabil 82(10):1461–1471
Minshall CT et al (2011) Safety and efficacy of heparin or enoxaparin prophylaxis in blunt trauma patients with a head abbreviated injury severity score >2. J Trauma 71(2):396–399. discussion 399–400
Modi NJ, Agrawal M, Sinha VD (2016) Post-traumatic subarachnoid hemorrhage: a review. Neurol India 64(Suppl):S8–S13. https://doi.org/10.4103/0028-3886.178030
Moen KG et al (2012) A longitudinal MRI study of traumatic axonal injury in patients with moderate and severe traumatic brain injury. J Neurol Neurosurg Psychiatry 83(12):1193–1200
Moen KG et al (2014) Traumatic axonal injury: the prognostic value of lesion load in corpus callosum, brain stem, and thalamus in different magnetic resonance imaging sequences. J Neurotrauma 31(17):1486–1496
Morales DL, Diaz-Daza O, Hayman LA. Brain Contusion Imaging. 2017 Nov 01, 2015 [cited 21.09.2017; Available from: http://emedicine.medscape.com/article/337782-overview - a1
Nagata K et al (2017) Early heparin administration after traumatic brain injury: prolonged cognitive recovery associated with reduced cerebral edema and neutrophil sequestration. J Trauma Acute Care Surg 83(3):406–412
Nakstad PH, Gjertsen O, Pedersen HK (2008) Correlation of head trauma and traumatic aneurysms. Interv Neuroradiol 14(1):33–38. https://doi.org/10.1177/159101990801400104
Nandigam RN et al (2009) MR imaging detection of cerebral microbleeds: effect of susceptibility-weighted imaging, section thickness, and field strength. AJNR Am J Neuroradiol 30(2):338–343
Naraghi L et al (2015) Is CT angiography of the head useful in the management of traumatic brain injury? J Am Coll Surg 220(6):1027–1031. https://doi.org/10.1016/j.jamcollsurg.2015.03.002
Narayan RK et al (2008) Progression of traumatic intracerebral hemorrhage: a prospective observational study. J Neurotrauma 25(6):629–639
Narum S et al (2016) Mortality among head trauma patients taking preinjury antithrombotic agents: a retrospective cohort analysis from a Level 1 trauma centre. BMC Emerg Med 16(1):29
Nishijima DK et al (2012) Immediate and delayed traumatic intracranial hemorrhage in patients with head trauma and preinjury warfarin or clopidogrel use. Ann Emerg Med 59(6):460–468. e1–7
Nishijima DK et al (2013) Risk of traumatic intracranial hemorrhage in patients with head injury and preinjury warfarin or clopidogrel use. Acad Emerg Med 20(2):140–145
Noguchi K et al (2000a) Comparison of fluid-attenuated inversion-recovery MR imaging with CT in a simulated model of acute subarachnoid hemorrhage. AJNR Am J Neuroradiol 21(5):923–927
Noguchi K, Seto H, Kamisaki Y, Tomizawa G, Toyoshima S, Watanabe N (2000b) Comparison of fluid-attenuated inversion-recovery MR imaging with CT in

a simulated model of acute subarachnoid hemorrhage. AJNR Am J Neuroradiol 21:923–927
Paiva WS et al (2013a) Bilateral acute epidural hematoma with good outcome. J Clin Diagn Res 7(11):2594–2595
Paiva WS, Andrade AF, Alves AC, Ribeiro IN, Teixeira MJ (2013b) Bilateral acute epidural hematoma with good outcome. J Clin Diagn Res 7:2594–2595. https://doi.org/10.7860/JCDR/2013/5709.3609
Paiva WS et al (2014) Computed tomography angiography for detection of middle meningeal artery lesions associated with acute epidural hematomas. Biomed Res Int 2014:413916. https://doi.org/10.1155/2014/413916
Pajic SS et al (2017) Trauma of the frontal region is influenced by the volume of frontal sinuses. A finite element study. Front Physiol 8:493
Pandey N, Mahapatra A, Singh PK (2014) Bilateral large traumatic hemorrhage of the basal ganglion. Asian J Neurosurg 9(4):240
Pandey S et al (2017) Bilateral traumatic intracranial hematomas and its outcome: a retrospective study. Indian J Surg 79(1):19–23. https://doi.org/10.1007/s12262-015-1416-3
Park JH et al (2009) Detection of traumatic cerebral microbleeds by susceptibility-weighted image of MRI. J Korean Neurosurg Soc 46(4):365–369
Parra MW et al (2013) Dabigatran bleed risk with closed head injuries: are we prepared? J Neurosurg 119(3):760–765
Peterson EC, Chesnut RM (2011) Talk and die revisited: bifrontal contusions and late deterioration. J Trauma 71(6):1588–1592
Phelan HA et al (2012) A randomized, double-blinded, placebo-controlled pilot trial of anticoagulation in low-risk traumatic brain injury: The Delayed Versus Early Enoxaparin Prophylaxis I (DEEP I) study. J Trauma Acute Care Surg 73(6):1434–1441
Phelan HA et al (2014a) Does isolated traumatic subarachnoid hemorrhage merit a lower intensity level of observation than other traumatic brain injury? J Neurotrauma 31(20):1733–1736
Phelan HA, Richter AA, Scott WW, Pruitt JH, Madden CJ, Rickert KL, Wolf SE (2014b) Does isolated traumatic subarachnoid hemorrhage merit a lower intensity level of observation than other traumatic brain injury? J Neurotrauma 31:1733–1736. https://doi.org/10.1089/neu.2014.3377
Post A et al (2015a) Traumatic brain injuries: the influence of the direction of impact. Neurosurgery 76(1):81–91
Post A, Hoshizaki TB, Gilchrist MD, Brien S, Cusimano M, Marshall S (2015b) Traumatic brain injuries: the influence of the direction of impact. Neurosurgery 76:81–91. https://doi.org/10.1227/NEU.0000000000000554
Provenzale J (2007) CT and MR imaging of acute cranial trauma. Emerg Radiol 14(1):1–12. https://doi.org/10.1007/s10140-007-0587-z
Quigley MR et al (2013a) The clinical significance of isolated traumatic subarachnoid hemorrhage. J Trauma Acute Care Surg 74(2):581–584
Quigley MR, Chew BG, Swartz CE, Wilberger JE (2013b) The clinical significance of isolated traumatic subarachnoid hemorrhage. J Trauma Acute Care Surg 74:581–584. https://doi.org/10.1097/TA.0b013e31827d6088
Ramesh VG et al (2017a) Vertex epidural hematoma: an analysis of a large series. Asian J Neurosurg 12(2):167–171
Ramesh VG, Kodeeswaran M, Deiveegan K, Sundar V, Sriram K (2017b) Vertex epidural hematoma: an analysis of a large series. Asian J Neurosurg 12:167–171. https://doi.org/10.4103/1793-5482.145555
Reddy S et al (2014) Incidence of intracranial hemorrhage and outcomes after ground-level falls in geriatric trauma patients taking preinjury anticoagulants and antiplatelet agents. Am Surg 80(10):975–978
Rinkel GJ, van Gijn J, Wijdicks EF (1993) Subarachnoid hemorrhage without detectable aneurysm. A review of the causes. Stroke 24(9):1403
Romero JM et al (2013a) Contrast extravasation on CT angiography predicts hematoma expansion and mortality in acute traumatic subdural hemorrhage. AJNR Am J Neuroradiol 34(8):1528–1534
Romero JM, Kelly HR, Delgado Almandoz JE, Hernandez-Siman J, Passanese JC, Lev MH, Gonzalez RG (2013b) Contrast extravasation on CT angiography predicts hematoma expansion and mortality in acute traumatic subdural hemorrhage. AJNR Am J Neuroradiol 34:1528–1534. https://doi.org/10.3174/ajnr.A3434
Rozsa L, Grote EH, Egan P (1989) Traumatic brain swelling studied by computerized tomography and densitometry. Neurosurg Rev 12(2):133–140
Ryan CG et al (2012a) Acute traumatic subdural hematoma: current mortality and functional outcomes in adult patients at a Level I trauma center. J Trauma Acute Care Surg 73(5):1348–1354
Ryan CG, Thompson RE, Temkin NR, Crane PK, Ellenbogen RG, Elmore JG (2012b) Acute traumatic subdural hematoma: current mortality and functional outcomes in adult patients at a Level I trauma center. J Trauma Acute Care Surg 73:1348–1354. https://doi.org/10.1097/TA.0b013e31826fcb30
Salvatori M, Kodikara S, Pollanen M (2012) Fatal subarachnoid hemorrhage following traumatic rupture of the internal carotid artery. Leg Med (Tokyo) 14(6):328–330. https://doi.org/10.1016/j.legalmed.2012.06.004
Samama MM (2011) The mechanism of action of rivaroxaban - an oral, direct Factor Xa inhibitor - compared with other anticoagulants. Thromb Res 127(6):497–504
Sarkar K et al (2014a) Computed tomography characteristics in pediatric versus adult traumatic brain injury. J Neurosurg Pediatr 13(3):307–314
Sarkar K, Keachie K, Nguyen U, Muizelaar JP, Zwienenberg-Lee M, Shahlaie K (2014b) Computed tomography characteristics in pediatric versus adult traumatic brain injury Journal of neurosurgery. Pediatrics 13:307–314. https://doi.org/10.3171/2013.12.PEDS13223

Sato T et al (2014) Traumatic basal subarachnoid hemorrhage suspected to have been caused by contrecoup cerebellar contusions: a case report. Leg Med (Tokyo) 16(2):92–94
Scheid R et al (2007) Comparative magnetic resonance imaging at 1.5 and 3 Tesla for the evaluation of traumatic microbleeds. J Neurotrauma 24(12):1811–1816
Schmidt L (2018) Doctoral Thesis under review. Eine Übersicht zu nicht-knöchernen Verletzungsfolgen nach Schädel-Hirn-Trauma mit einer retrospektiven Single-Center-Studie zur Abschätzung des Einflusses gerinnungshemmender Vor-Medikation am Beispiel des Klinikums der Universität München. Ludwig-Maximilians-Universität München, Germany
Schnabel RB et al (2012) Atrial fibrillation: its prevalence and risk factor profile in the German general population. Dtsch Arztebl Int 109(16):293–299
Scott G, Coats B (2015) Microstructural characterization of the pia-arachnoid complex using optical coherence tomography. IEEE Trans Med Imaging. https://doi.org/10.1109/TMI.2015.2396527
Scotti G et al (1977a) Evaluation of the age of subdural hematomas by computerized tomography. J Neurosurg 47(3):311–315
Scotti G, Terbrugge K, Melancon D, Belanger G (1977b) Evaluation of the age of subdural hematomas by computerized tomography. J Neurosurg 47:311–315. https://doi.org/10.3171/jns.1977.47.3.0311
Scudday T et al (2011) Safety and efficacy of prophylactic anticoagulation in patients with traumatic brain injury. J Am Coll Surg 213(1):148–153. discussion 153–4
Selariu E et al (2012a) Swirl sign in intracerebral haemorrhage: definition, prevalence, reliability and prognostic value. BMC Neurol 12:109
Selariu E, Zia E, Brizzi M, Abul-Kasim K (2012b) Swirl sign in intracerebral haemorrhage: definition, prevalence, reliability and prognostic value. BMC Neurol. 12:109. https://doi.org/10.1186/1471-2377-12-109
Servadei F, Picetti E (2014) Traumatic subarachnoid hemorrhage. World Neurosurg 82(5):e597–e598. https://doi.org/10.1016/j.wneu.2014.08.034
Servadei F et al (2002) Traumatic subarachnoid hemorrhage: demographic and clinical study of 750 patients from the European brain injury consortium survey of head injuries. Neurosurgery 50(2):261–267. discussion 267-9
Server A et al (2001) Post-traumatic cerebral infarction. Neuroimaging findings, etiology and outcome. Acta Radiol 42(3):254–260
Sharma DR, Gaillard APF. Subdural haemorrhage. 2018a [cited 2018 02/07/2018]; Available from: https://radiopaedia.org/articles/subdural-haemorrhage
Sharma DR, Gaillard APF (2018b) Subdural haemorrhage. Radiopaedia.org. https://radiopaedia.org/articles/subdural-haemorrhage. Accessed 02 July 2018 2018
Shimoda K et al (2014) Outcome and surgical management for geriatric traumatic brain injury: analysis of 888 cases registered in the Japan Neurotrauma Data Bank. World Neurosurg 82(6):1300–1306
Sigurdsson S et al (2012) Brain tissue volumes in the general population of the elderly: the AGES-Reykjavik study. NeuroImage 59(4):3862–3870. https://doi.org/10.1016/j.neuroimage.2011.11.024
Skaga NO et al (2008) Different definitions of patient outcome: consequences for performance analysis in trauma. Injury 39(5):612–622
Skandsen T et al (2010) Prevalence and impact of diffuse axonal injury in patients with moderate and severe head injury: a cohort study of early magnetic resonance imaging findings and 1-year outcome. J Neurosurg 113(3):556–563
Smith DH, Hicks R, Povlishock JT (2013) Therapy development for diffuse axonal injury. J Neurotrauma 30(5):307–323
Song SY et al (2016a) Delayed rebleeding of cerebral aneurysm misdiagnosed as traumatic subarachnoid hemorrhage. J Cerebrovasc Endovasc Neurosurg 18(3):253–257
Song SY, Kim DW, Park JT, Kang SD (2016b) Delayed rebleeding of cerebral aneurysm misdiagnosed as traumatic subarachnoid hemorrhage. J Cerebrovasc Endovasc Neurosurg 18:253–257. https://doi.org/10.7461/jcen.2016.18.3.253
Soon WC, Marcus H, Wilson M (2016) Traumatic acute extradural haematoma - Indications for surgery revisited. Br J Neurosurg 30(2):233–234. https://doi.org/10.3109/02688697.2015.1119237
Soustiel JF et al (2008) Perfusion-CT for early assessment of traumatic cerebral contusions. Neuroradiology 50(2):189–196
Southworth MR, Reichman ME, Unger EF (2013) Dabigatran and postmarketing reports of bleeding. N Engl J Med 368(14):1272–1274
Spektor S et al (2003) Low-dose aspirin prophylaxis and risk of intracranial hemorrhage in patients older than 60 years of age with mild or moderate head injury: a prospective study. J Neurosurg 99(4):661–665
Steyerberg EW et al (2008) Predicting outcome after traumatic brain injury: development and international validation of prognostic scores based on admission characteristics. PLoS Med 5(8):e165. https://doi.org/10.1371/journal.pmed.0050165. discussion e165
Stiell IG et al (2001) The Canadian CT Head Rule for patients with minor head injury. Lancet 357(9266):1391–1396
Struffert T, Axmann C, Reith W (2003) Schädel- und Hirntrauma. Radiologe 43(11):1001–1016
Su IC et al (2010) Differential CT features of acute lentiform subdural hematoma and epidural hematoma. Clin Neurol Neurosurg 112(7):552–556. https://doi.org/10.1016/j.clineuro.2010.03.001
Sullivan S et al (2015) White matter tract-oriented deformation predicts traumatic axonal brain injury and reveals rotational direction-specific vulnerabilities. Biomech Model Mechanobiol 14(4):877–896
Sweeney TE et al (2015a) Prediction of neurosurgical intervention after mild traumatic brain injury using the national trauma data bank. World J Emerg Surg 10:23

Sweeney TE, Salles A, Harris OA, Spain DA, Staudenmayer KL (2015b) Prediction of neurosurgical intervention after mild traumatic brain injury using the national trauma data bank. World J Emerg Surg 10:23. https://doi.org/10.1186/s13017-015-0017-6

Talbott JF et al (2014a) Calvarial fracture patterns on CT imaging predict risk of a delayed epidural hematoma following decompressive craniectomy for traumatic brain injury. AJNR Am J Neuroradiol 35(10):1930–1935

Talbott JF, Gean A, Yuh EL, Stiver SI (2014b) Calvarial fracture patterns on CT imaging predict risk of a delayed epidural hematoma following decompressive craniectomy for traumatic brain injury. AJNR Am J Neuroradiol 35:1930–1935. https://doi.org/10.3174/ajnr.A4001

Tamayo S et al (2015) Characterizing major bleeding in patients with nonvalvular atrial fibrillation: a pharmacovigilance study of 27 467 patients taking rivaroxaban. Clin Cardiol 38(2):63–68

Taylor CA et al (2017) Traumatic brain injury-related emergency department visits, hospitalizations, and deaths - United States, 2007 and 2013. MMWR Surveill Summ 66(9):1–16

Tian HL et al (2008) Risk factors related to hydrocephalus after traumatic subarachnoid hemorrhage. Surg Neurol 69(3):241–246. discussion 246

Tong WS et al (2011) Early CT signs of progressive hemorrhagic injury following acute traumatic brain injury. Neuroradiology 53(5):305–309

Tsutsumi S, Ono H, Yasumoto Y (2017) Immobile cerebral veins in the context of positional brain shift: an undescribed risk factor for acute subdural hemorrhage. Surg Radiol Anat 39(10):1063–1067. https://doi.org/10.1007/s00276-017-1837-8

van Gijn J, Rinkel GJ (2001) Subarachnoid haemorrhage: diagnosis, causes and management. Brain 124(Pt 2):249–278. https://doi.org/10.1093/brain/124.2.249

Vega MB et al (2015) Traumatic brain injury presenting with bilateral basal ganglia hemorrhage. Neurol Neurochir Pol 49(6):456–459

Verma RK et al (2013) Detecting subarachnoid hemorrhage: comparison of combined FLAIR/SWI versus CT. Eur J Radiol 82(9):1539–1545. https://doi.org/10.1016/j.ejrad.2013.03.021

Vieira RC et al (2016) Diffuse axonal injury: epidemiology, outcome and associated risk factors. Front Neurol 7:178

Vital RB et al (2016a) Spontaneous resolution of traumatic acute subdural haematomas: a systematic review. Neurocirugia (Astur) 27(3):129–135

Vital RB, Hamamoto Filho PT, Oliveira VA, Romero FR, Zanini MA (2016b) Spontaneous resolution of traumatic acute subdural haematomas: a systematic review. Neurocirugia (Asturias, Spain) 27:129–135. https://doi.org/10.1016/j.neucir.2015.05.003

Vos PE et al (2002) EFNS guideline on mild traumatic brain injury: report of an EFNS task force. Eur J Neurol 9(3):207–219

Vos PE et al (2012) Mild traumatic brain injury. Eur J Neurol 19(2):191–198

Wassef SN et al (2013) Traumatic intracranial hemorrhage in patients taking dabigatran: report of 3 cases and review of the literature. Neurosurgery 73(2):E368–E373. discussion E373-4

Wong GK et al (2011a) Neurological outcome in patients with traumatic brain injury and its relationship with computed tomography patterns of traumatic subarachnoid hemorrhage. J Neurosurg 114(6):1510–1515

Wong GK, Yeung JH, Graham CA, Zhu XL, Rainer TH, Poon WS (2011b) Neurological outcome in patients with traumatic brain injury and its relationship with computed tomography patterns of traumatic subarachnoid hemorrhage. J Neurosurg 114:1510–1515. https://doi.org/10.3171/2011.1.JNS101102

Wu Z et al (2010a) Evaluation of traumatic subarachnoid hemorrhage using susceptibility-weighted imaging. AJNR Am J Neuroradiol 31(7):1302–1310

Wu Z, Li S, Lei J, An D, Haacke EM (2010b) Evaluation of traumatic subarachnoid hemorrhage using susceptibility-weighted imaging. AJNR Am J Neuroradiol 31:1302–1310. https://doi.org/10.3174/ajnr.A2022

Yoganandan N et al (2009) Association of contact loading in diffuse axonal injuries from motor vehicle crashes. J Trauma 66(2):309–315

Yokobori S et al (2016a) Outcome and refractory factor of intensive treatment for geriatric traumatic brain injury: analysis of 1165 cases registered in the japan neurotrauma data bank. World Neurosurg 86:127–133 e1

Yokobori S et al (2016b) Outcome and refractory factor of intensive treatment for geriatric traumatic brain injury: analysis of 1165 cases registered in the Japan Neurotrauma Data Bank. World Neurosurg. 86:127–133.e121. https://doi.org/10.1016/j.wneu.2015.09.105

Yuh EL et al (2013) Magnetic resonance imaging improves 3-month outcome prediction in mild traumatic brain injury. Ann Neurol 73(2):224–235. https://doi.org/10.1002/ana.23783

Zwahlen RA et al (2007) Lateral impact in closed head injury: a substantially increased risk for diffuse axonal injury - a preliminary study. J Craniomaxillofac Surg 35(3):142–146

# Non-Accidental Injuries

Caren Landes and Sparsh Prasher

## Contents



## 1 Introduction

Abusive head trauma is the leading cause of fatal head injuries in children under the age of 2 years (Choudhary AK et al. 2018) with an annual incidence of 21 per 100,000 infants and an associated mortality of 30% (Trefan et al. 2016). It is reported that abusive head trauma causes more than 50% of significant brain injury cases (Choudhary AK et al. 2018) and accounts for approximately one-third of all deaths caused by non-accidental injury (Palusci et al. 2014).

The American Academy of Pediatrics states that “it is unequivocally clear that inflicted head injury is a relatively common and defined entity and that a differential diagnosis, including medical diseases that mimic Abusive Head Trauma/Shaken Baby Syndrome, can be evaluated by physicians objectively.”

C. Landes (✉) · S. Prasher
Alder Hey Children’s NHS Foundation Trust, Liverpool, UK
e-mail: caren.landes@alderhey.nhs.uk





M. Scaglione et al. (eds.), *Emergency Radiology of the Head and Spine*, Medical Radiology Diagnostic Imaging, https://doi.org/10.1007/978-3-030-91047-1_3

Imaging in abusive head trauma can be challenging, and its interpretation can cause anxiety amongst many Radiologists. It is true that imaging in abusive head trauma is a specialist subject but it is essential that all radiologists have an understanding of the imaging appearances and their implications.

In the first instance, it is important to have an appreciation of the terminology used.

Inflicted injury, non-accidental injury and physical abuse are all terms used to imply an injury that has not occurred as a result of an event where there is a clear and satisfactory account of the mechanism of injury. Abusive head trauma is an appropriate, inclusive term that allows for inflicted head injury caused by shaking, impact or both.

No single injury is pathognomonic of abusive head trauma (Choudhary AK et al. 2018). Abusive head trauma is a diagnosis that should be proposed where the imaging appearances are consistent with trauma but where there is no satisfactory account of the mechanism of injury or a medical explanation for the appearances. Other features, including spinal involvement, retinal haemorrhages and fractures, will also contribute to the final proposed diagnosis of abusive head trauma and a multidisciplinary team approach is essential in these cases.

The diagnosis of abusive head trauma cannot be made by the radiologist alone, and in some cases, it is beyond the remit of the clinicians to determine whether any explanations offered are satisfactory and the ultimate determination is made by the court.

In the United Kingdom, the standard document guiding imaging in suspected physical abuse is issued by the Royal College of Radiologists in conjunction with the Society and College of Radiographers (2018) and endorsed by the Royal College of Paediatrics and Child Health.

In 2009, the American Academy of Pediatrics published a policy statement on Diagnostic Imaging of Child Abuse indicating that the role of imaging in cases of child abuse is to identify the extent of physical abuse when abuse is present and to elucidate all imaging findings that point to alternative diagnoses (American Academy of Pediatrics Policy Statement 2009).

In 2008, the Royal College of Radiologists and the Royal College of Paediatrics and Child Health issued Standards for Imaging in Suspected Non Accidental Injury which were formally adopted by the European Society of Paediatric Radiologists. In 2017, the Royal College of Radiologists and the Society and College of Radiographers issued a revised document on The Radiological Investigation of Suspected Physical Abuse that has been endorsed by The Royal College of Paediatrics and Child Health and replaces the 2008 document.

The 2008 guidelines from the Royal College of Radiologists stressed that child protection should be everyone's responsibility (2008 RCR Standards) and laid out the imaging strategy in investigating suspected non-accidental injury. The 2017 document reinforced these principles. The UK guidance states that imaging should always include a full radiographic skeletal survey in children under 2 years old and a full radiographic skeletal survey and computed tomography (CT) head scan in children under 1 year old. Children who are older than 1 year and have external evidence of head trauma and/or abnormal neurological symptoms or signs should also have a CT head scan.

In order to justify any request for neuroimaging, the clinician must provide the radiologist with complete clinical information and the radiologist should be aware of any child protection concerns. The 2018 guidelines recommend that informed consent is acquired prior to any imaging being performed. It is the responsibility of the clinical team to acquire this consent, and it must be available for viewing by the radiographers and radiologists.

The United States document is less specific and states that all infants and children with suspected intracranial injury must undergo cranial CT, MRI or both with strategies directed towards the detection of all intracranial sequelae of abuse and neglect, with a thorough characterisation of the extent and age of the abnormalities (American Academy of Pediatrics Policy Statement 2009).

In order to provide more detailed guidance within this chapter, reference is made to the recommendations from the Royal College of Radiologists in the UK. This is not intended to exclude readers outside the UK or Europe but is intended to be a useful basis for imaging of suspected abusive head trauma anywhere in the world.

## 2 Mechanism of Injury

Head injury should be viewed as a dynamic process that is not limited to the time of impact but continues over time with sequelae felt many months/year down the line. It is helpful to categorise head injury into primary and secondary injuries.

Primary injuries are ones that occur at the time of the initial insult. These include skull fractures and intracranial haemorrhage.

Skull fractures typically occur as a result of translational forces applied to the skull following a fall from a height with an impact with a hard surface or as a result of a direct blow to the head.

These direct impact forces can also cause extraaxial haemorrhage and parenchymal contusion, both of which may be seen in older, independently mobile children as a result of accidental trauma.

Intracranial injuries may also occur as a result of rapid acceleration/deceleration forces applied to the brain and intracranial structures during shaking and may occur in the absence of external signs of head injury or skull fracture. The resulting triad of injuries of subdural haemorrhage, retinal haemorrhages and encephalopathy has been frequently reported (Wright JN 2017).

Secondary injuries occur hours/days after the initial trauma due to a combination of systemic and local effects triggered by the primary injury. This includes neural injury due to loss of autoregulation of perfusion pressure, hypotension, hypoxia, hypercapnia, oedema and brain herniation.

Infants appear to show particular susceptibility to brain injury as a result of abusive head trauma, and this is thought to be multifactorial; the head-to-body ratio is larger and less stable, the movement of the brain during acceleration and deceleration in an infant is greater, the skull is thinner and less protective, and the high water content means the brain is softer than in an older child where the white matter is more myelinated (Vazquez et al. 2014).

## 3 Imaging Strategy in Abusive Head Trauma

Imaging not only allows detection of the primary injury but also provides an insight into preventable factors that may cause secondary injury. This is important as secondary injuries can be preventable if recognised early. The 2018 Royal College of Radiologists guidance recognises this and recommends an immediate CT scan of the head as the first-line neuroimaging investigation. The advantage of CT is that it is widely available, allows rapid acquisition of images and has a high sensitivity for intracranial haemorrhage that require surgical intervention (Newberg et al. 2003). A multislice technique with a thickness of 0.8 mm, acquired from skull base to above the vertex with routine 3D surface reconstructed images employing bone and soft tissue windows for better appreciation of skull fractures and scalp soft tissue injuries, is recommended.

MRI is more sensitive than CT and can pick up areas of haemorrhage, ischaemia/infarction that were not evident on the initial CT in approximately 1 in 4 patients (Trefan et al. 2016). MRI of the head and spine should be performed at day 2 to 5 for all children when CT has shown intracranial haemorrhage and/or parenchymal brain injury and/or skull fracture (2018 RCR Guidelines) and in children in whom there are ongoing neurological symptoms or signs irrespective of an apparently normal initial CT scan.

The timescales for MR imaging are specifically defined in order to ensure that any areas of diffusion restriction are identifiable on the DWI sequences.

It is reported that diffusion restriction resolves within 5 days of the event, and there is a risk of pseudonormalisation if MR imaging is performed at 7 days. At this time, there is a risk that the DWI changes are no longer apparent but that the cor-

**Table 1** RCR 2018 Guidelines on Imaging in Suspected Physical Abuse recommended MRI sequences

| | |
|---|---|
| (**a**) Brain | |
| Sagittal | *T1W* |
| Axial | T1W, T2W, susceptibility-weighted imaging, diffusion-weighted imaging sequence |
| Coronal | Fluid attenuated inversion recovery (FLAIR) |
| (**b**) Spine | |
| Sagittal | T1W, T2W, short tau inversion recovery (STIR) |
| Axial | (T2W) and/or T1W as required |

responding changes on the other sequences are not yet evident (Van der Aa et al. 2013).

It is important that the MRI sequences performed identify pathology at any location within the intracranial space, including the extra-axial space and within the brain parenchyma. The sequences should also assist in narrowing the differential diagnoses.

The RCR 2018 recommended sequences for the brain are shown in Table 1a.

The RCR 2018 recommended sequences for the spine are shown in Table 1b.

Susceptibility-weighted imaging is very sensitive in the identification of blood products, and diffusion-weighted imaging may be the only sequence to demonstrate parenchymal injury secondary to ischaemia.

Post-gadolinium imaging is not part of the routine MR imaging protocol.

## 3.1 The Skull Vault and External Soft Tissues

### 3.1.1 Normal Anatomy and Development

In order to be able to identify pathology within the skull vault, it is important to have an understanding of the normal appearances of the paediatric skull vault.

The development of the skull is complex and variable.

The bones of the skull ossify in membrane and are separated by fibrous junctions called sutures and hyaline cartilage joints called synchondroses. During the first 4 years of life, the bones and junctions undergo growth and change.

Radiologists need to be aware of the appearance and location of the sutures in order to be able to recognise and identify fractures.

The frontal bone lies at the front of the skull. The parietal bones lie immediately posterior to the frontal bones, separated from each other in the midline by the sagittal suture and from the frontal bone by the coronal suture running transversely across the skull.

The occipital bone lies at the back of the skull and is divided from the parietal bones by the lambdoid sutures.

The sagittal suture meets the lambdoid sutures at the posterior fontanelle. Once the posterior fontanelle is closed, it is known as the lamda, so-called because it has the same shape as the Greek letter.

The anterior fontanelle is at the junction between the sagittal and coronal sutures.

The largest sutures—sagittal, coronal, lambdoid and squamosal sutures—are visible in childhood and are evident into adulthood.

| Suture | Age of closure |
|---|---|
| Metopic | 3–9 months |
| Sphenosquamosal | 6–10 years |
| Sphenofrontal | 15 years |
| Occipitomastoid | 16 years |
| Sagittal | 22 years |
| Coronal | 24 years |
| Lambdoid | 26 years |
| Squamosal | 60 years |
| Anterior Fontanelle | 12–18 months |
| Posterior Fontanelle | 2–3 months |

A number of other sutures are seen in infants and children including the innominate suture, the metopic suture in the midline of the frontal bone, the mendosal suture, the sphenosquamosal suture between the sphenoid bone and the squama of the temporal bone, the sphenofrontal suture and the occipitomastoid sutures (Fig. 1).

In addition to the sutures, there are a number of normal variants that can be seen on the imaging of the skull.

#### 3.1.1.1 Wormian Bones

Wormian bones are accessory bones found within the sutures of the skull, most commonly within

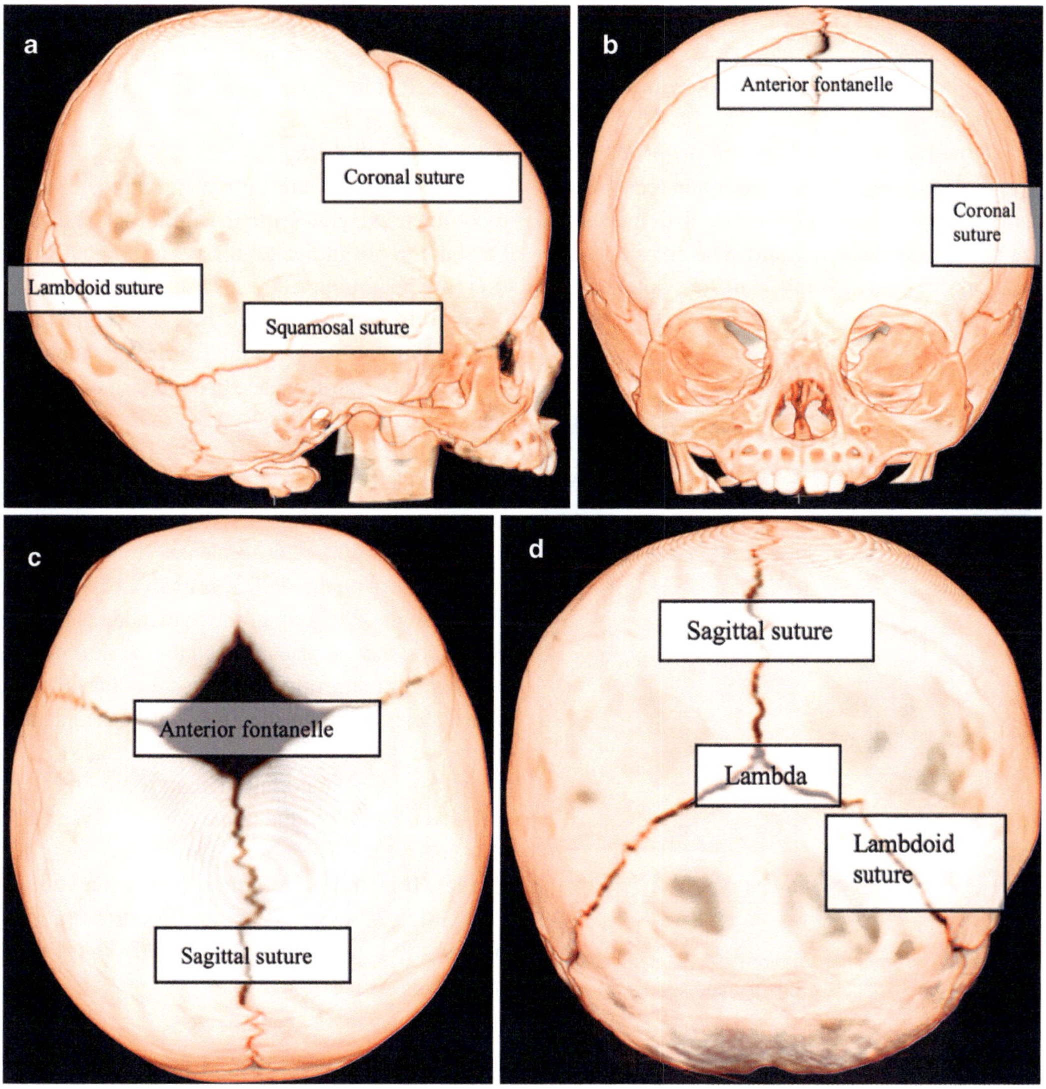


**Fig. 1** 3D reformatted views of the skull demonstrating the main sutures and fontanelles. (**a**) Lateral view of the skull. (**b**) Frontal view of the skull. (**c**) Superior view of the skull. (**d**) Posterior view of the skull

the posterior sagittal suture and the lambdoid sutures (Fig. 2).

It is generally accepted that normal patients may have up to 10 Wormian bones, but an abnormal number of Wormian bones are found in a number of syndromes including osteogenesis imperfecta, hypothyroidism, cleidocranial dysostosis, pyknodysostosis and trisomy 21.

The presence of an abnormal number of Wormian bones is particularly relevant in the context of suspected inflicted injury where a diagnosis of a bone fragility disorder may change the direction of any child protection proceedings.

#### 3.1.1.2 Accessory Sutures

The parietal and occipital bones have a number of ossification centres that fuse in foetal life but, rarely, the interval between the ossification centres partially persists giving rise to an accessory suture.

Accessory sutures typically extend from the lambdoid sutures, either into the parietal bones (most commonly) or into the occipital bones. They are typically short, bilateral and symmetrical.

The most commonly seen accessory sutures are seen in the parietal bones.

#### 3.1.1.3 Skull Fractures

Young children may present with an unexplained swelling to the scalp as a result of an unwitnessed or inflicted head injury.

In these cases, the most appropriate first-line investigation is an unenhanced volume CT scan of the head. This will demonstrate the soft tissue swelling and will enable identification of any bony and/or intracranial abnormality.

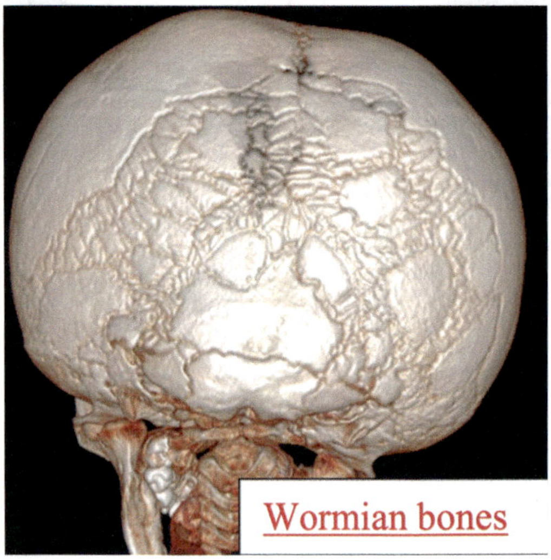


**Fig. 2** 3D Reformatted CT scan of the skull showing multiple Wormian bones within the lambdoid sutures

Linear skull fractures are the most commonly occurring types of skull fracture and most commonly affect the parietal bone (Fig. 3).

#### 3.1.1.4 Skull X-Ray

Skull radiographs are currently included in the recommended views for the initial skeletal survey but are not indicated for the initial investigation of a head injury.

Skull fractures are frequently seen in accidental trauma as a result of a fall from a height and an impact with a hard surface but can also occur as a result of a direct blow.

The RCR guidelines recommend AP and lateral views of the skull as part of the initial skeletal survey but it has been suggested that a volume CT scan of the head is sufficient to identify pathology that would be seen on the skull X-ray (Sharp et al. 2003; Whitby et al. 2004), and future amendments of the guidelines may obviate the need for the skull X-ray.

More complex fractures are also seen in both accidental and inflicted head trauma with branching and depressed skull fractures seen in both scenarios.

It should be recognised that some fractures traverse the bone in the plane of the CT scan and may be very difficult to define on the axial images. It is, therefore, imperative that a volume acquisition is acquired and a 3D reconstruction of the skull is reviewed when reporting a CT scan of the head (Figs. 4 and 5).

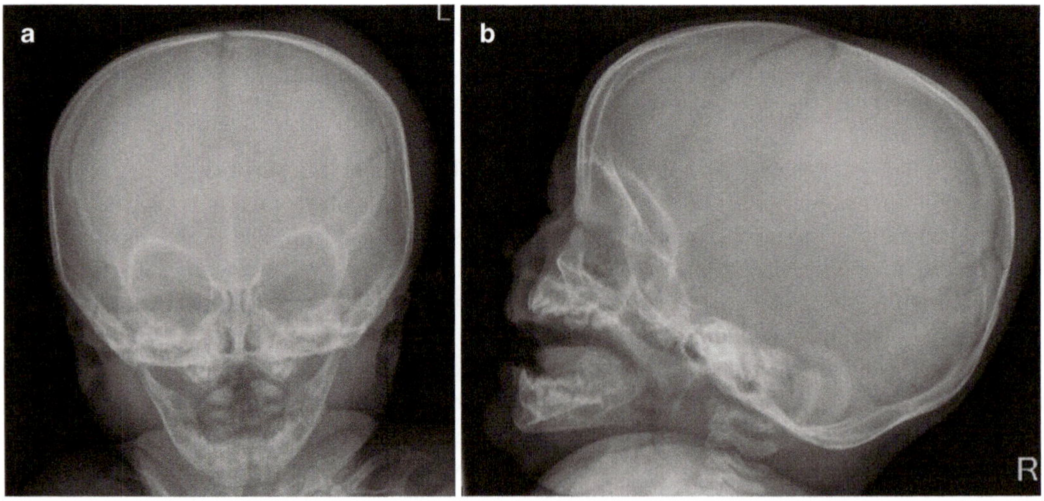


**Fig. 3** AP (**a**) and lateral (**b**) views of the skull demonstrating a linear fracture of the left parietal bone

# 4 Meningeal Anatomy and Intracranial Haemorrhage

## 4.1 Meningeal Anatomy

In order to understand the distribution and pattern of intracranial pathology, it is important to understand the anatomy of the intracranial layers and structures.

There are 3 layers of membrane between the skull and the cortex of the brain. These are the dura mater, the arachnoid mater and the pia mater and are known collectively as the meninges (Fig. 6).

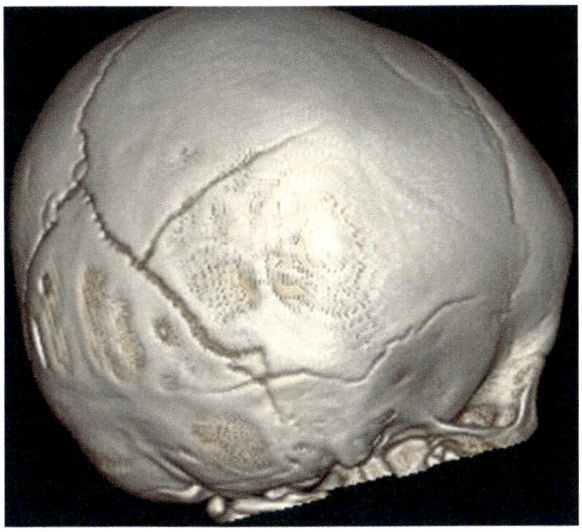

**Fig. 4** 3D reformatted CT scan demonstrating a right-sided parietal bone fracture

The dura mater is the outermost layer of the meninges. This is a tough layer that is closely related to the inner table of the skull. Beneath the dura mater is the arachnoid mater, and beneath this layer and overlying the brain is the pia mater.

There are potential spaces between the skull and the dura mater, known as the extradural space, and between the dura mater and the arachnoid mater, known as the subdural space.

The subarachnoid space is a CSF filled space between the arachnoid mater and the pia mater.

# 5 Intracranial Haemorrhage

Bleeding can occur in any, or all, of these potential and real spaces and it is helpful to understand these anatomical structures when reviewing the imaging and identifying the location of the haemorrhage.

## 5.1 Extradural Haematoma

Since the dura mater is closely applied to the inner aspect of the skull bones, bleeding in the extradural space typically distends the dura to give an "elliptical" shape making an acute angle with the skull bones. Extradural haemorrhage is also typically confined by the sutures of the skull.

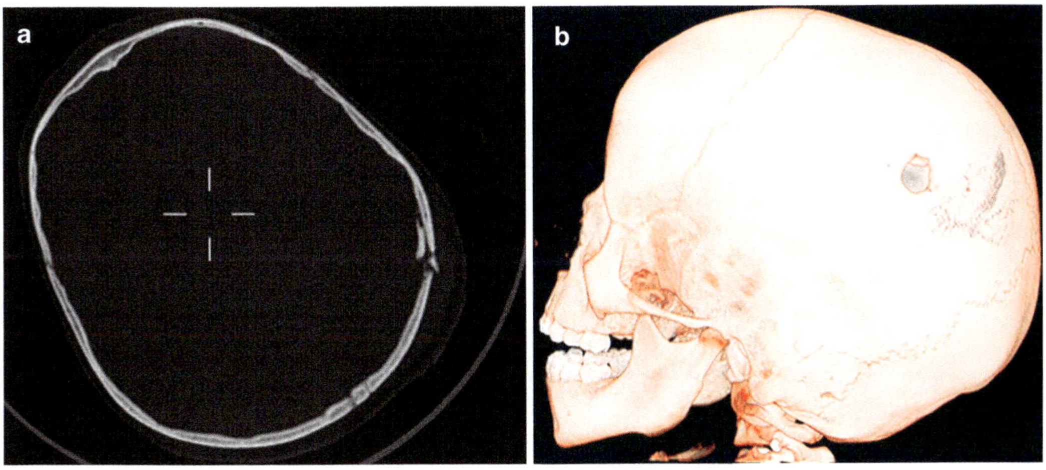


**Fig. 5** (**a**) Axial CT scan demonstrating a complex, depressed fracture of the left parietal bone. (**b**) 3D reformatted CT scan demonstrating the same complex, depressed fracture

## 5.2 Subdural Haematoma

Subdural bleeding is the most common intracranial haemorrhage seen in abusive head trauma and is seen in up to 90% of cases. It is thought to occur as a result of forceful shaking where a combination of rotation, acceleration and deacceleration forces causes rupture of the bridging veins transversing the subdural space. The result is collection of blood in the subdural space that appears, on imaging, as blood overlying the contour of the brain but not extending into the sulci.

The injured veins may thrombose and this can be seen on CT in 40–45% of cases (Wright JN 2017). These are typically seen at the vertex and are high attenuation on CT—described by some as "tadpole" shape due to the focal thrombus within the vein and a tail of more linear thrombus within the extravascular space. There is no reliable medical evidence that cerebral sinovenous thrombosis, hypoxic-ischaemic injury, vomiting or lumbar puncture are causes of abusive head trauma (consensus statement).

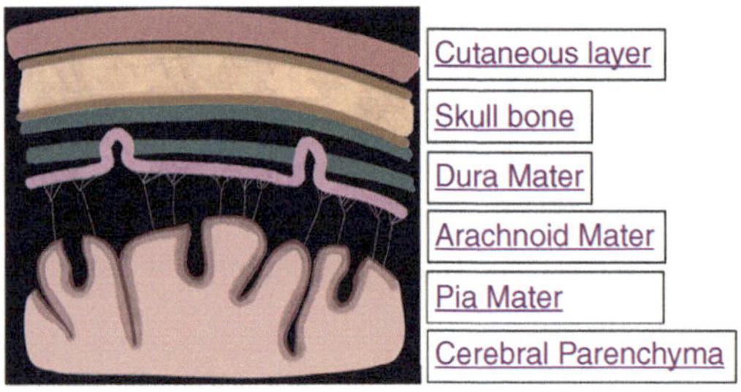


**Fig. 6** Diagrammatic representation of dural layers

Furthermore, disruption of the arachnoid mater results in the mixing of the subdural blood with CSF. On CT, this is manifested as blood of varying densities. Mixed attenuation haematomas and haematohygromas are more frequently seen in abusive head trauma than in accidental injury (Figs. 7, 8, and 9).

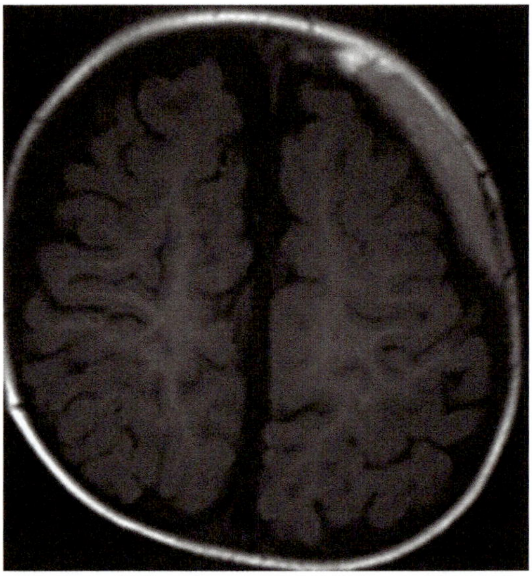

**Fig. 7** Axial T1W, T2W sequences demonstrate a subdural collection overlying the left frontal lobe with mild effacement of the underlying sulci. (**a**) Axial T1W sequence of the brain. (**b**) Axial T2W sequence of the brain. (**c**) Axial susceptibility-weighted imaging of the brain. Blooming artefact is demonstrated on the SWI sequences (axial plane) in keeping with a subdural haematoma (**c**)

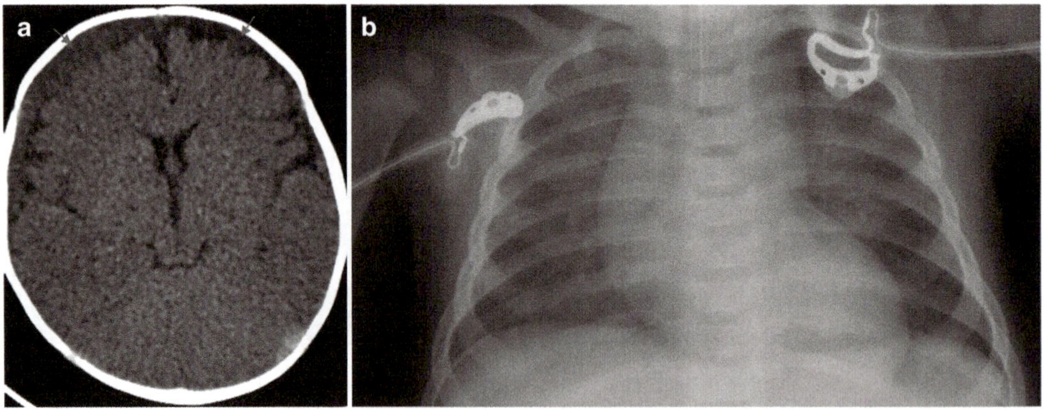


**Fig. 8** (**a**) Axial CT scan of the brain demonstrating bilateral subdural collections of mixed attenuation. (**b**) Chest X-ray of the same case revealed healing rib fractures of the posterior aspect of the left eighth and ninth ribs

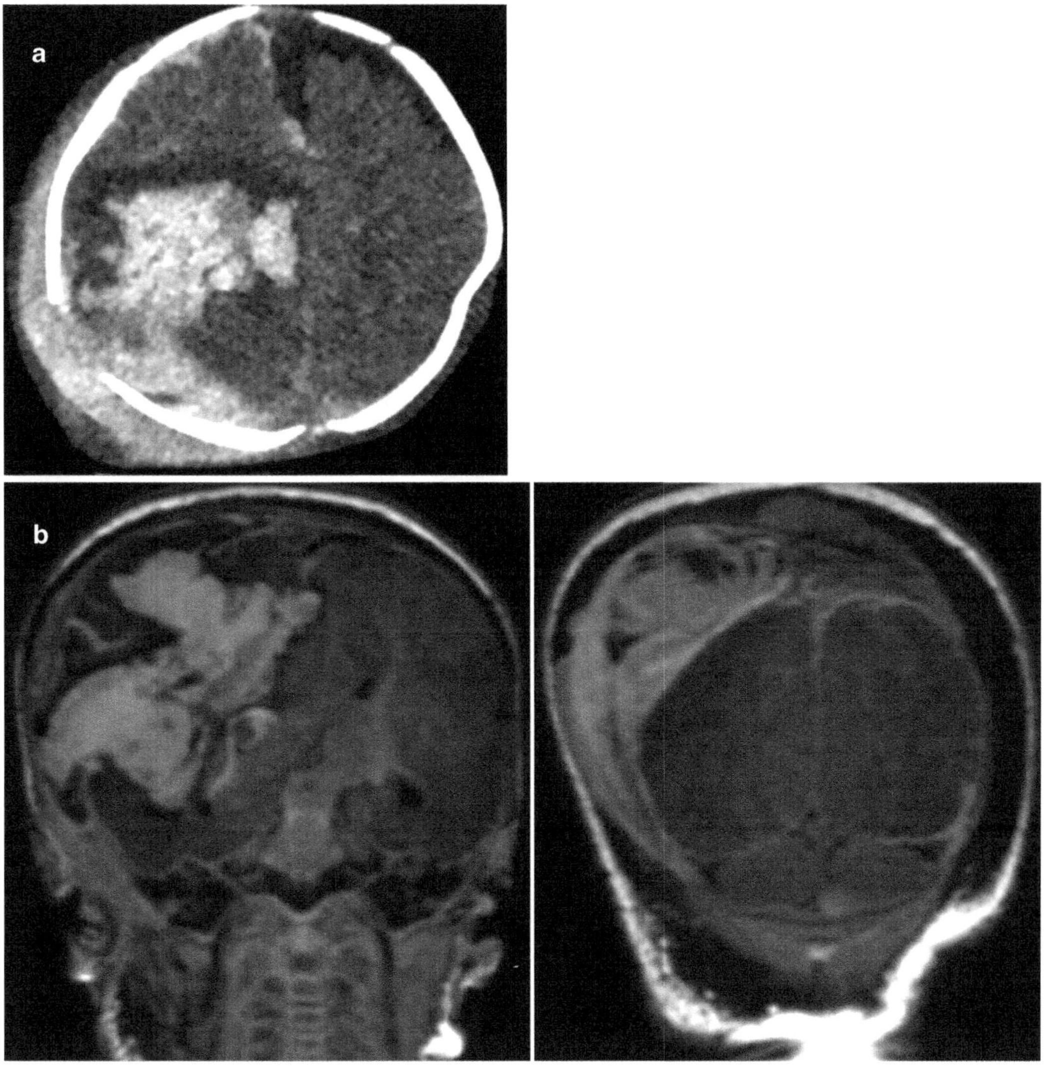


**Fig. 9** (**a**) Axial CT scan of the brain. (**b**) Coronal FLAIR sequence of the brain

There is a right parietal bone fracture. A large parenchymal haematoma is demonstrated in the right cerebral hemisphere within the central frontal and temporal lobes with surrounding oedema.

The cerebral parenchyma is partly herniating through a dural tear and the widely separated fracture.

There is intraventricular extension of the haemorrhage into the lateral ventricles and third ventricle.

Blood is also demonstrated within the sulci of the right frontal lobe in keeping with acute subarachnoid haemorrhage.

There is also an associated subdural haematoma. There is reduced grey-white matter differentiation and effacement of the sulcal-gyral pattern in keeping with brain swelling. Midline shift to the left is also demonstrated.

## 5.3 Subarachnoid Haemorrhage

Bleeding in the subarachnoid space extends into the sulci and basal cisterns and may be seen in the ventricular system. Subarachnoid haemorrhage is present in almost all fatal cases

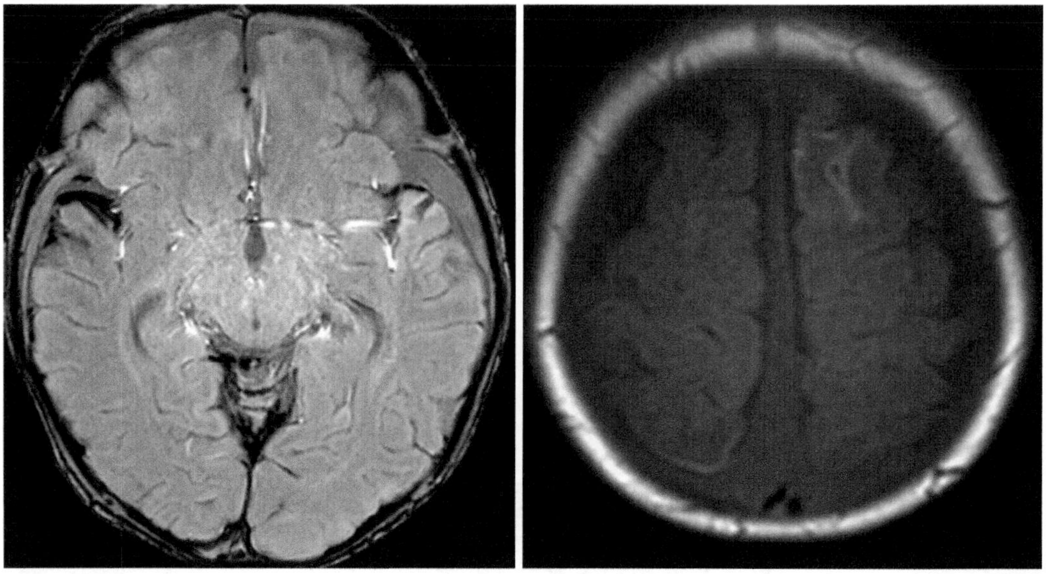

**Fig. 10** Axial susceptibility-weighted imaging and FLAIR sequence of the brain. Blooming artefact on the susceptibility-weighted imaging demonstrated in both sylvan fissures. High FLAIR signal in the sulci of the left frontal lobe. These features are in keeping with subarachnoid haemorrhage

of abusive head trauma. However, there is no evidence to suggest that it occurs more commonly than in accidental trauma (Vazquez et al. 2014) (Fig. 10).

## 5.4 Dating of Haemorrhage

It is accepted that high attenuation haemorrhage seen on CT, either as bridging vein thrombus or within an extra or intra-axial bleed, is less than 10 days of age the time of the scan (Wright JN 2017) but intracranial haemorrhage cannot be dated more specifically with either CT or MRI. It is, however, important to note that the converse cannot be assumed and that low-attenuation collections on CT are not necessarily older than 10 days of age (Sieswerda-Hoogendoorn et al. 2014).

It was previously considered that subdural haemorrhage of mixed attenuation was in keeping with multiple episodes of trauma or rebleeding into a chronic subdural haemorrhage. More recent evidence suggests that there are a number of factors that influence the imaging appearances of subdural bleeding including; degradation of haemoglobin, the degree of red cell hydration, the cell membrane integrity, the protein content of the clot, the concentration of red blood cells and the volume of CSF within the collection (Trefan et al. 2016). It is, therefore, very difficult to make assumptions about the dating of subdural collections from the imaging appearances alone and most expert Neuroradiologists would advise against attempts at dating intracranial haemorrhage other than in relation to the presence of high attenuation haemorrhage on CT. It is, therefore, advisable to avoid using terms such as acute or chronic in relation to the imaging appearances of intracranial haemorrhage.

## 5.5 Parenchymal Injury

Direct impact trauma may result in cerebral contusion and parenchymal laceration. This may be seen as focal haemorrhage or areas of low attenuation. Parenchymal haemorrhage can occur anywhere within the substance of the brain.

## 5.6 Cerebral Contusions

Contusions are the most common type of intra-axial injury and occur when sudden deacceleration causes the brain to impact against the skull or the falx cerebri/tentorium cerebelli. The most common areas are the inferior frontal lobes and the temporal lobes. Contusions manifest as focal areas of hyperdensity within the brain parenchyma that may be surrounded by low-attenuation oedema. Typically, these lesions and surrounding oedema increase in size over the 48 h following the primary injury.

## 5.7 Diffuse Axonal Injury

Sudden acceleration/deceleration (with/without rotational element), such as during shaking, produces shearing forces on the brain parenchyma—particularly at the interface of tissues of differing densities such as the junction of grey/white matter, corpus callosum, deep white matter, brainstem, periventricular and hippocampal regions. This results in axonal transection which may be partial or in severe cases complete.

In addition to the grey-white matter junction, diffuse axonal injury (DAI) may also involve the corpus callosum, brain stem and deep white matter.

Clinically, DAI manifests as loss of consciousness at the time of the injury that may progress to coma.

DAI, particularly in the absence of haemorrhage, is poorly discernible on CT initially but may become evident as areas of low attenuation with significant cerebral oedema as the pathology progresses.

On MRI, FLAIR is the sequence of choice and the injured areas demonstrate FLAIR hyperintensity.

Haemorrhagic DAI manifests as multifocal subcentimetre areas of microhaemorrhages typically at the grey-white matter junctions. On MRI, susceptibility-weighted imaging is very sensitive at detecting microhaemorrhages associated with diffuse axonal injury, which appear as, often multifocal, areas of low signal (Fig. 11).

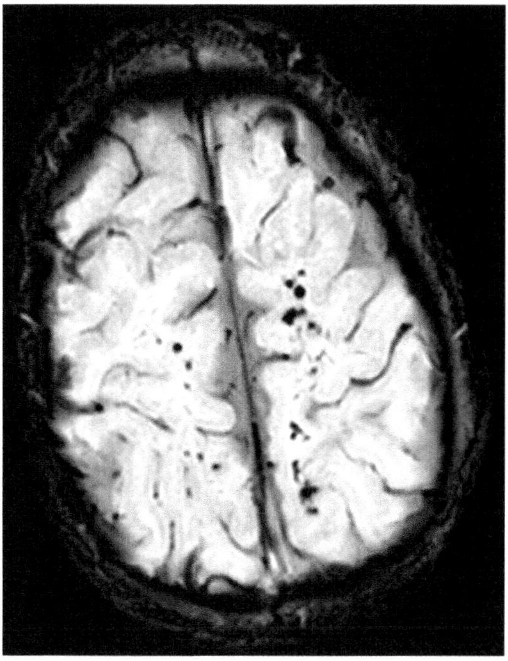

**Fig. 11** Axial susceptibility-weighted imaging demonstrating multifocal areas of low signal "blooming artefact" at the sites of multiple microhaemorrhages

## 5.8 Hypoxic-Ischaemic Injury

Parenchymal injuries may also occur as a result of ischaemia (Vazquez et al. 2014), where it is seen as loss of the normal grey-white matter differentiation with the extent of the injury being determined by the degree of hypoxia.

Prolonged seizure activity, aspiration or Injury to the brainstem or cervical spinal cord may cause central apnoea resulting in hypoxic-ischaemic injury to the brain. This is reportedly seen three times more frequently in abusive than accidental head trauma (Vazquez et al. 2014).

In light of this, it has been previously proposed that choking or acute life-threatening events may cause subdural haemorrhages, retinal haemorrhages or brain injury, but a study by Hansen et al. 2017. in 2016 determined that ALTEs are not supported as a causative mechanism for findings concerning for abusive head trauma (Hansen et al. 2017) (Fig. 12).

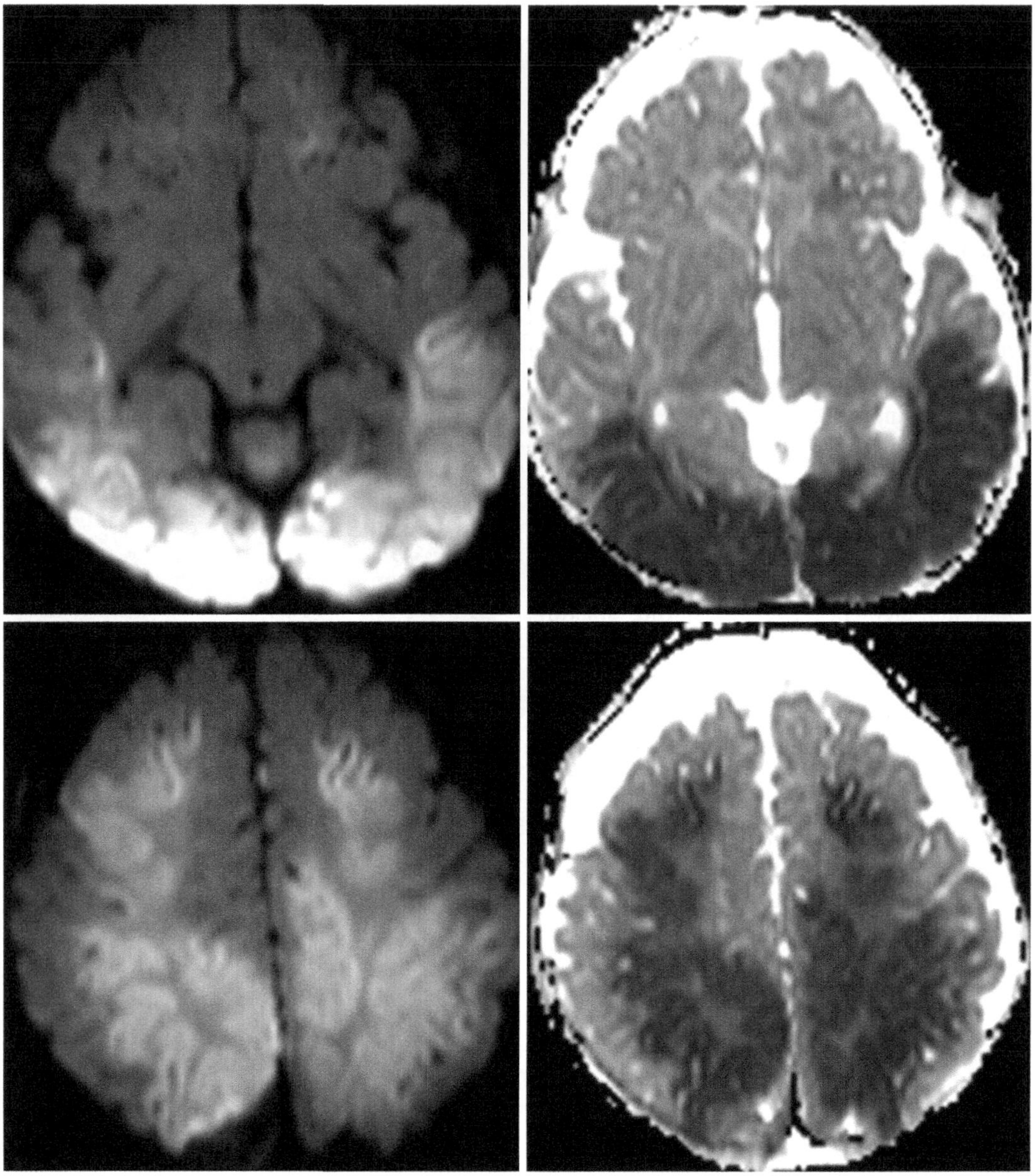

**Fig. 12** Axial DWI sequences. These is extensive bilateral symmetrical diffusion restriction within the cerebral hemispheres are in keeping with an acute hypoxic-ischaemic insult

### 5.8.1 Herniation

Herniation of brain parenchyma is rare in infants due to open fontanelles (anterior fontanelle closes by 9–18 months of age and posterior 1–2 months of age) and increased compliance of the skull.

### 5.8.2 Retinal Haemorrhage

Retinal haemorrhages are thought to occur due to vigorous repetitive forces or acceleration and deceleration that arise from shaking and/or direct impact. They are common in abusive head trauma—seen by ophthalmoscopy in up to 90% of patients.

In patients with abusive head trauma, retinal haemorrhages tend to be multiple and bilateral, and extend to the peripheries and involve multiple layers of the retina.

In contrast, retinal haemorrhages seen in accidental trauma tends to be limited to the posterior pole of the retina.

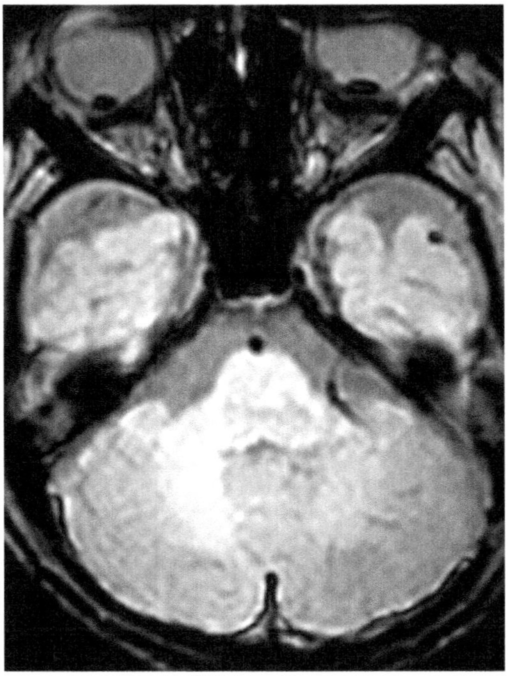

**Fig. 13** Four month old boy presented following an out of hospital arrest. CT demonstrated subdural haemorrhage. Axial susceptibility weighted sequences demonstrate low signal susceptibility artefact at the posterior aspects of both globes in keeping with retinal haemorrhages

Direct fundoscopy is the investigation of choice for diagnosis but high-grade retinal haemorrhages can be seen on cross-sectional imaging.

On CT, they appear as dense foci at the periphery of the globe.

MRI has a higher sensitivity compared to CT in detecting retinal haemorrhages, where they appear as foci of low signal (blooming artefact) on SWI (Gunda et al. 2019; Binenbaum and Forbes 2014) (Fig. 13).

## 5.9 Differential Diagnoses

The Association of American Pediatricians has recognised the importance of the multidisciplinary team approach in these cases with the diagnosis of abusive head trauma being made through a thorough history, physical examination, laboratory tests and imaging studies with the history being critically important in all cases.

For the radiologist, the interpretation of the imaging is entirely dependent on the accompanying clinical details and accidental trauma is probably the most important differential diagnosis to consider.

The presenting features of infants with inflicted head injury may be non-specific and can be initially interpreted as medical in origin. This can result in the underdiagnosis of head trauma (Wright JN 2017), with almost one-third of abusive head trauma cases initially missed by medical professionals and just over 25% of these cases diagnosed following the identification of additional injuries.

In 1 in 12 of the missed cases, misinterpretation of the radiology contributed to the misdiagnosis (Wright JN 2017).

It is therefore essential that, in the absence of a satisfactory account of the mechanism of injury or a medical explanation for the imaging findings, inflicted injury must be considered.

Differentiating between accidental and inflicted head injury is difficult but the evidence suggests that the presence of multiple areas of subdural haemorrhage over the convexity of the brain, interhemispheric haemorrhages, subdural haemorrhage within the posterior fossa, hypoxic-ischaemic injury and cerebral oedema are significantly associated with abusive head trauma (Trefan et al. 2016).

It has been reported that symmetrical, thin, diffuse subdural haemorrhage without associated mass effect is more common in accidental trauma (Wright JN 2017).

It is important to consider birth trauma as a cause for subdural haemorrhage but it should be noted that these have been shown to resolve by 4 weeks post-delivery (Whitby et al. 2018). There is no substantiation, at a time remote from birth, that an asymptomatic birth-related subdural haemorrhage can result in rebleed and sudden collapse (consensus statement).

Benign enlargement of subarachnoid spaces (BESS) is a common cause of macrocephaly in children under the age of 2 years. It is thought to arise from the mismatch between the reabsorption and production of CSF. On cross-sectional imaging, it manifests as increased subarachnoid spaces over the cerebral convexities. Spontaneous subdural bleeding has been reported in children with BESS due to disruption of bridging veins but this is rare (seen in approximately 6% of patients) and is usually an isolated imaging finding. Correlation with the clinical history and examination is essential and inflicted injury should always be considered within the differential diagnosis (Sieswerda-Hoogendoorn et al. 2012; Jenny C 2014).

## 6 Conclusion

Abusive head trauma is associated with significantly high mortality and morbidity.

The most common mechanism of injury is shaking and/or impact. This often causes subdural haematomas, cerebral contusions, diffuse axonal injuries and hypoxic-ischaemic injuries. Direct impact can cause skull fractures. Thin-slice volume CT of the head with 3D reconstructions is the first-line modality in the assessment of abusive head trauma and is indicated for all patients younger than 12 months who are being investigated for suspected inflicted injury.

MRI is reserved for patients who have CT evidence of intracranial injury or patients who have persistent neurological symptoms despite normal a CT scan of the head.

It is important to recognise that no injury pattern is pathognomonic for non-accidental injury and abusive head trauma can be difficult to diagnose especially in the face of inadequate, or even misleading, history from carers which can cause delayed or misdiagnosis as accidental trauma.

It is therefore essential that, in the absence of a clear and satisfactory account of the mechanism of injury or a medical explanation for the imaging findings, inflicted injury is considered.

## References


American Academy of Pediatrics Policy Statement on Diagnostic Imaging of Child Abuse (2009). https://doi.org/10.1542/peds.2009-0558

Binenbaum G, Forbes BJ (2014) The eye in child abuse: key points on retinal hemorrhages and abusive head trauma. Pediatr Radiol 44:S571–S577

Choudhary AK et al. (2018) Consensus statement on abusive head trauma in infants and young children. Pediatr Radiol 48:1048–1065

Gunda D et al (2019) Pediatric central nervous system imaging of nonaccidental trauma: beyond subdural hematomas. Radiographics 39:213–228

Hansen JB, Frazier T, Moffatt M, Zinkus T, Anderst JD. Evaluation of the Hypothesis That Choking/ALTE May Mimic Abusive Head Trauma. Acad Pediatr. 2017;17(4):362–67. https://doi.org/10.1016/j.acap.2016.10.002. Epub 2016 Dec 22. PMID: 28017711

Jenny C (2014) Alternate theories of causation in abusive head trauma: what the science tells us. Pediatr Radiol 44:S543–S547

Newberg AB, Alavi A. Neuroimaging in patients with head injury. Semin Nucl Med 2003;33:136–47

Palusci VJ, Covington TM (2014) Child maltreatment deaths in the U.S. National Child Death Review Case Reporting System. Child Abuse Negl 38(1):25–36

Sharp SR, Patel SM, Brown RE, Landes C, Newberg AB, Alavi A (2003) Neuroimaging in patients with head injury. Semin Nucl Med 33:136–147

Sieswerda-Hoogendoorn T et al (2012) Abusive head trauma part II: radiological aspects. Eur J Pediatr 171:617–623

Sieswerda-Hoogendoorn T, Postema FAM, Verbaan D, Majoie CB, van Rijn RR (2014) Age determination of subdural hematomas with CT and MRI: a systematic review. Eur J Radiol 83(7):1257–1268. https://doi.org/10.1016/j.ejrad.2014.03.015. Epub 2014 Apr 8

Society and College of Radiographers and The Royal College of Radiologists. The radiological investigation of suspected physical abuse in children, revised first edition, London: The Royal College of Radiologists; 2018

Trefan L, Houston R, Pearson G, et al. Epidemiology of Head Injury: a National Overview Arch Dis Child 2016;101:527–32

van der Aa NE, Benders MJ, Vincken KL, Groenendaal F, de Vries LS (2013) The course of apparent diffusion coefficient values following perinatal arterial ischemic stroke. PLoS One. 8(2):e56784. https://doi.org/10.1371/journal.pone.0056784

Vazquez E et al (2014) Imaging abusive head trauma: why use both computed tomography and magnetic resonance imaging? Pediatr Radiol 44:S589–S603

Whitby EH, Griffiths PD, Rutter S, Smith MF, Sprigg A, Ohadike P, Davies NP, Rigby AS, Paley MN (2004) Frequency and natural history of subdural haemorrhages in babies and relation to obstetric factors. Lancet 363(9412):846–851. https://doi.org/10.1016/S0140-6736(04)15730-9

Whitby EH, Griffiths PD, Rutter S, Smith MF, Sprigg A, Ohadike P, Davies NP, Rigby AS, Paley MN (2018) Head imaging in suspected non accidental injury in the paediatric population. In the advent of volumetric CT imaging, has the skull X-ray become redundant? Clin Radiol 73(5):449–453. https://doi.org/10.1016/j.crad.2017.11.027. Epub 2018 Mar 2

Wright JN (2017) CNS injuries in abusive head trauma. AJR Am J Roentgenol 208:991–1001

# Part II

# Brain: Non-traumatic Emergent Injuries (C. Çalli, Turkey – R. Basilico, IT)

# Acute Stroke: Parenchymal and Vessel Imaging

Sevcan Türk, Raffaella Basilico, and Cem Çalli

## Contents



## 1 Non-Contrast Computed Tomography

Computed tomography has been established as the most simple and readily available technique for the diagnosis and management of patients with acute stroke (Bouchez et al. 2017). CT-based techniques are preferred in acute stroke as the initial imaging study rather than MRI because of the availability and shorter scanning time. The second aim to use CT as the first modality is to exclude hemorrhage and stroke mimics since both the cause and treatment are different. tPA (tissue plasminogen activator) is the initial treatment in the acute ischemic stroke after the exclusion of the hemorrhagic stroke such as AVMs, hypertensive bleed, and hemorrhagic masses. (Lövblad et al. 2008) In the acute phase, CT has high accuracy for hemorrhage detection, with sensitivities and specificities of approximately 100%. However, SWI (susceptibility-weighted imaging) is the best modality of choice to demonstrate hemorrhage (Lansberg et al. 2000; Christopher 2017). The other objectives of acute ischemic stroke (AIS) imaging are to identify the best candidates for IV or IA treatments based on the extension of established infarct (core), the arterial occlusion (cloth) site, the presence of hemorrhage, collateral vascularization, and isch-

S. Türk · R. Basilico
Radiology Department, University of Michigan, Ann Arbor, MI, USA

C. Çalli (✉)
Department of Radiology, Ege University Medical School, Izmir, Turkey



M. Scaglione et al. (eds.), *Emergency Radiology of the Head and Spine*, Medical Radiology Diagnostic Imaging, https://doi.org/10.1007/978-3-030-91047-1_4

emic brain tissue (penumbra) (Vilelaa and Rowley 2017). CT sensitivity to detect acute ischemic stroke is found to be 12% in the first 3 h, less than 60% in the first 7 h, and 57–71% in the first 24 h (Lansberg et al. 2000; Vilelaa and Rowley 2017). Its sensitivity varies depending on the observers' experience. Astill and Agzarian showed that the discrepancy rate between neuroradiology faculty and trainee was 30% for acute stroke CT reports (Kidwell et al. 2004).

The classical NCCT early imaging findings in AIS are parenchymal hypodensity, cortical swelling, sulcal effacement, loss of grey-white matter differentiation, and hyperdense vascular structures. Parenchymal hypodensity is associated with vasogenic edema and irreversible injury (Fig. 1).

The Alberta Stroke Program Early CT score (ASPECTS) is the standard approach for quantifying the volume of early imaging changes involving middle cerebral artery (MCA) on NCCT (Fiebach 2004). The ASPECT score of the patient is one of the main selection criteria of treatment options by the AHA/ASA guidelines (Prakkamakul and Yoo 2017). The MCA territory is divided into 10 ASPECTS regions: caudate (C), insular ribbon (I), posterior limb of internal capsule (IC), lentiform nucleus (L), anterior inferior frontal cortex (M1), anterior temporal cortex (lateral to the insular ribbon; M2), posterior temporal cortex (M3), anterior superior MCA cortex (ACA-MCA border zone; M4), posterior frontal cortex (M5), and parietal cortex (M6) (Fig. 2) (Barber et al. 2000). The MCA territory is allotted 10 points. 1 point is subtracted for an area of early ischemic change for each of the defined regions. A normal CT scan has an ASPECTS

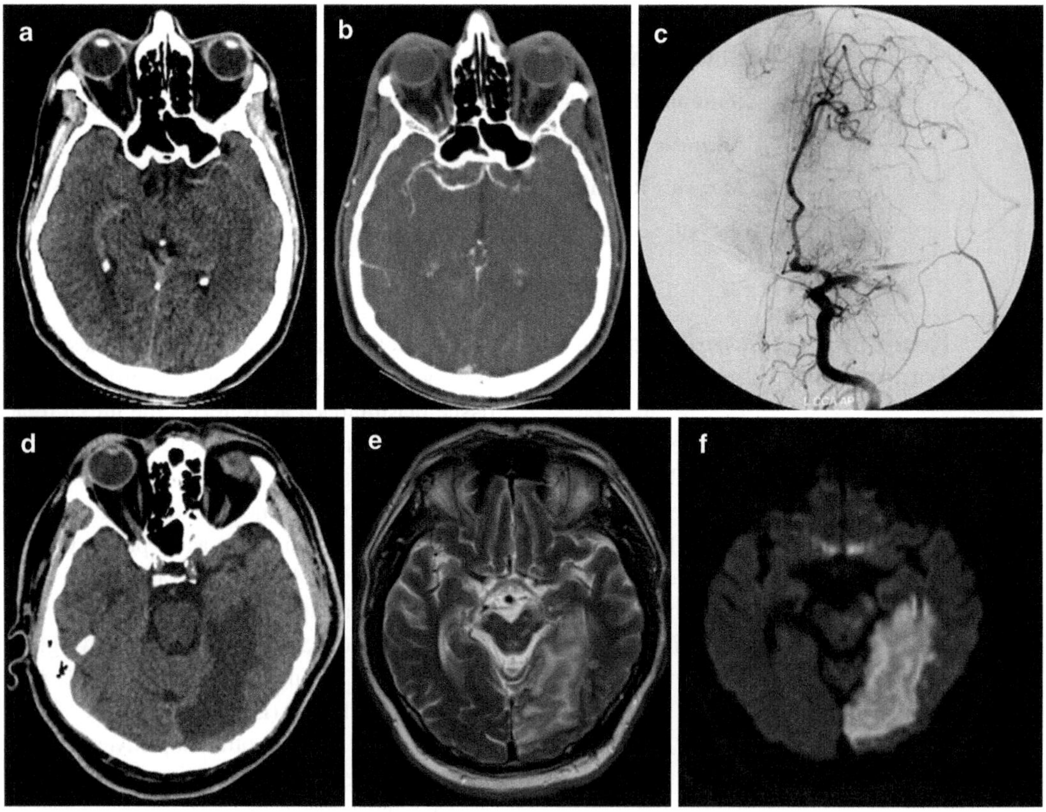


**Fig. 1** Stroke signs on NCCT: (**a**) Left-sided dens MCA sign, increased density on the left MCA M1 segment related to the acute thrombus in the lumen, (**b**) CTA image shows no contrast filling in the left M1, (**c**) DSA demonstrates thrombus on the left M1 segment, (**d**) parenchymal hypodensity and loss of grey-white matter differentiation are demonstrated in the left inferior temporal region in another stroke patient, (**e**) cortical swelling and sulcal effacement in the left inferior temporal region are seen on the T2-weighted image, (**f**) diffusion restriction in the same region is shown on DWI B1000 image

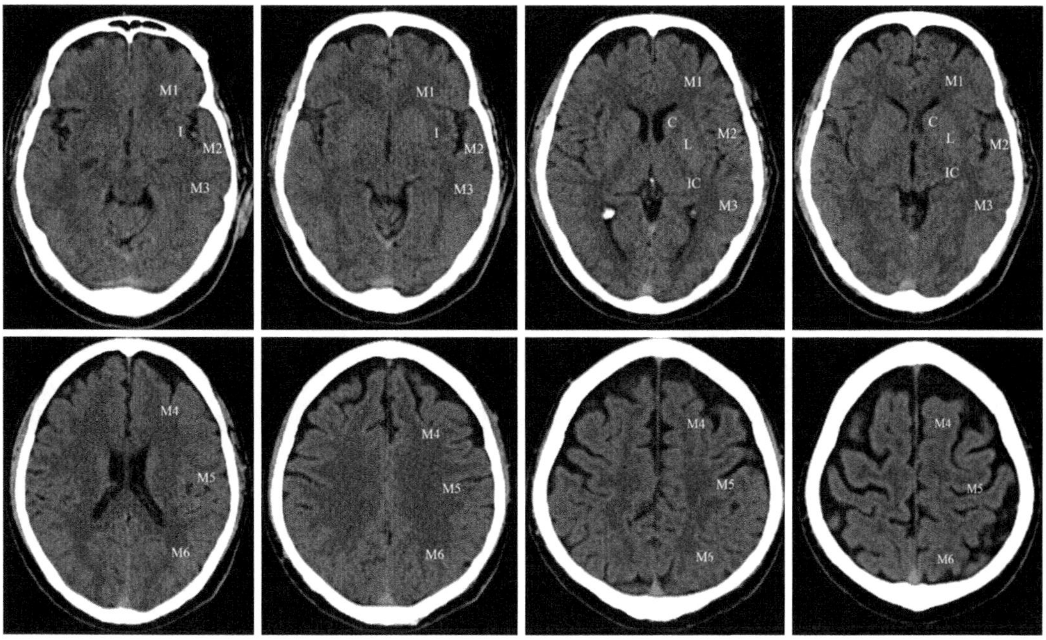


**Fig. 2** The MCA territory is divided into 10 ASPECTS regions: caudate (C), insular ribbon (I), posterior limb of internal capsule (IC), lentiform nucleus (L), anterior inferior frontal cortex (M1), anterior temporal cortex (lateral to the insular ribbon; M2), posterior temporal cortex (M3), anterior superior MCA cortex (ACA-MCA border zone; M4), posterior frontal cortex (M5), parietal cortex (M6)

value of 10 points (Fiebach 2004; Barber et al. 2000). 2018 Guidelines for the Early Management of Patients With Acute Ischemic Stroke regarding IAT recommended that patients who were candidates for endovascular treatment with a stent retriever should have ASPECTS at least 6, among other criteria (Prakkamakul and Yoo 2017). ASPECTS is a strong and consistent predictor of clinical outcome (Powers et al. 2018). The pc-ASPECTS system (Fig. 3) was defined for the posterior fossa similar to that of ASPECT score (Hill et al. 2014).

## 2 Computed Tomography Angiography

CTA is an ideal technique in the detection of large-vessel intracranial arterial stenosis or occlusion (Mendelow 2016). CTA acquisition during acute stroke evaluation is safe with regard to renal function and does not delay appropriate therapy delivery. Moreover, acute CTA acquisition helps to determine rapidly the vascular abnormalities, intracranial thrombus extent and location, vascular occlusion, and stenosis and helps define the appropriate treatment (Ehrlich et al. 2016) (Fig. 4). The ability to maintain cerebral parenchymal perfusion during states of ischemic insult depends largely on the capacity of the cerebral collateral circulation. It has been known that good collateral flow plays a major role in infarct size, recanalization rate, prognosis, and survival (Donahue et al. 2014). A study from Stefania Nannoni and colleagues showed that better collaterals are independently associated with minor early ischemic changes and lower clot burden (Nannoni et al. 2019). One study found the sensitivity of CTA to detect 50% or greater intracranial stenosis to be 97% and the specificity as 99% (Nguyen-Huynh et al. 2008). Multiphase CTA (mCTA) may be slightly better in the prediction of clinical outcome than single-phase CT angiography (sCTA) and perfusion CT (Menon et al. 2015). In a study, sCTA underestimated the collateral status when compared with mCTA. Shan-shan Lu et all also found that the ability of mCTA to predict 90-day modified

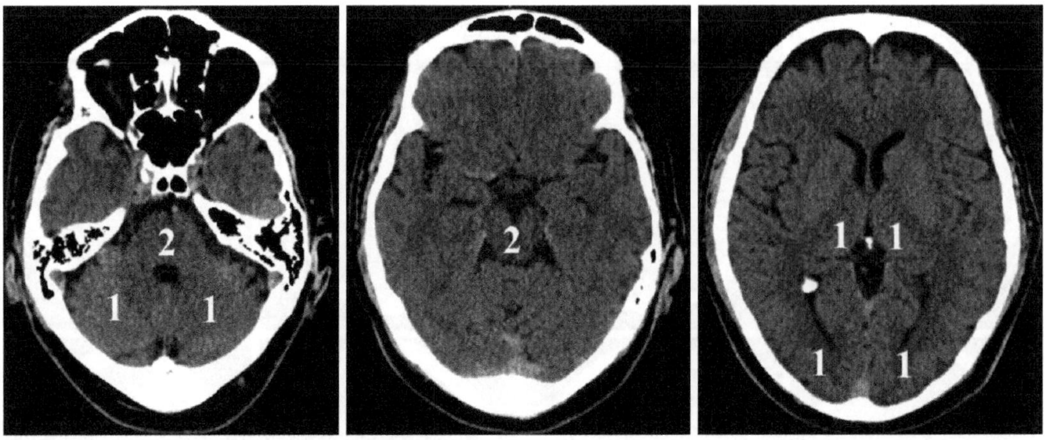


**Fig. 3** The posterior circulation Acute Stroke Prognosis Early CT Score (pc-ASPECTS). Acute ischemic changes in the left or right thalamus, cerebellum, or posterior cerebral artery territory are 1 point each; any part of midbrain or pons is 2 points. pc-ASPECTS 10 indicates a normal scan

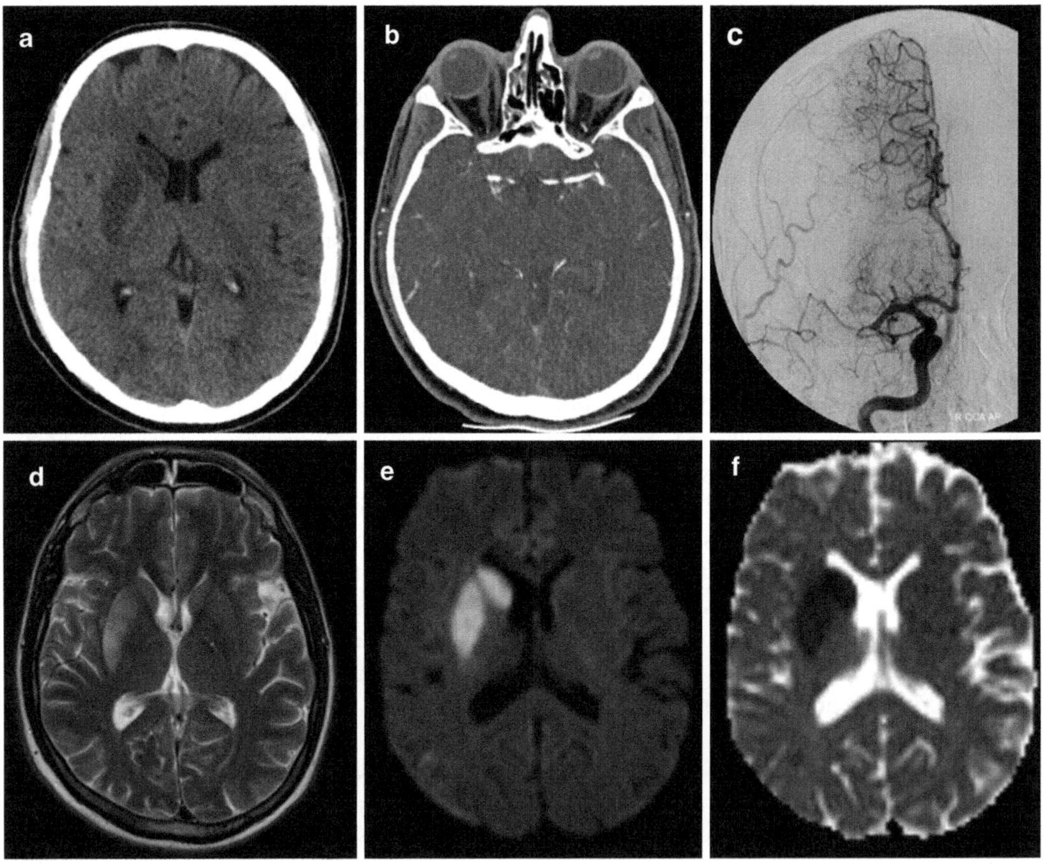


**Fig. 4** Acute ischemic stroke patient with NCCT, CTA, MRI, and DSA images, (**a**) NCCT shows parenchymal hypodensity and swelling on the right caudate head and putamen, (**b**) CTA demonstrates no contrast filling in the right M1 segment related to thrombus and gaze palsy is seen to the pathologic right side, (**c**) DSA shows no contrast filling in the right M1 segment, (**d**) swelling and edema are seen on the right caudate head and putamen on T2-weighted image, (**e**) diffusion restriction on the same region is seen on DWI B1000 image and ADC maps (**f**)

Rankin scale (mRS) score of 0–2 was comparable to CT perfusion (CTP), but better than sCTA. This finding is clinically relevant as collateral assessment by mCTA may be an alternative tool for CTP in AIS patients extending the 6-h time window for endovascular therapy (Shanshan et al. 2019). A noninvasive intracranial vascular study of some type is recommended during the initial imaging evaluation of the acute stroke patient, class 1A recommendation of stroke guideline (Prakkamakul and Yoo 2017).

## 3 Computed Tomography Perfusion Imaging

Perfusion imaging is recommended to estimate infarct core and penumbra in acute stroke patients (Prakkamakul and Yoo 2017). CTP maps are affected by the variations in heart rate, blood pressure, ejection fraction, rate of infusion, osmolality of IV contrast, rotation time, and temporal resolution of the scanner (González et al. 2013). CTP parameters are generated from time–concentration curves of contrast agents in each voxel: mean transit time (MTT), regional cerebral blood volume (rCBV), and regional cerebral blood flow (rCBF). The average time of the blood cell passage through the parenchyma represents MTT. rCBV reflects the blood volume for per unit of parenchyma (mL/100 g). rCBF is the ratio of rCBV/MTT. MTT is the most sensitive perfusion indicator of ischemia, where changes in rCBF and rCBV are found to be more specific for distinguishing penumbra from the ischemic core (Donahue et al. 2014). At-risk volume is defined as the volume with time to maximum of the residue function (Tmax) >6 s. The ischemic core is defined as the volume with relative cerebral blood flow <30% (Lee et al. 2019). In a study, CTP estimated ischemic core volumes were found to be substantially smaller than lesions on follow-up DWI at 24 h despite endovascular reperfusion within 2 h of imaging. However, volumetric CTP core overestimation was uncommon and not related to imaging-to-reperfusion time (Hoving et al. 2018). In another study of 37 MR CLEAN patients with large-vessel occlusions (LVOs) who did not receive endovascular treatment (EVT) or received EVT without substantial reperfusion in the acute setting, CTP at-risk volume predictions were found to frequently underestimate final infarct volume (FIV) (36%) (Lee et al. 2019). Penumbra refers to salvageable tissue with hypoperfusion. Ischemic core, on the other hand, is severely hypoperfused tissue that is destined to infarct. On CTP maps, the penumbra can be estimated by delayed MTT/TTP/Tmax/DT and with reduced CBF and CBV but still above a threshold, while infarct core can be delineated as under critical levels of the same CTP parameters (Bivard et al. 2011; Lin et al. 2013). Although there is still no universal consensus about the ideal thresholds for these perfusion maps to define penumbra and core, previous studies have validated that cerebral regions with CBF <40% of the contralateral normal tissue optimally represents infarct core, whereas regions with DT (delay time to the peak of the residual function) >2 s and CBF >40% of the contralateral normal tissue most accurately defines penumbra (Bivard et al. 2013). It has been shown that tissue perfusion measurements using CTP are prone to significant error (Schaefer et al. 2015; Copen et al. 2017a). CTP has no proven role in selecting patients for IV thrombolysis or endovascular therapy. Its roles should be limited to research patients who cannot get a diffusion-weighted MRI (González et al. 2013). Most believe that CTP-derived CBF maps cannot substitute for DWI in measuring the ischemic core (Copen et al. 2017b).

## 4 Conventional Magnetic Resonance Imaging

Conventional MR imaging is more sensitive and more specific than CT for the detection of acute cerebral ischemia within the first few hours after the onset of stroke (Srinivasan et al. 2006). However, conventional MRI sequences such as T1, T2, and fluid-attenuated inversion recovery (FLAIR) have low sensitivities (50%) for acute ischemia detection within the first 6 h after onset, whereas DWI was reported to have had high sensitivity and specificity, of 88–100% and 86–100%, respectively, in various studies (Srinivasan et al. 2006). Conventional MRI sequences become sensitive to ischemic changes only after a net increase in water content of the cerebral tissue and therefore can detect ischemia after 4–6 hof symptom onset. DWI, on the other hand, is sensitive to cytotoxic edema and can, therefore, provide the opportunity to determine the extent of ischemic injury even within the initial hours of ischemia (Arsava 2012).

Fluid-Attenuated Inversion Recovery Images.

On T2-weighted FLAIR imaging, the CSF signal is suppressed and the lesions appear bright as in T2WI, making cortical lesions and periventricular lesions visible (Mendelow 2016). However, 44.5% of stroke cases demonstrated FLAIR signal changes within 4.5 h (Emeriau et al. n.d.). Lesion size was a strong and independent predictor of lesion visibility in FLAIR sequence, increasing the odds that an acute ischemic lesion was identified on FLAIR imaging by about 7% per 10 mL lesion volume. FLAIR signal changes are subtle during the first 2–3 h of acute ischemia, especially in small ischemic lesions. Severe leukoaraiosis is a relevant confounding factor, which decreases the odds of acute ischemic lesions being detected on FLAIR images by 28% (Thomalla et al. 2011).

## 5 Diffusion-Weighted Imaging

DWI provides an early, distinct, and sensitive measure of both the size and location of ischemic brain lesions. DWI is sensitive to the movement of water molecules within the tissue, which is reduced in regions of cytotoxic edema during early ischemia (Heiss and Kidwell 2014). Diffusion restriction with reduced ADC has been observed as early as 30 min after the onset of ischemia. The ADC continues to decrease further and reaches a nadir at approximately 3–5 days. Thereafter, the ADC starts to increase again, and it returns to the baseline value at approximately 1–4 weeks (Srinivasan et al. 2006). Sensitivity of DWI is approximately 90% with an excellent inter-rater agreement (Simonsen et al. 2015). It has been reported that DWI lesion volumes of more than 70 mL are associated with poor outcome regardless of reperfusion treatment (Yoo et al. 2009). Moreover, DWI lesion volumes of more than 100 mL have been considered a malignant imaging profile associated with symptomatic ICH and poor outcome even after reperfusion (Albers et al. 2006). After endovascular thrombectomy, DWI reversal is more common; one-third of patients may experience DWI reversal more than 10 cc when reimaged within 12 h of ET. However, most of this is transient, with permanent DWI reversal commonly less than 5 mL (Inoue et al. 2014).

## 6 Susceptibility-Weighted Imaging (SWI)

SWI is a 3D gradient-echo T2* MR technique with enhanced sensitivity for paramagnetic substances, such as blood products, iron, and calcification (Haacke et al. 2004). Several studies have shown that SWI is superior to T2-weighted sequences in detecting cerebral microbleeds (Santhosh et al. 2009) (Fig. 5). However, there are controversies about the value of signs detected and their correlations with recanalization, ICH, functional outcome, and antiplatelet therapy in thrombolysis (Li et al. 2017). Moreover, the higher oxygen tension in the subarachnoid spaces and mixing of subarachnoid blood with CSF reduce the sensitivity of T2 and SWI for small amounts of SAH (Whang et al. 2015). SWI is also useful for the visualization of the penumbra by demonstrating prominent veins representing penumbral brain. Acute intra-arterial thrombus is seen as the presence of hypointensity from acute deoxyhemoglobin where the diameter of the hypointense vessel exceeds the contralateral vessel diameter (Halefoglu and Yousem 2018).

## 7 Magnetic Resonance Angiography

AIS patients in the carotid territory who are candidates for carotid endarterectomy (CEA) or stenting should undergo noninvasive imaging of

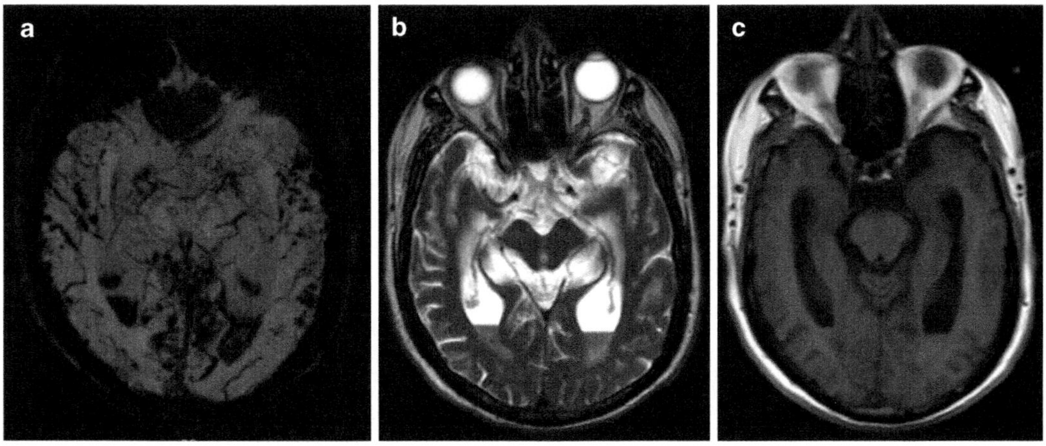


**Fig. 5** Patient with intraventricular hemorrhage (IVH) and amyloid angiopathy, (**a**) SWI image demonstrates microbleeds in temporal lobes and IVH as signal loss in temporal horns, (**b**) T2-weighted image of the same patient, intraventricular blood products are visible as dependent isointense material in occipital horns, (**c**) T1-weighted image shows isointense blood products in occipital horns, microbleeds are not visible

the cervical vessels routinely within 24 h of admission (Prakkamakul and Yoo 2017).

MRI-based selection for EVT was not found to be associated with improving functional outcome compared with CT-based selection, but it is suggested that MRA may be better at reducing the risk of symptomatic intracranial hemorrhage (Kim et al. 2019). In cerebrovascular diagnosis, MRA with contrast-enhanced (CE) or time-of-flight (TOF) methods are the standard approaches (Fig. 6). In CE-MRA, a rapid MR acquisition is timed to a bolus injection of contrast agent over a large field of view, permitting routine imaging of the vasculature from the aortic arch through to the branches of the circle of Willis. In TOF MRA, no contrast agent injection is required, and the vascular signal depends on the direction and velocity of blood flowing into the plane of imaging. The magnetization of protons in stationary tissue occurs through saturation by repeated low-flip-angle RF pulses, whereas protons in the vessels flowing into the tissue remain unsaturated and appear relatively bright. 3D TOF MRA gives superior spatial resolution than 2D and is less prone to signal loss from turbulent flow at sites of stenoses (Mendelow 2016). In a study, the specificity of the CEMRA was significantly higher than of TOF MRA: 0.99 versus 0.83, $P < 0.0001$ to show stenosis. The sensitivity, positive predictive value, negative predictive value, and accuracy were 0.98, 0.78, 0.99, and 0.89 versus 1, 0.98, 1, and 0.99 for the TOF MRA and CEMRA, respectively (Dhundass et al. 2019a). Another study showed that occlusion localization differed significantly on TOF MRA compared with DSA (*P* 0.001), while no significant difference was observed between DSA and CEMRA. Moreover, assessment of collaterals showed very good agreement between CEMRA and DSA (94.9% with *P* 0.25), but only fair agreement between TOF MRA and DSA (23.2% with *P* 0.001) (Boujan et al. 2018). A study showed that the area under curve of pial collateral grading based on TOF MRA was 0.830 (0.636–1.000; $P = 0.006$) with reference to DSA grading. The sensitivity and specificity were 0.700 and 0.933, respectively (Yuan et al. 2019). For the detection of carotid stenosis, CTA yields the best accuracy. However, CTA underestimated histological measurement by 2.4% (based on European Carotid Surgery Trial [ECST] methodology) and 11.9% (based on North American Symptomatic Carotid Endarterectomy Trial [NASCET] methodology) in a study, where MRA overestimated the histological measurement by 2.6% (ECST) and underestimated by 0.6% (NASCET). The study concludes

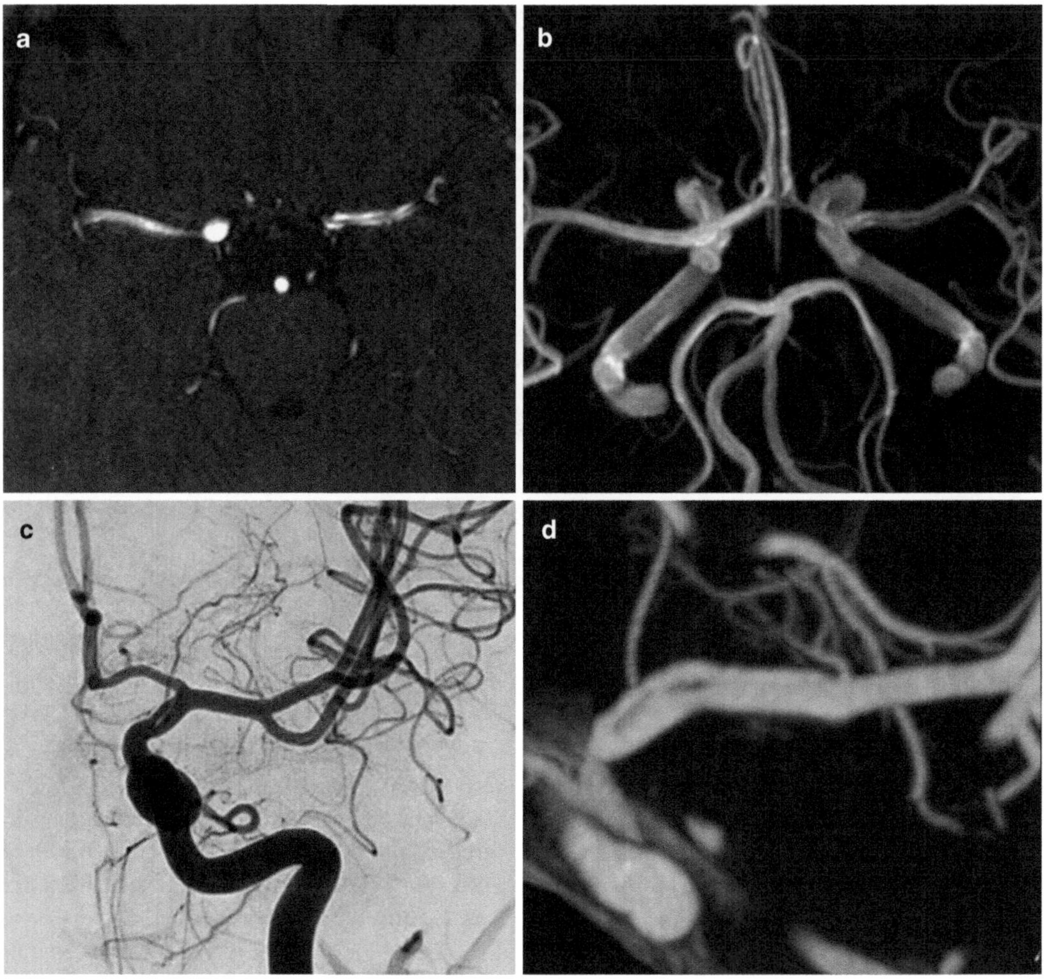


**Fig. 6** MRA, CTA, and DSA images of a stroke patient, (**a**) the contrast-enhanced (CE) and time-of-flight (TOF) MRA identify the dissection on the left MCA M1 segment, (**b**) 3D TOF MRA image demonstrates the intimal flap in the left MCA M1 segment, (**c**) DSA demonstrates the linear filling defect among the intimal flap, (**d**) hypodense intimal flip is seen on CTA MIP image

that CTA is more reliable than MRA for carotid stenosis measurement (Netuka et al. 2016). 3D TOF MRA is standard for arterial intracranial vascular imaging. Post-contrast 2D TOF MRA and post-contrast MRA are used for venous vascular imaging like sinus thrombosis. 3D TOF MRA is typically done at the carotid bifurcation only imaging where contrast-enhanced 2D TOF MRA is used for aortic arch to intracranial vascular imaging. One-stop shop MRI-neck MRA and intracranial MRA are beneficial for the detection of vascular stenosis, stroke volume, and perfusion studies for penumbra.

## 8 Magnetic Resonance Perfusion

Additional imaging beyond CT and CTA or MRI and MRA such as perfusion studies for selecting patients for mechanical thrombectomy in <6 h is not recommended. CTP or MRP studies are recommended beyond 6 h after stroke onset to discover salvageable brain tissue (Prakkamakul and Yoo 2017).

The most widely used technique is dynamic susceptibility contrast (DSC) imaging, which relies on the administration of a gadolinium-

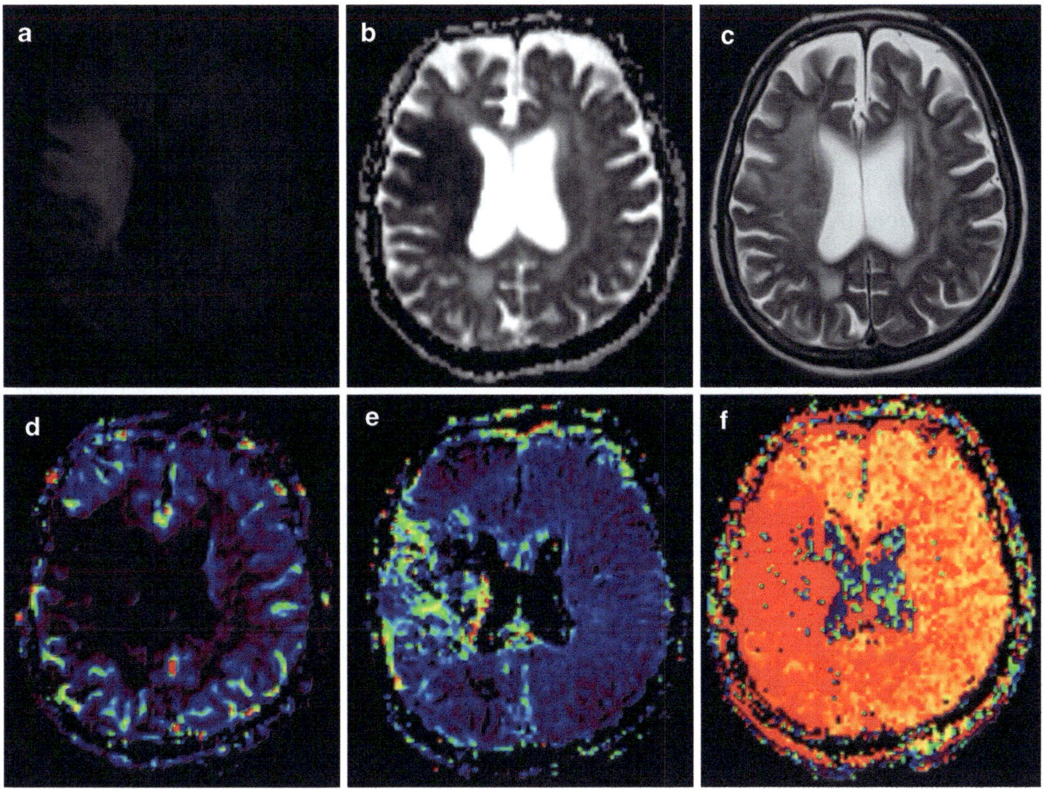


**Fig. 7** DWI, ADC, and MR perfusion maps of a patient with right MCA stroke: (**a** and **b**). DWI image shows diffusion restriction in the right frontal lobe, (**c**) T2-weighted image demonstrates cortical swelling and edema in the diffusion-restricted area in right frontal lobe, (**d**) CBV map shows decreased blood volume in the right frontal lobe, diffusion–perfusion mismatch is seen in the right posterior frontal lobe (penumbra), (**e**) MTT map shows increased blood transit time in the same region, (**f**) TTP map demonstrates increased blood flow time in the core and penumbra

based contrast agent. As the gadolinium passes through the large vessels, the capillaries, and then into the veins, there is local signal loss due to the T2 effects of the contrast. By rapidly imaging at multiple time points during contrast passage through the blood vessels, a time signal intensity curve is created. This then undergoes mathematical post-processing to yield perfusion maps of the brain (Bateman et al. 2017) (Fig. 7). DSC MR perfusion allows the visualization and quantification of the whole brain in less than a minute of acquisition time. However, the difficulty in determining absolute quantification, susceptibility artifacts (i.e., blood product, calcification, metal, air, and bone), and user dependence are the disadvantages of this technique (Essig et al. 2013).

Although CBV has been shown to offer good correlation with DWI and final infarct volume, it is rarely used in clinical practice for core infarct, as lesions are easier to identify on DWI, and DWI is less likely to miss small lesions (Schaefer et al. 2002).

In a meta-analysis for the nonviable/at-risk tissue, threshold was given as CBF $<12$ ml/100 g/min and $T_{max}$ 6 s. For the at-risk/not at-risk threshold quantitative CBF varied between 18 and 37.2 ml/100 g/min; MTT varied 1.78–8.1 s delay relative to the contralateral hemisphere; qualitative rCBF ranged from 0.58–0.61, regional mean transit time (rMTT) from 1.63 to 2.11, time to peak (TTP) from 4 to 7 s, and time to peak of the residue function ($T_{max}$) varied threefold from 1.45 to 5.46 s (56). Currently, the most widely utilized threshold to determine penumbral tissue is $T_{max}$ in the range of 4–6 s (Campbell and Macrae 2015).

In general, a mismatch volume of more than 20% is generally accepted as an indicator of penumbral presence. Moreover, the mismatch can persist to at least 48 h in some patients (Ma et al. 2015). Currently, there are insufficient data to support the routine use of PWI selection for reperfusion treatment within traditional time windows (Bateman et al. 2017). In selected patients with AIS within 6–24 h of last known normal who have LVO in the anterior circulation and meet other DAWN eligibility criteria, mechanical thrombectomy is reasonable (Prakkamakul and Yoo 2017). DAWN eligibility criteria are last seen well to emergency department arrival time 6–24 h, National Institutes of Health Stroke Scale (NIHSS) ≥10, presence of proximal anterior circulation large-vessel occlusion in the intracranial internal carotid artery or middle cerebral artery (segment 1/M1), clinical-core mismatch, baseline modified Rankin Scale score 0–1, life expectancy of >6 months, and ability to obtain consent (Dhundass et al. 2019b).

Quantitative CTP mismatch classification using relCBF and Tmax is similar to perfusion-diffusion MRI. The greater accessibility of CTP may facilitate generalizability of mismatch-based selection in clinical practice and trials (Campbell et al. 2012).

## References


Albers GW, Thijs VN, Wechsler L et al (2006) Magnetic resonance imaging profiles predict clinical response to early reperfusion: the diffusion and perfusion imaging evaluation for understanding stroke evolution (DEFUSE) study. Ann Neurol 60:508–517

Arsava EM (2012) The role of MRI as a prognostic tool in ischemic stroke. J Neurochem. 123(Suppl 2):22–28. https://doi.org/10.1111/j.1471-4159.2012.07940.x

Barber PA, Demchuk AM, Zhang J, Buchan AM (2000) Validity and reliability of a quantitative computed tomography score in predicting outcome of hyper-acute stroke before thrombolytic therapy. ASPECTS study group. Alberta stroke Programme early CT score. Lancet 355:1670–1674

Bateman M, Slater LA, Leslie-Mazwi T, Simonsen CZ, Stuckey S, Chandra RV (2017) Diffusion and perfusion MR imaging in acute stroke: clinical utility and potential limitations for treatment selection. Top Magn Reson Imaging 26:77–82

Bivard A, McElduff P, Spratt N et al (2011) Defining the extent of irreversible brain ischemia using perfusion computed tomography. Cerebrovasc Dis 31:238–245

Bivard A, Levi C, Spratt N, Parsons M (2013) Perfusion CT in acute stroke: a comprehensive analysis of infarct and penumbra. Radiology 267:543–550

Bouchez L, Sztajzel R, Vargas MI et al (2017) CT imaging selection in acute stroke. Eur J Radiol 96:153–161

Boujan XT, Neuberger XU, Pfaff XJ, Nagel XS, Herweh XC, Bendszus XM, Möhlenbruch XMA (2018) Value of contrast-enhanced mra versus time-of-flight mra in acute ischemic stroke MRI. AJNR Am J Neuroradiol. https://doi.org/10.3174/ajnr.A5771

Campbell BC, Macrae IM (2015) Translational perspectives on perfusion-diffusion mismatch in ischemic stroke. Int J Stroke 10:153–162

Campbell BC, Christensen S, Levi CR, Desmond PM, Donnan GA, Davis SM, Parsons MW (2012) Comparison of computed tomography perfusion and magnetic resonance imaging perfusion-diffusion mismatch in ischemic stroke. Stroke 43:2648–2653

Christopher SJ (2017) Astill and Marc J Agzarian, discrepancy rates in reporting of acute stroke CT. J Med Imaging Radiat Oncol 61(3):317–320

Copen WA, Yoo AJ, Rost NS et al (2017a) In patients with suspected acute stroke, CT perfusion-based cerebral blood flow maps cannot substitute for DWI in measuring the ischemic core. PLoS One 12:e0188891

Copen WA, Yoo AJ, Rost NS, Morais L'v T, Schaefer PW, Gonza'lez RG, Wu O (2017b) In patients with suspected acute stroke, CT perfusion-based cerebral blood flow maps cannot substitute for DWI in measuring the ischemic core. PLoS One. https://doi.org/10.1371/journal.pone.0188891

Dhundass S, Savatovskya J, Durona L, Fahedc R, Escalardc S, Michael Obadia D, Kevin Zuber E, Mettene MA, Mehdi Mejdoubi E, Blancc R, Sadika J-C, Collina A, Lecler A (2019a) Improved detection and characterization of arterial occlusion in acute ischemic stroke using contrast enhanced MRA. J Neuroradiol. https://doi.org/10.1016/j.neurad.2019.02.011

Dhundass S, Savatovsky J, Duron L, Fahed R, Escalard S, Obadia M, Zuber K, Metten MA, Mejdoubi M, Blanc R, Sadik JC, Collin A, Lecler A (2019b) Improved detection and characterization of arterial occlusion in acute ischemic stroke using contrast enhanced MRA. J Neuroradiol. https://doi.org/10.1016/j.neurad.2019.02.011

Donahue J, Sumer S, Wintermark M (2014) Assessment of collateral flow in patients with cerebrovascular disorders. J Neuroradiol 41(October 41 (4)):234–242

Ehrlich ME, Turner HL, Currie LJ, Wintermark M, Worrall BB, Southerland AM (2016) Safety of computed tomographic angiography in the evaluation of patients with acute stroke a single-center experience. Stroke. 47:2045–2050

Emeriau S, Serre I, Toubas O, Pombourcq F, Oppenheim C, Pierot L Can diffusion-weighted imaging–fluid-attenuated inversion recovery mismatch (positive diffusion-weighted imaging/negative fluid-attenuated inversion recovery) at 3 tesla identify patients with stroke at <4.5 hours? Stroke. n.d. https://doi.org/10.1161/STROKEAHA.113.001001

Essig M, Shiroishi MS, Nguyen TB, Saake M, Provenzale JM, Enterline D, Anzalone N, Dörfler A, Rovira À, Wintermark M, Law M (2013) Perfusion MRI: the five most frequently asked technical questions. AJR Am J Roentgenol 200(1):24–34. https://doi.org/10.2214/AJR.12.9543

Fiebach JB (2004) Stroke magnetic resonance imaging is accurate in hyperacute intracerebral hemorrhage: a multicenter study on the validity of stroke imaging. Stroke 35:502–506

González RG, Copen WA, Schaefer PW, Lev MH, Pomerantz SR, Rapalino O, Chen JW, Hunter GJ, Romero JM, Buchbinder BR, Larvie M, Hirsch JA, Gupta R (2013) The Massachusetts General Hospital acute stroke imaging algorithm: an experience and evidence based approach. J NeuroIntervent Surg 5:i7–i12. https://doi.org/10.1136/neurintsurg-2013-010715

Haacke EM, Xu Y, Cheng YC, Reichenbach JR (2004) Susceptibility weighted imaging (SWI). Magn Reson Med 52:612–618

Halefoglu AM, Yousem DM (2018 April 28) Susceptibility weighted imaging: clinical applications and future directions, world. J Radiol 10(4):30–45. https://doi.org/10.4329/wjr.v10.i4.30

Heiss W-D, Kidwell CS (2014 April) Imaging for prediction of functional outcome and assessment of recovery in ischemic stroke. Stroke 45(4):1195–1201. https://doi.org/10.1161/STROKEAHA.113.003611

Hill MD, Demchuk AM, Goyal M et al (2014) Alberta stroke program early computed tomography score to select patients for endovascular treatment: interventional Management of Stroke (IMS)-III trial. Stroke 45:444–449

Hoving JW, Marquering HA, Majoie CBLM, Yassi N, Sharma G, Liebeskind DS, van der Lugt A, Roos YB, van Zwam W, van Oostenbrugge RJ, Goyal M, Saver JL, Jovin TG, Albers GW, Davalos A, Hill MD, Demchuk AM, Bracard S, Guillemin F, Muir KW, White P, Mitchell PJ, Donnan GA, Davis SM, Campbell BCV (2018) Volumetric and spatial accuracy of computed tomography perfusion estimated ischemic core volume in patients with acute ischemic stroke. Stroke 49:00–00. https://doi.org/10.1161/STROKEAHA.118.020846

Inoue M, Mlynash M, Christensen S et al (2014) Early diffusion-weighted imaging reversal after endovascular reperfusion is typically transient in patients imaged 3 to 6 hours after onset. Stroke 45:1024–1028

Kidwell CS, Chalela JA, Saver JL, Starkman S, Hill MD, Demchuk AM et al (2004) Comparison of MRI and CT for detection of acute intracerebral hemorrhage. JAMA 292:1823–1830

Kim J-T, Cho B-H, Choi K-H, Park M-S, Kim BJ, Park J-M, Kang K, Lee SJ, Kim JG, Cha J-K, Kim D-H, Nah H-W, Park TH, Park S-S, Lee KB, Lee J, Hong K-S, Cho Y-J, Park H-K, Lee B-C, Yu K-H, Oh MS, Kim D-E, Ryu W-S, Choi JC, Kwon J-H, Kim W-J, Shin D-I, Yeo M-J, Sohn SIL, Hong J-H, Lee JS, Lee J, Bae H-J, Cho K-H (2019) Magnetic resonance imaging versus computed tomography angiography based selection for endovascular therapy in patients with acute ischemic stroke. Stroke 50:365–372. https://doi.org/10.1161/STROKEAHA.118.023173

Lansberg MG, Albers GW, Beaulieu C, Marks MP (2000) Comparison of diffusion-weighted MRI and CT in acute stroke. Neurology Apr 54(8):1557–1561

Lee S, Yoo AJ, Marquering HA, Berkhemer OA, Majoie CB, Dippel DWJ, Sheth SA (2019) For the MR CLEAN investigators, accuracy of "at risk" tissue predictions using CT perfusion in acute large vessel occlusions. J Neuroimaging 0:1–5. https://doi.org/10.1111/jon.12595

Li L, Liu M-S, Li G-Q, Zheng Y, Guo T-L, Kang X, Yuan M-T (2017) Susceptibility-weighted imaging in thrombolytic therapy of acute ischemic stroke. Chin Med J 130(20):2489–2497. https://doi.org/10.4103/0366-6999.216401

Lin L, Bivard A, Parsons MW (2013) Perfusion patterns of ischemic stroke on computed tomography perfusion. J Stroke 15:164–173

Lövblad KO, Altrichter S, Viallon M, Sztajzel R, Delavelle J, Vargas MI, El-Koussy M, Federspiel A, Sekoranja L (2008) Neuro-imaging of cerebral ischemic stroke. J Neuroradiol 35:197–209

Ma H, Wright P, Allport L et al (2015) Salvage of the PWI/DWI mismatch upto 48 h from stroke onset leads to favorable clinical outcome. Int J Stroke 10:565–570

Mendelow AD (2016) Stroke: pathophysiology, diagnosis, and management, 6th edn. Elsevier, Amsterdam

Menon BK, d'Esterre CD, Qazi EM, Almekhlafi M, Hahn L, Demchuk AM, Goyal M (2015) Multiphase CT angiography: a new tool for the imaging triage of patients with acute ischemic stroke. Radiology 275:510–520

Nannoni S, Sirimarco G, Cereda CW, Lambrou D, Strambo D, Eskandari A, Mosimann PJ, Wintermark M, Michel P (2019) Determining factors of better leptomeningeal collaterals: a study of 857 consecutive acute ischemic stroke patients. J Neurol. https://doi.org/10.1007/s00415-018-09170-3

Netuka D, Belšán T, Broulíková K, Mandys V, Charvát F, Malík J, Coufalová L, Bradáč O, Ostrý S, Beneš V. Detection of carotid artery stenosis using histological specimens: a comparison of CT angiography, magnetic resonance angiography, digital subtraction angiography and Doppler ultrasonography. Acta Neurochir 2016 Aug;158(8):1505–1514. doi: https://doi.org/10.1007/s00701-016-2842-0. Epub 2016 Jun 2. PMID: 27255656

Nguyen-Huynh MN, Wintermark M, English J et al (2008) How accurate is CT angiography in evaluating intracranial atherosclerotic disease? Stroke 39:1184–1188

Powers WJ, Rabinstein AA, Ackerson T, Adeoye OM, Bambakidis NC, Becker K, Biller J, Brown M, Demaerschalk BM, Hoh B, Jauch EC, Kidwell CS, Leslie-Mazwi TM, Ovbiagele B, Scott PA, Sheth KN, Southerland AM, Summers DV, Tirschwell DL, on behalf of the American Heart Association Stroke Council (2018) Guidelines for the early Management of Patients with Acute Ischemic Stroke. Stroke 2018(49):e46–e99

Prakkamakul S, Yoo AJ (2017) ASPECTS CT in acute ischemia: review of current data. Top Magn Reson Imaging. 26(3):103–112

Santhosh K, Kesavadas C, Thomas B, Gupta AK, Thamburaj K, Kapilamoorthy TR (2009) Susceptibility weighted imaging: a new tool in magnetic resonance imaging of stroke. Clin Radiol 64:74–83. https://doi.org/10.1016/j.crad.2008.04.022

Schaefer PW, Hunter GJ, He J et al (2002) Predicting cerebral ischemic infarct volume with diffusion and perfusion MR imaging. AJNR Am J Neuroradiol 23:1785–1794

Schaefer PW, Souza L, Kamalian S et al (2015) Limited reliability of computed tomographic perfusion acute infarct volume measurements compared with diffusion-weighted imaging in anterior circulation stroke. Stroke 46:419–424

Shan-shan L, Zhang X, Xiao-quan X, Cao Y-z, Zhao LB, Liu Q-H, Wu F-Y, Liu S, Shi H-B (2019) Comparison of CT angiography collaterals for predicting target perfusion profile and clinical outcome in patients with acute ischemic stroke. Eur Radiol. https://doi.org/10.1007/s00330-019-06027-9

Simonsen CZ, Madsen MH, Schmitz ML et al (2015) Sensitivity of diffusion- and perfusion-weighted imaging for diagnosing acute ischemic stroke is 97.5%. Stroke 46:98–101

Srinivasan A, Goyal M, Al Azri F, Lum C (2006) State-of-the-art imaging of acute stroke. RadioGraphics 26:S75–S95. https://doi.org/10.1148/rg.26si065501

Thomalla G, Cheng B, Ebinger M, Hao Q, Tourdias T, Wu O et al (2011) STIR and VISTA imaging investigators. DWI-FLAIR mismatch for the identification of patients with acute ischaemic stroke within 4.5 h of symptom onset (PRE-FLAIR): a multicentre observational study. Lancet Neurol 10:978–986. https://doi.org/10.1016/S1474-4422(11)70192-2

Vilelaa P, Rowley HA (2017) Brain ischemia: CT and MRI techniques in acute ischemic stroke. Eur J Radiol 96:162–172

Whang JS, Kolber M, Powell DK, Libfeld E (2015) Diffusion-weighted signal patterns of intracranial haemorrhage. Clin Radiol 70:909–916

Yoo AJ, Verduzco LA, Schaefer PW et al (2009) MRI-based selection for intraarterial stroke therapy: value of pretreatment diffusion-weighted imaging lesion volume in selecting patients with acute stroke who will benefit from early recanalization. Stroke 40:2046–2054

Yuan HW, Ji RJ, Wang AL, Lin YJ, Chen HF, Xu ZQ, Peng GP, Luo BY (2019) A grading scale for pial collaterals in middle cerebral artery total occlusion based on time-of-flight MR angiography source images. Magn Reson Med Sci. 18:62–69. https://doi.org/10.2463/mrms.mp.2018-0001

# Acute Stroke: Management

Frédéric Clarençon, Eimad Shotar, Raphaël Le Bouc, Romain Pasqualetto, Stéphanie Lenck, Kévin Premat, and Nader Sourour

## Contents



F. Clarençon (✉) · E. Shotar
Sorbonne University, Paris VI University, Paris, France

Department of Neuroradiology, Pitié-Salpêtrière Hospital, Paris, France
e-mail: frederic.clarencon@aphp.fr

R. Le Bouc
Department of Vascular Neurology, Pitié-Salpêtrière Hospital, Paris, France

R. Pasqualetto
Sorbonne University, Paris VI University, Paris, France

Neuro-Intensive Care Unit, Pitié-Salpêtrière Hospital, Paris, France

S. Lenck · K. Premat · N. Sourour
Department of Neuroradiology, Pitié-Salpêtrière Hospital, Paris, France



M. Scaglione et al. (eds.), *Emergency Radiology of the Head and Spine*, Medical Radiology Diagnostic Imaging, https://doi.org/10.1007/978-3-030-91047-1_5

**Abstract**

In the last years, we have faced a blooming of mechanical thrombectomy (MT). Numerous randomized controlled trials have shown the benefit of MT, combined with the best medical treatment, in the setting of acute ischemic stroke with large vessel occlusion. Thus, the management and triage of patients with acute ischemic stroke have become crucial in order to offer a swift recanalization to these patients. In this chapter, we will summarize the recent data of the literature on MT, review the indications and guidelines for MT, and discuss the different strategies for triage. We will also present the different techniques available for MT, and their respective safety and effectiveness.

## Abbreviations

| | |
|---|---|
| ADAPT | A direct aspiration first-pass technique |
| AHA | American Heart Association |
| AIS | Acute ischemic stroke |
| ASA | American Stroke Association |
| ASPECTS | Alberta Stroke Program Early CT Score |
| BMT | Best medical treatment |
| CSS | Comprehensive stroke center |
| ICA | Internal carotid artery |
| IV | Intravenous |
| LVO | Large vessel occlusion |
| MCA | Middle cerebral artery |
| MT | Mechanical thrombectomy |
| mRS | Modified Rankin Scale |
| mTICI score | Modified thrombolysis in cerebral infarction score |
| NIHSS | National Institutes of Health Stroke Scale |
| NNT | Number of patients needed to treat |
| RCT | Randomized controlled trial |
| tPA | Tissue plasminogen activator |

## 1 Recent Data on Mechanical Thrombectomy

Until 2015, all randomized controlled trials (RCTs) that have evaluated the effectiveness of mechanical thrombectomy (MT) in the setting of acute ischemic stroke (AIS) with large vessel occlusion (LVO) failed to demonstrate a benefit in terms of 3 months' neurological outcome compared with the best medical treatment (BMT) (Ciccone et al. 2013; Broderick et al. 2013; Kidwell et al. 2013). In 2015, five RCTs (Berkhemer et al. 2015; Jovin et al. 2015; Goyal et al. 2015; Campbell et al. 2015; Saver et al. 2015), with a close design, showed a strong benefit of MT in patients with LVO, associated with the BMT. Indeed, in these studies, the gap of good neurological outcome (i.e., modified Rankin Scale [mRS] score ≤2 at 3 months' follow-up) in favor of MT + BMT varied from 13.5 to 31%, and the number of patients needed to treat (NNT) to gain a patient with independency at 3-month follow-up ranged from 3 to 8. In most of the studies, the time window to start the MT procedure was 6 h, but some studies, selecting the patients with a small core infarct, extended the time window to 8 or even 12 h (REVASCAT (Jovin et al. 2015) and ESCAPE(Goyal et al. 2015) studies, respectively).

One could wonder what happened between the negative studies published in 2013 and the positive ones published in 2015. First, the patients' selection was more rigorous in the recent studies, which involved only patients with imaging-proven LVO. Second, all positive RCTs used the most recent MT devices, especially stent retrievers, while first-generation devices were used in previous RCTs. These methodological issues may explain the discrepancies between older and recent RCTs.

Since then, two additional RCTs have been published (Bracard et al. 2016; Mocco et al. 2016), confirming the results of the first five RCTs published in 2015.

## 2 Indications of Mechanical Thrombectomy

In 2015, the American Heart Association (AHA)/ American Stroke Association (ASA) published its recommendations concerning the indications of MT in the setting of AIS with LVO, based on the five above-mentioned RCTs published in 2015 in the New England Journal of Medicine (Powers et al. 2015). These recommendations specified that patients for whom MT was considered should receive IV thrombolysis if no contraindication is found. MT should be performed in patients ≥18 years, with an imaging proven LVO (M1 or ICA), with pre-MT mRS score ≤1, with a NIHSS (National Institutes of Health Stroke Scale) ≥6 and an ASPECTS (Alberta Stroke Program Early CT score) ≥6. MT should be initiated (groin puncture) within 6 h of symptom onset and performed with a stent retriever.

Recently, two RCTs have expanded the time window for mechanical thrombectomy in patients with an AIS due to LVO: the DWAN trial (Nogueira et al. 2018) and the DEFUSE 3 study (Albers et al. 2018).

The DAWN (*Clinical Mismatch in the Triage of Wake Up and Late Presenting Strokes Undergoing Neurointervention With Trevo*) trial (Nogueira et al. 2018) is a RCT that involved 206 patients and aimed at comparing MT associated with BMT vs BMT alone between 6 and 24 h from symptoms' onset (known symptoms' onset or last known well) in patients with AIS and LVO. Selection criteria, based on the core infarct volume, were as follows: infarct volume <31 ml in patients less than 80 years with a NIHSS ≥10 or infarct volume <51 ml in patients less than 80 years with a NIHSS ≥20 or infarct volume <21 ml in patients ≥80 years with a NIHSS ≥10. At 3 months' follow-up, good clinical outcome (i.e., mRS ≤ 2) was observed in 48.6% in the group MT + BMT vs 13.1% in the BMT group. Additionally, the NNT was close to 3 (2.8). For comparison purpose, the NNT for the exclusion treatment of ruptured intracranial aneurysms is 13 (Lanzino et al. 2013). It is noteworthy that about two-third of the patients included in the DWAN trial were wake-up strokes and that one-fourth were AIS with undetermined stroke onset.

Another recent study has expended the time window for MT: the DEFUSE3 trial (Albers et al. 2018). This study involved 182 patients from 38 centers from the United States. Patients with an AIS with LVO (proximal MCA or ICA occlusions), between 6 and 16 h after the symptom onset (or last known to be well) an initial infarct size of less than 70 ml, and a ratio of the volume of ischemic tissue on perfusion imaging to infarct volume of 1.8 or more, were randomized either for MT + BMT vs BMT alone. Results in terms of independency (mRS ≤2 at 3 months' follow-up) were better for the MT + BMT arm (45% vs 17%, $P < 0.001$). Additionally, the 90-day mortality rate was 14% in the endovascular therapy group and 26% in the medical therapy group ($P = 0.05$).

Since the publication of the DAWN and DEFUSE3 trials, AHA and ASA have updated their recommendations in 2018 (Powers et al. 2018), which now take into account a wider time window for MT, in selected patients, according to the above-described imaging criteria.

What DAWN and DEFUSE3 trials have in common is the patients' selection based on some form of mismatch. The mismatch is defined as the difference between hypoperfused and infarcted tissue and has many imaging and clinical surrogates. Identifying patients with symptomatic ischemic penumbra, at risk of evolution toward infarction, and amenable to tissue salvage by emergent LVO revascularization, is bound to be the cornerstone of patient selection for MT in the future.

## 3 Triage for Mechanical Thrombectomy

With the blooming of mechanical thrombectomy, due to the critical influence of the time to recanalization, triage of patients eligible for MT has become a crucial point. Indeed, the benefit of MT in terms of functional outcome decreases with time. For instance, it has been shown in the meta-analysis of Saver et al. that for every 4-min delay in emergency department door-to-reperfusion time, 1 of every 100 treated patients had a worse disability outcome, leading to no significant benefit of MT when initiated more than 7.3 h after the symptoms' onset (Saver et al. 2016). Thus, numerous strategies have been proposed and studied to improve the patient workflow and reduce, as much as possible, these critical times.

### 3.1 "Mothership" Vs "Drip and Ship"

Discrepancies in terms of equipment and facilities exist between the different hospitals in which patients with AIS associated with LVO may be managed. Indeed, some of them have both a neurovascular unit and an interventional neuroradiology department, in which MT can be performed. In these hospitals (called "comprehensive stroke centers"), the patients are directly sent to the angiography suite. This workflow is called the "*Mothership*" paradigm. In other hospitals (called "primary stroke centers"), no department of interventional neuroradiology is present. Thus, after neurological examination and imaging confirming the diagnosis of AIS with LVO, the patient will be transferred to another hospital in which MT will be performed. If the patient is admitted in the primary stroke center within the time window for IV thrombolysis, the tPA injection will be performed before the transfer to the comprehensive center. This workflow is called the "Drip and Ship" paradigm (Detraz et al. 2018).

In terms of safety, numerous non-randomized studies (Park et al. 2016a, b; Hiyama et al. 2016; Gerschenfeld et al. 2017) have shown no difference between the 2 paradigms on mortality rate, symptomatic hemorrhages, or intraoperative adverse events. Additionally, effectiveness of both paradigms, in terms of 3 months' neurological outcome, appears equivalent according to these non-randomized series (Park et al. 2016a, b; Hiyama et al. 2016; Gerschenfeld et al. 2017).

Interestingly, no RCT has compared the safety and the effectiveness of these two paradigms.

### 3.2 Clinical Scores

To improve the prehospital triage of patients who may benefit from MT, clinical scores may be used (Perez de la Ossa et al. 2014; Hastrup et al. 2016; Lima et al. 2016; Katz et al. 2015). This strategy may help to depict indirectly patients who may have LVO in order to refer them directly to a comprehensive stroke center. However, according to a recent publication, using published cut-offs of these scores for triage would result in a loss of opportunity for ≥20% of patients with LVO, who would be inappropriately sent to a center without neurointerventional angiography suite. On the contrary, using these cut-offs would result in sending patients inappropriately (false positive for LVO eligible to MT) to a comprehensive stroke center in 10% of the cases (Turc et al. 2016). To date, none of these scores can avoid performing cerebral imaging for triage.

### 3.3 Triage in Angiography Suite

Recently, some teams have proposed performing triage directly in the angiography suite (Ribo et al. 2018). Indeed, the recent advances in the cone-beam flat panel technology allow performing CT scan, CT angiography, and CT perfusion directly in the angio suite (van der Bom et al. 2012). This option may help avoiding loosing time during the different transfers of the patients. This "all-inclusive" option with C-arm CT acquisitions seems at a first glance very seducing since it reduces the delay between imaging acquisition and groin puncture and thus revascularization time (Ribo et al. 2017). However, this strategy for patients triage may have some limitations (Clarencon et al. 2018). Indeed, a consistent number of patients with no AIS (intraparenchymal hemorrhage, stroke mimic) or with AIS but no LVO may be screened in the angiography suite with this triage method, which may be a considerable source of disorganization for interventional neuroradiology departments, and may also be not cost-effective.

### 3.4 Perspectives

A perspective to improve the patient workflow is the use of an ambulance carrying a CT scan on which regular CT acquisition, as well as CTA and CT perfusion, could be performed (John et al. 2016). Preliminary experiences with such "*mobile stroke units*" have been described in different towns like Berlin (Ebinger et al. 2015) or Cleveland (Taqui et al. 2017). This strategy may help improving the patient transfer to the comprehensive stroke center (El-Ghanem et al. 2017). Telestroke management, mobile neuro-endovascular teams, or smart device applications may be other potential solutions to improve the patient workflow (El-Ghanem et al. 2017).

## 4 Technique(S)

### 4.1 Stent Retriever or Aspiration Catheter?

In most of the recent RCTs, the benefit of MT in AIS with LVO has been proven with stent retrievers (Berkhemer et al. 2015; Jovin et al. 2015; Goyal et al. 2015; Campbell et al. 2015; Saver et al. 2015). Fewer evidences are available concerning the effectiveness of aspiration with large bore catheters (Mocco et al. 2016). Stent retrievers are non-detachable stents, which will be opened in the clot in order to grab the clot within the stent retriever's mesh. Then, the stent retriever will be removed opened in the guiding catheter (Kang and Park 2017). In this technique, the clot is anchored in the stent retriever's mesh and withdrawn through the guiding catheter. To avoid fragmentation of the clot during removal, and thus the risk of clot migration in the same and/or another territory, flow arrest with balloon guiding catheters or combination of stent retriever with aspiration catheter close to the thrombus may be used (cf *infra*).

Based on mTICI (modified thrombolysis in cerebral infarction) score (Zaidat et al. 2013) grading (Table 1), a 77% recanalization rate (mTICI 2b or 3) has been reported with stent retrievers (Campbell et al. 2016).

An alternative strategy is the contact aspiration. This technique consists in navigating a large bore catheter in contact with the clot and to aspirate the clot, either by manual aspiration or by means of an aspiration pump (Fig. 1). ADAPT (a direct aspiration first-pass technique) is a variant of the aspiration technique, which consists in using aspiration thrombectomy as the first-line treatment with the possibility of adjuvant treatment if recanalization is not initially achieved. Fewer evidences are available for the effectiveness of aspiration/ADAPT for the management of AIS with LVO. Effectiveness of the aspiration technique in terms of recanalization (TICI 2b-3) has been reported ranging from 65 to 89% (Wei et al. 2017); the one of ADAPT technique from 76% to 97% (Wei et al. 2017). Good 3 months' clinical outcome with the aspiration technique has been reported ranging from 38 to 78% (Wei et al. 2017) and from 39 to 84% with the ADAPT technique (Wei et al. 2017) .Interestingly a benchtop study has shown that the ADAPT technique was responsible for fewer distal emboli, compared with stent retriever thrombectomy technique (Chueh et al. 2016).

The THERAPY trial (Mocco et al. 2016) was the sole RCT that compared MT performed with the ADAPT technique + BMT vs BMT alone. This study did not show significant difference between the two treatment strategies (38% vs

**Table 1** Modified thrombolysis in cerebral infarction (mTICI) score(Zaidat et al. 2013)

| |
|---|
| Grade 0: No perfusion |
| Grade 1: Antegrade reperfusion past the initial occlusion, but limited distal branch filling with little or slow distal reperfusion |
| Grade 2<br>• Grade 2a: Antegrade reperfusion of less than half of the occluded target artery previously ischemic territory (e.g., in one major division of the middle cerebral artery (MCA) and its territory)<br>• Grade 2b: Antegrade reperfusion of more than half of the previously occluded target artery ischemic territory (e.g., in two major divisions of the MCA and their territories) |
| Grade 3: Complete antegrade reperfusion of the previously occluded target artery ischemic territory, with absence of visualized occlusion in all distal branches |

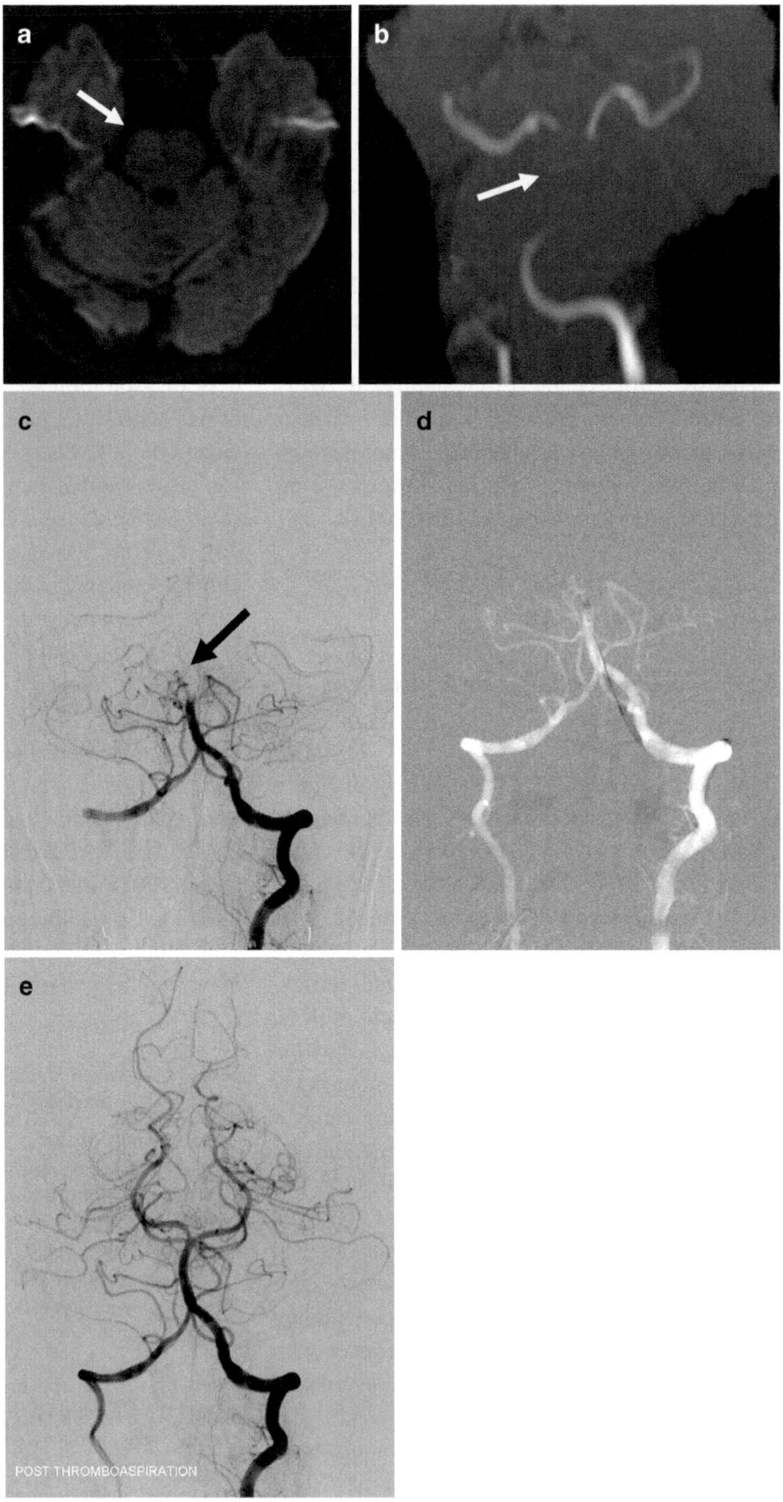


**Fig. 1** A 63-year-old female with sudden onset of left hemiplegia. NIHHSS = 12. (**a**) MRI diffusion-weighted image, axial slice, showing a faint hyperintense signal located on the right aspect of the pons (arrow). (**b**) 3D time-of-flight MR angiography demonstrating an occlusion of the mid- and distal aspects of the basilar artery (arrow). (**c**) Left vertebral artery digital subtraction angiography (DSA) in anteroposterior (AP) projection confirming the occlusion of the basilar artery, distally to the origin of the antero-inferior cerebellar arteries (arrow). (**d**) Road map from the left vertebral artery in AP projection. Navigation of a large bore catheter (0.068″) close to the occlusion site. After a 90s aspiration, the catheter is removed under aspiration with a pump. (**e**) Left vertebral artery DSA in AP projection at the end of the procedure. Complete recanalization of the basilar artery is seen, after one aspiration pass. The procedure, from the groin puncture to the final DSA run, lasted 15 min

30%, $P = 0.52$) but the study was prematurely stopped (108 patients enrolled; 692 patients planed for inclusion) after the publication of the results of the MR CLEAN trial (Berkhemer et al. 2015).

Only one RCT has compared the ADAPT technique vs the stent retriever technique: the ASTER trial (Lapergue et al. 2017). The results of this study showed no statistically significant difference in terms of recanalization rate or good clinical outcome between the two techniques. A non-significant trend toward a lower complication rate (emboli in a new territory, symptomatic hemorrhage) was observed in the group treated by the ADAPT technique.

### 4.2 Balloon Guiding Catheters

Balloon guiding catheters (BGCs) are guiding catheters with a balloon mounted at their tip. The balloon is inflated during the retrieval of the stent retriever in order to obtain flow arrest and to reduce the risk of emboli migration either in the same territory or in another one. A number of benchtop studies have shown the benefit of using BGCs to reduce distal emboli during MT and to obtain more effective revascularization (Chueh et al. 2013; Mokin et al. 2016). Numerous clinical studies have also shown a benefit in terms of angiographic and clinical outcomes with the use of BGCs in MT (Nguyen et al. 2014; Velasco et al. 2016). In a recent meta-analysis, it has been shown that patients treated with BGCs had higher odds of first-pass recanalization and higher rates of TICI 3 or TICI 2b/3 recanalizations (Brinjikji et al. 2018). Additionally, patients treated with BGCs had a higher rate of 3 months' good neurological outcome (59.7% vs 43.8%) and a lower mortality rate (13.7% vs 24.8%). Mean procedure time was also significantly shorter for patients treated with BGCs (weighted mean difference: −7.7 min, 95% CI − 9.0 to −6.4) (Brinjikji et al. 2018). It is however noteworthy that no RCT has proven the superiority of BGCs in MT over the other techniques.

### 4.3 Combined Technique

Numerous series have studied a technique combining aspiration catheter and stent retriever for clot removal (Delgado Almandoz et al. 2016) (Fig. 2). Various names have been given to this technique with faint variations: Solumbra (Delgado Almandoz et al. 2016), ARTS (aspiration-retriever technique for stroke) (Massari et al. 2016), SAVE (Stent retriever Assisted Vacuum-locked Extraction) (Maus et al. 2018).

Recently, a technique combining stent retriever + aspiration catheter + balloon guiding catheter (the so-called "PROTECT" [PRoximal balloon Occlusion TogEther with direCt Thrombus aspiration] technique) has been described, with promising results (Maegerlein et al. 2018). Finally, a RCT comparing BGC associated with intermediate catheter and stent retriever vs BGC with stent retriever alone has recently been performed (the "ASTER2" trial, ClinicalTrial NCT03290885); the results of this study will soon be published.

## 5 Safety of Mechanical Thrombectomy

The safety of MT has been proven, and regarding adverse events, many RCTs have proven that patients who underwent MT with BMT vs BMT alone did not have significantly higher mortality or symptomatic intracranial hemorrhage rates (Barral et al. 2018).

Mortality rate in patients treated by MT has been reported ranging from 9% to 21% (Berkhemer et al. 2015; Jovin et al. 2015; Goyal et al. 2015; Campbell et al. 2015; Saver et al. 2015), which is not significantly higher than in patients with LVO who received the BMT (Marmagkiolis et al. 2015).

A meta-analysis has found a symptomatic intracranial hemorrhage rate of 5.6% in patients treated by MT (range: 0–7.7%), which is quite similar to the one of medical treatment (5.2%) (Hao et al. 2017). However, the rate of asymptomatic intracranial hemorrhage is higher in

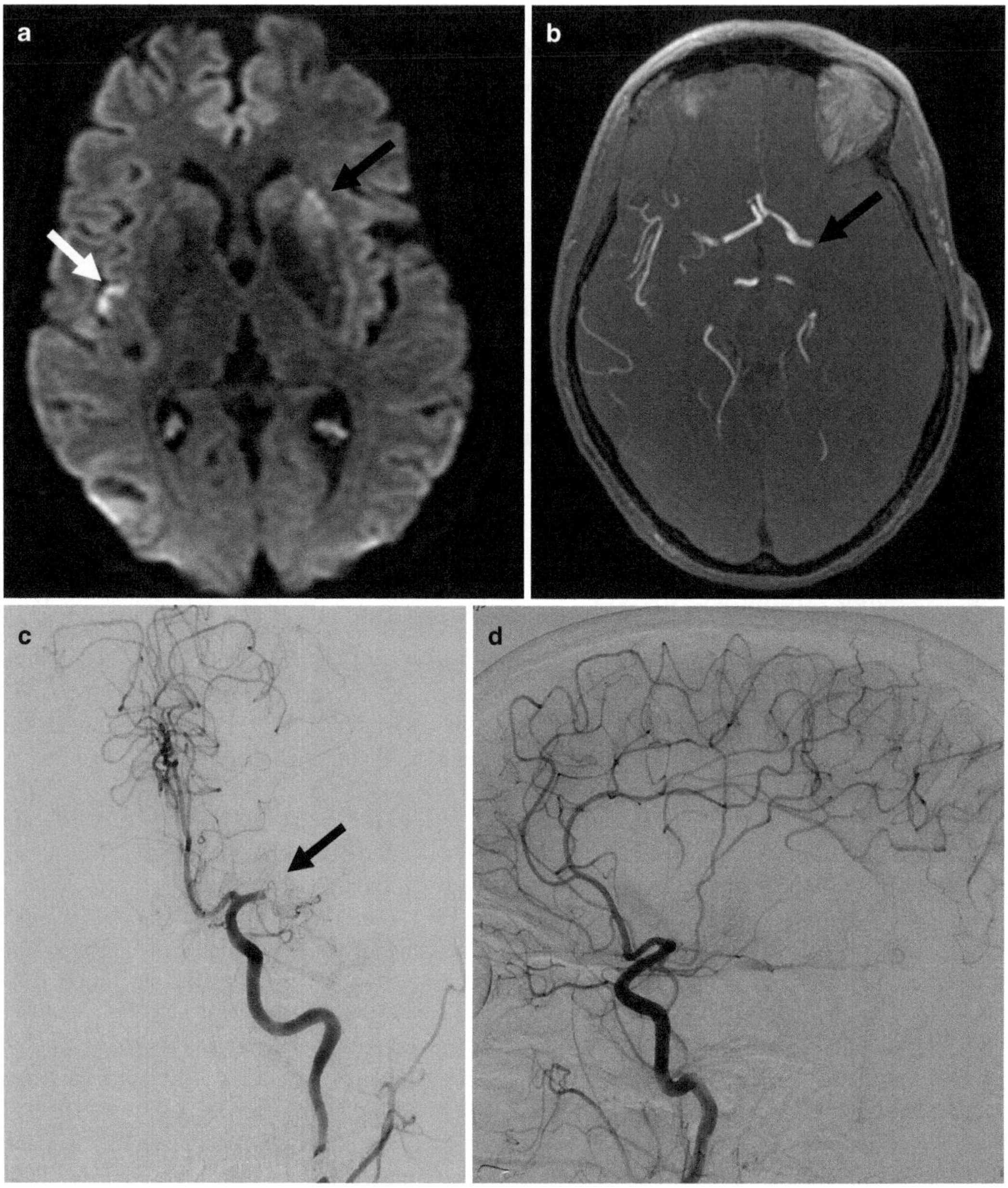


**Fig. 2** A 47-year-old female presenting a sudden onset of right hemiplegia and aphasia (NIHSS = 24). (**a**) MRI diffusion-weighted image, axial slice, showing a slight hyperintense signal on the right insula (white arrow) and of the left caudate nucleus (black arrow). (**b**) 3D time-of-flight MR angiography demonstrating an occlusion of the left MCA (M1 segment). Left internal carotid artery (ICA) DSA in AP (**c**) and lateral (**d**) projections showing an occlusion of the M1 segment (**c**, arrow) with hypoperfusion of the whole left MCA territory (**d**). (**e**) Road map from the left ICA with the aspiration catheter positioned in M1 (black arrow) and the stent retriever opened in the thrombus (white arrowhead). (**f**) Retrieval of the stent retriever inside the aspiration catheter under aspiration (black arrow, aspiration catheter's tip; white arrowhead, stent retriever). On control DSA in AP (**g**) and lateral (**h**) projection, complete recanalization of the left MCA territory is seen (mTICI3)

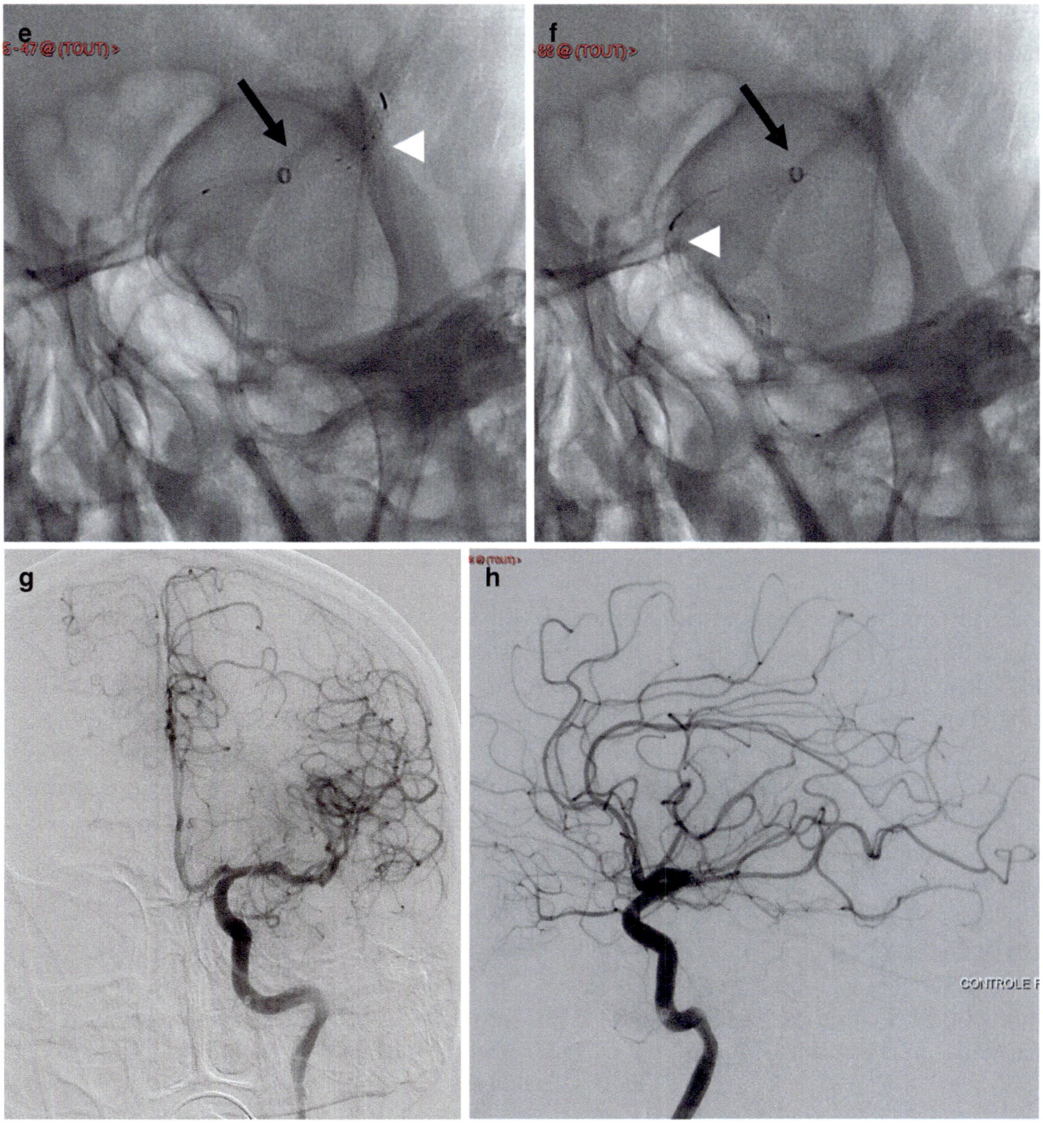


**Fig. 2** (continued)

patients treated by MT compared with BMT (28% vs 13.9%) (Hao et al. 2017). The perforation rate (with either the microguide wire, the microcatheter, or the stent retriever) in MT has been reported ranging from 0% to 4.9% in the first RCTs (Berkhemer et al. 2015; Jovin et al. 2015; Goyal et al. 2015; Campbell et al. 2015; Saver et al. 2015).

Migration of emboli in another territory (for instance migration in an embolus in the anterior cerebral artery during an MCA thrombectomy) may also occur during MT and may worsen the patient's clinical condition. They have been reported occurring as frequently as in about 10% of the cases (Chalumeau et al. 2018).

Another complication that may occur after MT is a groin hematoma. Groin hematomas may be observed in about 5% of the cases (Chivot et al. 2018). Most of these hematomas are ≤5 cm and do not require surgical treatment and/or blood transfusion. They are not more frequently observed in patients who received IV tPA, or those previously treated with antiplatelet therapy. Interestingly, groin hematomas are not more frequent when the puncture is ipsilateral to the inferior limb's neurological deficit (Chivot et al. 2018).

## 6 Effectiveness of Mechanical Thrombectomy

Effectiveness of MT in terms of recanalization (mTICI 2b-3) has been reported ranging from 58.7% to 100% in the recent RCTs (Berkhemer et al. 2015; Jovin et al. 2015; Goyal et al. 2015; Campbell et al. 2015; Saver et al. 2015). The pooled estimate of patients with mTICI 2b–3 after MT was 71% (95% CI: 62–79%). These RCTs also demonstrated a significant improvement in terms of neurological outcome (mRS scores 0–2 at 3 months) in patients treated with MT: OR = 2.14, 95% CI: 1.72–2.67 ($P < 0.00001$) (Barral et al. 2018).

Only three studies (REVASCAT (Jovin et al. 2015), ESCAPE (Goyal et al. 2015), and THRACE (Bracard et al. 2016)) reported the results of Barthel index scores and showed the superiority of MT + BMT over BMT alone (scores of 95–100 at 3 months, OR: 2.43, 95% CI) (Barral et al. 2018).

However, it is noteworthy that MT has no significant impact on survival rate (OR: 0.82, 95% CI: 0.62–1.07) (Barral et al. 2018).

## 7 Questions Yet to be Answered

### 7.1 Is Intravenous Thrombolysis Still Necessary in Combination with Mechanical Thrombectomy?

In all the RCTs demonstrating the effectiveness of MT, endovascular treatment was associated with the BMT, being most of times the IV thrombolysis. One could wonder if IV thrombolysis is really required in combination with MT. Indeed, IV tPA could potentially be responsible for higher intracranial hemorrhage rates and may worsen puncture site complications. Additionally, IV thrombolysis may lead to a clot fragmentation, which could be responsible for more challenging MT procedures with numerous distal emboli to remove instead of one proximal thrombus.

Results from non-randomized studies are contradictory. Indeed, some series have clearly shown the benefit of additional IV thrombolysis in combination with MT (Goyal et al. 2018). Others found no clinical benefit in combining MT with IV thrombolysis (Coutinho et al. 2017; Kass-Hout et al. 2014).

Additionally, symptomatic hemorrhages and groin puncture complication rates are not statically higher in patients treated by MT and IV thrombolysis.

The only RCT that compared BMT alone vs MT, the Synthesis-Expansion trial (Ciccone et al. 2013), was in disfavor of MT. However, in this study, numerous endovascular procedures were not performed with the most recent MT devices, such as stent retrievers.

More evidences on the benefit of pre-MT IV thrombolysis are yet to be provided, through RCTs using the most recent MT devices.

### 7.2 Distal Occlusions

In the RCTs, most of the occlusion sites were proximal (i.e., ICA terminus or proximal M1). Only limited data on the effectiveness of MT in distal occlusions are thus available. In the above-mentioned RCTs that proved the benefit of MT in LVO (Berkhemer et al. 2015; Jovin et al. 2015; Goyal et al. 2015; Campbell et al. 2015; Saver et al. 2015; Bracard et al. 2016; Mocco et al. 2016), the rate of patients included with a M2 occlusion ranged from 1% to 14.3%.

No RCT has evaluated the benefit of MT in M2 occlusions. According to a recent meta-analysis (Saber et al. 2018), recanalization after MT in M2 occlusions is obtained in 81% of the cases, with no significant difference with the recanalization rate in M1 occlusions. Good clinical outcome is obtained in 56.2% of the cases for MT in M2 occlusions, which is significantly higher than in M1 occlusions (Saber et al. 2018). However, it is noteworthy that patients with a M1 occlusion usually have a poorer initial condition than those with a M2 occlusion (Bhogal et al. 2017). Additionally, MT in M2 occlusions may be associated with a higher risk of vessel perforation due to vessel fragility (Mokin et al. 2017) and an increased risk of symptomatic intracranial hemorrhage (Saber et al. 2018).

Finally, it should be mentioned that only short retrospective case series (Uno et al. 2018) are available on the effectiveness of MT in anterior cerebral arteries occlusions, and no series has been published on PCA occlusions treated by MT. No RCTs studying the effectiveness of MT + BMT vs BMT alone are available for these specific occlusion sites.

### 7.3 Basilar Artery Occlusions

To date, no RCT has demonstrated the superiority of MT combined with the BMT over the BMT alone in patients with basilar artery occlusion (BAO). A systematic review of the literature showed a recanalization rate ranging from 44 to 100% (average 80%) and a good 3 months' clinical outcome from 20 to 58% (average 43%) in patients with BAO treated by MT. A recent meta-analysis (Gory et al. 2016) showed a 3 months' favorable outcome in 42% of the patients and a mortality rate of 30%. Symptomatic intracranial hemorrhage rate in this meta-analysis was 4%. Predictors of mortality in patients treated by MT for BAO were mainly age ≥60 years, a high initial NIHSS at admission, and absence of successful recanalization (Gory et al. 2018). Two prospective RCTs (BASICS [NCT01717755] and Best [NCT02441556] trials) are currently ongoing, comparing MT + BMT vs BMT alone in order to prove definitively the effectiveness of MT in BAO.

### 7.4 Anesthesia for Mechanical Thrombectomy

The best strategy for anesthesia (i.e., general anesthesia, conscious sedation, or local anesthesia) in MT is still debated. A first meta-analysis from the recent RCTs (Ouyang et al. 2016) showed evidences of a better outcome in patients treated under conscious sedation vs general anesthesia. However, these results were biased since no randomization was performed on this criterion. Additionally, one could wonder that patients in worse condition at admission, who will usually have the worse clinical outcome at follow-up, were more frequently treated under general anesthesia due to an agitation or a comatose state. Three RCTs (Schonenberger et al. 2016; Lowhagen Henden et al. 2017; Simonsen et al. 2018) have been published, comparing general anesthesia vs non-general anesthesia MT. In all these 3 RCTs, no significant difference was observed in terms of clinical outcome between the two techniques. Interestingly, these studies were all mono-centric.

## 8 Conclusion

In recent years, MT has radically changed the management of patients with AIS secondary to LVO. Numerous evidences have been gathered on its safety and effectiveness and have shown its superiority compared with the BMT alone. Time window for MT has been recently expanded for patients with a small core infarct.

Numerous questions have yet to be answered, especially for distal occlusions or basilar artery occlusions.

## References

Albers GW, Marks MP, Kemp S, Christensen S, Tsai JP, Ortega-Gutierrez S et al (2018) Thrombectomy for stroke at 6 to 16 hours with selection by perfusion imaging. N Engl J Med 378:708–718

Barral M, Boudour S, Viprey M, Giroudon C, Aulagner G, Schott AM et al (2018) Stent retriever thrombectomy for acute ischemic stroke: a systematic review and meta-analysis of randomized controlled trials, including thrace. Rev Neurol (Paris) 174:319–326

Berkhemer OA, van Zwam WH, Dippel DW, Investigators MC (2015) Stent-retriever thrombectomy for stroke. N Engl J Med 373:1076

Bhogal P, Bucke P, AlMatter M, Ganslandt O, Bazner H, Henkes H et al (2017) A comparison of mechanical thrombectomy in the m1 and m2 segments of the middle cerebral artery: a review of 585 consecutive patients. Interv Neurol 6:191–198

Bracard S, Ducrocq X, Mas JL, Soudant M, Oppenheim C, Moulin T et al (2016) Mechanical thrombectomy after intravenous alteplase versus alteplase alone after stroke (THRACE): a randomised controlled trial. Lancet Neurol 15:1138–1147

Brinjikji W, Starke RM, Murad MH, Fiorella D, Pereira VM, Goyal M et al (2018) Impact of balloon guide catheter on technical and clinical outcomes: a systematic review and meta-analysis. J Neurointerv Surg. 10:335–339

Broderick JP, Tomsick TA, Palesch YY (2013) Endovascular treatment for acute ischemic stroke. N Engl J Med 368:2432–2433

Campbell BC, Mitchell PJ, Kleinig TJ, Dewey HM, Churilov L, Yassi N et al (2015) Endovascular therapy for ischemic stroke with perfusion-imaging selection. N Engl J Med 372:1009–1018

Campbell BC, Hill MD, Rubiera M, Menon BK, Demchuk A, Donnan GA et al (2016) Safety and efficacy of solitaire stent thrombectomy: individual patient data meta-analysis of randomized trials. Stroke 47:798–806

Chalumeau V, Blanc R, Redjem H, Ciccio G, Smajda S, Desilles JP et al (2018) Anterior cerebral artery embolism during thrombectomy increases disability and mortality. J Neurointerv Surg. https://doi.org/10.1136/neurintsurg-2018-013793

Chivot C, Deramond H, Bouzerar R, Yzet T (2018) Safety and efficacy of femoral artery closure with the femoseal device after cerebral thrombectomy using an 8 french sheath. Eur J Vasc Endovasc Surg 55:730–734

Chueh JY, Kuhn AL, Puri AS, Wilson SD, Wakhloo AK, Gounis MJ (2013) Reduction in distal emboli with proximal flow control during mechanical thrombectomy: a quantitative in vitro study. Stroke 44:1396–1401

Chueh JY, Puri AS, Wakhloo AK, Gounis MJ (2016) Risk of distal embolization with stent retriever thrombectomy and adapt. J Neurointerv Surg. 8:197–202

Ciccone A, Valvassori L, Investigators SE (2013) Endovascular treatment for acute ischemic stroke. N Engl J Med 368:2433–2434

Clarencon F, Rosso C, Degos V, Shotar E, Rolla-Bigliani C, Samson Y et al (2018) Triage in the angiography suite for mechanical thrombectomy in acute ischemic stroke: not such a good idea. AJNR Am J Neuroradiol 39:E59–E60

Coutinho JM, Liebeskind DS, Slater LA, Nogueira RG, Clark W, Davalos A et al (2017) Combined intravenous thrombolysis and thrombectomy vs thrombectomy alone for acute ischemic stroke: a pooled analysis of the swift and star studies. JAMA Neurol 74:268–274

Delgado Almandoz JE, Kayan Y, Young ML, Fease JL, Scholz JM, Milner AM et al (2016) Comparison of clinical outcomes in patients with acute ischemic strokes treated with mechanical thrombectomy using either solumbra or adapt techniques. J Neurointerv Surg. 8:1123–1128

Detraz L, Ernst M, Bourcier R (2018) Stroke transfer and its organizational paradigm : review of organizational paradigms and the impact on outcome. Clin Neuroradiol. https://doi.org/10.1007/s00062-018-0715-z

Ebinger M, Kunz A, Wendt M, Rozanski M, Winter B, Waldschmidt C et al (2015) Effects of golden hour thrombolysis: a prehospital acute neurological treatment and optimization of medical care in stroke (phantom-s) substudy. JAMA Neurol 72:25–30

El-Ghanem M, Al-Mufti F, Thulasi V, Singh IP, Gandhi C (2017) Expanding the treatment window for ischemic stroke through the application of novel system-based technology. Neurosurg Focus 42:E7

Gerschenfeld G, Muresan IP, Blanc R, Obadia M, Abrivard M, Piotin M et al (2017) Two paradigms for endovascular thrombectomy after intravenous thrombolysis for acute ischemic stroke. JAMA Neurol 74:549–556

Gory B, Eldesouky I, Sivan-Hoffmann R, Rabilloud M, Ong E, Riva R et al (2016) Outcomes of stent retriever thrombectomy in basilar artery occlusion: an observational study and systematic review. J Neurol Neurosurg Psychiatry 87:520–525

Gory B, Mazighi M, Labreuche J, Blanc R, Piotin M, Turjman F et al (2018) Predictors for mortality after mechanical thrombectomy of acute basilar artery occlusion. Cerebrovasc Dis 45:61–67

Goyal M, Demchuk AM, Menon BK, Eesa M, Rempel JL, Thornton J et al (2015) Randomized assessment of rapid endovascular treatment of ischemic stroke. N Engl J Med 372:1019–1030

Goyal N, Tsivgoulis G, Frei D, Turk A, Baxter B, Froehler MT et al (2018) Comparative safety and efficacy of combined ivt and mt with direct mt in large vessel occlusion. Neurology 90:e1274–e1282

Hao Y, Zhang Z, Zhang H, Xu L, Ye Z, Dai Q et al (2017) Risk of intracranial hemorrhage after endovascular treatment for acute ischemic stroke: systematic review and meta-analysis. Interv Neurol. 6:57–64

Hastrup S, Damgaard D, Johnsen SP, Andersen G (2016) Prehospital acute stroke severity scale to predict large artery occlusion: design and comparison with other scales. Stroke 47:1772–1776

Hiyama N, Yoshimura S, Shirakawa M, Uchida K, Oki Y, Shindo S et al (2016) Safety and effectiveness of drip, ship, and retrieve paradigm for acute ischemic stroke: a single center experience. Neurol Med Chir (Tokyo) 56:731–736

John S, Stock S, Cerejo R, Uchino K, Winners S, Russman A et al (2016) Brain imaging using mobile ct: current status and future prospects. J Neuroimaging 26:5–15

Jovin TG, Chamorro A, Cobo E, de Miquel MA, Molina CA, Rovira A et al (2015) Thrombectomy within 8 hours after symptom onset in ischemic stroke. N Engl J Med 372:2296–2306

Kang DH, Park J (2017) Endovascular stroke therapy focused on stent retriever thrombectomy and direct clot aspiration: historical review and modern application. J Korean Neurosurg Soc 60:335–347

Kass-Hout T, Kass-Hout O, Mokin M, Thesier DM, Yashar P, Orion D et al (2014) Is bridging with intravenous thrombolysis of any benefit in endovascular therapy for acute ischemic stroke? World Neurosurg 82:e453–e458

Katz BS, McMullan JT, Sucharew H, Adeoye O, Broderick JP (2015) Design and validation of a prehospital scale to predict stroke severity: Cincinnati prehospital stroke severity scale. Stroke 46:1508–1512

Kidwell CS, Jahan R, Gornbein J, Alger JR, Nenov V, Ajani Z et al (2013) A trial of imaging selection and endovascular treatment for ischemic stroke. N Engl J Med 368:914–923

Lanzino G, Murad MH, d'Urso PI, Rabinstein AA (2013) Coil embolization versus clipping for ruptured intracranial aneurysms: a meta-analysis of prospective controlled published studies. AJNR Am J Neuroradiol 34:1764–1768

Lapergue B, Blanc R, Gory B, Labreuche J, Duhamel A, Marnat G et al (2017) Effect of endovascular contact aspiration vs stent retriever on revascularization in patients with acute ischemic stroke and large vessel occlusion: the aster randomized clinical trial. JAMA 318:443–452

Lima FO, Silva GS, Furie KL, Frankel MR, Lev MH, Camargo EC et al (2016) Field assessment stroke triage for emergency destination: a simple and accurate prehospital scale to detect large vessel occlusion strokes. Stroke 47:1997–2002

Lowhagen Henden P, Rentzos A, Karlsson JE, Rosengren L, Leiram B, Sundeman H et al (2017) General anesthesia versus conscious sedation for endovascular treatment of acute ischemic stroke: the AnStroke trial (anesthesia during stroke). Stroke 48:1601–1607

Maegerlein C, Monch S, Boeckh-Behrens T, Lehm M, Hedderich DM, Berndt MT et al (2018) Protect: proximal balloon occlusion together with direct thrombus aspiration during stent retriever thrombectomy - evaluation of a double embolic protection approach in endovascular stroke treatment. J Neurointerv Surg. 10:751–755

Marmagkiolis K, Hakeem A, Cilingiroglu M, Gundogdu B, Iliescu C, Tsitlakidou D et al (2015) Safety and efficacy of stent retrievers for the management of acute ischemic stroke: comprehensive review and meta-analysis. JACC Cardiovasc Interv 8:1758–1765

Massari F, Henninger N, Lozano JD, Patel A, Kuhn AL, Howk M et al (2016) Arts (aspiration-retriever technique for stroke): initial clinical experience. Interv Neuroradiol 22:325–332

Maus V, Behme D, Kabbasch C, Borggrefe J, Tsogkas I, Nikoubashman O et al (2018) Maximizing first-pass complete reperfusion with save. Clin Neuroradiol 28:327–338

Mocco J, Zaidat OO, von Kummer R, Yoo AJ, Gupta R, Lopes D et al (2016) Aspiration thrombectomy after intravenous alteplase versus intravenous alteplase alone. Stroke 47:2331–2338

Mokin M, Setlur Nagesh SV, Ionita CN, Mocco J, Siddiqui AH (2016) Stent retriever thrombectomy with the cover accessory device versus proximal protection with a balloon guide catheter: in vitro stroke model comparison. J Neurointerv Surg. 8:413–417

Mokin M, Fargen KM, Primiani CT, Ren Z, Dumont TM, Brasiliense LBC et al (2017) Vessel perforation during stent retriever thrombectomy for acute ischemic stroke: technical details and clinical outcomes. J Neurointerv Surg. 9:922–928

Nguyen TN, Malisch T, Castonguay AC, Gupta R, Sun CH, Martin CO et al (2014) Balloon guide catheter improves revascularization and clinical outcomes with the solitaire device: analysis of the north american solitaire acute stroke registry. Stroke 45:141–145

Nogueira RG, Jadhav AP, Haussen DC, Bonafe A, Budzik RF, Bhuva P et al (2018) Thrombectomy 6 to 24 hours after stroke with a mismatch between deficit and infarct. N Engl J Med 378:11–21

Ouyang F, Chen Y, Zhao Y, Dang G, Liang J, Zeng J (2016) Selection of patients and anesthetic types for endovascular treatment in acute ischemic stroke: a meta-analysis of randomized controlled trials. PLoS One 11:e0151210

Park MS, Yoon W, Kim JT, Choi KH, Kang SH, Kim BC et al (2016a) Drip, ship, and on-demand endovascular therapy for acute ischemic stroke. PLoS One 11:e0150668

Park MS, Lee JS, Park TH, Cho YJ, Hong KS, Park JM et al (2016b) Characteristics of the drip-and-ship paradigm for patients with acute ischemic stroke in South Korea. J Stroke Cerebrovasc Dis 25:2678–2687

Perez de la Ossa N, Carrera D, Gorchs M, Querol M, Millan M, Gomis M et al (2014) Design and validation of a prehospital stroke scale to predict large arterial occlusion: the rapid arterial occlusion evaluation scale. Stroke 45:87–91

Powers WJ, Derdeyn CP, Biller J, Coffey CS, Hoh BL, Jauch EC et al (2015) 2015 American heart association/American stroke association focused update of the 2013 guidelines for the early management of patients with acute ischemic stroke regarding endovascular treatment: a guideline for healthcare professionals from the American heart association/American stroke association. Stroke 46:3020–3035

Powers WJ, Rabinstein AA, Ackerson T, Adeoye OM, Bambakidis NC, Becker K et al (2018) 2018 guidelines for the early management of patients with acute ischemic stroke: a guideline for healthcare professionals from the American heart association/American stroke association. Stroke 49:e46–e110

Ribo M, Boned S, Rubiera M, Tomasello A, Coscojuela P, Hernandez D et al (2017) Direct transfer to angiosuite to reduce door-to-puncture time in thrombectomy for acute stroke. J Neurointerv Surg. https://doi.org/10.1136/neurintsurg-2017-013038.

Ribo M, Boned S, Rubiera M, Tomasello A, Coscojuela P, Hernandez D et al (2018) Direct transfer to angiosuite to reduce door-to-puncture time in thrombectomy for acute stroke. J Neurointerv Surg. 10:221–224

Saber H, Narayanan S, Palla M, Saver JL, Nogueira RG, Yoo AJ et al (2018) Mechanical thrombectomy for acute ischemic stroke with occlusion of the m2 segment of the middle cerebral artery: a meta-analysis. J Neurointerv Surg 10:620–624

Saver JL, Goyal M, Bonafe A, Diener HC, Levy EI, Pereira VM et al (2015) Stent-retriever thrombectomy after intravenous t-pa vs. T-pa alone in stroke. N Engl J Med 372:2285–2295
Saver JL, Goyal M, van der Lugt A, Menon BK, Majoie CB, Dippel DW et al (2016) Time to treatment with endovascular thrombectomy and outcomes from ischemic stroke: a meta-analysis. JAMA 316:1279–1288
Schonenberger S, Uhlmann L, Hacke W, Schieber S, Mundiyanapurath S, Purrucker JC et al (2016) Effect of conscious sedation vs general anesthesia on early neurological improvement among patients with ischemic stroke undergoing endovascular thrombectomy: a randomized clinical trial. JAMA 316:1986–1996
Simonsen CZ, Yoo AJ, Sorensen LH, Juul N, Johnsen SP, Andersen G et al (2018) Effect of general anesthesia and conscious sedation during endovascular therapy on infarct growth and clinical outcomes in acute ischemic stroke: a randomized clinical trial. JAMA Neurol 75:470–477
Taqui A, Cerejo R, Itrat A, Briggs FB, Reimer AP, Winners S et al (2017) Reduction in time to treatment in prehospital telemedicine evaluation and thrombolysis. Neurology 88:1305–1312
Turc G, Maier B, Naggara O, Seners P, Isabel C, Tisserand M et al (2016) Clinical scales do not reliably identify acute ischemic stroke patients with large-artery occlusion. Stroke 47:1466–1472
Uno J, Kameda K, Otsuji R, Ren N, Nagaoka S, Maeda K et al (2018) Mechanical thrombectomy for acute anterior cerebral artery occlusion. World Neurosurg. https://doi.org/10.1016/j.wneu.2018.08.196
van der Bom IM, Mehra M, Walvick RP, Chueh JY, Gounis MJ (2012) Quantitative evaluation of c-arm ct cerebral blood volume in a canine model of ischemic stroke. AJNR Am J Neuroradiol 33:353–358
Velasco A, Buerke B, Stracke CP, Berkemeyer S, Mosimann PJ, Schwindt W et al (2016) Comparison of a balloon guide catheter and a non-balloon guide catheter for mechanical thrombectomy. Radiology 280:169–176
Wei D, Mascitelli JR, Nistal DA, Kellner CP, Fifi JT, Mocco JD et al (2017) The use and utility of aspiration thrombectomy in acute ischemic stroke: a systematic review and meta-analysis. AJNR Am J Neuroradiol 38:1978–1983
Zaidat OO, Yoo AJ, Khatri P, Tomsick TA, von Kummer R, Saver JL et al (2013) Recommendations on angiographic revascularization grading standards for acute ischemic stroke: a consensus statement. Stroke 44:2650–2663

# Nontraumatic Intracranial Hemorrhage

Merve Gürsoy, Raffaella Basilico, and Cem Çalli

## Contents



## 1 Nontraumatic Intracranial Hemorrhage

Nontraumatic intracranial hemorrhage (ICH) accounts for 10–15% of all strokes. Although the incidence of ischemic stroke is decreasing globally, the incidence of ICH is increased in older adults in association with the use of oral anticoagulants (Flaherty et al. 2007; Bejot et al. 2013). In addition, there has been significant improvement in the management of and treatments for ischemic stroke, whereas the same is not applicable to ICH, which is still associated with high mortality and morbidity. ICH case fatality rate in the first month exceeds 50%, and only 20% of the survivors achieve full functional recovery within 6 months (van Asch et al. 2010).

Nontraumatic (spontaneous) ICH may be linked to many causes, and it is important to know the anatomic localization of the bleeding in order to reveal the underlying cause. The term ICH refers to bleeding into the brain parenchyma. However, bleeding may also extend to the subarachnoid space, subdural space, intraventricular space, or rarely to the epidural space. ICH can be classified as deep, lobar, and posterior fossa according to its localization. Deep ICH is the most common type, whereas posterior fossa is the rarest localization of ICH. Localization of the bleeding, patient's age, and clinical history (use

M. Gürsoy
Faculty of Medicine, Department of Radiology, Izmir Katip Celebi University, Izmir, Turkey

R. Basilico
Department of Neuroscience, Imaging and Clinical Sciencfves, Ss Annunziata Hospital "G. d'Annunzio" University, Chieti, Italy

C. Çalli (✉)
Department of Radiology, Ege University Medical School, Izmir, Turkey



M. Scaglione et al. (eds.), *Emergency Radiology of the Head and Spine*,
Medical Radiology Diagnostic Imaging, https://doi.org/10.1007/978-3-030-91047-1_6

of oral anticoagulants, hypertension, etc.) help narrow down the list of differential diagnoses that may be the cause of bleeding. The most common causes of nontraumatic ICH are hypertension and cerebral amyloid angiopathy (CAA) in older adults, and vascular anomaly and venous thrombosis in younger patients.

The first clinical manifestation of ICH is a sudden focal neurologic deficit which changes depending on the localization of the bleeding and frequently coexists with decreased level of consciousness, headache, and seizure. Hematomas expand in a few hours, and the clinical presentation progressively worsens in one-third of the patients with ICH (Delcourt et al. 2012). Therefore, prompt neuroimaging is critical. It was shown that the expansion of bleeding could be demonstrated better in patients who promptly undergo imaging (Fujii et al. 1998). Moreover, since the clinical findings of ischemic stroke and ICH are similar, neuroimaging is needed to distinguish between these 2 entities and to reveal the underlying cause.

## 2 Neuroimaging of ICH

Noncontrast computed tomography (CT), magnetic resonance imaging (MRI), and digital subtraction angiography (DSA) are frequently used to diagnose patients suspected of having ICH and to understand the cause of the condition.

### 2.1 Computed Tomography

Noncontrast CT is the primary imaging method of choice since it can be performed rapidly, showing bleeding with high sensitivity, and it is easily accessible in an emergency room setting. Noncontrast CT can both show the presence of bleeding and help evaluate the localization and size of the bleeding, presence of intraventricular hemorrhage as well as edema and mass effect that coexist with the hemorrhage. Blood may appear hyperdense on CT within a few minutes after extravasating from the vessel. Approximately after the third day, attenuation values of the clot start to drop and it becomes isodense within a few weeks (Fig. 1). Therefore, while CT and MRI can show acute bleeding with similar sensitivity, MRI is superior to CT in showing chronic bleeding (Kidwell et al. 2004). In intraparenchymal hemorrhage, a hypodense area is observed around the hyperdense bleeding and it is caused by the serum from the retracted clot. The mentioned hypodensity reaches its maximum on day 5 with added vasogenic edema. Chronic hematomas appear as hypodense areas. Residual hypodensity, calcification, or slit-like lesions can be observed or there can be no signs on CT scans after the hemorrhage (Kreel et al. 1991).

CT angiography (CTA) is routinely performed at many centers along with CT in patients who are clinically suspected of having ICH or following the demonstration of hemorrhage with CT. CTA is especially recommended for young patients who have lobar hemorrhage without history of hypertension (Hemphill 3rd et al. 2015). In this patient group, CTA can help identify the cause of bleeding by showing vascular anomalies that frequently cause hemorrhage. Moreover, CTA may show the presence of "spot sign" on source images. Spot sign is defined as foci enhancement of 1–2 mm size in hematoma and implies active bleeding. Presence of a spot sign is an independent predictor of hematoma expansion and poor prognosis (Fig. 2) (Wada et al. 2007; Demchuk et al. 2012). Early hemostatic therapy (recombinant factor VIIa) was shown to potentially improve the prognosis of ICH by preventing the expansion of hematomas. However, the importance of spot sign in terms of showing which patients can benefit from hemostatic therapy and its exact role in treatment management remains to be demonstrated.

### 2.2 Magnetic Resonance Imaging

MRI is more sensitive than CT, especially for hemorrhages localized in the brain stem and posterior fossa as well as microbleeds associated with cerebral amyloid angiopathy (CAA) and hypertension. Appearance of blood on MRI is more complex than on CT scans, and the findings

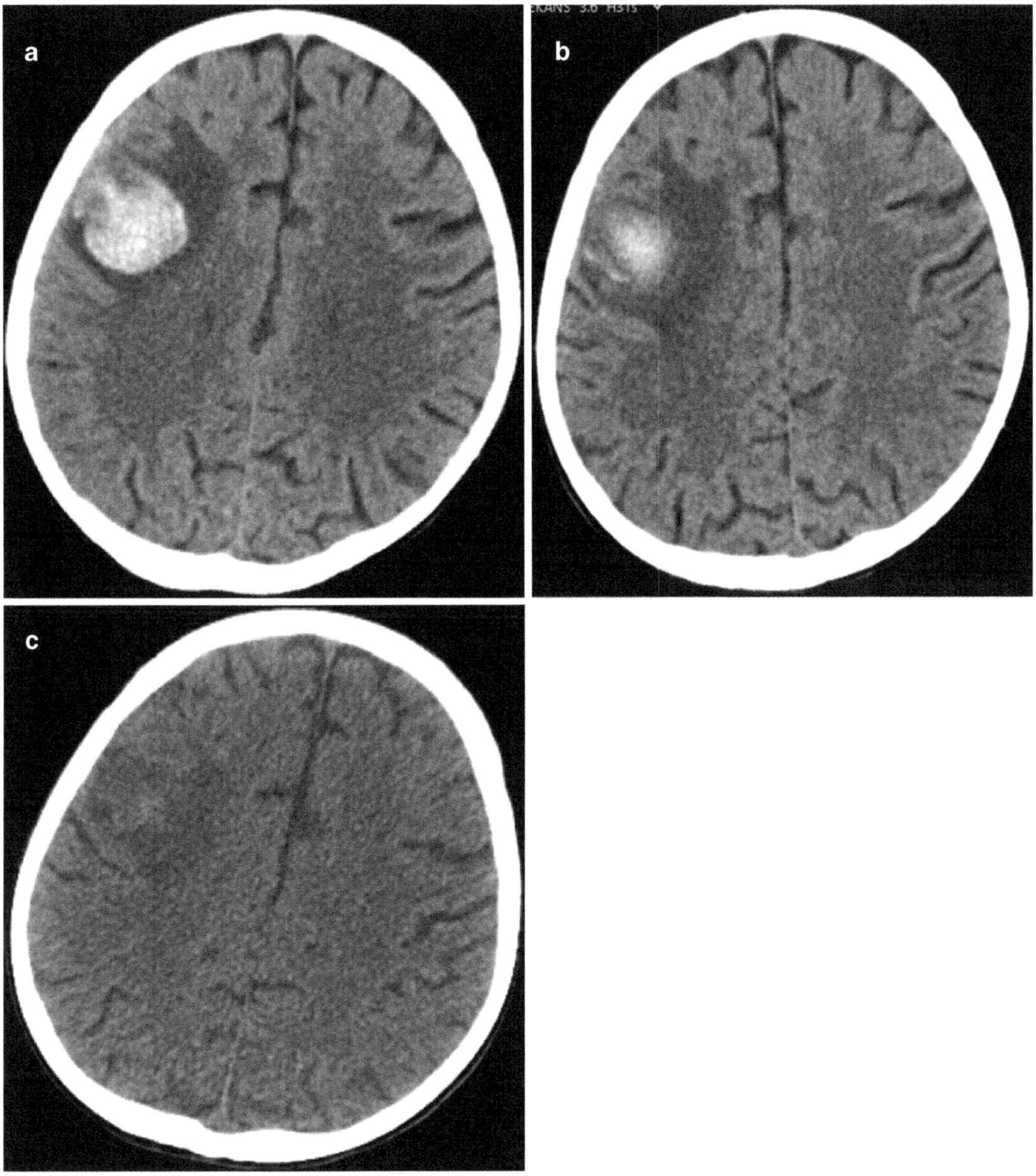


**Fig. 1** Left frontal acute hematoma. (**a**) Hematoma appears hyperdense on first admission. (**b**) The density of hematoma decreases on day eighth with increasing diameter of peripheral edema. (**c**) On day 19th, the hematoma is almost isodense to cerebral parenchyma with continuation of peripheral edema

of imaging vary depending on the stage of bleeding and MRI sequence (Table 1). The variability of the findings depending on stage stem from the transformation of blood products from oxyhemoglobin to hemosiderin and ferritin.

Susceptibility-weighted imaging (SWI) is a modality that combines T2* imaging and phase information to detect products that change the intensity of the local magnetic field (Haacke et al. 2009). Blood products such as ferritin and hemosiderin have paramagnetic nature that changes the intensity of an external magnetic field and they appear as signal loss on SWI. SWI is significantly superior to the standard gradient recalled echo (GRE) sequence in detecting hemorrhage in the brain (Wycliffe et al. 2004).

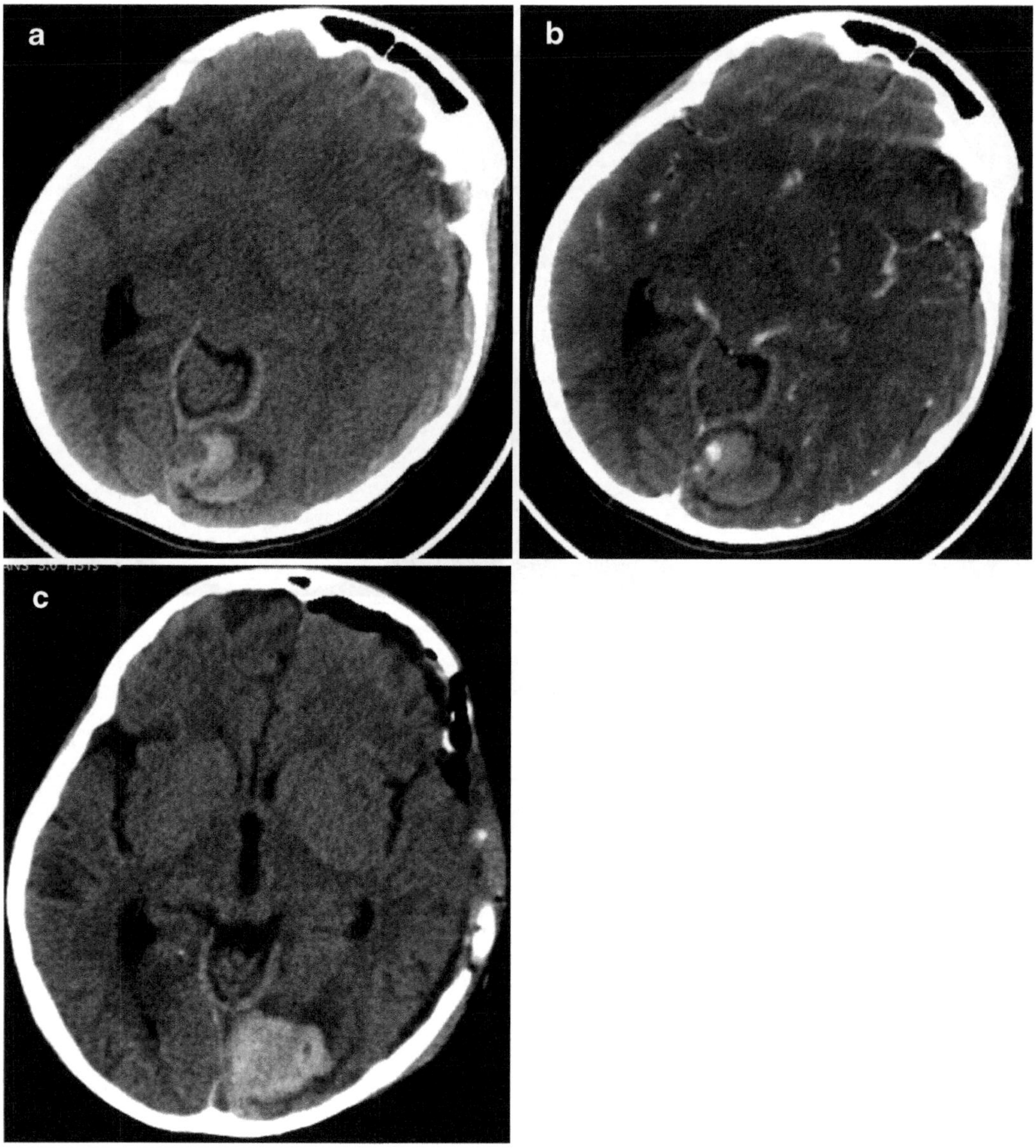


**Fig. 2** Hematoma and the "Spot sign". (**a**) Left occipital hematoma is depicted on pre-contrast CT image. (**b**) CTA in the same session shows nodular focal enhancement inside the hematoma, so called "Spot sign" which predicts further hematoma growth. (**c**) CT examination after 2 days proves the increase in size of the hematoma

Another method that is used in neurovascular imaging and that employs a GRE sequence is time-of-flight MR angiography (TOF MRA). It utilizes flow-related enhancement. TOF MRA has high sensitivity for evaluating flow dynamics and detecting vascular lesions, and it does not require a contrast, which is the best advantage of this method.

MRI with diffusion-weighted imaging (DWI) is highly useful in detecting hemorrhagic transformation of ischemic stroke. The location and size of the infarct underlying the bleeding which can be overlooked in noncontrast CT can be clearly determined with DWI. However, emergency MRI cannot be performed in many cases due to limited time, costs, and patients who cannot tolerate the test.

**Table 1** MRI Signal Characteristics and CT appearance of Different Stages of Intracranial Hemorrhage (Figs. 3, 4, 5, and 6)

| Stage | Phase of hemoglobin | CT | T1WI | T2WI |
|---|---|---|---|---|
| Hyperacute (<12 h) | Oxyhemoglobin | High density (high protein) | Isointense to hypointense | Hyperintense with hypointense rim |
| Acute (12 h to 3 days) | Deoxyhemoglobin | High density (high protein) | Isointense | Hypointense |
| Early subacute (3–7 days) | Intracellular methemoglobin | High density (high protein) | Hyperintense | Hypointense |
| Late subacute (7–14 days) | Extracellular methemoglobin | Isodense (absorption of high protein) | Hyperintense | Hyperintense |
| Chronic (>2 weeks) | Hemosiderin and ferritin | Low density (atrophy) | Hypointense | Hypointense |

*MRI* magnetic resonance imaging, *CT* computed tomography, *T1WI* T1-weighted image, *T2WI* T2-weighted image

Hypointense Isointense Hyperintense

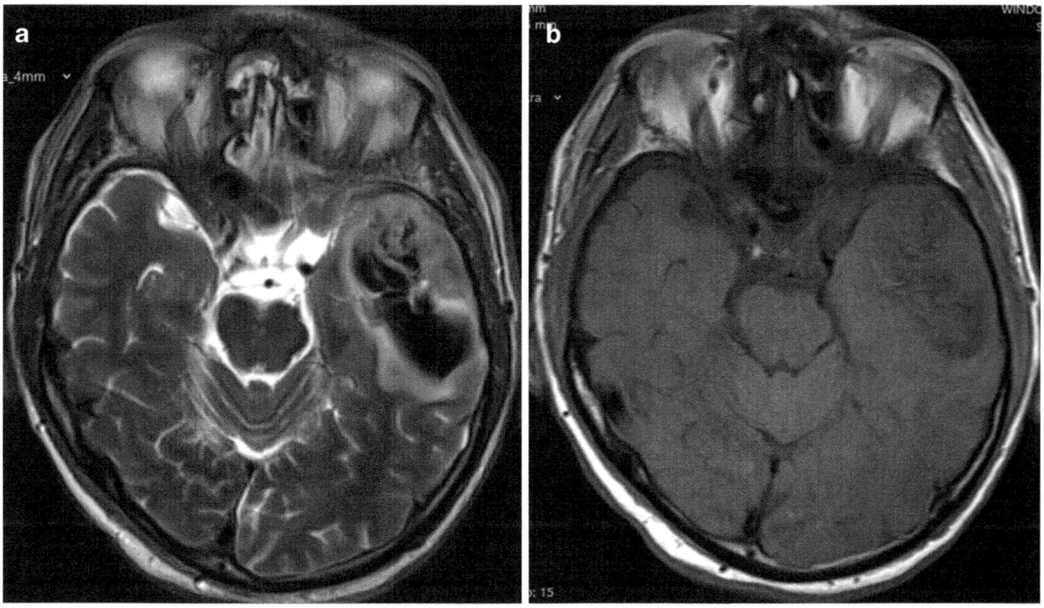


**Fig. 3** Acute hematoma. (**a**) T2W image depicts hypointensity and (**b**) T1W image shows iso-hypointensity in left temporal acute stage hematoma

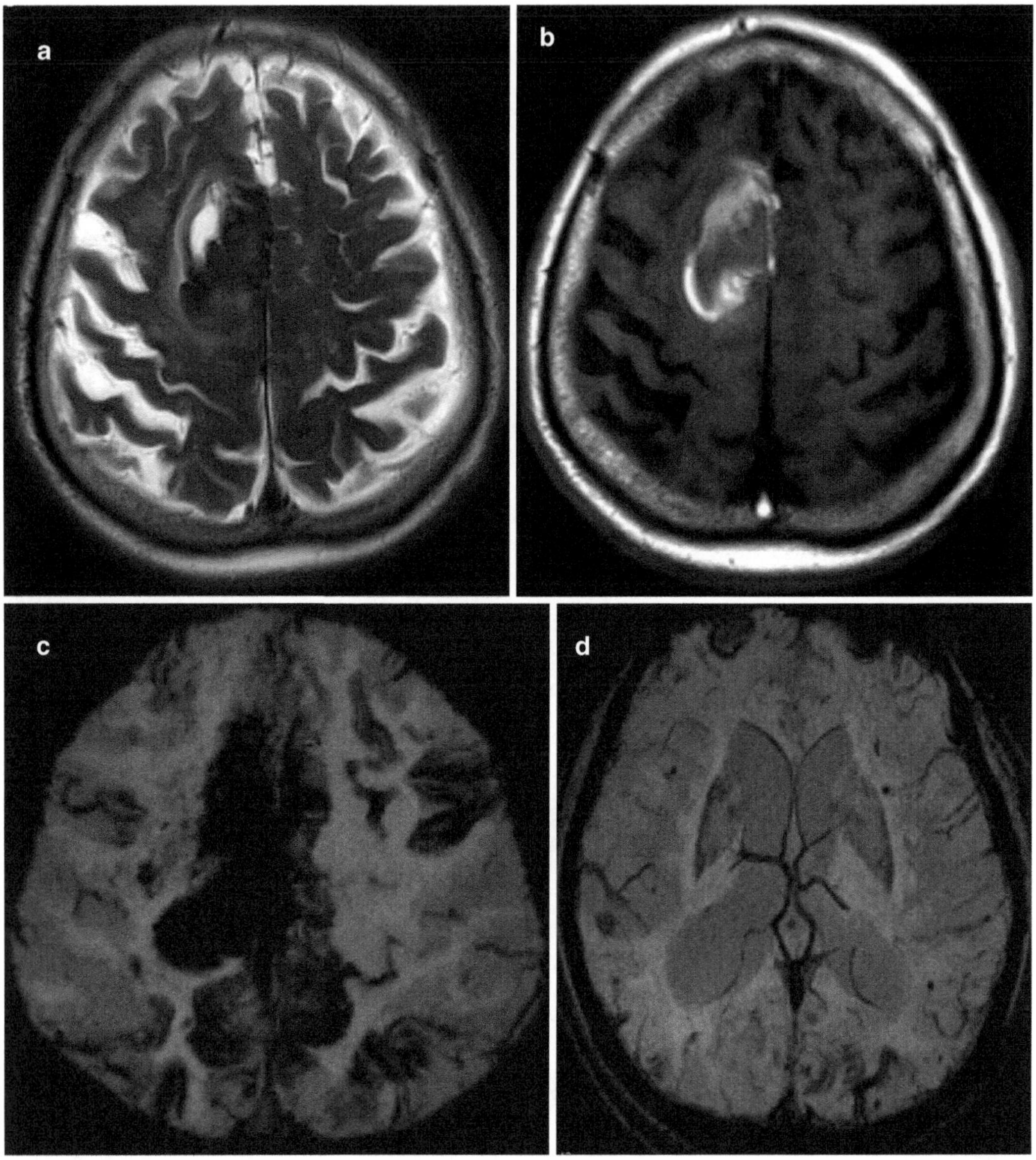


**Fig. 4** Early subacute hematoma. The right frontal lobar hematoma reveals hypointensity on T2W image (**a**) and peripheral hyperintensity on T1W image (**b**). (**c**) SWI image shows marked hypointensity in the lesion as well as multiple subcortical nodular and sulcal hypointensities consistent with CAA. (**d**) SWI image at more caudal level does not reveal microbleeds in basal ganglia

## 2.3 Digital Subtraction Angiography

Despite the advanced examination methods and developments in neuroimaging, digital subtraction angiography (DSA) is still used in certain patients to identify the cause of ICH. It was shown that the localization of bleeding, patient's age, and history of hypertension were important factors that had an impact on the possibility of detecting vascular anomalies with cerebral angiography in nontraumatic (spontaneous) ICH (Xhu et al. 1997). DSA is recommended for patients under 45 who do not have history of

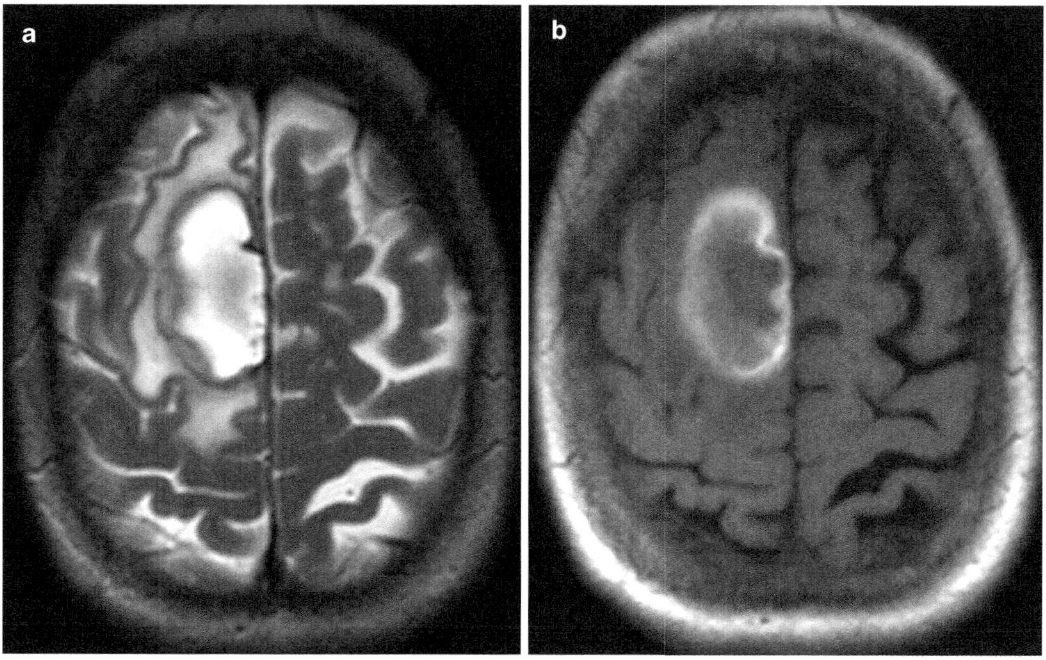


**Fig. 5** Late subacute hematoma. Right frontal lobar hematoma shows hyperintensity on both T2W (**a**) and T1W images (**b**)

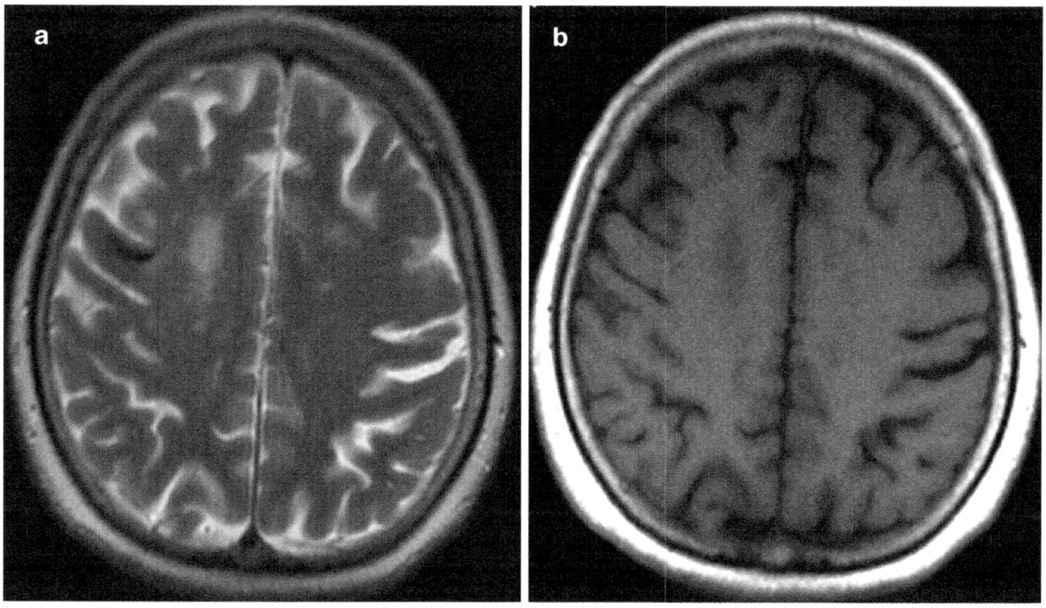


**Fig. 6** Chronic hematoma. There is a linear hypointensity at right frontal subcortical white matter on T2W image (**a**), which is also hypointense on T1W image (**b**)

hypertension and have lobar hemorrhage if the cause of bleeding cannot be identified with noninvasive methods or for patients above 45 if the cause of bleeding cannot be identified with SWI and contrast MRI.

## 3 Causes of Nontraumatic Intracerebral Hemorrhage

ICH is traditionally classified as traumatic and nontraumatic (spontaneous), wherein nontraumatic ICH is classified as primary and secondary depending on the cause of hemorrhage. The term primary ICH is used for CAA and hypertension that involve cerebral small vessels and primary ICHs constitute the majority of nontraumatic ICHs (78–88%) (Foulkes et al. 1988). In addition, secondary ICH encompasses hemorrhages with an apparent underlying cause such as coagulopathy, vascular lesion, tumor, or venous sinus thrombosis (Table 2). Therefore, knowing the localization of hemorrhage (lobar, deep, posterior fossa), clinical history (hypertension, use of oral anticoagulants), and patient's age is essential to narrow down this considerably long list of differential diagnoses.

**Table 2** Classification of nontraumatic intracranial hemorrhage according to causes

| Causes | Characteristics |
|---|---|
| *Primary* | |
| Hypertension | Most common reason, deep location, clinical history of hypertension |
| Amyloid angiopathy | Lobar, cortical-subcortical location, older patients, high recurrence |
| *Secondary* | |
| Vascular malformations<br>• Cavernous angioma.<br>• Arteriovenous malformation. | Young adults, need for imaging studies such as CTA/MRA and DSA |
| Venous thrombosis | Noncompliance with arterial distribution, bleeding near the dural venous sinus or deep cerebral vein, empty delta sign. |
| Nontraumatic subarachnoid hemorrhage | Ruptured aneurysm, the most severe headache in patient's life, sulcal hyperintensity on FLAIR is sensitive but not specific. |
| Coagulopathy<br>• Use of anticoagulants.<br>• Congenital (antithrombin III, protein C, protein S, von Willebrand, factor VII, IX, VII deficiency).<br>• Acquired (thrombocytopenia, DIC, uremia, MM, leukemia). | Most commonly associated with use of anticoagulants. The clinical history is important to prevent continued bleeding. |
| Neoplasm<br>• Primary (grade III, IV astrocytoma).<br>• Metastasis. | Mostly malign, contrast-enhanced MRI is useful for diagnosis. Recurrence of hemorrhage is common. |
| Hemorrhagic transformation of ischemic stroke | DWI is useful in demonstrating the ischemia underlying bleeding. |
| Vasculitis/vasculopathy | Serological examination of CSF or brain biopsy is required for certain diagnosis. |
| Infection | Other signs of infection (fever, elevated ESR, and CRP), hemorrhage due to vasculitis, coagulopathy, septic embolism, or microbial aneurysm. |
| Alcohol and drugs<br>• Cocaine.<br>• Amphetamine. | Due to acute (drugs) or chronic (alcohol) elevation of hypertension. Concomitant pathologies (aneurysm, AVM) may be present in drug-associated ICH. |

*MRI* magnetic resonance imaging, *DSA* digital subtraction angiography, *DWI* diffusion-weighted imaging, *DIC* disseminated intravascular coagulopathy, *MM* multiple myeloma, *CSF* cerebrospinal fluid, *ESR* erythrocyte sedimentation rate, *CRP* C-reactive protein, *ICH* intracranial hemorrhage

## 3.1 Primary Nontraumatic Intracranial Hemorrhage

### 3.1.1 Hypertension

Chronic hypertension is the leading cause of primary ICH. Long-term hypertension causes reactive hyperplasia in the deep-penetrating arterioles that originate from the anterior, middle, or posterior cerebral arteries and basilar artery in the brain. This leads to lipohyalinosis and fibrinoid necrosis on arteriole walls. As a result of these degenerative changes, compliance decreases, and the arteriole becomes prone to rupture. It was previously thought that hemorrhages due to hypertension originated from microscopic aneurysms that are called Charcot-Bouchard aneurysms. However, it was then understood that such hemorrhages were extravascular clots that stemmed from endothelial damage or subadventitial hemorrhages (Fisher 1971).

Hypertensive ICH is typically observed in the putamen and internal capsule (60–65%), thalamus (15–25%), and pons (5–10%) (Osborn 1994). Localization of hemorrhage reflects the watershed areas of the affected deep perforating arteries. Lobar location is rarer and accounts for 10% of the cases. It is thought that lobar hemorrhage can stem from CAA which can be observed with hypertension especially in older patients (Pantoni 2010). Neuroimaging shows other signs of hypertension in the brain in addition to hemorrhage due to hypertension (Fig. 7). Although small arterioles are generally beyond the resolution of MRI, their complex effects on the brain can still be visualized. The key MRI findings associated with small vessel disease consist of cerebral microbleeds and leukoaraiosis (white matter changes). Cerebral microbleeds appear as small, homogenous, and round- or oval-shaped hypointense foci on images obtained by T2*-weighted GRE and SWI. Leukoaraiosis appears

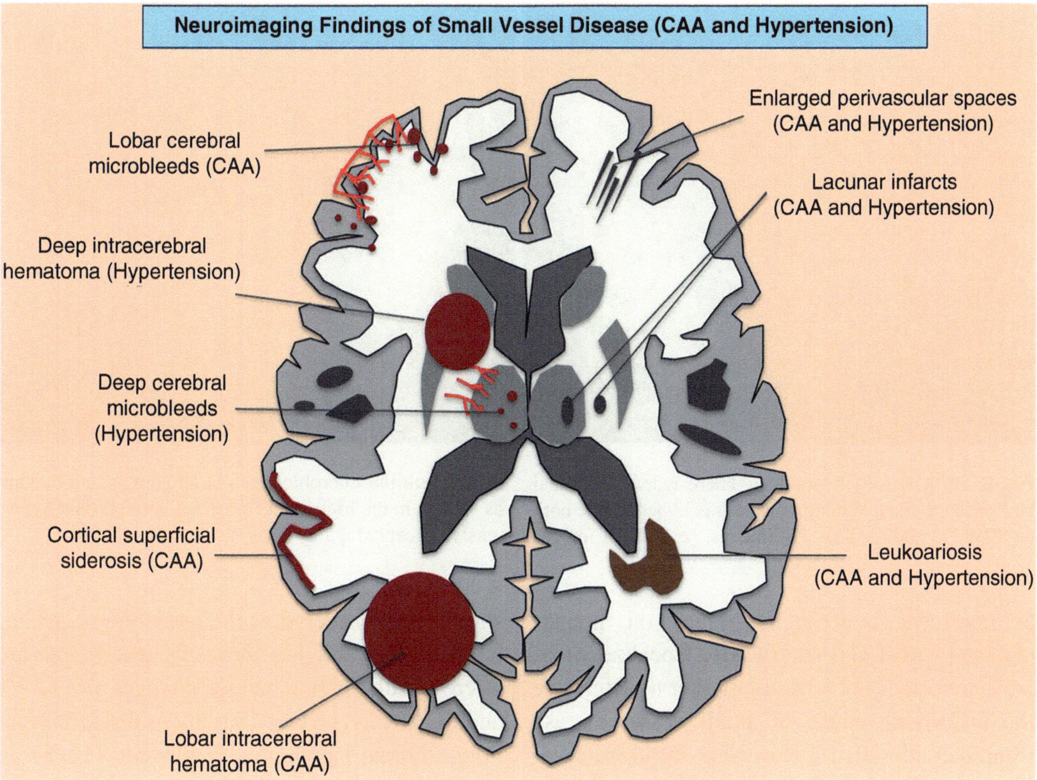


**Fig. 7** Schematic drawing shows neuroimaging findings of small vessel disease. *CAA*: cerebral amyloid angiopathy

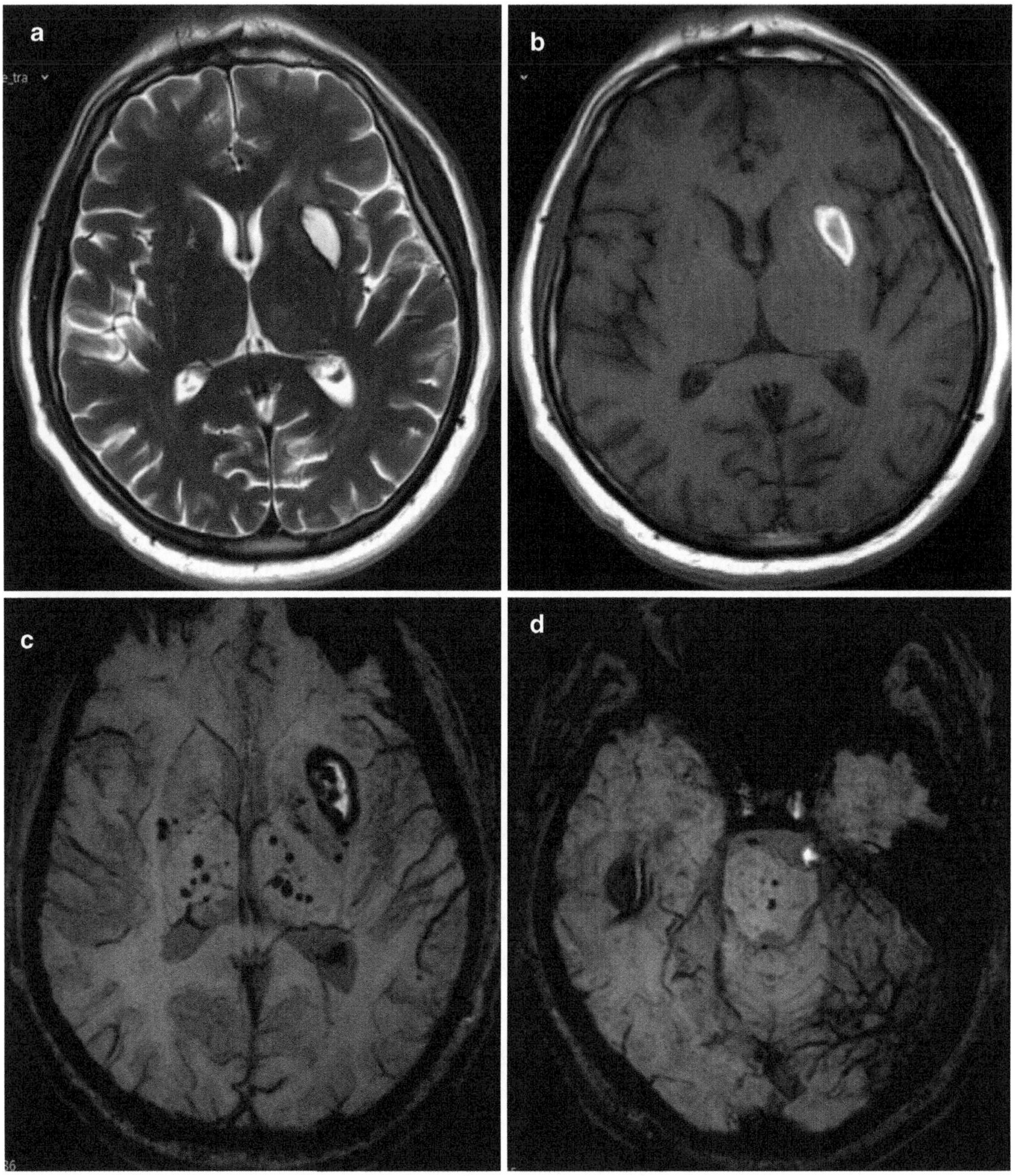


**Fig. 8** Hypertensive hematoma. There is left putaminal late subacute focal hematoma which is hyperintense both on T2W (**a**) and on T1W (**b**) images. (**c**, **d**) SWI images depict multiple microbleeds in basal ganglia and thalami as well as in the brainstem consistent with chronic hypertensive encephalopathy

as confluent hyperintense areas on images obtained with T2WI and FLAIR. Localization of leukoaraiosis is not a useful marker to determine the underlying cause of small vessel disease (Smith et al. 2010). However, localization of cerebral microbleeds is useful in determining the underlying cause of hemorrhage. Hypertension should be considered as the underlying cause of hematoma in patients above 45, when there are microvascular white matter changes on T2W1 and FLAIR as well as deep microbleeds at locations of basal ganglia and brainstem (Fig. 8). In addition, lobar microbleeds are strongly associated with CAA. Another neuroimaging finding in small vessel disease is lacunar infarcts. While lacunar infarcts associated with hypertension are localized in deep gray matter like in microbleeds, lacunar infarcts linked to CAA are localized in centrum semiovale and lobar regions.

More than one in three intraparenchymal hematomas expand within 24–36 h. It was shown that the possibility of hematoma expansion was higher in those who underwent the first CT sooner, used oral anticoagulants, and had larger hematomas (Brott et al. 1997). Therefore, it should be kept in mind that the mass effect, which is lower initially, will also increase with expanding hematoma and increasing edema.

### 3.1.2 Cerebral Amyloid Angiopathy

CAA is a small vessel disease in which progressive β-amyloid protein build-up is observed on the walls of superficial small and mid-sized vessels in the leptomeninges and cerebral cortex. The affected vessels exhibit wall thickening, microaneurysms, and fibrinoid degeneration. The vessels become prone to rupture and luminal occlusion can also be observed in vessels. ICH develops when the vessel ruptures, whereas ischemia and leukoencephalopathy develop when there is occlusion.

The prevalence of CAA increases with age (particularly >60 years), but most of these patients are asymptomatic. Autopsy studies have shown that more than 70% of the asymptomatic population older than 90 had CAA (Tanskanen et al. 2012).

The definitive diagnosis of CAA is made by histopathological examination of the tissue. However, neuroimaging is critical, since such histopathological examination is not possible most of the time. Therefore, Boston criteria that include imaging findings were described in order to standardize the diagnosis of CAA (Table 3) (Knudsen et al. 2001). While CAA can be asymptomatic with cerebral microbleeds and white matter changes, it can also lead to symptomatic ICH. Cerebral microbleeds associated with CAA typically have cortical and subcortical localization unlike the deep localization in hypertension.

**Table 3** Boston criteria for the diagnosis of CAA in patients with intracranial hemorrhage

| Category | Description |
|---|---|
| Definite CAA | Postmortem examination<br>• Lobar, cortical, or corticosubcortical hemorrhage.<br>• Severe CAA.<br>• Absence of another cause. |
| Probable CAA with supporting pathology | Clinical data and pathologic tissue<br>• Lobar, cortical, or corticosubcortical hemorrhage.<br>• Some amyloid deposition in specimen.<br>• Absence of another cause. |
| Probable CAA | Clinical data and MRI<br>• Multiple lobar, cortical, or corticosubcortical hemorrhages.<br>• Age >55 years.<br>• Absence of another cause. |
| Possible CAA | Clinical data and MRI<br>• Single lobar, cortical, or corticosubcortical hemorrhage.<br>• Age >55 years.<br>• Absence of another cause. |

*CAA* cerebral amyloid angiopathy, *MRI* magnetic resonance imaging

In general, there are multiple hemorrhages that tend to recur. CAA should be considered in patients older than 55 who have microbleeds localized in the cortical and corticomedullary junction without history of hypertension. CAA-related ICH accounts for 5–20% of all nontraumatic ICHs (Maia et al. 2007). Symptomatic parenchymal hemorrhage most frequently occurs in the frontal and parietal lobes, cortex, and subcortical regions and extends to the subarachnoid and rarely to the subdural space. Hemorrhage can also be observed in the cerebellum, although rare. Symptomatic hemorrhages are larger than microbleeds (>5 mm). Another rare sign associated with CAA is cortical superficial siderosis. It is a progressive disease caused by chronic recurrent subarachnoid hemorrhage and is characterized by the deposition of hemosiderin on pial surfaces of the central nervous system (CNS). The imaging shows hypointensity, especially marked in SWI, covering the surface of the brain (Fig. 4).

It was shown that hypertension, higher number of cerebral microbleeds, and anticoagulant use increased the risk of hemorrhage in CAA (Rosand et al. 2000; Greenberg et al. 2004). Therefore, the risks and benefits should be assessed, and the treatment should be personalized in patients who need to use anticoagulants for some other reason.

## 3.2 Secondary Nontraumatic Intracranial Hemorrhage

### 3.2.1 Vascular Malformations

Vascular malformations represent a large group of pathologies including arteriovenous malformation (AVM), cavernous malformation (CM), dural arteriovenous fistulas (dAVFs), developmental venous anomaly (DVA), and capillary telangiectasia. DVA and capillary telangiectasia are common, but they frequently do not cause hemorrhage, whereas AVM and CM have a higher potential to cause hemorrhage. In addition, dAVF rarely causes bleeding.

Vascular malformation is the most common cause of nontraumatic ICH in young adults (Shahi and Warlow 2001). CTA can detect the underlying vascular malformation with 90% accuracy, after the presence of ICH has been demonstrated using CT (Romero et al. 2009; Yeung et al. 2009). The abnormal vessels can be directly visualized, similar to MRA. DSA is generally used to identify and treat small lesions that are not visible on CT and MRI.

**AVM:** AVM stems from abnormal connections between the arteries and veins. AVM consists of one or more feeding arteries, a bundle of blood vessels where the arterial blood is shunted called the nidus and enlarged draining veins. There may be an aneurysm in the feeding arteries and nidus. The feeding artery originates from the internal carotid artery or vertebrobasilar system. One in three ICHs occur due to AVM in young adults. AVMs that have not ruptured have 2–4% risk of hemorrhage per year, and this risk increases in recurrent hemorrhages (Al-Shahi and Warlow 2001). There are many morphological factors that are associated with hemorrhage in AVMs. It was shown that increasing age, deep brain localization, and exclusive deep venous drainage were independent predictors of hemorrhage in AVM (Stapf et al. 2006).

AVMs are generally asymptomatic, and they are detected incidentally on CT and MRI scans performed for other reasons. Noncontrast CT and MRI can generally detect an unruptured AVM. Enlarged draining veins can appear as slightly hyperdense areas in serpentine configuration on a noncontrast CT scan. This is generally accompanied by calcification and encephalomalacia surrounding the AVM. Contrast-enhanced CT may show curvilinear vascular structures with marked contrast uptake. MRI typically shows curvilinear flow voids in feeding arteries and draining veins. The nidus and enlarged vascular structures can be clearly visualized using CTA and MRA (particularly time-resolved enhanced MRA and CTA). When hemorrhage occurs in AVM, the bleeding may hinder the visualization of the AVM (Fig. 9). Calcification and enlarged vessels in the vicinity of the bleed may assist the diagnosis. In addition, small AVMs, especially when they are localized near the dural venous sinus, may not be visible on CT and MRI scans (since draining veins will travel a shorter path). Therefore, the definitive diagnosis of AVMs is made using DSA. However, a negative result from the first angiogram should not rule out an AVM, since the mass effect from the hematoma may prevent the visualization of small AVMs. Therefore, a second evaluation should be considered after the mass effect is removed, if there is clinical suspicion.

Transcatheter embolization, surgery, and stereotactic radiosurgery are used in the treatment of AVMs. A grading system has been described by Spetzler and Martin in order to predict the surgical outcome in AVMs. With this grading system, AVMs were classified and graded according to size, localization, and pattern of venous drainage (Table 4). A higher score means that the estimated surgical outcome is worse (Spetzler and Martin 1986).

**CM:** CMs are lesions that consist of thin-walled dilated venous channels lined by a single layer of endothelial cells. These vascular lesions

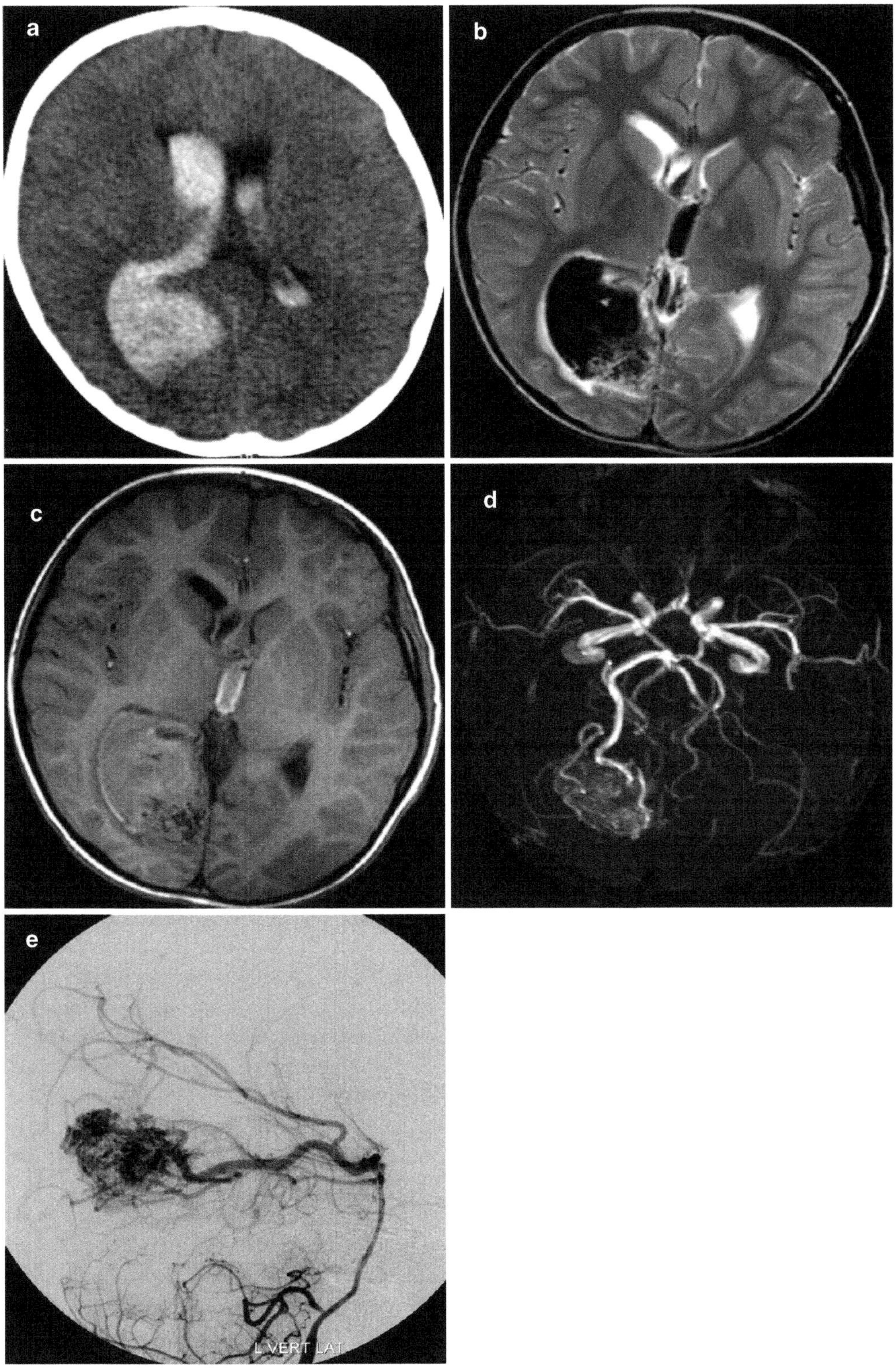


**Fig. 9** AVM hemorrhage. (**a**) Noncontrast CT shows right occipital acute hematoma with extension to the ventricles. Hematoma is hypointense on T2W (**b**) and isointense on T1W (**c**) images. Note that subtle signal voids at the posterior aspect of the hematoma are seen. (**d**) 3D TOF MRA reveals abnormal arterial structures inside the hematoma consistent with AVM. Right posterior cerebral artery is dilated as the major feeding artery. (**e**) DSA proves the presence of an AVM

**Table 4** Spetzler-Martin grading scale for arteriovenous malformations[a]

| Graded Feature | Points Assigned |
|---|---|
| *Size of AVM* | |
| Small (<3 cm) | 1 |
| Medium (3 to 6 cm) | 2 |
| Large (>6 cm) | 3 |
| *Eloquence of adjacent brain* | |
| No | 0 |
| Yes | 1 |
| *Venous drainage* | |
| Superficial only | 0 |
| Deep | 1 |

[a]Grade = size + eloquence + venous drainage
Data from Spetzler RF, Martin NA. A proposed grading system for arteriovenous malformation. J Neurosurg 1986;65:476e83

do not contain glial or neural tissue. CMs can be sporadic or familial. While there is a single lesion in the sporadic type, the familial type has multiple lesions. CMs can be associated with DVA or occur independently. Although CMs can be present at any region in the brain, they are generally located in the supratentorial region. CMs are generally asymptomatic and they are detected by chance on imaging tests performed for another indication, or patients present with an acute focal neurologic deficit or seizure due to hemorrhage. The annual hemorrhage rate of CMs is 2.5% per patient-year. Several risk factors (younger age, female sex, deep location, size, multiplicity, associated DVA, etc.) were defined for hemorrhage in CM in various studies. However, the results are controversial. The most well-known risk factor, among others, is history of CM hemorrhage (Gross and Du 2017). Hemorrhage rates for unruptured CMs are ranging from 0.4% to 0.6% per patient-year in the literature. Those for ruptured CM vary from 4.5% to 22.9% per patient-year (Gross and Du 2017).

CMs generally appear on CT scans as small, round-, or oval-shaped isodense lesions containing high-density areas. Edema and mass effect are not usually observed in the absence of hemorrhage. MRI should be the imaging method of choice in the diagnosis of CM. CMs are typically surrounded by a hypointense rim due to hemosiderin on T1WI and T2WI. The hypointense rim is more marked on SWI. In addition, sometimes, small CMs can only be visualized using the SWI sequence (Fig. 10). The signal at the center of the lesion varies depending on the stage of hemorrhage but it is generally a heterogenous signal (popcorn pattern) with hyperintense areas on T1WI and T2WI. There is usually a slight contrast uptake on postcontrast series. However, a contrast agent is mainly administered to detect a coexisting DVA. 8–33% of CM cases also have DVA (Rammos et al. 2009). Detection of a DVA is particularly useful for diagnosing CM, which is difficult to visualize in the presence of a hematoma. CMs are not visible on catheter angiography, which is not used for the diagnosis. Asymptomatic CMs are generally followed up in a conservative fashion. Surgical excision of the lesion or stereotactic radiosurgery is recommended for symptomatic cases due to the fact that recurrent hemorrhages may lead to permanent neurologic deficits. For patients who are planned to undergo surgery, a contrast-enhanced MRI should be performed before the treatment in order to detect an accompanying DVA and due to the risk of postoperative venous infarction.

**dAVF:** dAVF refers to an abnormal connection between the meningeal artery and meningeal vein or lumen of the dural venous sinus. It frequently occurs secondary to dural sinus thrombosis. On the other hand, dAVF may also be idiopathic, posttraumatic, secondary to craniotomy, or due to hormonal changes (pregnancy, use of oral contraceptives). It constitutes 10–15% of all intracranial vascular malformations (Newton and Cronqvist 1969). dAVF is most frequently observed at the cavernous sinus level or the cribriform plate or sigmoid sinus (Zipfel et al. 2009).

Clinical signs of dAVF depend on the localization of the lesion and the pattern of venous drainage (Tsai et al. 2004; Lucas Cde et al. 2006). The most distinct clinical presentation is observed in dAVFs that drain into the cavernous sinus. Proptosis, chemosis, ophthalmoplegia, and loss

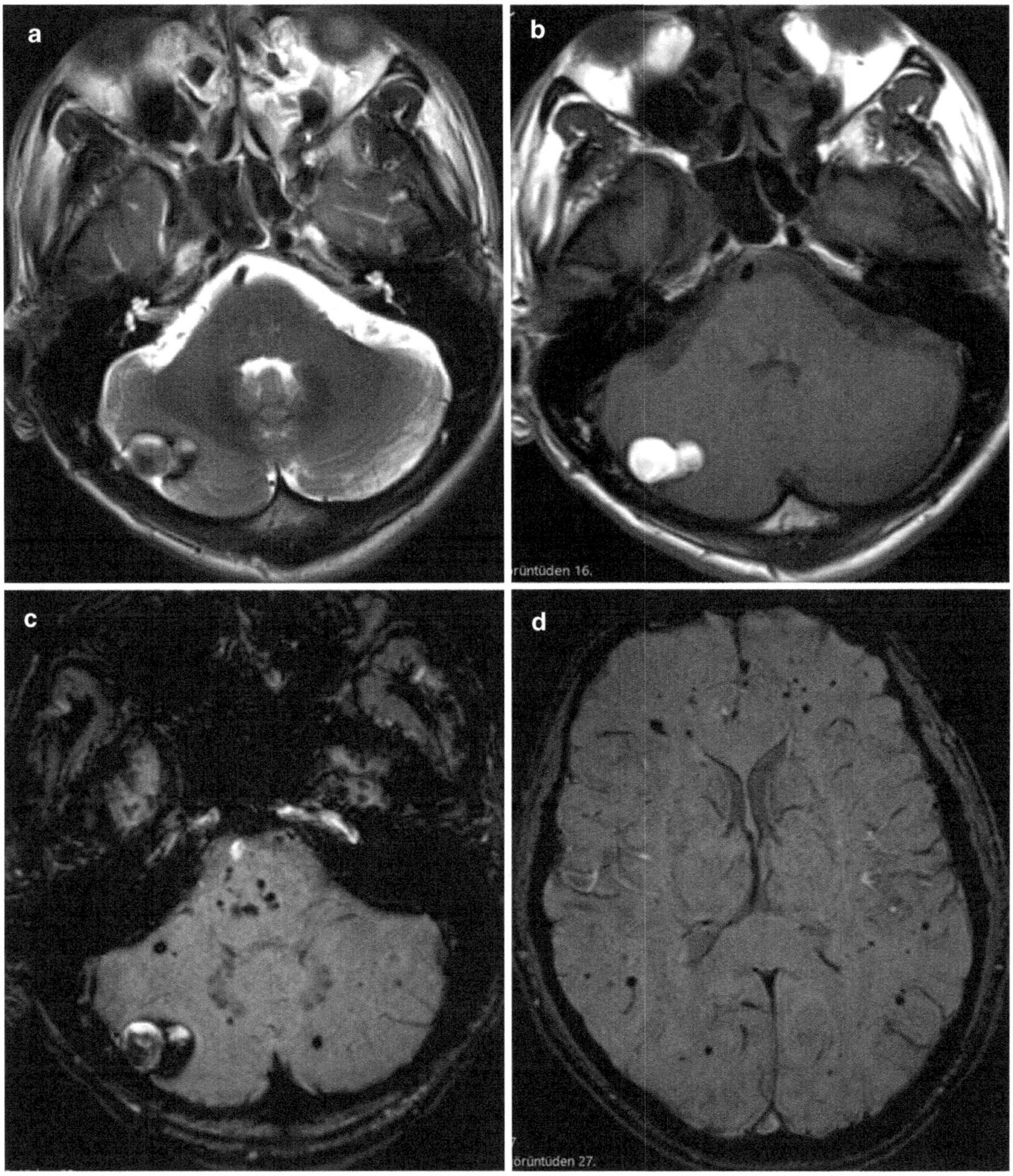


**Fig. 10** Cavernoma. There is right cerebellar early subacute hematoma which is hypointense on T2W image (**a**) and also hyperintense on T1W image (**b**). (**c**, **d**) SWI images depict multiple tiny hypointense lesions representing multiple cavernomas, which cannot be detected on conventional images

of vision are typically observed. In addition, dAVFs in the transverse sigmoid junction typically exhibit pulsatile tinnitus. Headache secondary to venous hypertension and dementia as a result of cerebral hypoxia can also be observed. dAVF rarely causes bleeding. Hemorrhage stems from the increased pressure due to retrograde venous flow causing the rupture of parenchymal veins. Petrosal or straight sinus location, leptomeningeal venous drainage, and presence of varix in the draining vein increase the risk of hemorrhage.

dAVFs may appear completely normal on CT and MRI in the absence of dural venous sinus thrombosis, dilated cortical veins, hydrocephaly, or ICH. Tortuous feeding arteries, venous sinus occlusion, enlarged cortical veins can be clearly visualized on CTA and MRA/MR venography (MRV). DSA is the gold standard in diagnosis. A selective angiogram encompassing the bilateral internal carotid arteries, external carotid, and vertebral artery should be obtained. DSA can provide the diagnosis of the lesion in addition to the characterization of the arterial feeding vessels and pattern of venous drainage as well as enabling endovascular treatment of many lesions. Various grading systems were proposed for the grading of dAVFs. The Cognard and Borden classifications, based on the pattern of venous drainage, are the most commonly used systems (Cognard et al. 1995; Borden et al. 1995). A higher grade means more aggressive presentation and higher risk of hemorrhage (Table 5).

### 3.2.2 Venous Thrombosis

Venous thrombosis accounts for 0.5–1% of all strokes in the adult population (Saposnik et al. 2011). The incidence thereof is higher in the pediatric population and females (Coutinho et al. 2012). There are many risk factors that play a role in the etiology of venous thrombosis including thrombophilia (genetic or acquired), oral contraceptive use, pregnancy, dehydration (diarrhea in children), head trauma, malignancy, and infections. Clinical signs are not specific to venous thrombosis. The diagnosis may be delayed since symptoms such as headaches, seizures, papilledema, and focal neurologic deficits can be present in various pathologies. Headaches and papilledema, which can be observed in 40% of the patients, are associated with increased intracranial pressure.

39% of all venous thrombosis events are associated with hemorrhage (Ferro et al. 2004). It was shown that some factors such as pregnancy, thrombosis of a large sinus, and hypertension at admission were associated with intracerebral hemorrhage and poor prognosis (Kumral et al. 2012). Venous thrombosis should be considered as the underlying cause, especially when ICH is localized in certain regions such as the temporal lobe, parasagittal frontal or parietal lobe, bilateral thalami, and internal capsule. Noncontrast CT is the first diagnostic procedure as in all patients who present with nonspecific neurological symptoms. However, CTV or MRI/MRV should be

**Table 5** Classification systems for cerebral dAVFs

| Cognard classification | | Borden classification | |
|---|---|---|---|
| Type | Description | Type | Description |
| Type I | Anterograde drainage into venous sinus | Type I | Anterograde drainage into the dural sinus/ meningeal vein |
| Type II | Drainage into a sinus but with insufficient antegrade venous drainage and reflux. | Type II | Anterograde drainage into dural sinus and retrograde drainage into cortical veins |
| • Type IIa | Retrograde venous drainage into sinüs | Type III | Isolated retrograde drainage into cortical veins |
| • Type IIb | Retrograde venous drainage into cortical veins | | |
| • Type IIa + IIb | Retrograde venous drainage into sinus and cortical veins | | |
| Type III | Direct cortical venous drainage without ectasia | | |
| Type IV | Direct cortical venous<br>Drainage with venous<br>Ectasia >5 mm and 3 times larger than the diameter of the draining vein | | |
| Type V | Drainage into the spinal perimedullary veins | | |

performed promptly in the presence of findings that are suggestive of venous thrombosis on noncontrast CT scans. Indirect signs of venous thrombosis such as hemorrhage, if present, and brain edema can be observed on noncontrast CT images. Thrombosed dural venous sinus or cortical vein (cord sign) can appear hyperdense. However, this classical finding is not observed in most of the cases. Venous thrombosis should be suspected in case of hemorrhage or edema near the dural venous sinus or deep cerebral vein. The most common direct sign on CTV is a filling defect in the dural venous sinus, also known as the "empty delta sign" (Poon et al. 2007). The sensitivity of CTV for detecting venous thromboses is higher for the dural venous sinuses than for the cortical veins. On the other hand, open dural sinuses appear as flow voids on MRI scans. Loss of flow void or abnormal signals imply thrombosis and detection would be more successful when imaging plane is perpendicular to the direction of blood flow. Signal intensity of the clot varies in time, similar to a hematoma, and should be confirmed with different sequences (Leach et al. 2006). SWI is highly beneficial in detecting subtle clots that are not visible with other sequences. MRV can detect a blood clot and help evaluate recanalization and collateral status with high accuracy (Fig. 11). Although TOF MRV does not require the use of a contrast agent (particularly important in patients with renal failure), which is an important advantage, it is necessary to be careful about pitfalls. Particularly on 2D TOF MRV, signal loss due to in-plane flow or hypoplastic/aplastic venous sinus can mimic thrombosis (Rollins et al. 2005). Filling defect can be directly visualized using postcontrast MRV. However, it should also be remembered that chronic thrombosis may exhibit contrast uptake on MRV, thereby leading to the interpretation of the sinus as normal, which is a false-negative result (Dmytriw et al. 2018).

### 3.2.3 Nontraumatic Subarachnoid Hemorrhage

The most common cause of subarachnoid hemorrhage (SAH) is trauma, whereas the most common cause of nontraumatic SAH is a ruptured aneurysm (nearly 85%). In addition to aneurysms, amyloid angiopathy, venous thrombosis, and vascular anomalies can also cause spontaneous SAH. Aneurysmal SAH is a very severe clinical presentation with a mortality rate ranging from 18% to 67% (Connolly et al. 2012; van Gijn et al. 2007). It also has high morbidity, wherein only one-third of the patients achieve full recovery after treatment. The classic clinical presentation of aneurysmal SAH is sudden onset of (within 1 min.) severe headache described as "the worst headache of my life" by the patients (Ducros and Bousser 2013). In addition, photophobia, seizures, vomiting, neck stiffness, and changes in consciousness can also be observed. The first imaging modality used in diagnosis is noncontrast CT. Lumbar puncture is recommended when noncontrast CT result is negative, for patients who are clinically suspected of having SAH (sudden onset and severe headache). Sensitivity of noncontrast CT for detecting SAH reaches up to 100% when performed within the first 6 h after the onset of symptoms (Carpenter et al. 2016; Perry et al. 2011). Sensitivity decreases with time and drops down to less than 90% within the first 72 h. Fissures and/or basal cisterns appear hyperdense on noncontrast CT scans. Pattern of bleeding provides information about the localization of the aneurysm. For instance, presence of blood in the interhemispheric fissure and lateral ventricle suggests anterior communicating artery aneurysm, whereas blood in the Sylvian fissure suggests middle cerebral artery aneurysm. Blood frequently extravasates to the brain parenchyma (30%) and ventricles (>50%) other than the subarachnoid space after the aneurysm ruptures, whereas subdural hemorrhage is rare (<5%). Vascular examination should be performed to determine the underlying cause after a patient has been diagnosed with SAH. DSA is the gold standard for determining the cause of hemorrhage and planning the treatment (Fig. 12). DSA is invasive, risky, and time-consuming; therefore, it has been replaced by CTA. Saccular aneurysms appear on CTA as round-shaped lesions filled with contrast forming a sac protruding from the vessel wall. Saccular aneurysms that cause SAH are fre-

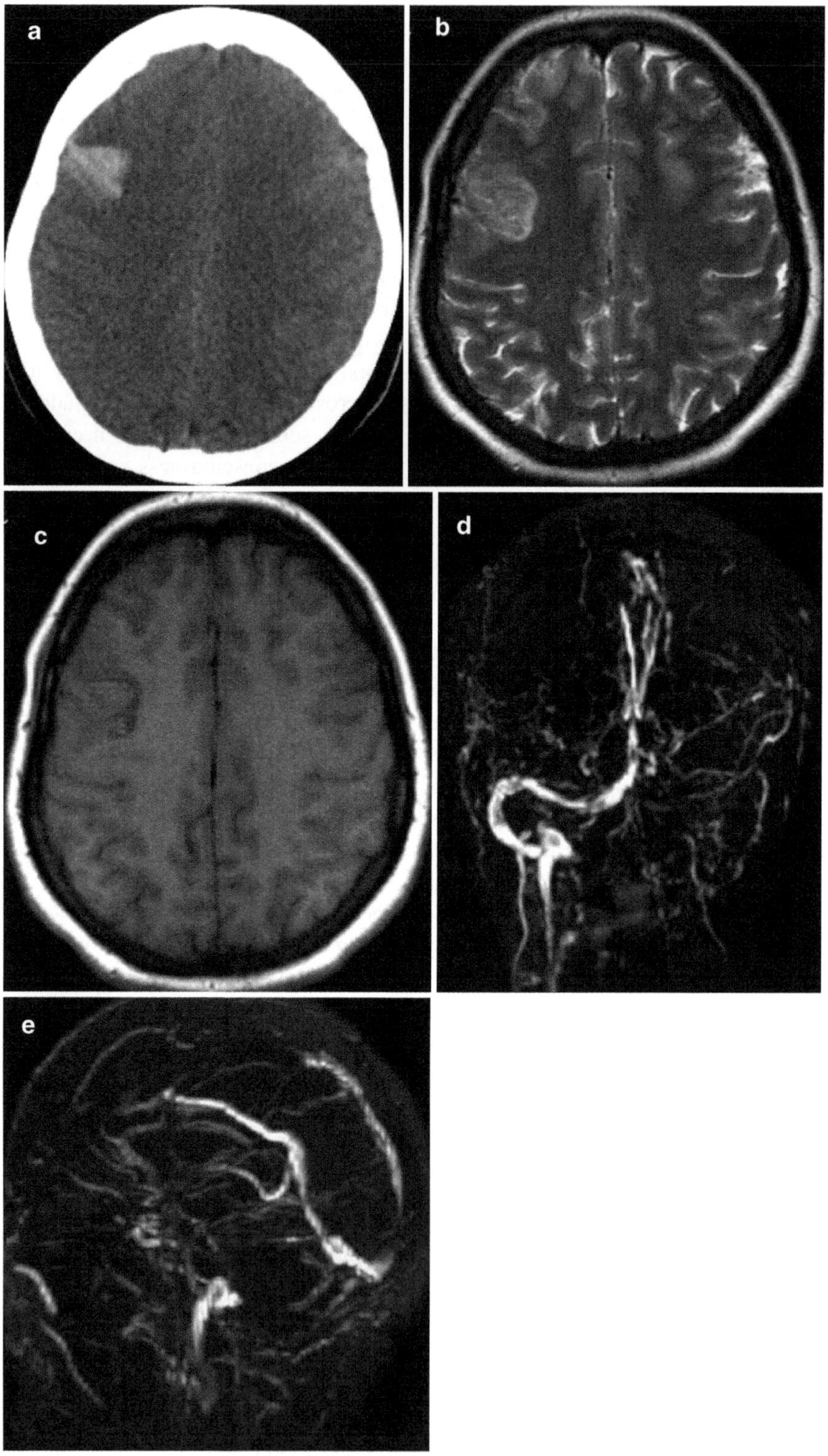


**Fig. 11** Dural venous sinus thrombosis. (**a**) Noncontrast CT shows right frontal acute hematoma. (**b**, **c**) T2W and T1W images depict the hematoma as well as cortical thickening and edema on the left hemisphere. (**d**, **e**) MR venography shows partial occlusion of the superior sagittal sinus and total occlusion on the left transverse and sigmoid sinuses

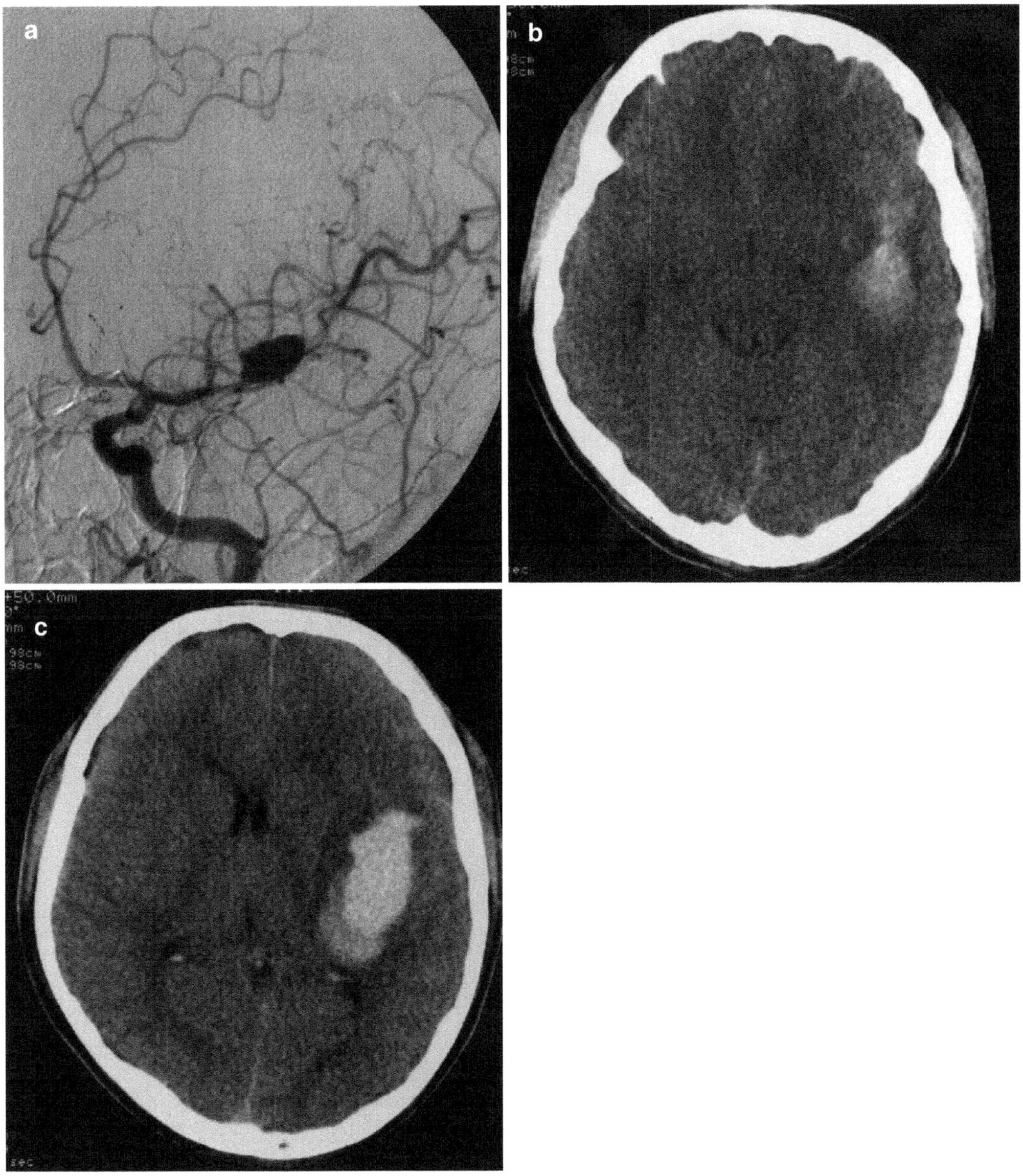


**Fig. 12** Aneurysm. (**a**) DSA reveals an aneurysm on the left middle cerebral artery bifurcation which caused both intracerebral hematoma and subarachnoid hemorrhage on the left cerebral hemisphere (**b**, **c**)

quently localized at the bifurcation of major arteries in the Willis polygon. The risk of rupture is especially higher for aneurysms larger than 10 mm. DSA should be preferred when noncontrast CT and CTA are negative. CTA or DSA can be repeated or an MRI/MRA can be performed when DSA is also negative. However, the clinical presentation prevents performing an MRI in many patients. It was shown that aneurysms could be detected in 10% of such patients, when DSA was repeated several weeks later. Increased cerebrospinal fluid (CSF) signal intensity on FLAIR is sensitive but not specific for SAH (Fig. 13). Conditions that cause sulcal hyperintensity on FLAIR are shown in Table 6.

Aneurysms are repaired using 2 methods: neurosurgical clipping or endovascular coiling. Endovascular coiling was shown to provide better

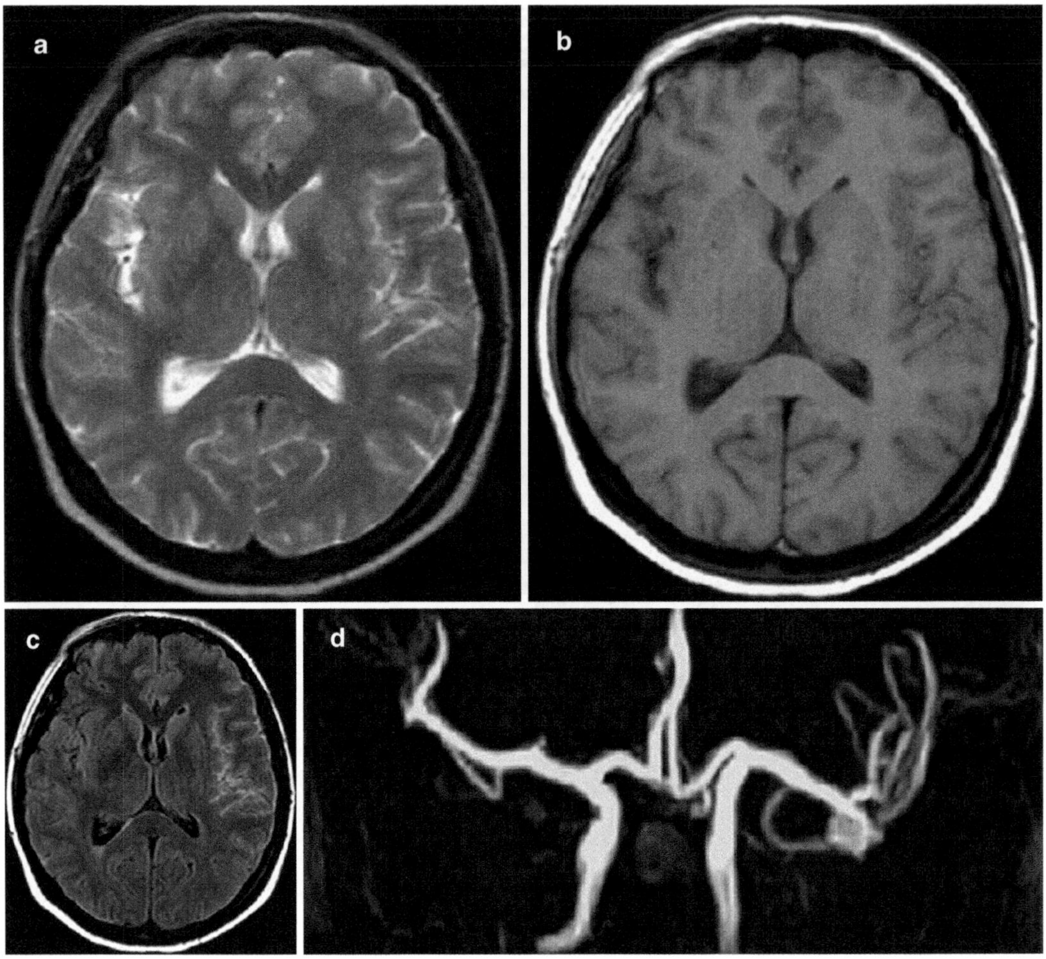


**Fig. 13** Subarachnoid hemorrhage. (**a**, **b**) T2W and T1W images look normal whereas FLAIR image (**c**) depicts sulcal hyperintensity on the left hemisphere, consistent with SAH. (**d**) 3D TOF MRA shows left middle cerebral artery bifurcation aneurysm

**Table 6** Differential diagnosis of subarachnoid FLAIR hyperintensity

| Differential diagnosis of subarachnoid FLAIR hyperintensity |
|---|
| Subarachnoid hemorrhage |
| Meningitis |
| Leptomeningeal carcinomatosis |
| Leptomeningeal melanomatosis |
| Acute stroke |
| Moyamoya disease |
| Fat-containing lesions (lipoma, ruptured dermoid cyst) |
| Hyperoxygenation therapy |
| Artifacts (CSF flow artifact, magnetic susceptibility artifact, motion artifact, vascular pulsation artifact |

outcomes. However, it is not possible to perform endovascular coiling in every patient. Treatment selection depends on the localization and size of the aneurysm, general condition of the patient, and experience of the clinician. The most severe complication of SAH is rebleeding, which is mostly seen within the first 6 h, with a mortality rate of 8–23% (Larsen and Astrup 2013). A late complication of SAH is cerebral vasospasm, which mostly occurs within the first 10 days and may lead to cerebral infarction. Incidence of cerebral vasospasm is directly proportional to the amount of blood in the subarachnoid space at the time of diagnosis.

### 3.2.4 Coagulopathy

Coagulopathies can be acquired (anticoagulants, idiopathic thrombocytopenic purpura, disseminated intravascular coagulation, alcoholism, etc.) or genetic (hemophilia A and B, von Willebrand factor deficiency, etc.). They account for 10–20% of all nontraumatic ICHs (Ciura and Romero 2014). Acquired coagulopathies constitute the majority of all coagulopathies. The epidemiology of the causes of ICH keeps changing due to the administration of more aggressive therapies for hypertension and increased use of anticoagulants, wherein the incidence of hemorrhages due to oral anticoagulant use is also increased (Flaherty et al. 2007). Currently, the most common cause of hemorrhages due to coagulopathy is medication.

It was proposed that anticoagulants alone did not cause ICH but increased the bleeding volume in patients who were predisposed to bleeding (e.g., CAA and hypertensive arteriopathy). Studies showed that hematoma expansion, hematoma volume, and mortality were higher in patients who used anticoagulants than those who did not (Horstmann et al. 2013; Flibotte et al. 2004). Nonoral anticoagulants pose a higher risk of ICH than oral anticoagulants. In addition, advanced age, hypertension, and use of multiple anticoagulants increase the risk of bleeding. While hemorrhages due to anticoagulants may have intraparenchymal, subdural, epidural, or subarachnoid localization, they most frequently have intraparenchymal and lobar localization. This reflects the probable contribution of CAA to the risk of intracerebral hemorrhage in the elderly.

### 3.2.5 Neoplasm

Hemorrhages associated with neoplasms constitute 10% of all ICHs. It was found in autopsy series that nearly half of all intracranial neoplasms exhibited histopathological bleeding. However, most microscopic bleeds do not manifest with clinical signs. Brain tumors that exhibit bleeding may be primary or metastatic tumors. The primary brain tumor that most frequently causes ICH is glioblastoma, and metastatic tumors that most frequently manifest with bleeding are bronchogenic carcinomas, choriocarcinoma, melanoma, thyroid carcinoma, and renal cell carcinoma. Tumors that cause bleeding are usually malignant. On the other hand, it should be remembered that benign tumors such as meningioma, pituitary adenoma, and vestibular schwannoma may also lead to ICH.

It is not always possible to show that a tumor is the underlying cause of hemorrhage on noncontrast CT. However, edema that is more than expected and rather heterogenous appearance of the hematoma should raise suspicion. Features that help differentiate intratumoral bleeding from primary ICH are more clearly visible on MRI. Hemorrhagic neoplasms appear more heterogenous than benign causes of bleeding due to the coexistence of blood products and tumor tissues (Destian et al. 1989). Another difference is observed in the amount of edema, mass effect, and persistence. Intratumoral hemorrhages exhibit more edema and mass effect and they persist for a long time or become worse. The hemosiderin ring around the hematoma is incomplete and irregular, and even not visible sometimes, in neoplastic hemorrhages (Atlas et al. 1987). In addition, in neoplasic hemorrhages, the expected signal change in the bleeding over time may prolong. Hypointensity observed on T2WI in the acute or early subacute phase may continue longer than 1 week. Postcontrast series are also highly beneficial in showing tumors that are the underlying cause of bleeding. Presence of contrast uptake in the nonhemorrhagic areas of the mass or observing multiple lesions particularly in metastatic disease is helpful for making a diagnosis (Fig. 14). Of note, subacute hematomas can also exhibit slight contrast uptake. However, contrast uptake due to neoplasms is more nodular and thicker. Sometimes a large hematoma or a small tumor makes it harder to visualize an underlying mass. MRI follow-up is recommended in such cases, if a tumor is suspected (e.g., large amount of edema and mass effect) (Ciura and Romero 2014).

### 3.2.6 Hemorrhagic Transformation of Ischemic Stroke

Hemorrhagic transformation of ischemic stroke refers to bleeding into the arterial infraction area.

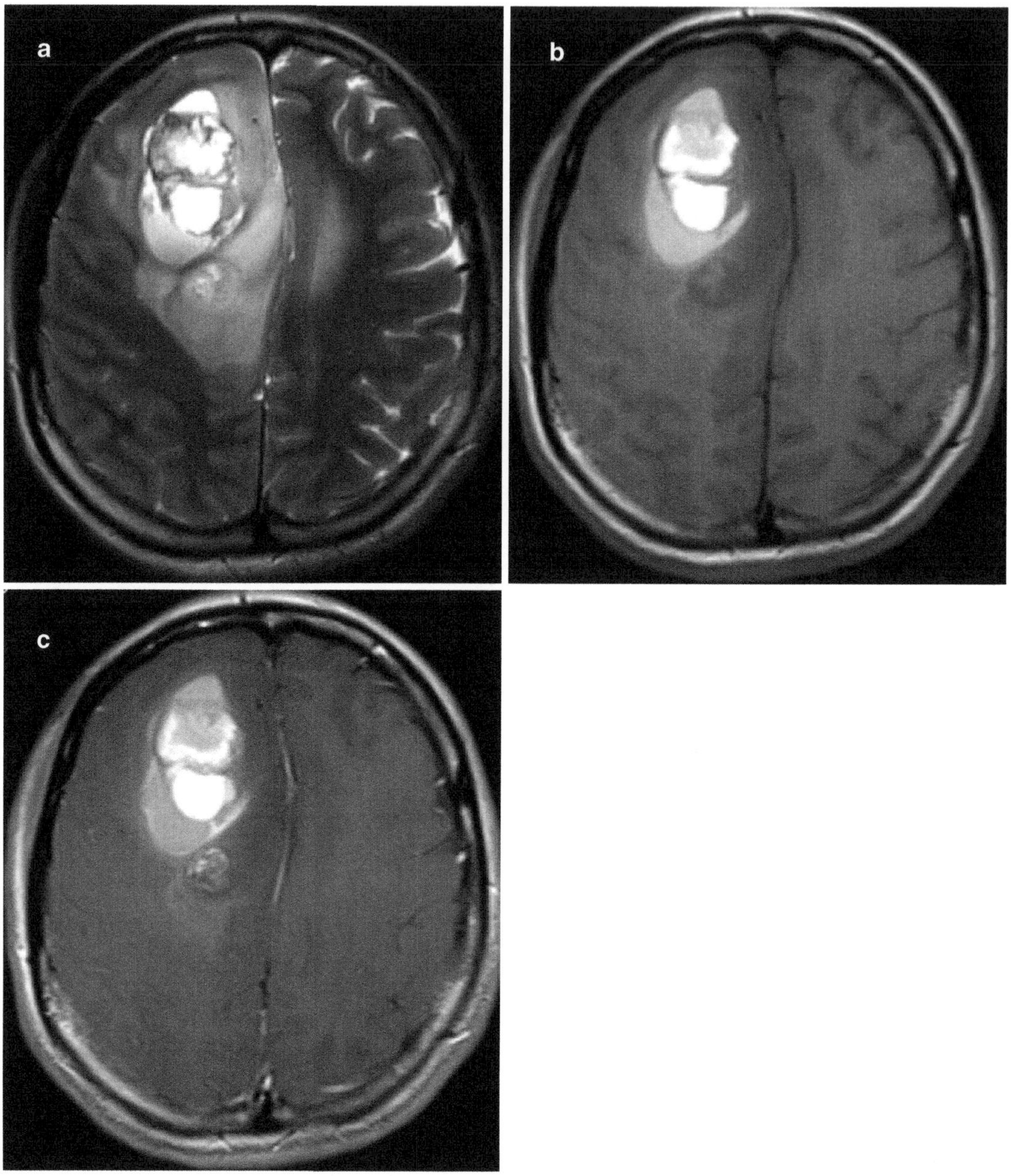


**Fig. 14** Tumoral hemorrhage. A patient with bronchial carcinoma. (**a**, **b**) T2W and T1W images demonstrate a right frontal subacute hematoma with prominent peripheral edema. (**c**) Postcontrast image depicts focal smaller enhancing lesion at the posterior aspect of the hematoma consistent with metastasis

One-third of all ischemic infarcts exhibit hemorrhagic transformation (Hart and Easton 1986). One of the leading causes of hemorrhagic transformation is thrombolytic therapy. 6–12% of the patients who receive thrombolytic therapy develop hemorrhagic transformation. Hemorrhagic transformation after thrombolytic therapy generally occurs in the early phase (first 48 h), whereas spontaneous hemorrhages can be observed up to 2 weeks after ischemia. Apart from thrombolytic therapy, hypertension, hyperglycemia, use of oral anticoagulants, advanced age, and severe infarcts are other factors that lead to increased risk of hemorrhagic transformation (Aviv et al. 2009;

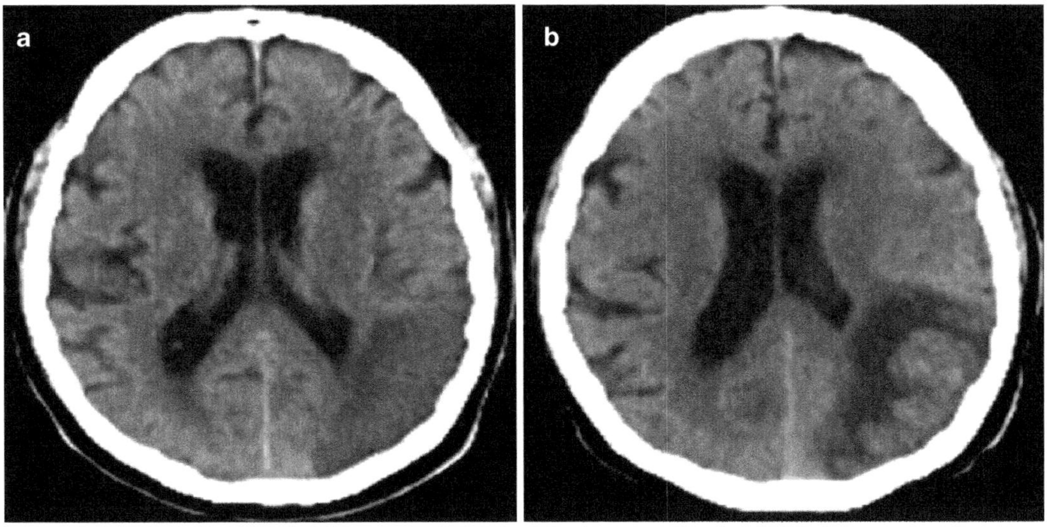


**Fig. 15** (**a**) Noncontrast CT shows acute infarction at the posterior temporal lobe. (**b**) 3 days later, hyperdense areas consistent with hemorrhage occurred in the infarcted area. Hemorrhagic transformation

Lansberg et al. 2007a). Hemorrhage can be petechial or parenchymal. Petechial hemorrhages do not usually have a clinical sign; they are detected in imaging and create gyriform low signal on T2*-weighted sequences. CT findings are even more unspecific with punctate hyperdensities in gray matter. Parenchymal hemorrhages have a more severe clinical presentation. In case of parenchymal hemorrhage, it may be difficult to distinguish between hemorrhagic transformation of ischemic infarct and other causes of intraparenchymal hemorrhage. A large area of cytotoxic edema around the hematoma and signal change compatible with a specific arterial feeding area on CT and MRI should raise suspicion (Fig. 15). In addition, DWI and SWI are also highly beneficial in the diagnosis. It is important to demonstrate an infarct area with low ADC along with a low-signal bleeding area on SWI.

Imaging findings that reflect the risk of hemorrhage in patients with ischemic stroke have been defined. A large hypodense area that reflects the infarction area on CT, hyperdense middle cerebral artery (MCA) sign, and prolonged period between stroke onset and initial imaging were associated with a high risk of hemorrhage (Chen et al. 2016; Lansberg et al. 2007b). It was also shown that a high blood–brain barrier permeability and hypoperfusion status on perfusion CT were associated with hemorrhagic transformation (Suh et al. 2019). It was demonstrated that a higher baseline DWI lesion volume on MRI meant a higher risk of bleeding to the same extent (Lansberg et al. 2007a).

### 3.2.7 Vasculitis/Vasculopathy

Vasculitis is the inflammation of blood vessel walls. As a result of inflammation, the vessel wall becomes thicker, luminal narrowing, or occlusion occurs or the vessel ruptures due to necrosis of the blood vessel wall. Therefore, ischemic symptoms due to occlusion or ICH due to blood vessel rupture is observed in vasculitis. Nearly 11% of the patients with CNS vasculitis develop ICH. The hemorrhage is frequently parenchymal, but it can also have subarachnoid and rarely subdural localization (Rehman 2000).

Vasculitis is diagnosed based on clinical findings, laboratory tests, and radiologic imaging due to the challenges in biopsy. Patients usually present with nonspecific symptoms such as headache, seizures, and focal neurologic deficits. Increased sedimentation rate and elevated CRP values according to the laboratory tests suggest inflammation. Imaging findings can be direct or indirect in CNS vasculitis. Direct findings of vessel involvement are thickening of the vessel wall and intramural contrast uptake, whereas indirect findings are luminal narrowing of the vessel and resulting ischemia, as well as perfusion abnormalities and ICH. The gold standard imaging modality in the diagnosis of CNS vasculitis is DSA. The specified inflammatory changes classically cause segmental cerebral vein stenosis and enlargement on angiography. However, the most commonly employed modality in patients with suspected vasculitis is MRI/MRA. The sensitivity of MRA for the diagnosis of large artery vasculitis reaches up to 100%, whereas DSA is superior to MRA in detecting pathologies of the small arteries (Pipitone et al. 2008; Garg 2011). Therefore, DSA should be performed when MRI + MRA is negative in patients suspected of having CNS vasculitis in order to rule out or diagnose small vessel involvement (Abdel Razek et al. 2014).

Moyamoya disease is a progressive vaso-occlusive disease of the distal internal carotid artery and its proximal branches (proximal anterior and middle cerebral arteries). As a result of occlusion, the lenticulostriate arteries and other perforating arteries become enlarged and form collateral vessel networks (puff of smoke). The term "Moyamoya syndrome" is used if there is an underlying cause (sickle cell anemia, neurofibromatosis type I, Down syndrome). MRI particularly shows ischemic lesions with watershed appearance and MRA shows lenticulostriate collateral veins and stenosis in the supraclinoid ICA. The disease generally manifests with cerebral ischemia in children, whereas hemorrhage is more prominent in the adult population. Hemorrhage is generally secondary to collateral vein rupture. Intraventricular hemorrhage is common, wherein intraparenchymal or subarachnoid hemorrhage can also be observed. Another cause of hemorrhage is the rupture of an anterior choroidal artery aneurysm, which is common in Moyamoya disease. The rate of rebleeding and infraction was shown to be higher in hemorrhage due to Moyamoya disease as compared to primary ICH (Nah et al. 2012).

Reversible cerebral vasoconstriction syndrome (RCVS) is characterized by thunderclap headache and manifests with vasoconstriction in multiple cerebral arteries. In addition, the patients may also have ischemic or hemorrhagic stroke and focal neurologic deficits. Vascular examination shows multifocal segmental constrictions in cerebral veins. Unlike other vasculopathies, these findings disappear within less than 3 months. Hemorrhages associated with RCVS can be isolated convexity SAH or intraparenchymal (Fig. 16). RCVS-associated hemorrhages were reported to be more prevalent in females and those with migraine type headaches (Ducros et al. 2010). Distinguishing RCVS from CNS vasculitis is essential for both administering the suitable treatment and predicting the prognosis. When RCVS is accurately diagnosed, unnecessary use of steroids and immunosuppressive agents, which are used to treat CNS vasculitis, would be prevented and the related side effects would be avoided. Elimination of the stimulus that triggers the syndrome would generally be sufficient to treat RCVS. In addition, compared to CNS vasculitis, RCVS does not require a biopsy to diagnose, the clinical picture is not progressive, and RCVS is more benign (Ducros et al. 2007; Marder et al. 2012).

### 3.2.8 Infection

Cerebral infections rarely cause ICH. However, it is critical to determine the infectious agent that causes ICH in order to start a specific treatment as soon as possible. Infectious agents cause hemorrhage via various mechanisms. These consist of vasculitis (as a result of the inflammatory reaction caused by the infectious agent on the vessel wall) and vessel wall necrosis, coagulopathy (thrombocytopenia, DIC, hemophagocytic syndrome), septic emboli, and microbial aneurysm rupture (Radwan and Sawaya 2011).

Infection should be considered, although rare, in the differential diagnosis of ICH in patients who do not have risk factors such as hypertension, who have negative angiography results and clinical (fever) and laboratory (leukocytosis, elevated sedimentation rate, and CRP) findings consistent with infection. CT and MRI may show bilateral multifocal hemorrhage foci secondary to septic emboli. Septic emboli should be suspected especially in the presence of bacterial endocarditis, miliary tuberculosis, and cryptococcal infec-

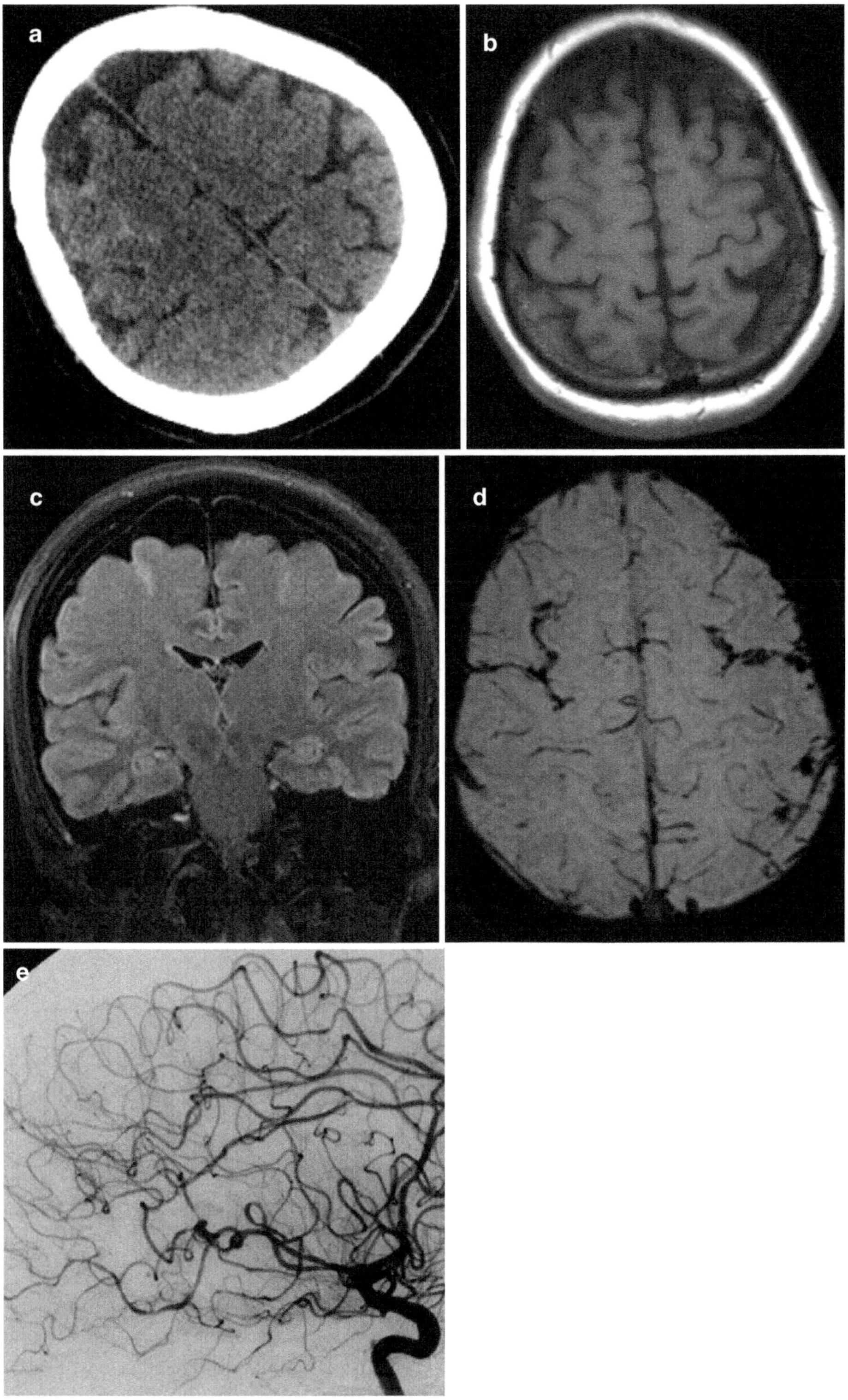


**Fig. 16** RCVS. (**a**) Noncontrast CT shows right frontal sulcal SAH in a young woman. T1W image looks normal (**b**) whereas FLAIR image (**c**) demonstrates sulcal hyperintensity on the right frontal region. (**d**) SWI much better demonstrates SAH in bilateral frontal sulci as sulcal hypointensities. (**e**) DSA shows beaded appearance and multiple focal stenotic areas in the distal branches of anterior and middle cerebral arteries

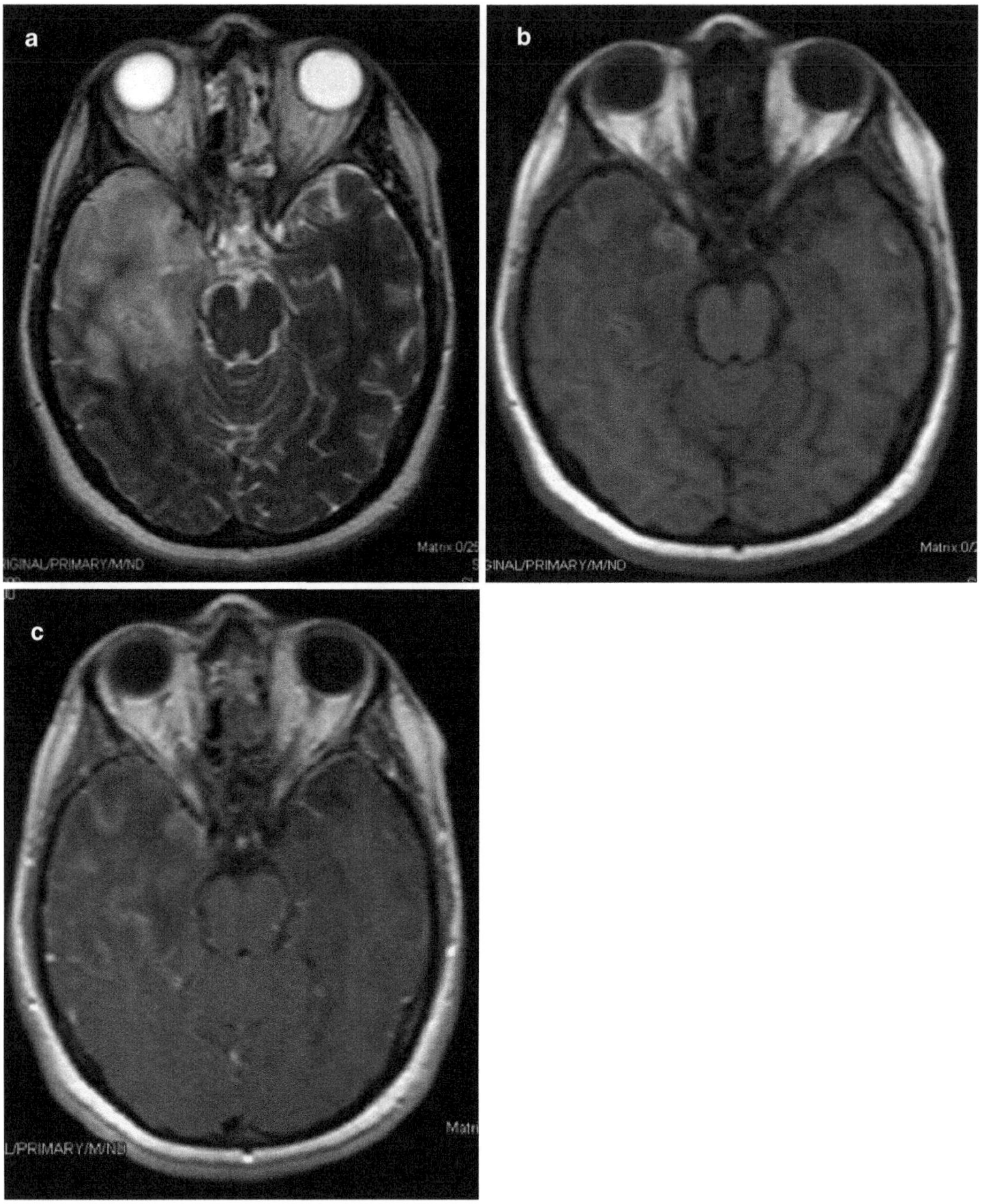


**Fig. 17** Hemorrhagic infectious encephalitis. (**a**) T2W image displays hyperintense lesion on the right temporal lobe which is diagnosed as herpes encephalitis. (**b**) Noncontrast T1W image demonstrates hyperintense foci inside the lesion consistent with hemorrhage. (**c**) On postcontrast image, heterogenous enhancement of the lesion is depicted

tion. The agent that most frequently causes microbial aneurysms is *S. aureus*, which commonly affects the distal branches of the middle cerebral artery. Pathologically, vessel wall inflammation, destruction of the muscularis and elastic lamina, subintimal fibrosis, and intimal hyperplasia can be observed. All these changes predispose the vein to rupture and SAH occurs. Herpes simplex virus (HSV) is the most common cause of encephalitis. HSV typically leads to necrotizing encephalitis that involves the temporal lobe, insula, and cingulate gyrus (Fig. 17).

Frequently, hemorrhage occurs secondary to necrosis. Hemorrhage is usually petechial. Intracranial hematoma formation is rarer (Argyriou et al. 2006). The mortality rate of HSV encephalitis ranges between 50 and 70%, wherein the prognosis is known to be worse in patients who have hemorrhage.

The most common causes of ICH in patients infected with HIV are neoplasms associated with HIV (primary CNS lymphoma, metastatic Kaposi's sarcoma) and opportunistic infections such as toxoplasmosis. However, ischemic lesions are more common than hemorrhages in patients with HIV (Pinto 1996).

### 3.2.9 Alcohol and Drugs

Alcohol is an important risk factor for ICH, and the risk is directly proportional to the amount of alcohol consumed. People who consume more than 40 g of alcohol per day (1 drink is defined as 12 g of alcohol) have a 4.6-fold increased risk of ICH in comparison with nondrinkers (Juvela et al. 1995). The risk increases up to 11.3-fold if alcohol consumption exceeds 120 g/day. ICH related to alcohol consumption is probably associated with the chronic increase in blood pressure due to alcohol. In addition, impaired hemostasis, decreased circulating levels of clotting factors produced by the liver, and DIC are other mechanisms that contribute to the pathophysiology of ICH. Hemorrhages may have intraparenchymal or subarachnoid localization (O'Connor et al. 2005).

Hemorrhages linked to drug abuse frequently occur due to sympathomimetic drugs (cocaine and amphetamine). Less frequently, opioids and cannabis may also cause ICH. Sympathomimetic drugs, especially cocaine and amphetamine, lead to a 9.6-fold increased risk of hemorrhage (Petitti et al. 1998). Whether the stroke is ischemic or hemorrhagic depends on the form of cocaine used. The hydrochloride form is more closely associated with hemorrhagic stroke and ICH than the alkaloidal form. In addition, it was shown that 41% of the patients with ICH associated with drug abuse also had coexisting pathologies such as an underlying aneurysm or AVM (Levine et al. 1991). Therefore, an angiography should be performed to detect underlying vascular malformations in drug users. In ICH associated with drug abuse, acute increase in blood pressure leads to hemorrhage unlike in the case of alcohol use. Moreover, cocaine is thought to cause hemorrhage by triggering the development of cerebral vasculitis or hemorrhagic transformation of ischemic infarct. It was shown that ICHs associated with cocaine use frequently had subcortical localization and more frequently had intraventricular extension and a poor prognosis.

## References


Abdel Razek AA, Alvarez H, Bagg S, Refaat S, Castillo M (2014) Imaging spectrum of CNS vasculitis. Radiographics 34:873–894

Al-Shahi R, Warlow C (2001) A systematic review of the frequency and prognosis of arteriovenous malformations of the brain in adults. Brain 124:1900e26

Argyriou A, Tsota I, Solomou E, Marangos M, Kalogeropoulou C, Petsas T et al (2006) Intracerebral haemorrhage as a rare complication of HSV-1 meningoencephalitis: case report and review of the literature. Scand J Infect Dis 1:63–66

Atlas SW, Grossman RI, Gomori JM et al (1987) Hemorrhagic intracranial malignant neoplasms: spin-echo MR imaging. Radiology 164:71–77

Aviv RI, D'Esterre CD, Murphy BD et al (2009) Hemorrhagic transformation of ischemic stroke: prediction with CT perfusion. Radiology 250:867e77

Bejot Y, Cordonnier C, Durier J et al (2013) Intracerebral haemorrhage profiles are changing: results from the Dijon population-based study. Brain 136:658–664

Borden JA, Wu JK, Shucart WA (1995) A proposed classification for spinal and cranial dural arteriovenous fistulous malformations and implications for treatment. J Neurosurg 82:166–179

Brott T, Broderick J, Kothari R et al (1997) Early hemorrhage growth in patients with intracerebral hemorrhage. Stroke 28:1e5

Carpenter CR, Hussain AM, Ward MJ et al (2016) Spontaneous subarachnoid hemorrhage: a systematic review and meta-analysis describing the diagnostic accuracy of history, physical examination, imaging, and lumbar puncture with an exploration of test thresholds. Acad Emerg Med 23:963–1003

Chen G, Wang A, Zhao X, Wang C, Liu L, Zheng H, Wang Y, Cao Y, Wang Y (2016) Frequency and risk factors of spontaneous hemorrhagic transformation following ischemic stroke on the initial brain CT or MRI: data from the China National Stroke Registry (CNSR). Neurol Res 38:538–544

Ciura VA, Romero JM (2014) Nontraumatic acute intraparenchymal hemorrhage: algorithm for workup and differential diagnosis. Semin Roentgenol 49:112–126

Cognard C, Gobin YP, Pierot L et al (1995) Cerebral dural arteriovenous fistulas: clinical and angiographic correlation with a revised classification of venous drainage. Radiology 194:671–680

Connolly ES, Rabinstein AA, Carhuapoma JR et al (2012) Guidelines for the management of aneurysmal subarachnoid hemorrhage: a guideline for healthcare professionals from the American Heart Association/American Stroke Association. Stroke 43:1711–1737

Coutinho JM, Zuurbier SM, Aramideh M, Stam J (2012) The incidence of cerebral venous thrombosis: a cross-sectional study. Stroke 43:3375–3377

Delcourt C, Huang Y, Arima H, Chalmers J, Davis SM, Heeley EL et al (2012) Hematoma growth and outcomes in intracerebral hemorrhage: the INTERACT1 study. Neurology 79:314–319

Demchuk AM, Dowlatshahi D, Rodriguez-Luna D et al (2012) Prediction of haematoma growth and outcome in patients with intracerebral haemorrhage using the CT-angiography spot sign (PREDICT): a prospective observational study. Lancet Neurol 11:307–314

Destian S, Sze G, Krol G et al (1989) MR imaging of hemorrhagic intracranial neoplasms. Am J Roentgenol 152:137–144

Dmytriw AA, Song JSA, Yu E, Poon CS (2018) Cerebral venous thrombosis: state of the art diagnosis and management. Neuroradiology 60:669–685

Ducros A, Bousser MG (2013) Thunderclap headache. BMJ 346:e8557

Ducros A, Boukobza M, Porcher R et al (2007) The clinical and radiological spectrum of reversible cerebral vasoconstriction syndrome. A prospective series of 67 patients. Brain 130:3091–3101

Ducros A, Fiedler U, Porcher R et al (2010) Hemorrhagic manifestations of reversible cerebral vasoconstriction syndrome: frequency, features, and risk factors. Stroke 41:2505–2511

Ferro JM, Canhao P, Stam J et al (2004) Prognosis of cerebral vein and dural sinus thrombosis: results of the International Study on Cerebral Vein and Dural Sinus Thrombosis (ISCVT). Stroke 35:664e70

Fisher CM (1971) Pathological observations in hypertensive cerebral hemorrhage. J Neuropathol Exp Neurol 30:536–550

Flaherty ML, Kissela B, Woo D et al (2007) The increasing incidence of anticoagulant-associated intracerebral hemorrhage. Neurology 68:116–121

Flibotte JJ, Hagan N, O'donnell J et al (2004) Warfarin, hematoma expansion, and outcome of intracerebral hemorrhage. Neurology 63:1059–1064

Foulkes MA, Wolf PA, Price TR, Mohr JP, Hier DB (1988) The stroke data Bank: design, methods, and baseline characteristics. Stroke 19:547–554

Fujii Y, Takeuchi S, Sasaki O et al (1998) Multivariate analysis of predictors of hematoma enlargement in spontaneous intracerebral hemorrhage. Stroke 29:1160–1166

Garg A (2011) Vascular brain pathologies. Neuroimaging Clin N Am 21:897–926

Greenberg SM, Eng JA, Ning M, Smith EE, Rosand J (2004) Hemorrhage burden predicts recurrent intracerebral hemorrhage after lobar hemorrhage. Stroke 35:1415–1420

Gross BA, Du R (2017) Hemorrhage from cerebral cavernous malformations: a systematic pooled analysis. J Neurosurg 126:1079–1087

Haacke EM, Mittal S, Wu Z, Neelavalli J, Cheng YC (2009) Susceptibility-weighted imaging: technical aspects and clinical applications, part 1 AJNR. Am J Neuroradiol 30:19–30

Hart RG, Easton JD (1986) Hemorrhagic infarcts. Stroke 17:586–589

Hemphill JC 3rd, Greenberg SM, Anderson CS et al (2015) Guidelines for the management of spontaneous intracerebral hemorrhage: a guideline for healthcare professionals from the American Heart Association/American Stroke Association. Stroke 46:2032–2060

Horstmann S, Rizos T, Lauseker M et al (2013) Intracerebral hemorrhage during anticoagulation with vitamin K antagonists: a consecutive observational study. J Neurol 260:2046–2051

Juvela S, Hillbom M, Palomaki H (1995) Risk factors for spontaneous intracerebral hemorrhage. Stroke 26:1558–1564

Kidwell CS, Chalela JA, Saver JL et al (2004) Comparison of MRI and CT for detection of acute intracerebral hemorrhage. J Am Med Assoc 292:1823–1830

Knudsen KA, Rosand J, Karluk D et al (2001) Clinical diagnosis of cerebral amyloid angiopathy: validation of the Boston criteria. Neurology 56(4):539

Kreel L, Kay R, Woo J, Wong HY, Nicholls MG (1991) The radiological (CT) and clinical sequelae of primary intracerebral haemorrhage. Br J Radiol 64: 1096–1100

Kumral E, Polat F, Uzunkopru C, Calli C, Kitis O (2012) The clinical spectrum of intracerebral hematoma, hemorrhagic infarct, non-hemorrhagic infarct, and non-lesional venous stroke in patients with cerebral sinus-venous thrombosis. Eur J Neurol 19:537–543

Lansberg MG, Thijs VN, Bammer R et al (2007a) Risk factors of symptomatic intracerebral hemorrhage after tPA therapy for acute stroke. Stroke 38:2275e8

Lansberg MG, Albers GW, Wijman CA (2007b) Symptomatic intracerebral hemorrhage following thrombolytic therapy for acute ischemic stroke: a review of the risk factors. Cerebrovasc Dis 24:1e10

Larsen CC, Astrup J (2013) Rebleeding after aneurysmal subarachnoid hemorrhage: a literature review. World Neurosurg 79:307–312

Leach JL, Fortuna RB, Jones BV, Gaskill-Shipley MF (2006) Imaging of cerebral venous thrombosis: current techniques, spectrum of findings, and diagnostic pitfalls. Radiographics 26:S19–S41

Levine SR, Brust JC, Futrell N et al (1991) A comparative study of the cerebrovascular complications of cocaine: alkaloidal versus hydrochloride—a review. Neurology 41:1173–1177

Lucas Cde P, Caldas JG, Prandini MN (2006) Do leptomeningeal venous drainage and dysplastic venous dilation predict hemorrhage in dural arteriovenous fistula? Surg Neurol 66(Suppl 3):S2–S5. discussion S5-6

Maia LF, Mackenzie IR, Feldman HH (2007) Clinical phenotypes of cerebral amyloid angiopathy. J Neurol Sci 257:23–30

Marder CP, Donohue MM, Weinstein JR et al (2012) Multimodal imaging of reversible cerebral vasoconstriction syndrome: a series of 6 cases. AJNR Am J Neuroradiol 33:1403–1410

Nah HW, Kwon SU, Kang DW et al (2012) Moyamoya disease-related versus primary intracerebral: hemorrhage location and outcomes are different. Stroke 43:1947–1950

Newton TH, Cronqvist S (1969) Involvement of dural arteries in intracranial arteriovenous malformations. Radiology 93:1071–1078

O'Connor AD, Rusyniak DE, Bruno A (2005) Cerebrovascular and cardiovascular complications of alcohol and sympathomimetic drug abuse. Med Clin North Am 89:1343–1358

Osborn AG (1994) Diagnostic neuroradiology. Mosby, St. Louis, MO

Pantoni L (2010) Cerebral small vessel disease: from pathogenesis and clinical characteristics to therapeutic challenges. Lancet Neurol 9:689–701

Perry JJ, Stiell IG, Sivilotti ML et al (2011) Sensitivity of computed tomography performed within six hours of onset of headache for diagnosis of subarachnoid haemorrhage: prospective cohort study. BMJ 343: d4277

Petitti DB, Sidney S, Quesenberry C et al (1998) Stroke and cocaine or amphetamine use. Epidemiology 9:596–600

Pinto AN (1996) AIDS and cerebrovascular disease. Stroke 27:538–543

Pipitone N, Versari A, Salvarani C (2008) Role of imaging studies in the diagnosis and follow-up of large-vessel vasculitis: an update. Rheumatology (Oxford) 47:403–408

Poon CS, Chang J-K, Swarnkar A, Johnson MH, Wasenko J (2007) Radiologic diagnosis of cerebral venous thrombosis: pictorial review. Am J Roentgenol 189:S64–S75

Radwan W, Sawaya R (2011) Intracranial haemorrhage associated with cerebral infections: a review. Scand J Infect Dis 43:675–682

Rammos S, Maina R, Lanzino G (2009) Developmental venous anomalies: current concepts and implications for management. Neurosurgery 65:20e9

Rehman HU (2000) Primary angiitis of the central nervous system. J R Soc Med 93:586–588

Rollins N, Ison C, Reyes T, Chia J (2005) Cerebral MR venography in children: comparison of 2D time-of-flight and gadolinium enhanced 3D gradient-echo techniques. Radiology 235:1011–1017

Romero JM, Artunduaga M, Forero NP et al (2009) Accuracy of CT angiography for the diagnosis of vascular abnormalities causing intraparenchymal hemorrhage in young patients. Emerg Radiol 16:195–201

Rosand J, Hylek EM, O'Donnell HC et al (2000) Warfarin associated hemorrhage and cerebral amyloid angiopathy: a genetic and pathologic study. Neurology 55:947e51

Saposnik G, Barinagarrementeria F, Brown RD, Bushnell CD, Cucchiara B, Cushman M, deVeber G, Ferro JM, Tsai FY (2011) On behalf of the American Heart Association stroke council and the council on epidemiology and prevention. Diagnosis and management of cerebral venous thrombosis: a statement for healthcare professionals from the American Heart Association/American Stroke Association. Stroke 42:1158–1192

Shahi R, Warlow C (2001) A systematic review of the frequency and prognosis of arteriovenous malformations of the brain in adults. Brain 124:1900e26

Smith EE, Nandigam KR, Chen YW et al (2010) MRI markers of small vessel disease in lobar and deep hemispheric intracerebral hemorrhage. Stroke 41:1933–1938

Spetzler RF, Martin NA (1986) A proposed grading system for arteriovenous malformations. J Neurosurg 65:476e83

Stapf C, Mast H, Sciacca R et al (2006) Predictors of hemorrhage in patients with untreated brain arteriovenous malformation. Neurology 66:1350e5

Suh CH, Jung SC, Cho SJ, Kim D, Lee JB, Woo DC, Oh WY, Lee JG, Kim KW (2019) Perfusion CT for prediction of hemorrhagic transformation in acute ischemic stroke: a systematic review and meta-analysis. Eur Radiol 29:4077–4087

Tanskanen M, Makela M, Myllykangas L et al (2012) Prevalence and severity of cerebral amyloid angiopathy: a population-based study on very elderly Finns (Vantaa 85+). Neuropathol Appl Neurobiol 38:329–336

Tsai LK, Jeng JS, Liu HM et al (2004) Intracranial dural arteriovenous fistulas with or without cerebral sinus thrombosis: analysis of 69 patients. J Neurol Neurosurg Psychiatry 75:1639–1641

van Asch CJ, Luitse MJ, Rinkel GJ et al (2010) Incidence, case fatality, and functional outcome of intracerebral haemorrhage over time, according to age, sex, and ethnic origin: a systematic review and meta-analysis. Lancet Neurol 9:167–176

van Gijn J, Kerr R, Rinkel G (2007) Subarachnoid haemorrhage. Lancet 369:306–318

Wada R, Aviv RI, Fox AJ et al (2007) CT angiography "spot sign" predicts hematoma expansion in acute intracerebral hemorrhage. Stroke 38:1257–1262

Wycliffe ND, Choe J, Holshouser B et al (2004) Reliability in detection of hemorrhage in acute stroke by a new three-dimensional gradient recalled echo susceptibility-weighted imaging technique compared to computed tomography: a retrospective study. J Magn Reson Imaging 20:372–377

Xhu XL, Chan MS, Poon WS (1997) Spontaneous intracranial hemorrhage: which patients need diagnostic cerebral angiography? Stroke 28:1406–1409

Yeung R, Ahmad T, Aviv RI et al (2009) Comparison of CTA to DSA in determining the etiology of spontaneous ICH. Can J Neurol Sci 36:176–180

Zipfel GJ, Shah MN, Refai D et al (2009) Cranial dural arteriovenous fistulas: modification of angiographic classification scales based on new natural history data. Neurosurg Focus 26:E14

# Emergent CNS Infections, Inflammations, and Tumors

Ferdinando Caranci, Domenico Cicala, Fabio Tortora, Federico Donnarumma, Pasquale Guerriero, Emiliano Barbieri, and Luca Brunese

## Contents




F. Caranci (✉) · F. Donnarumma · P. Guerriero
E. Barbieri · L. Brunese
Department of Medicine and Health Sciences, University of Molise, Campobasso, Italy
e-mail: ferdinando.caranci@unimol.it

D. Cicala
Pediatric Neuroradiology, Santobono-Pausilipon Children's Hospital, Naples, Italy

F. Tortora
Department of Precision Medicine, School of Medicine, "Luigi Vanvitelli" University of Campania, Naples, Italy



**Abstract**

Patients with central nervous system (CNS) neoplasms are potentially subjected to develop many neurologic complications of their disease or its treatment. The central and peripheral nervous systems can be also significantly affected by systemic malignancies.

These neuro-oncologic conditions are common and represent a significant cause of mor-




M. Scaglione et al. (eds.), *Emergency Radiology of the Head and Spine*, Medical Radiology Diagnostic Imaging, https://doi.org/10.1007/978-3-030-91047-1_7

bidity and hospital admission, not rarely at risk for serious, timely, and life-threatening events.

Early diagnosis and timely treatment are required to ensure the best possible outcome, prolonging survival, and improving the quality of life; appropriate management may preserve neurologic function and may be life-saving.

Neuroimaging evaluation represents a critical point in management of these patients, being helpful and often essential to define the diagnosis. Noncontrast head computed tomography (CT) is often the preferred imaging modality for the first examination of acute patients, due to speed and availability. Magnetic resonance imaging (MRI) is superior in identifying lesions and related features, characterizing them, and detecting the associated complications in order to obtain a more complete diagnosis.

Central nervous system infections still have a great impact in terms of severity, affecting all age groups; they may represent a real medical emergency because of the consequent complications and fatal outcome if not diagnosed and treated promptly.

The role of diagnostic imaging is fundamental, because CT and MR imaging have had a great impact on the diagnosis and management of CNS infections together with the physical examination and laboratory investigations, especially in identifying and narrowing the differential diagnosis and monitoring the therapeutic response.

The relevant literature concerning all of these topics is summarized in this chapter.

## 1 Neuro-Oncologic Emergencies

### 1.1 Introduction

Patients with central nervous system (CNS) neoplasms are potentially subjected to develop many neurologic complications of their disease or its treatment. The central and peripheral nervous systems can be also significantly affected by systemic malignancies.

These neuro-oncologic conditions are common and represent a significant cause of morbidity and hospital admission, not rarely at risk for serious, timely, and life-threatening events. Neurologic signs and symptoms occur in about 15% of cancer patients over the course of treatment and are present in approximately 30% to 50% of oncologic patients presenting to the emergency department or requiring neurologic consultation (Giglio and Gilbert 2010; Schiff et al. 1998a, b). Furthermore, with increasing life expectancy of cancer patients, these emergencies will be more frequently encountered.

Neurologic conditions are commonly due to the tumor's direct effects on the nervous system, such as hydrocephalus, cerebral edema, and increased intracranial pressure, seizures, spinal cord compression, and leptomeningeal metastases.

Indirect effects may develop as a result of systemic cancer-related conditions, which may secondarily involve the brain, the spinal cord, and the peripheral nervous system. These complications include paraneoplastic encephalitis, infectious disease, and cerebrovascular disease.

In addition, various treatment modalities can damage the nervous system and are also associated with various neurologic complications and emergencies.

Neurocritical multidisciplinary team must be able to promptly recognize these emergencies, which, when untreated, may result in irreversible injury to nervous system.

Early diagnosis and timely treatment are required to ensure the best possible outcome, prolonging survival, and improving the quality of life; appropriate management may preserve neurologic function and may be life-saving.

Neuroimaging evaluation represents a critical point in the management of these patients, being helpful and often essential to define the diagnosis. Noncontrast head computed tomography (CT) is often the preferred imaging modality for the first examination of acute patients, due to speed and availability. Magnetic resonance imaging (MRI) is superior in identifying lesions and related features, characterizing them, and detecting the associated complications in order to obtain a more complete diagnosis.

## 1.2 Edema and Cerebral Herniation

The development of elevated intracranial pressure (ICP) syndrome is a frequent complication and emergency in neuro-oncologic patients, which can rapidly result in irreversible neurologic deficits and death.

Primary or secondary CNS neoplasms are often associated with edema and resultant mass effect, which may lead to a progressive increase in ICP, brain tissue displacement, and ultimately herniation.

Peritumoral edema is a significant cause of morbidity and mortality in patients with CNS neoplasms; it is typically vasogenic (Kaal and Vecht 2004), caused by inflammatory reaction around the neoplasms and blood–brain barrier (BBB) disruption resulting in increased vascular permeability.

Patients with cerebral tumor present with signs and symptoms related to tumor mass and increased intracranial pressure; clinical status may be more heterogeneous, ranging from vague symptoms to severe and life-threatening conditions. Localized neurologic symptoms are variable and related to the tumor mass locations; they may include seizures, hemiparesis, hemisensory deficits, aphasia and/or dysphasia, ataxia, cranial nerve palsies, endocrine dysfunction, and visceral dysfunction (Baldwin et al. 2012; Forsyth and Posner 1993).

Typical nonfocal symptoms of increased intracranial pressure include headache, nausea, vomiting, diplopia from abducens nerve palsies, and mental status decline; clinical onset is usually subtle or insidious, although associated intratumoral hemorrhage or obstructive hydrocephalus may cause a more dramatic presentation, with acute onset and severe mental status alteration, resulting in lethargy or obtundation. Bradycardia and hypertension are late findings, generally following a decline in consciousness status (Jo and Schiff 2017; Forsyth and Posner 1993; Damek 2010; Pater et al. 2014). Evidence of papilledema at ophthalmologic examination may be helpful to support clinical suspicion in early diagnosis (Jo and Schiff 2017; Forsyth and Posner 1993).

Peritumoral vasogenic edema exacerbates signs and symptoms related to mass effect and increased intracranial pressure. Furthermore, over the CNS neoplastic course, patients often develop worsening of vasogenic edema due to tumor progression, intratumoral hemorrhage, radiation effects, and other systemic complications or comorbidities.

Progressive vasogenic edema and/or massive tumor growth can lead to acute cerebral herniation, especially when rapid increment of ICP occurs, due to the development of an intracranial pressure gradient (Gower et al. 1987; Coburn and Rodriguez 1998). Herniation is characterized by a rapid decline in clinical status and depression in the level of consciousness; in this case, an emergency decompressive craniotomy may be life-saving.

Brain MRI provides a better characterization of edema and mass effect than CT examination, although the latter is preferable in the acute stage and unstable patients. In MRI studies, edema is clearly visible as areas of hyperintensity on T2 and fluid-attenuated inversion recovery (FLAIR) sequences because of high water content, associated with effacement of the cortical sulci and compression of the ventricular system, due to tumoral mass effect (Fig. 1). Disruption of the BBB is visualized as areas of parenchymal enhancement in post-contrast T1-weighted sequences (Kaal and Vecht 2004; Walker and Kapoor 2007; Jo and Schiff 2017).

Intracranial brain herniation syndrome includes various types related to mass location, characterized by a typical spectrum of imaging findings and clinical signs (Coburn and Rodriguez 1998; Katabathina et al. 2013); it is often associated with secondary complications such as hydrocephalus, vascular compression, and ischemic and/or hemorrhagic tissue damage.

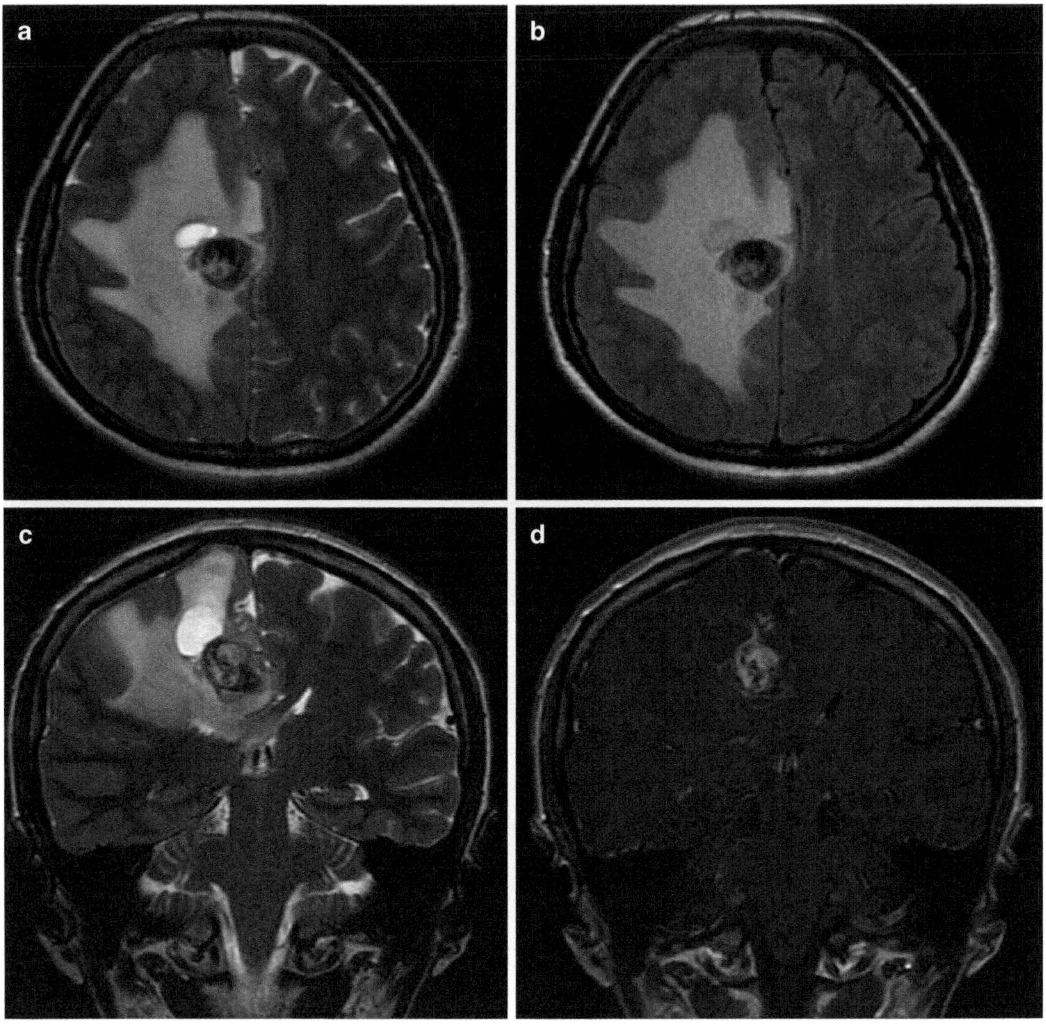


**Fig. 1** Neoplastic edema and mass effect. Axial T2-weighted (**a**) and FLAIR-weighted images (**b**) and coronal T2-weighted (**c**) and *gadolinium*-enhanced T1-weighted images (**d**) show right frontal metastatic lesion of breast cancer with large amount of perilesional vasogenic edema, effacement of the cortical sulci, compression of ventricular system, and incipient subfalcine herniation; inhomogeneous lesional enhancement is observed on post-contrast T1-weighted sequences

In *subfalcine herniation*, which can occur as a consequence of large frontal lobe masses, cingulate gyrus is displaced under the falx (Fig. 2); it can lead to hydrocephalus due to obstruction of the foramina of Monro and compression of the anterior cerebral artery (Jo and Schiff 2017; Pater et al. 2014; Lin and Avila 2017; Marino et al. 2006; Stevens et al. 2012).

Massive temporal tumors and/or edema could evolve in *descending transtentorial herniation*, in which uncus and parahippocampal gyrus displace inferiorly through the tentorial incisura (Fig. 3); the herniating lobe may cause compression of the midbrain against the opposite tentorial incisura, compression of the ipsilateral third cranial nerve, and contralateral corticospinal tract resulting in oculomotor palsy and motor impairment in the same side of supratentorial lesion (Kernohan's notch phenomenon); herniation may also cause compression of the posterior cerebral artery that can cause occipital infarct; the suprasellar cistern can be obliterated,

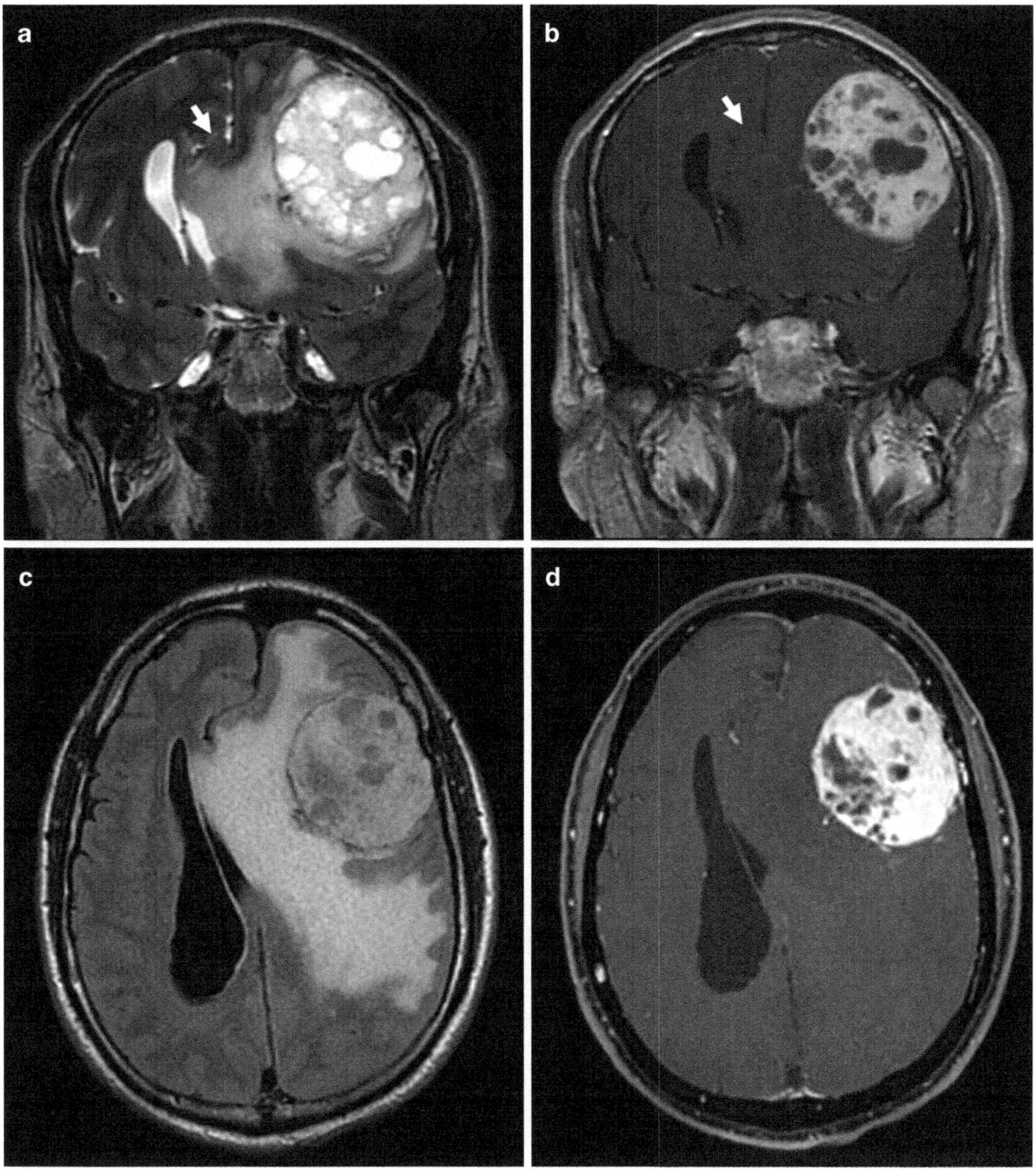


**Fig. 2** Subfalcine herniation. Coronal T2-weighted (**a**) and *gadolinium*-enhanced T1-weighted images (**b**) and axial FLAIR-weighted (**c**) and *gadolinium*-enhanced T1-weighted images (**d**) show left frontal meningioma causing displacement and compression of frontal lobe and ventricular system, vasogenic edema, and subfalcine herniation of the cingulate gyrus

with secondary compression of the optic chiasm and neighboring vascular structures (Jo and Schiff 2017; Pater et al. 2014; Lin and Avila 2017; Marino et al. 2006; Stevens et al. 2012).

*Tonsillary herniation* in spinal canal may occur in cases of large tumor involving posterior fossa, more frequently in pediatric patients (Fig. 4). Cerebellar tonsils are pushed inferiorly through the foramen magnum. Obstructive hydrocephalus may result from secondary occlusion of the fourth ventricle and its apertures. Obliteration of cisterna magna and brainstem

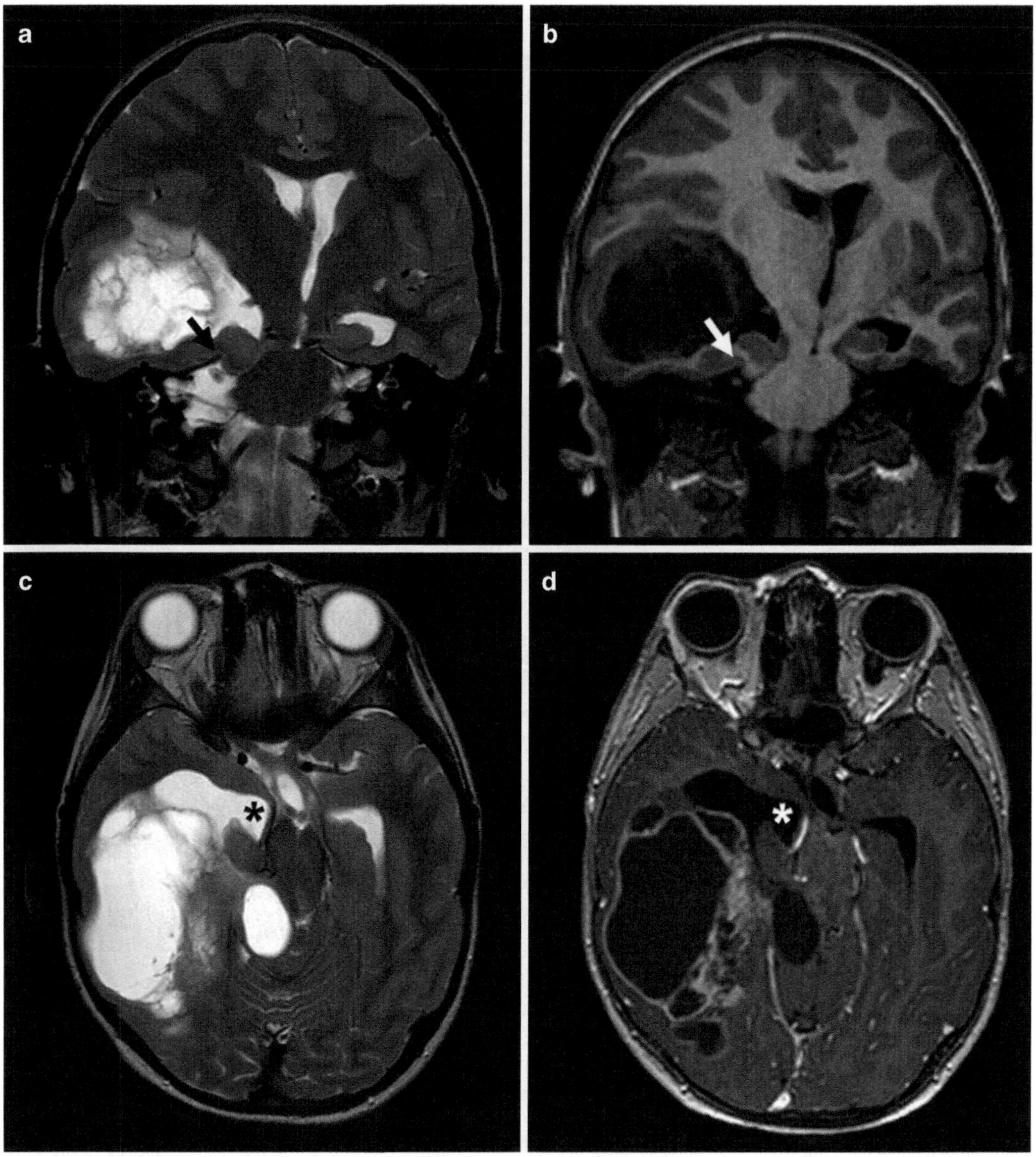


**Fig. 3** Descending transtentorial herniation. Neoplastic intracerebral mass of right temporal lobe causing mass effect and descending transtentorial herniation of medial temporal lobe through the tentorial incisura (arrow), as shown in coronal T2-weighted (**a**) and T1-weighted MR images (**b**). Axial T2-weighted (**c**) and *gadolinium-enhanced* T1-weighted MR images (**d**) demonstrate uncal herniation across the tentorial incisura (asterisk), compressing the brainstem and the optic chiasm in suprasellar cistern

compression may also occur, affecting the respiratory centers. Sometimes, posterior fossa mass effect can lead to *ascending transtentorial herniation* of cerebellum and midbrain (Jo and Schiff 2017; Damek 2010; Pater et al. 2014; Lin and Avila 2017; Stevens et al. 2012).

Besides the evaluation of tumoral mass and edema, neuroimaging can detect displacement of intracranial structures, midline shift, and ventricular compression (Coburn and Rodriguez 1998; Stevens et al. 2012). Identification of the type of herniation is critical to define the type of emergency treatment. Management of ICP and

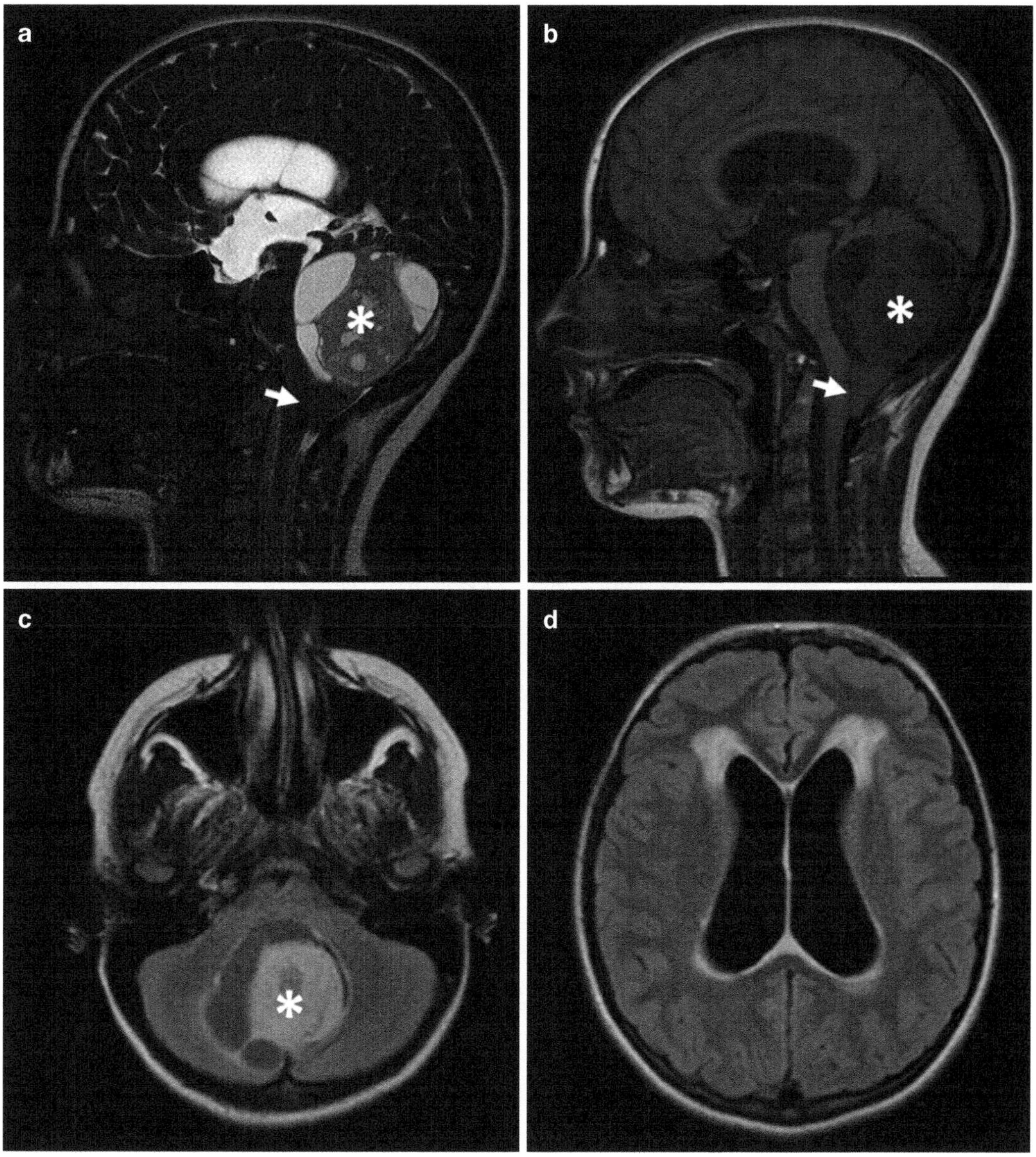


**Fig. 4** Tonsillar herniation. Neoplastic lesion into the fourth ventricle (asterisk) causes inferior descent of the cerebellar tonsils below the foramen magnum (arrow), detectable on midsagittal T2-weighted (**a**) and T1-weighted MR images (**b**); occlusion of the *cerebral aqueduct with* secondary obstructive hydrocephalus and prominence of the floor of third ventricle in suprasellar cistern are observed. Axial FLAIR-weighted MR images (**c** and **d**) show obliteration of pontocerebellar cistern, enlargement of supratentorial ventricles, and periventricular white matter hyperintensities around the frontal ventricular horns, due to periventricular transependymal edema

edema includes high-dose corticosteroids administration and osmotherapy; urgent surgical debulking or decompression is often required for the treatment of herniation.

### 1.3 Hemorrhage

Intracerebral hemorrhage (ICH) is not rarely a complication of CNS tumors, also because of the increased risk of bleeding in cancer patients (Lulla et al. 2011; Navi et al. 2010).

Approximately 1–10% of all spontaneous intracranial hemorrhages are due to bleeding from brain tumors (Iwama et al. 1992; Fewel et al. 2003; Little et al. 1979). ICH as onset of brain tumors accounts approximately in 0.5–3.5% of cases; it is the main finding of clinical status at diagnosis of about 40% of all brain tumors with hemorrhage (Iwama et al. 1992).

Various types of brain tumors may cause hemorrhage. Commonly, intratumoral hemorrhage occurs in approximately 5% of patients with high-grade gliomas, especially in glioblastoma (Lulla et al. 2011; Navi et al. 2010; Li et al. 2014; Barkovich and Atlas 1988; Ryken et al. 2014; Schettino et al. 2017); during the tumor growth, rapid progression and hypervascular setting of neoplasms are characterized by the development of numerous immature new vessels, which may be responsible for angiorrhexis and hemorrhagic stroke. However, some low-grade neoplasms may also have intratumoral hemorrhage (Lulla et al. 2011; White et al. 2008): some authors reported increased rate of hemorrhage in pilocytic astrocytoma compared to glioblastoma [20, 27, 28]. Bleeding depends also on some tumor's intrinsic properties, such as oligodendroglioma, which shows hemorrhage in 7–14% of cases (Iwama et al. 1992; Lieu et al. 1999; Wakai et al. 1982). Furthermore, tumoral hemorrhage occurs in about 9% of metastatic intracranial tumors; among them, choriocarcinoma, melanoma, lung, papillary thyroid, and renal cell cancer are the most prone to hemorrhage (Iwama et al. 1992; Lieu et al. 1999).

Hemorrhage may be caused by hemodynamic and structural changes in vascular network near and inside the tumoral mass, such as vascular necrosis and proliferation of fragile vessels supplying the growing tumor (Lulla et al. 2011; Iwama et al. 1992; Lieu et al. 1999). Bleeding may also occur as a consequence of surgical procedures or radiation-induced vascular damage. Risk factors include hypertension, treatment with antiangiogenic agents, thrombocytopenia, and coagulopathy.

Although not always symptomatic, the presence of intratumoral hemorrhage should be suspected in CNS tumor patients demonstrating new onset or worsening of intracranial hypertension symptoms, focal neurologic deficits or seizures, or sudden deterioration of clinical status (Lulla et al. 2011; Iwama et al. 1992).

Intracerebral hemorrhage may represent an emergency in the clinical course of cancer patients. At neuroradiological evaluation, bleeding often intensifies tumor volume and the amount of peripheral edema zone and space-occupying effect, resulting in new appearance or worsening of hydrocephalus, intracranial hypertension syndrome, or brain hernias. CT scan is an excellent and easily available modality for detecting acute blood products, which appear as hyperdense areas within or around the tumoral mass. MRI is more sensitive in detecting subtle blood products in the brain and within the tumor, especially on gradient recall echo (GRE) or susceptibility-weighted imaging (SWI) sequences (Fig. 5) (Kaal and Vecht 2004; Walker and Kapoor 2007; Jo and Schiff 2017; Haacke et al. 2004; Law 2009). Contrast-enhanced CT or MRI can be helpful to discriminate areas of cancerous tissue as solid-enhancing portion (Destian et al. 1989; Schrader et al. 2000).

Sometimes, unexplained hemorrhage may be the presentation of an unknown CNS tumor; irregularly shaped hemorrhages with conspicuous peripheral edema and mass effect, without the typical characteristics of hypertensive hemorrhage, may be suggestive of an underlying neoplasm; and other MRI features that may guide the clinical suspect include significant contrast enhancement and atypical clot evolution with time (Li et al. 2014; Clarke et al. 2010).

Delayed imaging within 6–12 weeks after the onset may be helpful in detecting the presence of an occult neoplasm, because of potential camouflage by recent blood products.

The acute management of intratumoral hemorrhage does not differ significantly from the spontaneous type. Treatment depends on the volume and the location of hemorrhagic

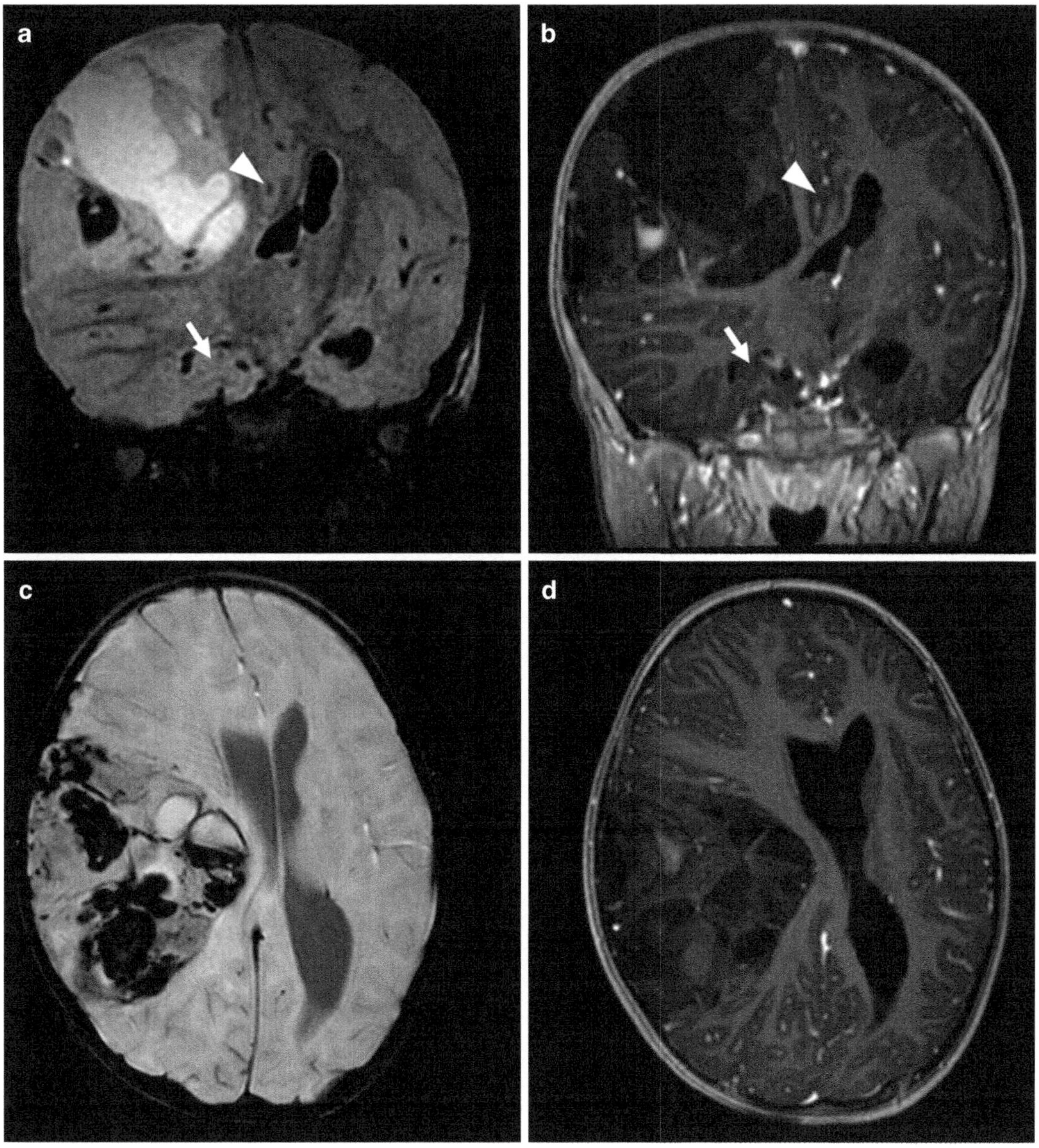


**Fig. 5** Intratumoral hemorrhage. Massive hemispheric desmoplastic infantile ganglioglioma with intralesional hemorrhage, which intensifies the mass effect: Coronal FLAIR-weighted (**a**) and *gadolinium*-enhanced T1-weighted images (**b**) show incipient subfalcine herniation (arrowhead) and transtentorial herniation (arrow); axial SWI-weighted (**c**) and *gadolinium*-enhanced T1-weighted (**d**) show fluid level due to intratumoral hemorrhage, well detectable on SWI image as low signal intensity areas

collection and clinical status of the patient; it includes corticosteroids and medication used for edema, blood pressure control, and treatment of coagulopathy; in some cases, surgical decompressive intervention or tempestive tumoral excision may be necessary for survival.

## 1.4 Hydrocephalus

Hydrocephalus is a not uncommon complication in CNS tumors. It may be classified into two different subtypes, obstructive and communicating.

Obstructive or noncommunicating hydrocephalus is a result of the obstruction to the CSF flow through ventricular system caused by a structural lesion such as neoplasm.

Communicating hydrocephalus results from impairment of CSF reabsorption, as in case of an obstruction of the arachnoid granulations. In cancer patients, it is most commonly caused by malignant seeding or infiltration of the leptomeninges, called "leptomeningeal carcinomatosis (LMC)" and described below. Nonobstructive hydrocephalus may be also caused by impairment of venous drainage due to sinus venous thrombosis, subarachnoid hemorrhage, or infectious meningitis.

Acute obstructive hydrocephalus is one of the major emergencies in patients with CNS tumor, frequently due to an obstacle to the flow of cerebrospinal fluid (CSF) in the ventricular system.

Obstructive hydrocephalus is common in pediatric oncologic patients, in which most tumors are located in the infratentorial compartment, in contrast to that observed in the adult population.

Clinical onset of posterior fossa tumors in children presents with signs and symptoms of hydrocephalus in 80% of cases (Lulla et al. 2011; Bognar et al. 2003). Medulloblastoma, ependymoma, and pilocytic astrocytoma are common pediatric CNS tumors of posterior cranial fossa, frequently showing compression or extension in the fourth ventricle and leading to obstructive supratentorial hydrocephalus (Fig. 6a–d).

Tumors in the pineal region can also present with obstructive hydrocephalus due to compression of cerebral aqueduct or third ventricle, resulting in dilatation of the bilateral lateral ventricles and downward herniation (Fig. 6e–h) (Lin and Avila 2017).

Obstructive hydrocephalus can be also a result of an intraventricular tumor, such as ependymoma, choroid plexus papilloma, intraventricular meningioma, and cystic non-neoplastic lesions (Spennato et al. 2016), which may cause obstruction at different levels of the ventricular system; for example, subependymal giant cell astrocytoma, commonly associated with tuberous sclerosis complex, is typically located near the foramina of Monro, potentially leading to hydrocephalus (Fig. 6i–n). Massive hemispheric lesion can entrap a lateral ventricle, resulting in an isolated dilatation of that ventricle, frequently associated with uncal herniation (Lin and Avila 2017).

*Extra-axial tumors such as meningioma or masses of sellar/suprasellar region can also present with obstructive hydrocephalus due to external compression of ventricular system* (Fig. 7).

Sometimes, obstructive hydrocephalus may present in cases of m*assive infiltrative intra-axial tumor, such as d*iffuse intrinsic pontine gliomas, generally as a delayed feature due to neoplastic volume and progression.

In adult patients, hydrocephalus is generally caused by massive leptomeningeal carcinomatosis or metastatic intraventricular diffusion.

Diagnosis of acute hydrocephalus should be considered in patient who presents intracranial hypertension syndrome with altered mental status, headache, vomiting, diplopia, and lateral gaze palsy due to sixth cranial nerve dysfunction and papilledema on fundoscopic examination.

The clinical presentation in younger children and infants can be subtle, ranging between irritability, macrocephaly, and tense anterior fontanelle to severe lethargy, bradycardia, and hypertension.

Acute hydrocephalus is a life-threatening emergency. Quickly detection and treatment can prevent a poor prognostic evolution.

CT or MRI examinations can provide a prompt evaluation of findings of obstructive hydrocephalus, which typically include ventriculomegaly proximal to the site of obstruction, periventricular transependymal edema, and effacement of the cortical sulci.

Differently from the communicating type, in patients with obstructive hydrocephalus a lumbar puncture is potentially unsafe because of the increasing risk of herniation and death (Lin and Avila 2017). For this reason, lumbar puncture is

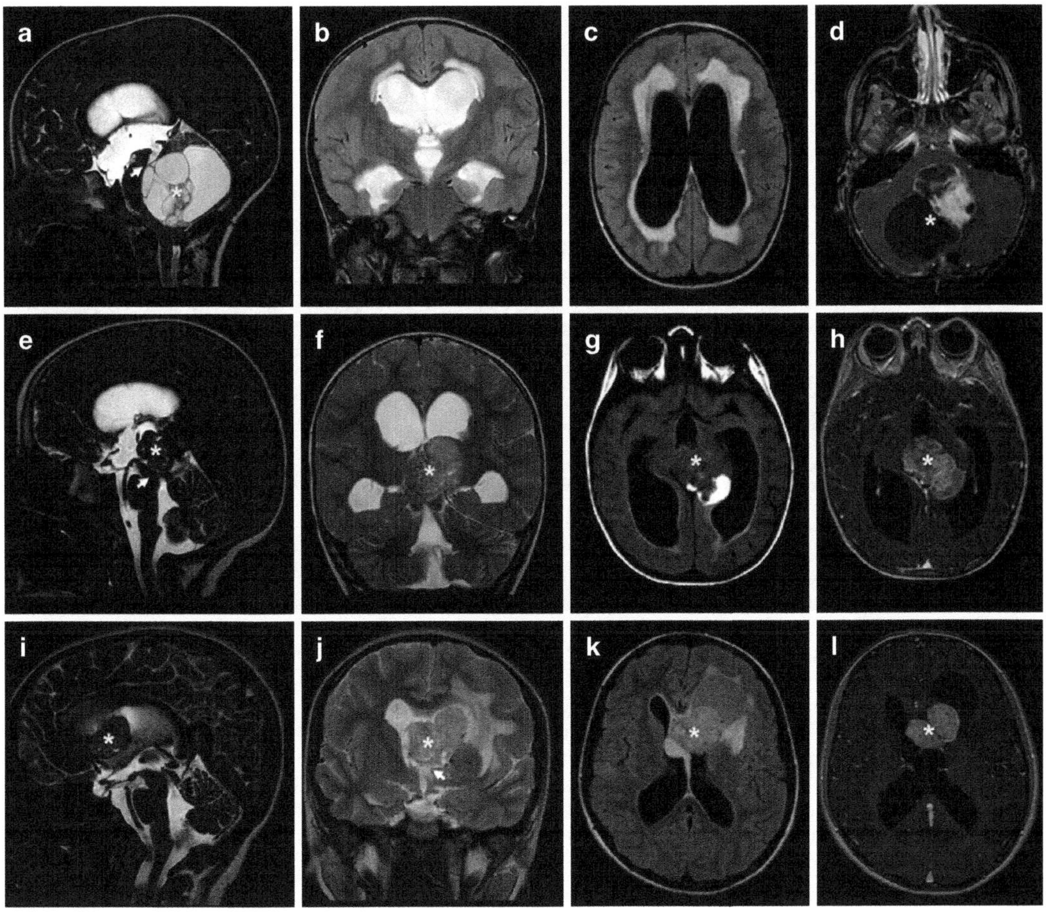


**Fig. 6** Obstructive hydrocephalus. Midsagittal T2-weighted DRIVE, coronal T2-weighted, axial FLAIR-weighted, and axial *gadolinium*-enhanced T1-weighted MR images show neoplastic masses (asterisk) causing obstruction at different levels (arrow) of the ventricular system. (**a–d**) Massive posterior fossa lesion occupies the fourth ventricle causing obstruction of the CSF egress at the lower segment of the aqueduct; secondary obstructive supratentorial hydrocephalus with prominence of the floor of third ventricle in suprasellar cistern, significant enlargement of the lateral ventricles, and periventricular transependymal edema are also visible. (**e–h**) Tumor in the pineal region causes aqueductal stenosis resulting in similar obstructive hydrocephalus. (**i–l**) Subependymal giant cell astrocytoma (SEGA) in patient affected by tuberous sclerosis results in bilateral obstruction of Monro foramen and asymmetric dilation of the lateral ventricles; note the entrapment of the left frontal horn characterized by different CSF fluid signal and sectorial periventricular edema

not recommended as intermediate step in the management of obstructive hydrocephalus, which needs prompt decompressive procedures (Gower et al. 1987; Lin and Avila 2017).

Many neurosurgical options can be performed to improve CSF flow, such as an emergency endoscopic ventriculostomy, ventricular shunting aqueductoplasty, septostomy, and tumor debulking and/or excision.

### 1.5 Leptomeningeal Carcinomatosis

Leptomeningeal carcinomatosis is a debilitating complication of malignancy, often occurring in the course of advanced disease. Cancer cells disseminate throughout the subarachnoid space, resulting in multifocal seeding on pia and arachnoid mater, which is most prominent in the

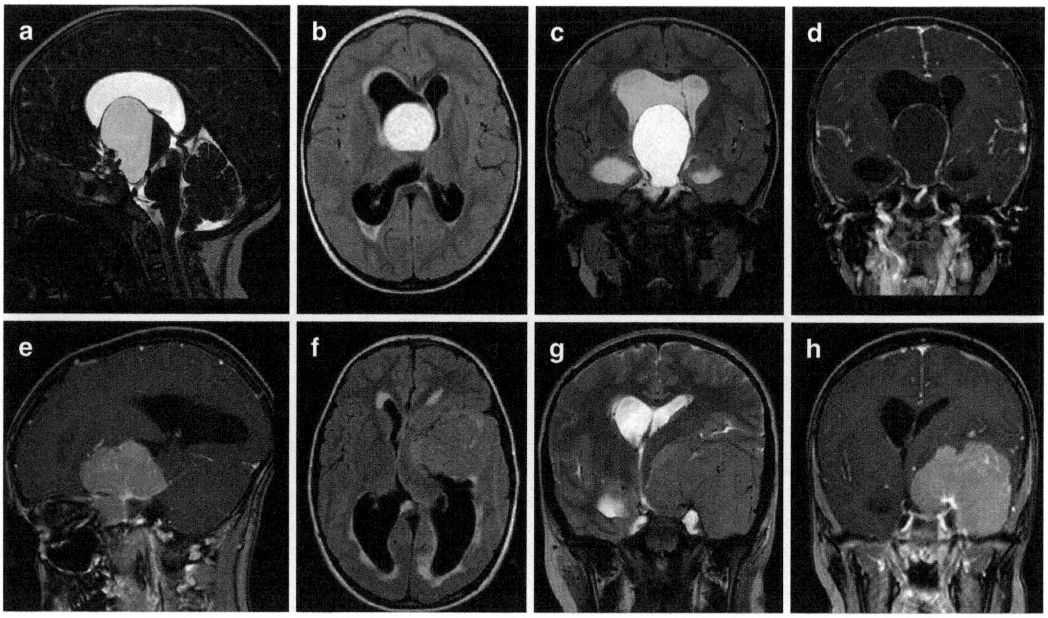


**Fig. 7** Hydrocephalus due to external compression of ventricular system. (**a–d**) Midsagittal T2-weighted DRIVE, axial FLAIR-weighted, coronal T2-weighted, and *gadolinium*-enhanced T1-weighted MR images show suprasellar neoplastic masses with massive cystic component and fluid level, causing obliteration of third ventricle and asymmetric obstruction of foramen of Monro with prevalent dilation of the right ventricle. (**e–h**) Sagittal *gadolinium*-enhanced T1-weighted, axial FLAIR-weighted, coronal T2-weighted, and *gadolinium*-enhanced T1-weighted MR images show large anterior clinoid meningioma causing displacement of temporal and frontobasal regions, with displacement and compression of frontal horn of ipsilateral ventricle, third ventricle, and Monro foramina resulting in obstructive hydrocephalus

skull base, cauda equina, and dorsal surface of spinal cord, because of gravitational effects. It causes multifocal neurologic symptoms and often results in a communicating type hydrocephalus (Jo and Schiff 2017; Chamberlain et al. 2014; Groves 2011; Clarke et al. 2010).

Metastatic involvement of the leptomeninges occurs most commonly in patients with hematologic malignancies (5%–15%) including lymphoma and leukemia, followed by solid tumors (1%–5%) such as breast cancer, lung cancer, and melanoma. Metastatic meningitis also occurs in patients with primary brain tumor (1–2%), especially medulloblastoma, ependymoma, high-grade gliomas, pineoblastomas, choroid plexus carcinoma, and primary CNS lymphoma (Giglio and Gilbert 2010; Jo and Schiff 2017; Baldwin et al. 2012; Katabathina et al. 2013; Chamberlain et al. 2014; Groves 2011; Clarke et al. 2010; Wassertrom et al. 2006; Chamberlain 1997). Furthermore, leptomeningeal seeding is reported in about 8–20% of autopsy in cancer patients (Giglio and Gilbert 2010; Glass et al. 1979). Malignant cells spread to the subarachnoid space mainly by hematogenous dissemination or direct extension from adjacent structures (Giglio and Gilbert 2010; Baldwin et al. 2012; Katabathina et al. 2013; Clarke et al. 2010; Chamberlain 1997).

Simultaneous occurrence of signs and symptoms affecting multiple areas of the neuraxis in a patient with cancer is highly suggestive of diffuse meningeal disease (Giglio and Gilbert 2010; Katabathina et al. 2013).

Patients may present multifocal symptoms reflecting multilevel nervous system involvement, such as headache and encephalopathy by hemisphere involvement, multiple cranial neuropathies, weakness, radicular pain, and bowel and bladder dysfunction due to spinal or nerve root involvement (Giglio and Gilbert 2010; Jo and Schiff 2017; Baldwin et al. 2012; Groves

2011; Clarke et al. 2010; Chamberlain 1997). In the initial phase, patients may also develop transitory normal pressure hydrocephalus with typical apraxic gait, incontinence, and confusion. Progressively, symptoms of increased intracranial pressure may appear when CSF flow obstruction occurs (Lin and Avila 2017; De la Fuente and DeAngelis 2014).

Diagnosis is made by CSF cytology and is supported by neuroimaging.

Before performing CSF analysis, gadolinium-enhanced MRI of the entire neuraxis should be performed to stage the extent of leptomeningeal involvement and guide management. It is also indicated in order to detect the presence of concurrent brain lesions and signs of increased intracranial pressure, in which case lumbar puncture is contraindicated (Giglio and Gilbert 2010; Katabathina et al. 2013).

In these last cases and when no malignant cells are detected in the fluid samples, MR imaging may provide strong support for diagnosis of leptomeningeal carcinomatosis; it is positive in approximately 95% of cases (Katabathina et al. 2013; Clarke et al. 2010; Passarin et al. 2015; Straathof et al. 1999).

MRI findings suggestive of LMC include meningeal enhancement in the cerebral sulci, cerebellar folia, basal cisterns, and cauda equina, which may be linear or nodular; enhancement of the ependymal surface of ventricles, cranial and spinal nerves, and hydrocephalus is also demonstrated (Fig. 8) (Katabathina et al. 2013; Groves 2011; Clarke et al. 2010; Sze et al. 1989).

Detection of malignant cells in the CSF samples remains the gold standard for diagnosis, with a specificity of about 95% and sensitivity of 50% (Enting 2005). Another purpose of the

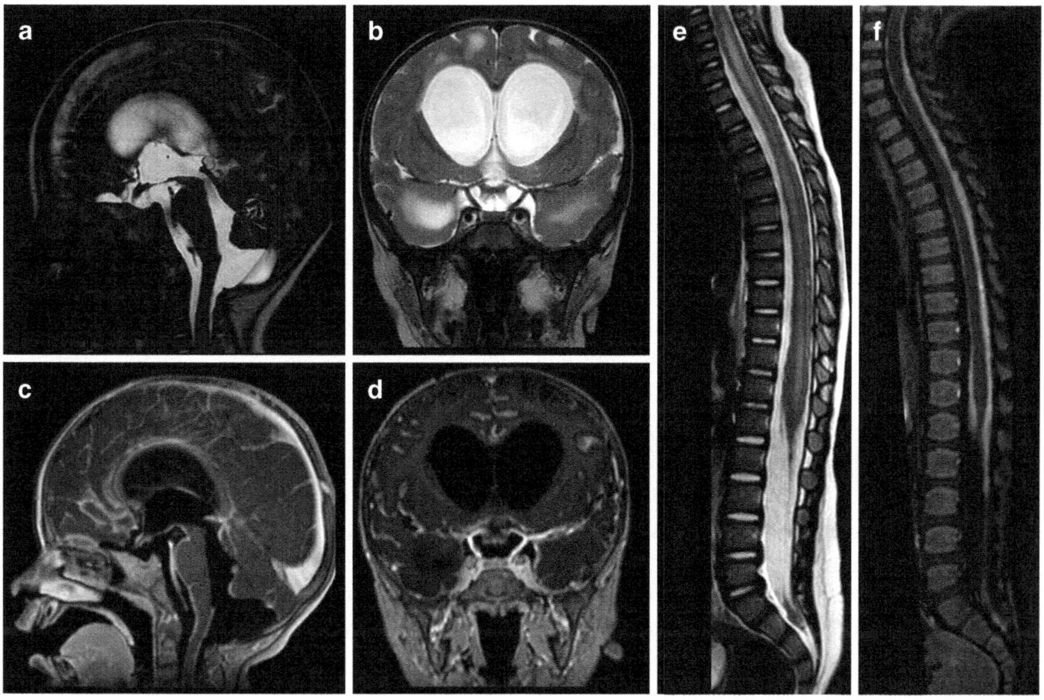


**Fig. 8** Leptomeningeal carcinomatosis. Brain T2-weighted (**a** and **b**) and *gadolinium*-enhanced T1-weighted images on sagittal and coronal planes (**c** and **d**) show diffuse leptomeningeal enhancement along the *pial surface* of the brain stem and basal cisterns, ventricular ependymal *surfaces*, cerebral sulci, and cerebellar folia, resulting in hydrocephalus. Spinal sagittal T2-weighted (**e**) and *gadolinium*-enhanced fat-suppressed T1-weighted images (**f**) show diffuse infiltrative thickening along the pial surface of the spinal cord with nodular thickening at the cauda equina and deposit of enhancing material in the thecal sac; diffuse pathological signal intensity of the spinal cord, due to consequent congestion and compression phenomena

lumbar puncture is to assess the potential benefits of ventricular decompression procedures in the patients to relieve the symptoms, in order to define the therapeutic strategies (Lin and Avila 2017).

Treatment is challenging and only palliative; the decision to initiate a therapy should be made according to prognostic implications. Median survival of LM is about 4–6 weeks for untreated patients, improving by 1–3 months in treated patients (Jo and Schiff 2017; Groves 2011; Clarke et al. 2010).

Treatment modality includes radiotherapy, systemic chemotherapy, or intrathecal chemotherapy. Patients showing an improvement in neurologic symptoms of hydrocephalus following CSF drainage could be candidate to surgery, in order to perform ventriculoperitoneal shunt (Lin and Avila 2017; De la Fuente and DeAngelis 2014).

## 1.6 Spinal Cord Compression

Spinal cord compression is a critical complication, which occurs in approximately 5% of cancer patients (Baldwin et al. 2012; Scott 2015; Bach et al. 1990; Schiff et al. 1998a, b; Elefante et al. 2012; Elefante et al. 2013); it is mostly due to spinal involvement of disseminated cancer-causing metastatic epidural spinal cord compression. More rarely, compression syndrome occurs in patients with intramedullary spinal tumors (astrocytomas and myxopapillary ependymoma), intradural extramedullary tumors (schwannomas, neurofibromas, dermoid, leptomeningeal metastases), or primary epidural tumors (sarcomas, neuroblastomas).

Lung, breast, and prostate cancer, lymphoma, and multiple myeloma are the most common primary source of underlying bone metastases (Jo and Schiff 2017; Scott 2015; McCurdy and Shanholtz 2012; Mak et al. 2011; Spinazze et al. 2005).

The vertebral column is the most common site for osseous metastases; the thoracic spine is most commonly involved (70%), followed by lumbar (20%) and cervical (10%) segments (Jo and Schiff 2017; Baldwin et al. 2012; Scott 2015; Spinazze et al. 2005).

Malignant spinal compression arises by 2 mechanisms.

Spread by means of a hematogenous route typically occurs via the Boston venous plexus to the vertebral body; consequent phenomena of invasion and bone destruction lead to vertebral collapse and its posterior displacement, in turn leading to invasion and outgrowth into the epidural space.

Tumors affecting the paraspinal region, such as lymphoma and neuroblastoma, could directly invade the spinal canal through the vertebral foramen with secondary growth of tumoral epidural masses, compressing the spinal cord (Jo and Schiff 2017; Baldwin et al. 2012; Katabathina et al. 2013; Scott 2015; Schiff et al. 1998a, b; Hammack 2012).

Spinal cord compression is a medical and/or surgical emergency that should be promptly evaluated to avoid severe morbidity due to potential irreversible deficits, such as paralysis and sphincter dysfunction. If not treated, it could lead to cord edema followed by ischemia and irreversible cord infarction (Baldwin et al. 2012; Sun and Nemecek 2010).

Early recognition of suspect signs and symptoms and timely diagnostic confirmation are imperative, since an appropriate management and urgent treatment can significantly improve the chance of neurologic recovery until complete remission of deficits.

Patient's pretreatment neurologic status is the most important prognostic factor for functional recovery (Jo and Schiff 2017; Bach et al. 1990). Furthermore, loss of ambulation has been shown to be an independent poor prognostic factor, also related to increment in hospital length of stay and costs (Scott 2015; Savage et al. 2014).

New onset back pain is the most common presenting symptom, followed by weakness and motor deficits, sensory loss, bladder, and bowel abnormalities related to autonomic dysfunction; the latter generally occurs later in the course of disease (Jo and Schiff 2017; McCurdy and Shanholtz 2012; Hammack 2012). Metastatic solid tumors may present with acute paraparesis or quadraparesis due to spinal cord compression (Lulla et al. 2011; Klein et al. 1991).

When spinal cord compression is clinically suspected, patients should be further evaluated with urgent spine imaging. MR imaging is the most reliable imaging modality for diagnosis (93% sensitivity and 97% specificity) (Schiff et al. 1998a, b; Baldwin et al. 2012), also useful for planning of radiotherapy and surgical resection. The entire spine should be imaged, in order to detect multilevel involvement (Katabathina et al. 2013; Cook et al. 1998).

Imaging findings include collapsed vertebral bodies and a spinal or paraspinal soft tissue mass, which is generally hypointense on T1-weighted MRI sequences and hyperintense on T2-weighted sequences and enhances with gadolinium (Fig. 9); displacement and compression of the thecal sac and spinal cord; increased T2 signal of cord indicative of edema, venous congestion, or ischemia (Katabathina et al. 2013; Hammack 2012; Cicala et al. 2013; Li and Poon 1988; Crocker et al. 2011; Caranci et al. 2018).

Multidetector CT is an acceptable alternative for diagnosis when MRI is contraindicated; nevertheless, it is not accurate enough to define the tumoral tissue, and intracanalar and paraspinal region and extent of spinal cord involvement (Schiff et al. 1998a, b; Hammack 2012).

When anamnestic history of neoplasm is not known, differential diagnosis between benign compression fractures and pathologic fractures can be challenging; some MR findings are helpful to establish the cause of vertebral collapse. Findings suggestive of metastatic fracture are evidence of a focal epidural or paraspinal mass, convex posterior border of the vertebral body, pedicle or posterior element involvement, and evidence of similar lesions at other spinal levels. Findings reported as suggestive of benign

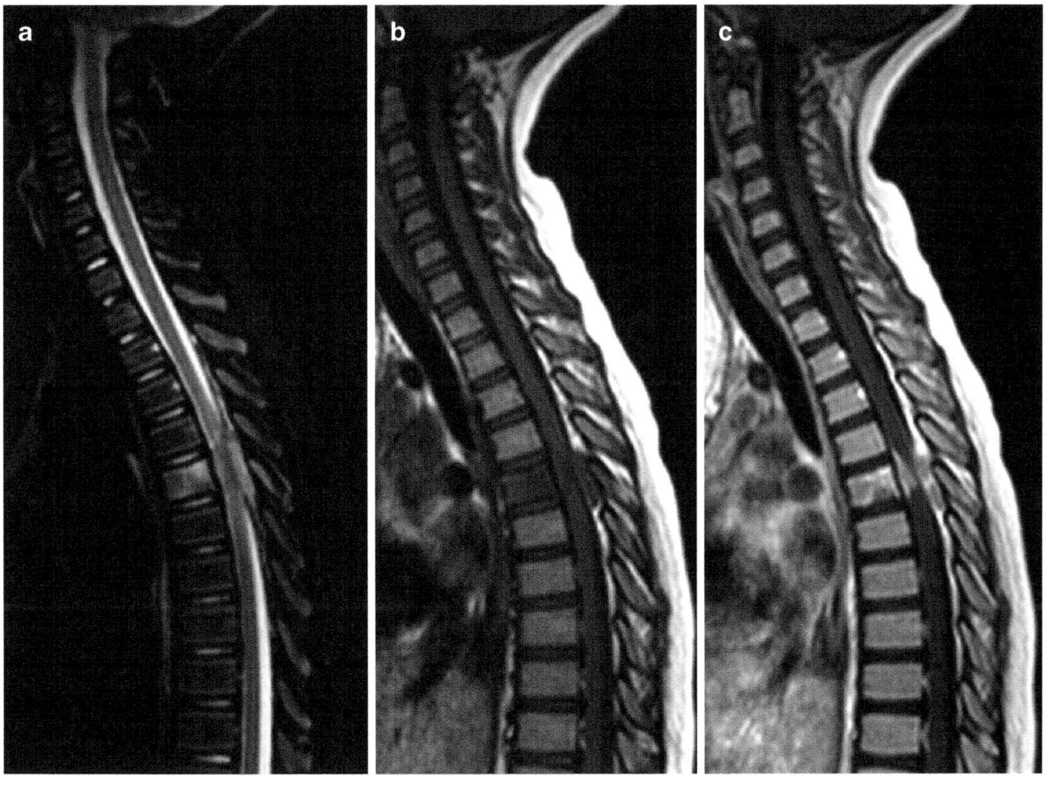


**Fig. 9** Spinal compression. Sagittal T2-weighted fat-suppressed (**a**), T1-weighted (**b**), and *gadolinium*-enhanced T1-weighted (**c**) of the cervicothoracic spine show Ewing sarcoma involving D5 body with extensive extradural extension and circumferential epidural mass resulting in spinal compression

compression fracture include retropulsion of a posterior bone fragment, presence of an intravertebral fluid collection and intravertebral vacuum cleft sign, and evidence of multiple compression fractures (Cicala et al. 2013; Thawait et al. 2013).

Available treatment options, although sometimes palliative, are based on preservation of neurologic function and pain control (Jo and Schiff 2017; Baldwin et al. 2012; Scott 2015; Witham et al. 2006). Other clinical comorbidities and cancer-related systemic conditions dictate the treatment choice, while neoplasm histology does not (Katabathina et al. 2013; Scott 2015).

Immediate treatment with high-dose corticosteroid should be the initial management of spinal cord compression in order to reduce vasogenic edema and local inflammation, followed by emergent surgical decompression, radiation therapy, or a combination of these options. Chemotherapy has a limited role in emergency treatment; it is an available option for selected chemosensitive tumors such as lymphoma and seminoma, without malignant compression (Jo and Schiff 2017; Baldwin et al. 2012; Hammack 2012).

Urgent decompressive spine surgery within less than 24 h from the time of diagnosis, followed by regional radiation therapy, is the most effective treatment to avoid loss of ambulatory ability.

## 1.7 Seizures and Status Epilepticus

Seizures are common and potentially devastating complications in patients with primary and secondary CNS tumors. They may occur as presenting signs in approximately 25% of patients (Lulla et al. 2011; Ullrich 2009; Lacy et al. 2012; Van Breemen et al. 2007) or during the course of CNS cancer disease.

Risk for the development of seizures is related to the pathologic type and anatomic location of brain tumors (Lin and Avila 2017; Lulla et al. 2011; Lacy et al. 2012; Van Breemen et al. 2007).

Seizures occur more frequently in patients with supratentorial tumors, especially those cortically based type, with the involvement of leptomeninges and located in the temporal lobes or the motor cortex, compared with deep lesions in the basal ganglia or white matter.

Seizures occur in approximately 60% of patients with primary brain tumors and in 25% of those with metastatic tumors (Lacy et al. 2012; Maschio 2012).

Low-grade gliomas are more epileptogenic than high-grade type, with a seizure incidence of approximately 60–85% versus 30–60% (Lin and Avila 2017; Lacy et al. 2012; Lote et al. 1998).

Glioneuronal tumors exhibit intrinsic strong tendency to trigger seizures (Jo and Schiff 2017; Baldwin et al. 2012). Ganglioglioma is the most common neoplasm resulting in focal epilepsy; other epileptogenic low-grade tumors include dysembryoplastic neuroepithelial tumor (DNET), pleomorphic xanthoastrocytoma, and oligodendroglioma (Lulla et al. 2011; Ogiwara et al. 2010). Among secondary tumors, melanoma and other hemorrhagic metastases show the highest risk of seizures (Oberndorfer et al. 2002).

Epilepsy as clinical onset may result from cortical irritability due to structural abnormality and tumor infiltration of normal structures, surrounding edema, and presence of tumor-related blood products.

Seizures are typically partial and localization-related, which may or not be secondarily generalized; they often resolve without any intervention.

Neuroimaging evaluation may be required depending on the presence of focal neurologic deficits and other symptoms; it sometimes may facilitate an earlier diagnosis (Lulla et al. 2011; Ullrich 2009).

During the clinical course of known CNS tumor, patients may develop seizures or change in the seizure pattern due to structural changes of lesion, such as enlarging, hemorrhage, or worsening edema or mass effect of the tumor; seizures also may occur as complications of treatment, due to radiation damage phenomena or scar formation at the surgical site (Lin and Avila 2017; Lulla et al. 2011). MR evaluation and electroencephalogram (EEG) are often recommended to investigate lesions, structural changes, and epileptogenic foci in order to define the most effective management (Lulla et al. 2011; Ullrich 2009).

MRI is better than CT in revealing brain masses, edema, and mass effect, hemorrhage, and other finding suggestive of tumor progression or complications; it may also detect structural changes related to seizures, such as foci of restricted diffusion in the cortical mantle.

Most seizures are focal in onset and self-limited.

Although uncommon, seizures in cancer patients could rapidly generalize and evolve into status epilepticus, becoming a critical neurologic emergency with prolonged seizure or more seizures occurring without a return to baseline in between events.

Status epilepticus is a critical emergency, with a higher risk of death and a mortality rate approximately of 20% (Baldwin et al. 2012).

Differently from general population, refractory seizures of status epilepticus in patients with CNS cancer are frequently caused by structural changes in neoplastic mass related to tumor progression, rather than medication noncompliance phenomena (Baldwin et al. 2012; Lin and Avila 2017).

Furthermore, sometimes status epilepticus may have nonconvulsive seizures, but only subtle clinical signs such as eye deviation or motor twitching.

Therefore, MR evaluation and EEG are indicated to confirm clinical suspect and provide the diagnosis in patients with altered mental status after a seizure. Prompt diagnosis and treatment are mandatory to avoid morbidity related to prolonged convulsive seizures (Baldwin et al. 2012).

Seizures may also occur in patients with systemic cancer, due to other different mechanisms such as treatment complication, posterior reversible encephalopathy syndrome (PRES), or paraneoplastic limbic encephalitis; treatment-related metabolic derangements (hyponatremia, hypoglycemia), infections, chemotherapy, and other medications may also result in appearance of epileptic syndrome, triggered by lowering of the seizure threshold from brain tumor (Lin and Avila 2017; Lulla et al. 2011; Lacy et al. 2012).

The management of convulsive seizures in cancer patients includes antiepileptic drugs such as benzodiazepines, phenytoin, phenobarbital, and valproic acid (Lin and Avila 2017; Brophy et al. 2012).

Surgical resection could be a valid therapeutic option for refractory seizures in patients with several types of low-grade tumors, such as temporal lobe DNET (Lacy et al. 2012; Luyken et al. 2003).

## 1.8 Paraneoplastic Neurologic Emergencies

Paraneoplastic disorders are immune-related and nonmetastatic conditions that may occur in patients with cancer (Martel et al. 2014).

Paraneoplastic limbic encephalitis is a rare syndrome, probably underdiagnosed, difficult to detect as often misdiagnosed as a psychiatric disorder. It is recognized as a clinically and immunobiologically heterogeneous group of disorders, which may present in patients with brain tumors, caused by activation of humoral autoimmunity: antibodies are produced in response to antigens secreted by the tumor, but they cross-react with normal components of the central or peripheral nervous system causing various neurological findings.

Paraneoplastic antibodies related to limbic encephalitis include anti-Hu, anti-GABA receptor, anti-NMDA receptor, and anti-voltage-gated potassium channels antibodies, but the spectrum of autoantibody-associated variants continues to evolve (Baldwin et al. 2012; Lin and Avila 2017).

Heterogeneous clinical entities include progressive subacute syndromes that could be managed in ambulatory settings, such as anti-Hu antibody sensory neuronopathy.

Sometimes, disorders are more acute and potentially devastating, requiring emergent treatment. Clinical presentation of paraneoplastic limbic encephalitis includes confusion, neuropsychiatric symptoms, autonomic dysfunction, and seizures, sometimes evolving in critical conditions such as status epilepticus and respiratory distress (Scott 2015).

It may also present as an isolated neurologic syndrome or as a more widespread neurologic syndrome such as paraneoplastic encephalomyelitis (Baldwin et al. 2012).

Early diagnosis and management are mandatory to avoid irreversible damage to neural tissue.

The differential diagnoses include primary psychiatric disorders in early stages, HSV encephalitis, temporal lobe epilepsy, and toxic and metabolic encephalopathies (Baldwin et al. 2012; Law 2009; Scott 2015).

Diagnostic evaluation should include MR imaging and serum and CSF tests. Brain MR may detect typical but not constant T2 and FLAIR hyperintensity in the mesial temporal lobes in paraneoplastic limbic encephalitis. Findings can be indistinguishable from HSV encephalitis; hemorrhage is generally not present, and mass effect is less pronounced (Cakirer et al. 2002).

Diffuse cerebellar hemispheric enlargement or widespread abnormalities can be seen in encephalomyelitis. However, normal MRI studies are not uncommon. Atrophic evolution can be detected in chronic cases (Jo and Schiff 2017; Damek 2010).

Serum and CSF tests are performed in order to reveal evidence of inflammation, antibodies titers, their binding targets, and the presence of cross-reactivity, using immunohistochemical techniques.

The treatment of neurologic paraneoplastic syndromes consists of a combination of different approaches, including tumor removal, immunosuppressive therapies aiming at the removal of auto-antibodies with IVIG, and plasmapheresis and seizure management (Baldwin et al. 2012; Lin and Avila 2017; Law 2009; Scott 2015).

## 1.9 Meningitis–Encephalitis

Infections can occur in CNS cancer population either de novo or as a result of immunosuppressed status, the latter responsible for significant susceptibility to develop opportunistic fungal, parasitic, and viral infections. CNS infection occurs most common in patients with hematologic malignancies than primary tumors (Jo and Schiff 2017; Pruitt 2003).

Diagnosis requires a careful clinical history, neuroimaging evaluation, and other tests. It is important to detect neuroimaging suggestive findings in order to make a prompt diagnosis and a correct therapy. Brain neuroimaging is useful to detect abscess, meningeal enhancement, and focal or multifocal lesions. In some cases, it may be helpful to suggest etiology: Diffuse encephalitis is likely viral, whereas cerebral ischemic lesions suggest varicella vasculitis or bacterial or fungal endocarditis. It is also recommended prior to lumbar puncture to rule out mass lesions. Nevertheless, CT and MR studies cannot make a definitive diagnosis, thus requiring CSF analysis and other tests (Jo and Schiff 2017; Baldwin et al. 2012; Damek 2010; Pruitt 2003).

Patients with CNS cancer show a lower threshold for post-procedural bacterial meningitis, such as after a lumbar puncture. It may be a challenging diagnosis since neutropenic patients may not present with evident clinical sign and may lack CSF pleocytosis (Lin and Avila 2017; Pruitt 2003).

Viral encephalitis also occurs in cancer patients due to their frequent immunosuppressed status, caused by several pathogenic agents. Human herpes virus 6 (HHV6) causes a limbic encephalitis; herpes simplex also may cause encephalitis in the cancer immunosuppressed population (Lin et al. 2017).

Clinical suspicion in a patient with fever and altered mental status may be supported by a concerning MRI findings (Cakirer et al. 2002); diagnosis is made by CSF PCR analysis.

Varicella reactivation should be considered in the immunocompromised patient with suspected encephalitis associated with arterial ischemic stroke lesions, due to small or large-vessel vasculopathy. It can also cause a meningitis and myelitis (Lin and Avila 2017; Nagel and Gilden 2013).

Progressive multifocal leukoencephalopathy (PML) is a devastating demyelinating condition potentially fatal, caused by reactivated JC virus infection in immunosuppressed patients (Lin and Avila 2017).

Fungal and parasitic agents may be also responsible of CNS infection in immunocompromised individuals, such as cryptococcosis or aspergillosis and cerebral toxoplasmosis.

## 1.10 Cerebrovascular Complications

Cancer patients are at increased risk of cerebrovascular diseases, such as arterial ischemic stroke, intracerebral hemorrhage, and cerebral venous thrombosis. In addition to typical risk factors for stroke, several direct and indirect effects of cancer status and treatment must be considered (Giglio and Gilbert 2010; Lin and Avila 2017; Lulla et al. 2011; Law 2009).

Acute ischemic stroke can occur in tumoral patients due to several *pathogenetic* mechanisms: hypercoagulable state secondary to release of mucin, cytokines, or other procoagulant molecules (most commonly in adenocarcinoma); obstruction of small vessels secondary to hyperviscosity (multiple myeloma, polycythemia vera, some types of leukemia); embolism from tumoral mass (e.g., mixoma, lung carcinoma) or aggregates of fibrin on normal heart valves (e.g., nonbacterial thrombotic endocarditis in patients with adenocarcinoma); direct tumor infiltration of the blood vessel wall (e.g., intravascular diffuse large B-cell lymphoma); and subsequent arterial occlusion.

Vascular compression may also be due to mass effect from a large intracranial mass: massive edema and midline shift can occlude the anterior cerebral arteries; uncal transtentorial herniation may result in posterior cerebral artery occlusion, due to its compression close to the tentorial incisura.

Furthermore, cerebral venous thrombosis may represent another possible manifestation of cancer-related hypercoagulability, as well as a consequence of the procoagulant effect of several medications, such as the anti-estrogen tamoxifen. Sometimes, venous thrombosis may result by direct compression or invasion of cerebral sinuses from meningioma or extra-axial metastases (Bang et al. 2011).

Finally, increased risk of stroke may result from effects of chemotherapy and radiation-induced endothelial vascular damage (including Moyamoya syndrome, vascular malformations, and vascular stenosis) and from infections secondary to the weakened immune system (Giglio and Gilbert 2010; Lin and Avila 2017; Lulla et al. 2011; Ullrich et al. 2007).

Clinical presentations of ischemic stroke in tumoral patients range from transient ischemia to acute events with neurological deficits, to diffuse cerebrovascular disease.

Several patterns of stroke may be detected on neuroradiological examination, frequently with multiple embolic lesions involving different vascular territories and showing various ages (Jo and Schiff 2017; Bang et al. 2011; Navi and Segal 2009). CT and MRI examinations and related angiographic and venographic techniques reveal ischemic lesions and vascular occlusion.

The management of stroke in the cancer population is similar to that of conventional stroke patients, aimed at correction of risk factors and identifiable stroke pathologic mechanisms, assisted by antiplatelet therapy compatibly with frequent contraindications such as recent major surgery. Anticoagulation is the primary treatment in venous sinus thrombosis.

Hemorrhagic stroke may present in different patterns in neoplastic patients such as intracerebral hemorrhage (ICH) and subarachnoid hemorrhage (SAH), more frequently due to hemorrhagic conversion of tumoral mass (as described above) and to complication of thrombocytopenia and coagulopathy, rarely as consequences by rupture of intratumoral vascular malformations. Pituitary apoplexy is a rare complication of pituitary adenomas, caused by acute hemorrhage and/or infarction of parenchymal tissue.

Like ischemic stroke, several types of tumor such as hematologic malignancies, certain chemotherapeutic agents, and radiation vasculopathy lead to increased risk of hemorrhagic events in cancer population (Lulla et al. 2011). ICH is reported as the most common form of stroke in patients with hematologic malignancies.

On CT or MR images, multiple hemorrhagic lesions in atypical location and the presence of enhancing soft tissue masses may suggest the presence of cerebral tumoral lesions.

The management depends on the site and size of hemorrhage, clinical status, and risk factors for the patients. The first priority is the correction of coagulation abnormalities and thrombocytopenia. Indication for surgical decompressive intervention is the development of herniation due to massive edema; hydrocephalus due to intraventricular extension of the ICH may require external ventricular drainage.

## 1.11 Iatrogenic Neurologic Emergencies

Neurologic complications of cancer treatment can occur following radiotherapy, chemotherapy, and as a consequence of medications and surgical procedures.

Iatrogenic neurotoxic complication includes a broad range of clinical manifestations, which differ in pathogenetic mechanisms, severity, and prognosis, frequently with progressive course; sometimes, complication of therapies may present acute onset or evolution with potential devastating sequelae, requiring timely diagnosis and prompt management.

Neurologic complications may occur during the course of radiation therapy (RT), caused by a combination of vascular damage and damage to glia, mainly oligodendrocytes.

Radiation-related CNS complications are classified based on the timing of tissue injury, related to potential reversibility of symptoms (Giglio and Gilbert 2010; Jo and Schiff 2017; Giglio and Gilbert 2003; Elefante et al. 2003; D'Amico et al. 2003).

Acute encephalopathy (less than 1 month) can develop immediately or days after starting RT, probably caused by inflammation, injury to capillaries, and leakage with edema; it is generally steroid-responsive. There is no specific imaging finding associated with early injury to the brain (Ricard et al. 2012).

Early-delayed injuries (1–6 months) are due to multifactorial pathogenesis including altered capillary permeability and edema, radiation-induced demyelination, inflammation, and radionecrosis. This condition occurs in approximately 20% of patients with glioblastoma, treated by combined management including radiotherapy and temozolomide.

Patients may develop transient neurologic deterioration and worsening of tumor-related symptoms or somnolence syndrome. Brain MRI findings may include increased vasogenic edema, mass effect, and contrast enhancement, mimicking tumor progression; this is a phenomenon referred to as "pseudoprogression." These changes are generally reversible and tend to respond to treatment with corticosteroids (Giglio and Gilbert 2010; Lacy et al. 2012; Ricard et al. 2012; Brandsma et al. 2008).

Complications occurring more than 6 months from completion of radiation therapy are termed late injury. It is believed to be caused by a combination of small- and medium-sized vessel damage, demyelination, damage to oligodendrocytes, and immune reaction from antigens released by damaged glial cells.

Neuroimaging shows permanent diffuse and bilateral white matter abnormalities (leukoencephalopathy) and atrophy, which are typically best identified on MRI as central and periventricular white matter hyperintensity on T2-w and FLAIR sequences with relative sparing of subcortical U fibers, dilated ventricles, and signs of cortical atrophy (Fig. 10) (Lulla et al. 2011; Soussain et al. 2009).

These findings are associated with a clinical spectrum ranging from mild cognitive impairment to severe dementia (Giglio and Gilbert 2010; Ricard et al. 2012; Chi et al. 2008). Risk factors are radiation dose, brain volume receiving

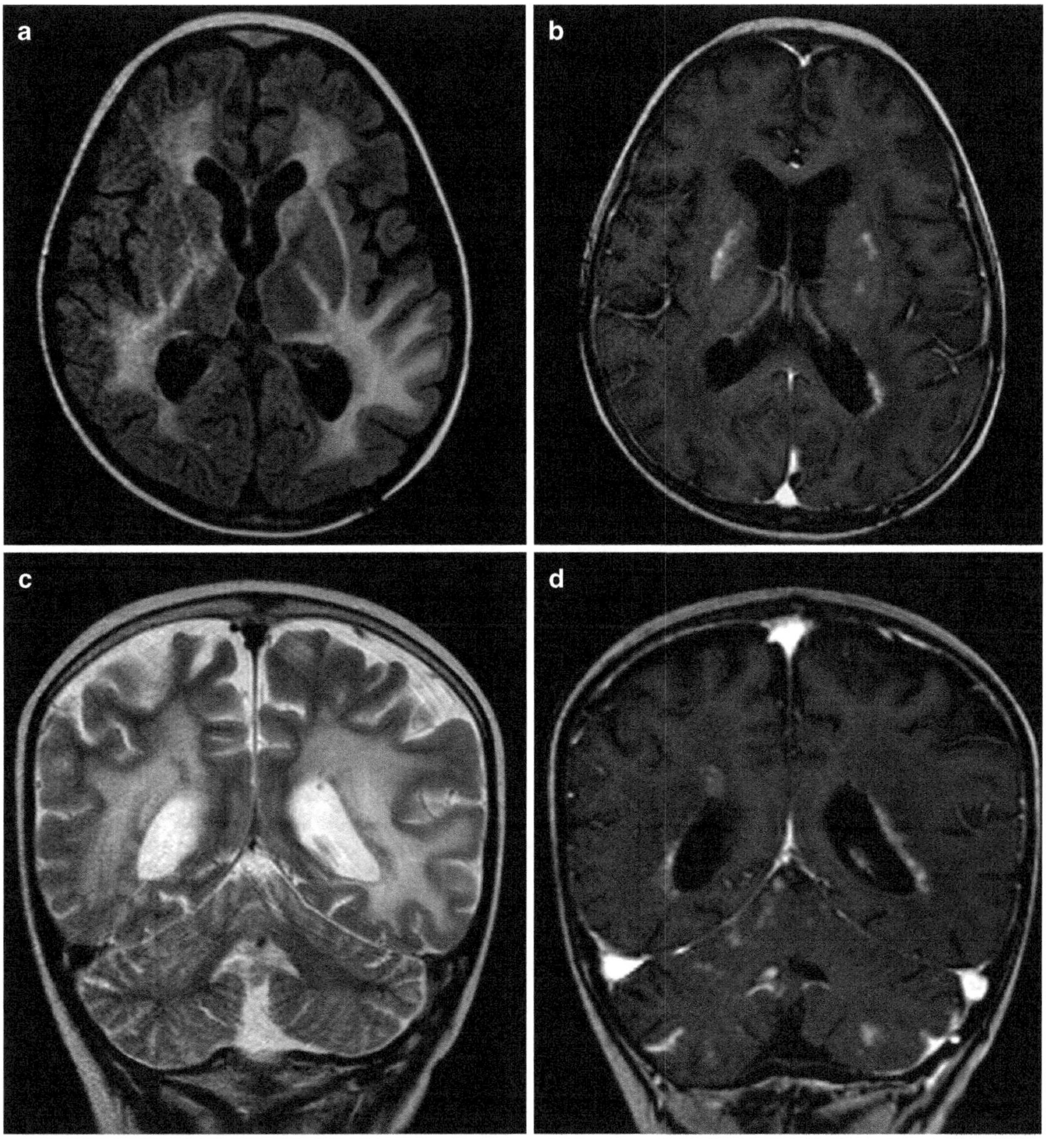


**Fig. 10** Radiotherapy-induced white matter injury. Axial FLAIR-weighted (**a**), *gadolinium*-enhanced T1-weighted (**b**), coronal T2-weighted (**c**), and *gadolinium*-enhanced T1-weighted images (**d**) show radiation-induced leukoencephalopathy, characterized by diffuse abnormal signal of the deep white matter with the involvement of periventricular regions, centrum semiovale and corona radiata, and external and internal capsules. Small foci of patchy parenchymal enhancement are seen in the periventricular, capsular, and cerebellar white matter, suggestive of radiation necrosis

radiation, older age, and combined treatment with chemotherapy (Chi et al. 2008). There are no effective therapies to treat this irreversible and severe condition.

Focal areas of radiation necrosis may be seen on MR studies on the end state; they might be difficult to be distinguished from tumor progression (pseudoprogression) (Giglio and Gilbert 2010; Jo and Schiff 2017). Imaging may show lesions with surrounding vasogenic edema, mass effect, and increased heterogeneous enhancement, with typical "soap bubble" appearance, suggesting radiation necrosis. Perfusion MRI can be helpful, suggesting that areas of increased perfusion are indicative of tumor tissue, while decreased perfusion is suggestive of radiation necrosis phenomena.

Steroid therapy and bevacizumab have variable benefits in this condition. Surgery may be necessary to exclude definitive tumor progression confirming the diagnosis, as well as a therapeutic option in several symptomatic cases (Giglio and Gilbert 2010; Scott 2015).

Late-delayed myelopathy and permanent cranial neuropathies and plexopathies may be also seen during the late course of radiation therapy. Additional late complications include cerebrovascular events, endocrinopathies, optic toxicities, and secondary malignancies, such as meningiomas, gliomas, and nerve sheath tumors (Fig. 11).

Several chemotherapeutic and biologic agents can result in neurotoxicity and clinical syndrome, whose severity and reversibility depends on dose, duration, and modality of administration, concomitant morbidities, and medications.

Neurologic complications are relatively rare and generally nonemergent; more frequent conditions include peripheral neuropathy and mild encephalopathy; seizures, myelopathy, neuropsychiatric syndrome, cerebellar syndrome, aseptic meningitis, and stroke can also occur.

Some cytotoxic agents may cause specific clinical syndromes, such as cerebellar encephalopathy by cytarabine neurotoxicity, aseptic meningitis by intrathecal methotrexate, or stroke events by bevacizumab (Giglio and Gilbert 2010; Jo and Schiff 2017; Scott 2015).

Chemotherapeutic agents may also be responsible for neutropenia and infection and electrolyte abnormalities, increasing the susceptibility to the onset of seizures and other neurologic complications (Lulla et al. 2011).

Neurological chemotherapy-induced emergencies are relatively rare and may be due to prolonged convulsions, up to the epileptic status.

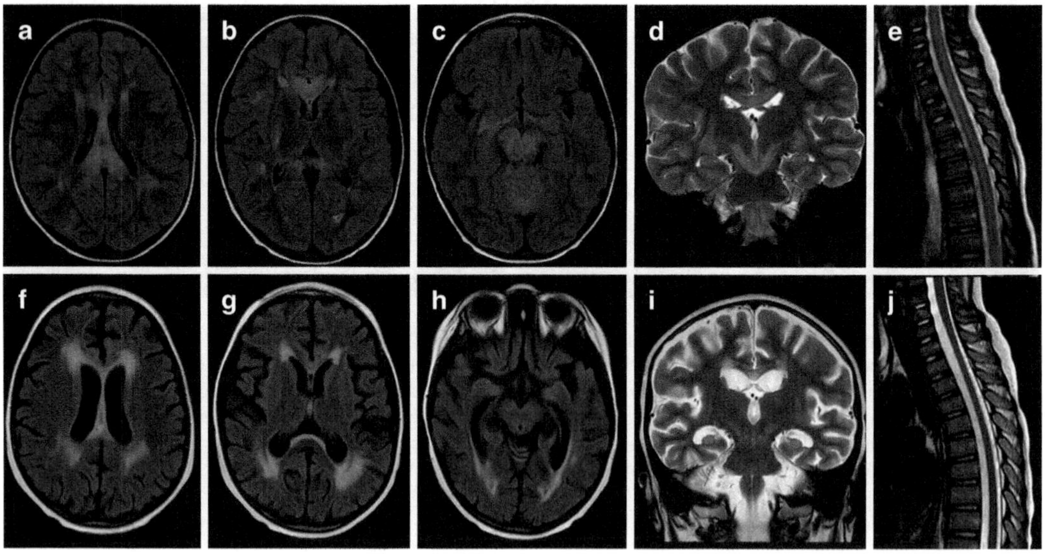


**Fig. 11** Chemotherapy-induced white matter injury. Evidence of leukoencephalopathy on axial FLAIR-weighted and coronal T2-weighted images of the brain and of myelopathy on sagittal T2-weighted scan of the spinal cord. In the acute phase (**a–d**), swelling and abnormal signal are observed in the corpus callosum, external capsule, midbrain, and spinal cord (**e**), due to edema; abnormal hyperintensity is also seen at subcortical white matter. After 3 months, symmetric deep and periventricular white matter abnormalities with sparing of subcortical U fibers, dilated ventricles, and cortical sulci due to atrophic evolution of the white matter injury are demonstrated (**f–i**); mild spinal cord thinning is also observed (**j**)

Posterior reversible encephalopathy syndrome (PRES) is a complication associated with certain chemotherapeutic medications, both cytotoxic and biologic (e.g., cisplatin and bevacizumab) (Lin and Avila 2017; Lulla et al. 2011). Patients may present seizures, hypertension, cortical blindness, headache, and altered mental status. Pathophysiology is probably related to failure of cerebrovascular self-regulation mechanisms.

MRI is helpful for the diagnosis and should be promptly performed. It shows typical findings of FLAIR/T2 cortical/subcortical hyperintensities due to edema, with predominant but not exclusive involvement of posterior parietal and occipital lobes and cerebellar lobes at junction of vascular "watershed zones"; rare variants may involve brainstem or basal ganglia. Generally, DWI shows elevated diffusion, but, although rare, restriction abnormalities may be found; petechial hemorrhages are frequently seen (Lulla et al. 2011; Tortora et al. 2015; Battipaglia et al. 2012; Fischer and Schmutzhard 2017) (Fig. 12).

PRES alterations are potentially but not always reversible. Prompt diagnosis is critical to avoid bad outcome. Management strategies include withdrawal of the offending agent and blood pressure management.

## 2 CNS Infections

### 2.1 Introduction

Central nervous system (CNS) infections still have a great impact in terms of severity, affecting all age groups, especially the pediatric range; they may represent a real medical emergency because of the consequent complications and fatal outcome if not diagnosed and treated promptly.

Moreover, HIV infection, the emergence of multidrug-resistant strains, and widespread immigration have changed the diagnosis and imaging of CNS infections (Aiken 2010).

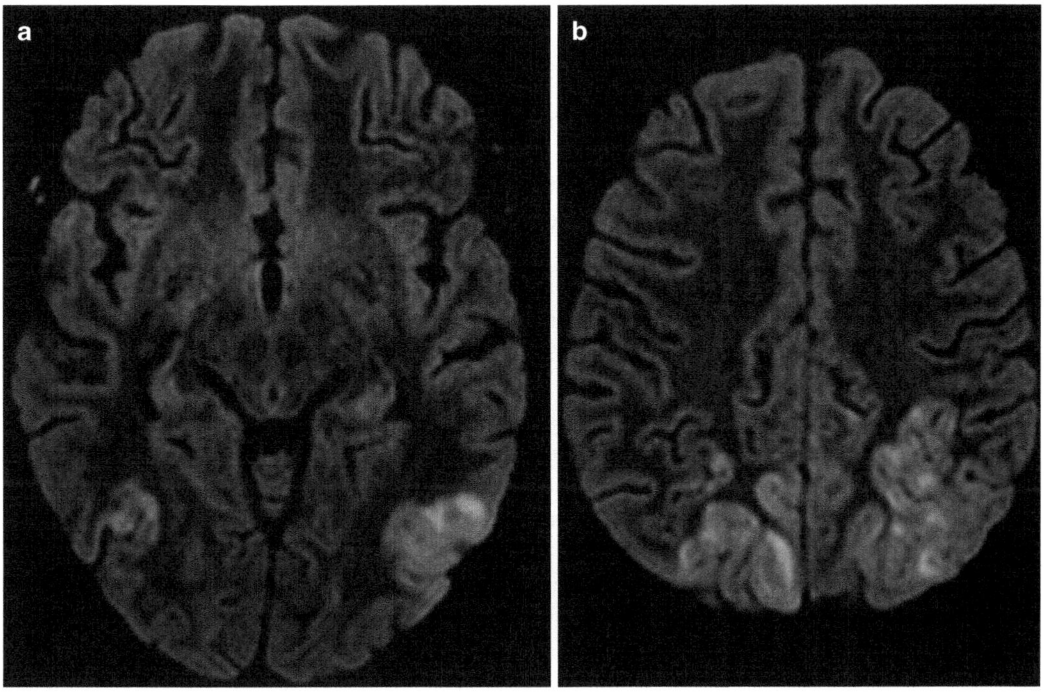


**Fig. 12** PRES. Axial FLAIR-weighted images at the planes of temporal lobes (**a**) and parietal convexities (**b**) show bilateral vasogenic edema involving cortical/subcortical regions at posterior watershed zones

The role of diagnostic imaging is fundamental, together with the physical examination and laboratory investigations; therefore, the neuroradiologist plays a crucial role in identifying and narrowing the differential diagnosis of CNS infection and monitoring the therapeutic response (Aiken 2010).

Computed tomography (CT) is often the first imaging study for the evaluation of suspected CNS infection because of its widespread availability and rapid assessment of emergencies and complications; magnetic resonance imaging (MRI) is the study of choice for further characterization of CNS infection, and it is more sensitive for the identification of meningitis, empyema, ventriculitis, and complications (Aiken 2010).

## 2.2 Meningitis

The meninges offer poor resistance to infections and are an excellent breeding ground for germs. Meningitis is divided into two categories: pachymeningitis affecting the dura mater and leptomeningitis affecting the arachnoid, pia, and liquor. Pachymeningitis is rarer and has predominantly bacterial etiology, while leptomeningitis has a predominantly viral etiology.

Neuroradiological examinations are mainly used to monitor complications and outcomes of the pathology.

*Viral meningitis* is among the most common CNS infections, mainly affecting the children; the main etiologic agents are enteroviruses (90% of cases) (Logan and MacMahon 2008).

The diagnosis is based on clinical (fever, vomiting, headache, signs of meningeal irritation) and laboratory findings (liquor examination). The prognosis is good: They are self-limiting infections.

Neuroimaging is often negative; sometimes, MRI can demonstrate altered signal of the cerebrospinal fluid (CSF) in the subarachnoid spaces and mild enhancement of the meningeal spaces involved by inflammation (Vaswani et al. 2014).

*Bacterial meningitis* represents an emergency condition being characterized by high mortality and high rate of disability. The most common etiologic agents are Haemophilus influenzae, Streptococcus pneumoniae, and Neisseria meningitidis (Adriani et al. 2015). Symptoms in older children and adults are characterized by fever, headache, neck stiffness, disorientation, and altered state of consciousness that goes from hibernation to coma. The diagnosis is entirely based on the analysis of the liquor; neuroradiology plays a remarkable role in the complications of meningitis (abscess collections, extra-axial empyema, hydrocephalus, vascular thrombosis, infarctions; Fig. 13). Post-gadolinium and FLAIR sequences are most sensitive for detecting abnormal meningeal enhancement and subarachnoid space disease, respectively (Fig. 14) (Singer et al. 1998; Pagliano et al. 2017).

Tuberculous meningitis is the most common presentation of neurotuberculosis, occurring by contiguity of nearby infected sites or by hematogenous diffusion from remote infections.

Clinical manifestations of tuberculosis are nonspecific and inconstant; fever, convulsions, meningism, and focal neurological deficits may occur.

It usually presents as a long-standing insidious process with exuberant inflammation of the basilar meninges and an obliterative vasculopathy of the basal penetrating vessels. Most infarcts are thus seen in the basal ganglia and internal capsule (Bernaerts et al. 2003).

The common imaging triad consists of basal meningeal enhancement, hydrocephalus, and cerebral infarction (Fig. 15) (Bernaerts et al. 2003).

## 2.3 Empyema

*Subdural empyema* is a medical emergency usually requiring neurosurgical intervention; it may be a complication of meningitis, or extend from sinusitis or mastoiditis, or recent surgery and trauma (Aiken 2010).

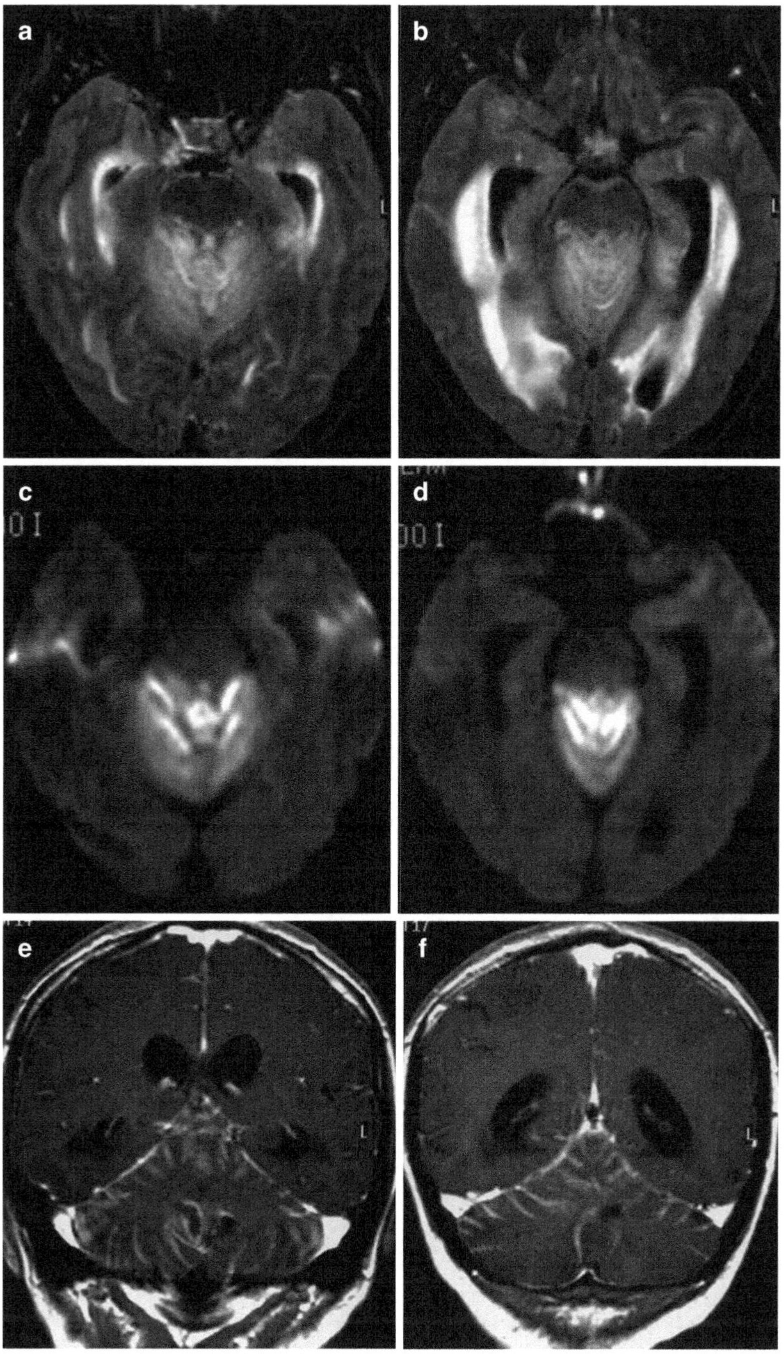


**Fig. 13** Bacterial meningitis (type B Streptococcus Pneumoniae). (**a** and **b**) FLAIR axial sections: temporal horn dilation with transependymal edema, associated with cortico-leptomeningeal hyperintense signal involving the cerebellar convexity. (**c** and **d**) DWI axial sections: The viscous pus filling the cerebellar sulci restricts strongly. (**e** and **f**) T1-w axial sections after intravenous contrast medium injection: diffuse linear cerebellar sulcal enhancement

CT, often used acutely, is useful in defining the extent and degree of mass effect; however, small subdural empyemas can be missed on CT, especially when located along the inner table of the skull (Nathoo et al. 1999).

MRI shows an extra-axial semilunar collection with hypointense signal on T1-w images (brighter than CSF due to its proteinaceous content and inflammatory debris), hyperintense on T2-w images, with reduced diffusion, marked

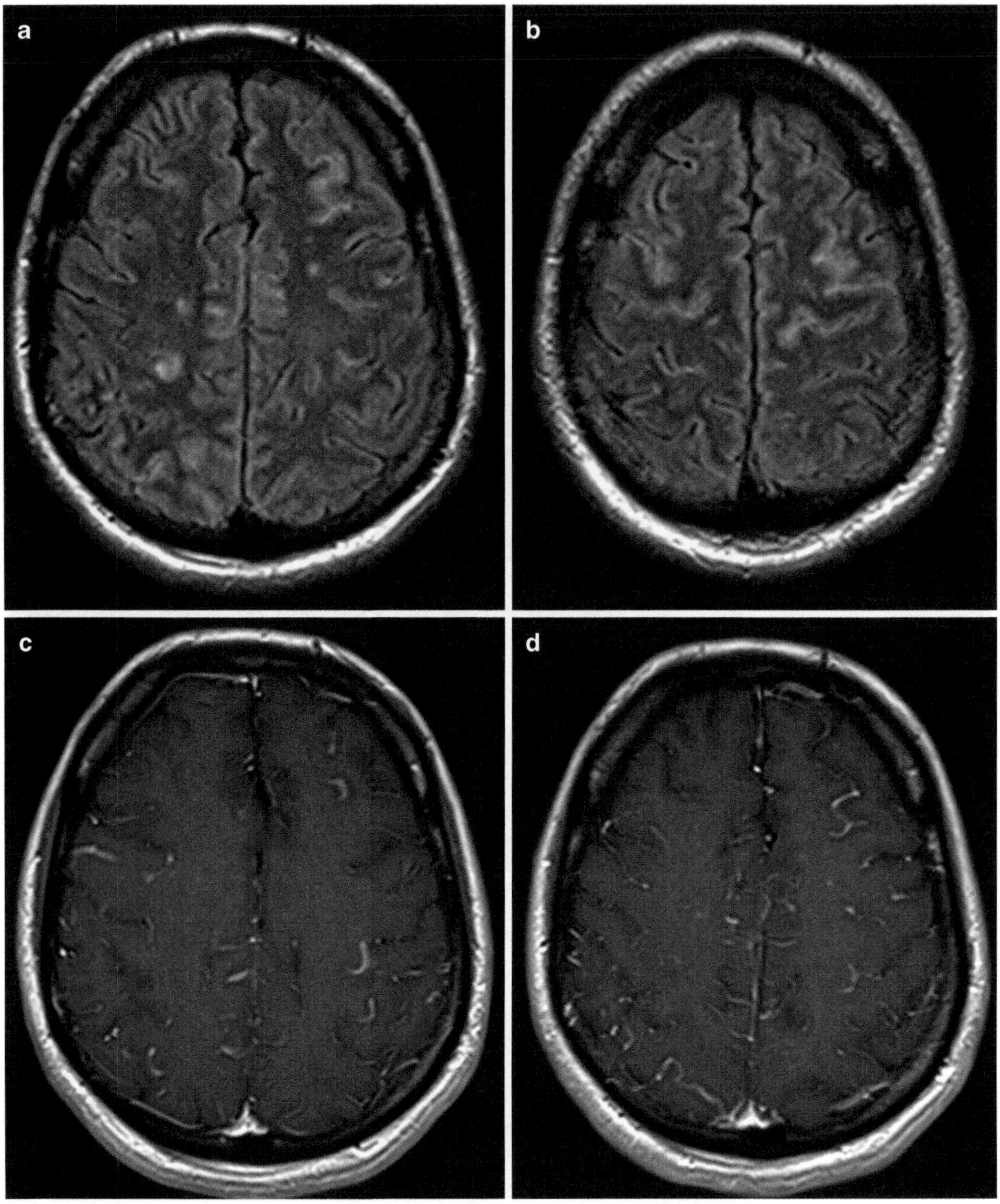


**Fig. 14** Bacterial meningitis. (**a** and **b**) FLAIR sections on axial plane; (**c** and **d**) T1-w sections after intravenous contrast medium injection. Cortico-leptomeningeal hyperintense signal involving the brain convexity, with diffuse linear sulcal enhancement

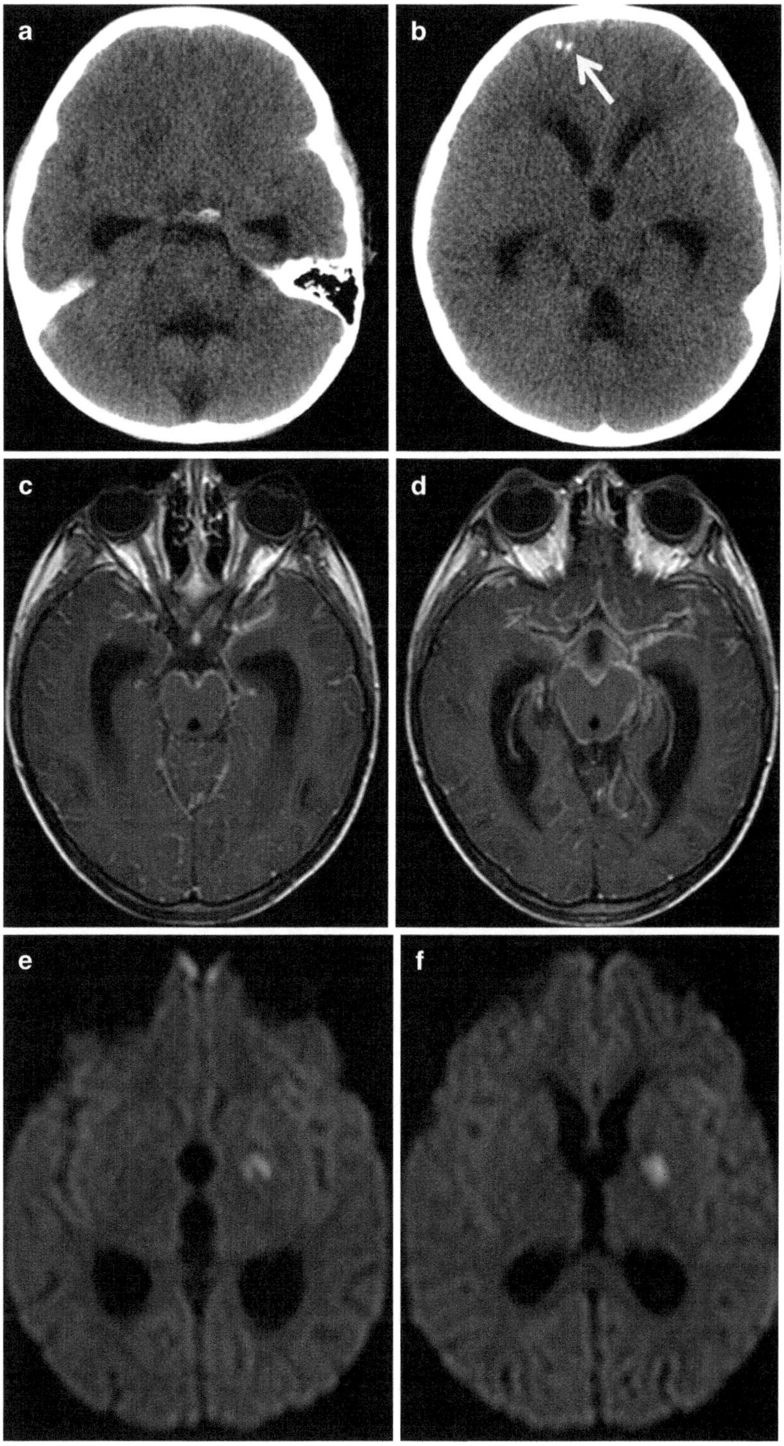


**Fig. 15** Tuberculous meningitis. (**a** and **b**) CT sections: acute obstructive hydrocephalus with dilated temporal horns and effacement of the Sylvian fissures; note the presence of two calcified healed granulomas (arrow) in the right frontal cortex. (**c** and **d**) T1-w axial sections after intravenous contrast medium injection: diffuse enhancing exudates involving the basilar cisterns and sulci, most striking in the Sylvian fissures. (**e** and **f**) DWI axial sections: presence of lacunar infarction in the left internal capsule with restricted diffusion

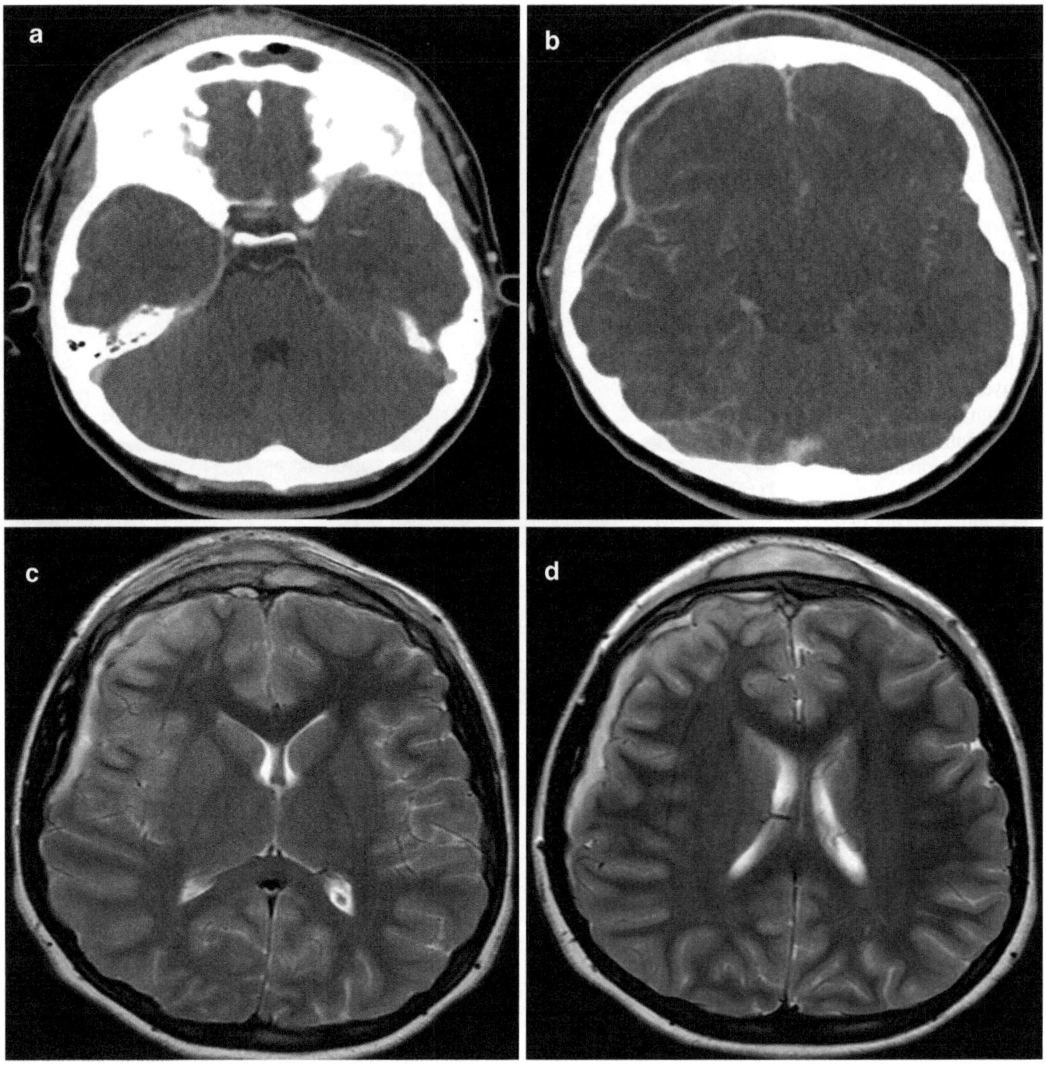


**Fig. 16** Subdural empyema. (**a** and **b**) CT scan after contrast medium injection. Frontal sinusitis with adjacent extracranial abscess collection; presence of a right hypodense frontotemporal semilunar collection, with marked enhancement of the inflamed dura. (**c** and **d**) T2-w axial sections. The extra-axial hyperintense semilunar collection is well delineated; note the edema of the underlying compressed brain parenchymal (arrow)

enhancement of the inflamed dura on post-contrast images, and edema of the underlying brain parenchyma (Fig. 16) (Aiken 2010; De Divitiis and Elefante 2012).

*Epidural empyema* is a purulent collection localizes outside the dura, most commonly extending from the paranasal sinuses; etiology includes recent surgery, trauma, and mastoiditis.

CT and MRI demonstrate a lentiform collection tacked down at the sutures, possibly crossing the midline, unlike subdural collections, with similar signal characteristics (Figs. 17 and 18) (Aiken 2010).

## 2.4 Viral Encephalitis

Encephalitis is a diffuse infective or inflammatory process of the brain, typically of viral origin; nonviral causes of infectious encephalitis include bacterial, fungal, parasitic, and rickettsial etiology (Rath et al. 2012).

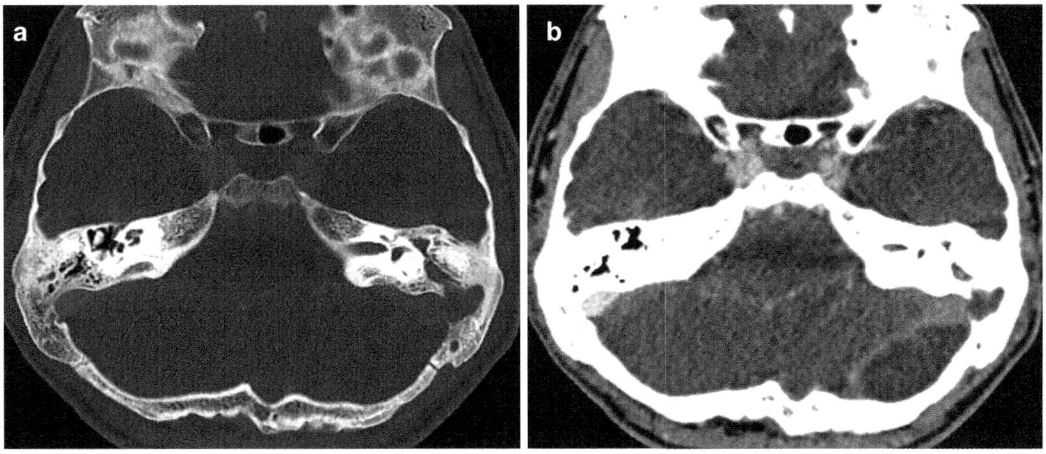


**Fig. 17** Epidural empyema. (**a**) CT scan (bone window): presence of abnormal soft tissue attenuation in the left right mastoid air cells (acute mastoiditis) with erosion of the sigmoid plate. (**b**) CT scan after contrast medium injection: presence of a large left epidural hypodense collection, with thrombosis of the left lateral and sigmoid sinuses (arrow)

Imaging plays a role in the diagnosis of encephalitis when combined with the medical history (febrile course, headache, altered level of consciousness), serologic studies, and cerebrospinal fluid (CSF) analysis (Rath et al. 2012).

### 2.4.1 Herpes Simplex Encephalitis

The type 1 (90% of cases) and type 2 herpes simplex (HS) virus are the main etiological agents of viral encephalitis, with an incidence of 1.4 cases per 100.000 inhabitants, therefore constituting the main cause of adverse outcomes of encephalitis.

The type 1 HS encephalitis represents a devastating necrotizing encephalitis resulting from reactivation of latent HSV-1 infection within the trigeminal ganglion; the infection spreads intracranially along meningeal branches of the trigeminal nerve, thus explaining the predilection for the temporal lobe (Aiken 2010).

The onset may be fulminating and progressive, in the latter case with a particularly insidious course characterized by headache, fever, generalized malaise, fatigue, irritability, and rarely convulsions; thereafter, signs of focal and progressive neurological deficit appear, together with disorders of consciousness and seizures.

Neuroradiological imaging is essential for the diagnosis of herpetic encephalitis. This severe acute necrotizing encephalitis affects bilaterally, but not symmetrically the brain, mostly involving the medial and basal frontotemporal regions.

CT may be normal in the early phase; when performed 48–72 h after the onset of symptoms, it is able to show a cortical–subcortical hypodense area due to edema (Fig. 19a and b) with hyperdense nuclei due to hemorrhagic extravasation; after 1 week, a necrotic damage may result (Zimmerman et al. 1980).

MRI performed at an early stage can demonstrate an extensive edematous hyperintense area on T2- weighted (w) images in the affected regions (medial temporal lobe, insular cortex, cingulate gyrus, inferior frontal lobe; Fig. 20). The basal ganglia are rarely involved in HSE, which helps to distinguish this disease process from other encephalitis; therefore, when insular and subinsular involvement is noted but the signal abnormality abruptly stops at the lateral putamen, HSE should be considered (Rath et al. 2012).

DWI is variable, but areas of reduced diffusion from cytotoxic edema have been demonstrated as one of the earliest findings (Fig. 19c and d). Hyperintense nuclei on T1-w images or abnormal susceptibility on gradient-echo

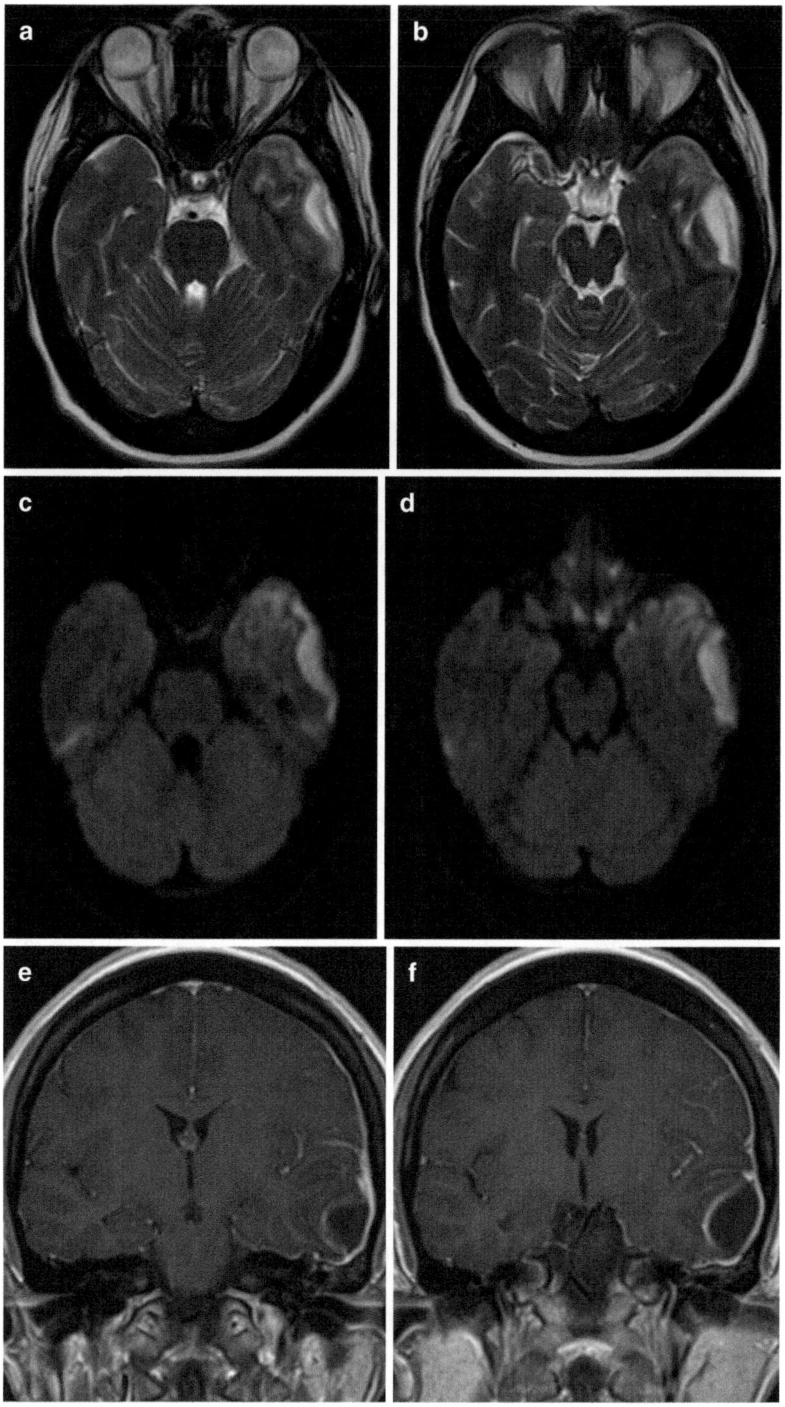


**Fig. 18** Epidural empyema (from Cryptococcus meningitis). (**a** and **b**) T2-w axial sections; (**c** and **d**) DWI axial sections; (**e** and **f**) T1-w coronal sections after intravenous contrast medium injection. Presence of a left temporal biconvex lentiform epidural fluid collection with restricted diffusion and enhancing rim, associated with unilateral diffuse pachymeningeal and leptomeningeal enhancement

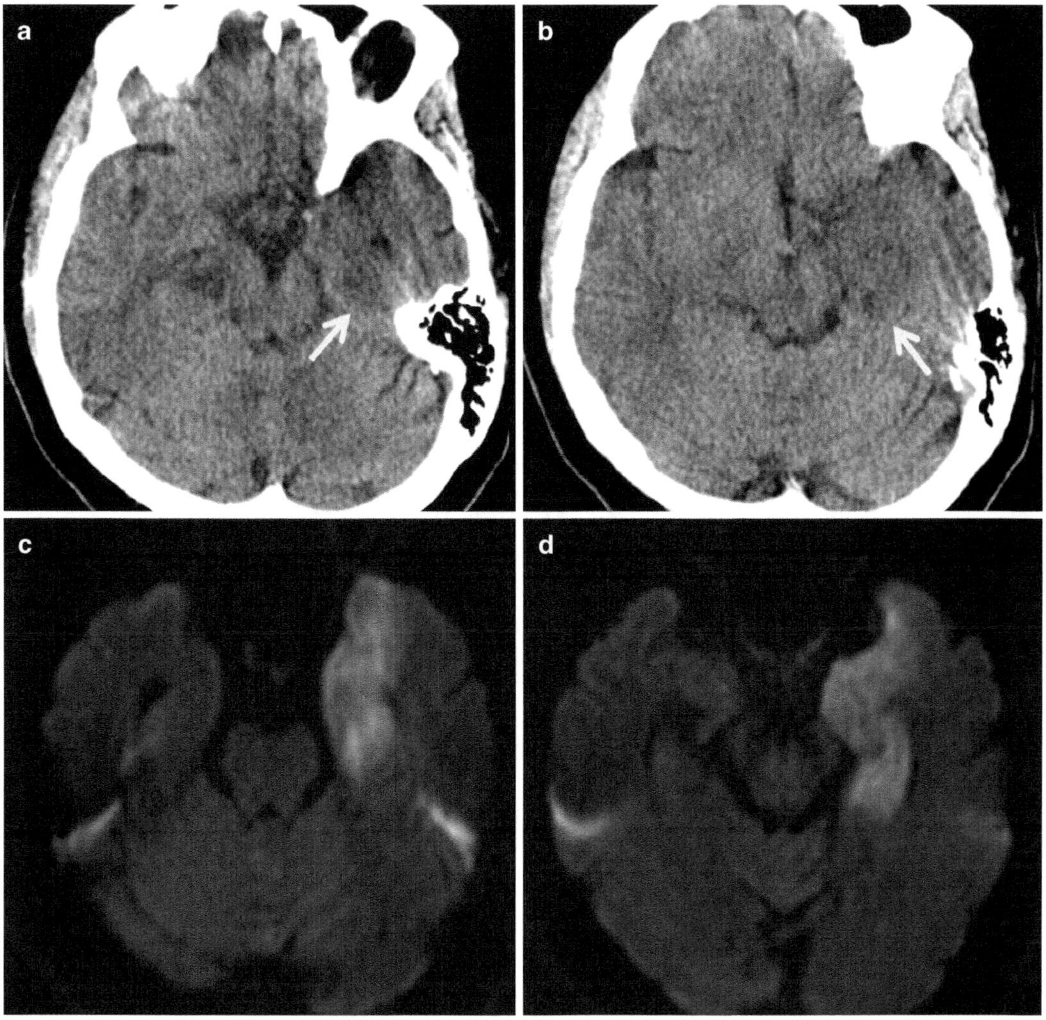


**Fig. 19** Herpes encephalitis. (**a** and **b**) CT sections: presence of an ill-defined low-attenuation area in the left medial temporal lobe. (**c** and **d**) DWI axial sections: The same case shows restricted diffusion in the anterior and medial temporal lobe cortex

sequences from subacute hemorrhage if some bleeding areas have already been established can be associated; intravenous (iv) contrast medium injection in subacute phases can show variable grades of enhancement (gyriform, anular, leptomeningeal, widespread).

MR spectroscopy (MRS) can show reduced NAA, elevated choline compounds, and sometimes elevated lactate (Rath et al. 2012).

Treatment is immediately initiated in presence of clinical suspicion and consistent imaging findings with HSE, as it decreases mortality rates from 70% to 20–30% (Rath et al. 2012).

### 2.4.2 Other Viral Encephalitis

The *encephalitis by the varicella-zoster virus* (VZV), belonging to the herpes virus family, derives from viral reactivation in elderly

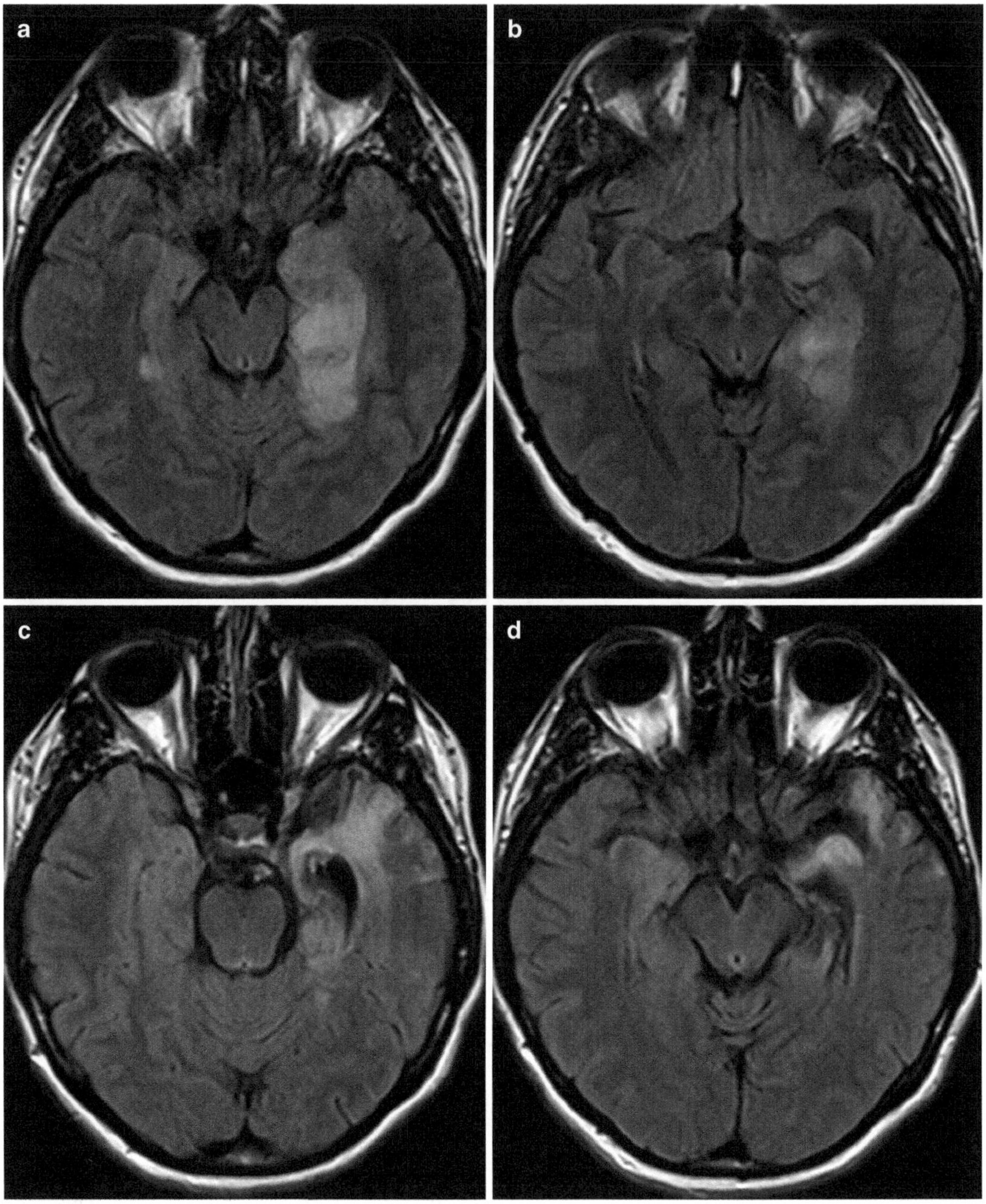


**Fig. 20** Herpes encephalitis. (**a** and **b**) FLAIR axial sections: presence of gyral swelling with indistinct gray-white interfaces in the left anterior medial temporal lobe, associated with a small hyperintense area in the right hippocampus. (**c** and **d**) FLAIR axial sections: gliotic evolution of the affected areas with consensual dilation of the temporal horn

individuals whose cell-mediated immunity to VZV has declined or in immunosuppressed patients.

The CNS complications of VZV reactivation are described as meningoencephalitis and, in a predominant way, vasculopathy. Typically, both large-vessel and small-vessel arteries are involved, often presenting with acute stroke or transient ischemic attacks. Imaging show multiple areas of high signal on T2-w images, classically involving the gray-white junction, and/or deep and superficial infarcts, some with associated hemorrhage.

Less frequently, VZV vasculopathy results in aneurysm formation, subarachnoid or parenchymal hemorrhage, vascular ectasia, or dissection (Rath et al. 2012).

Following infection with zoster or cytomegalovirus, an immune-mediated encephalitis called Bickerstaff encephalitis may develop, whose pathogenetic mechanism seems to be common with many other immunomediated conditions (Bulakbasi and Kocaoglu 2008; Odaka et al. 2001). MRI can show a transitory involvement of the brainstem and basal ganglia, characterized by the presence of a hyperintense T2-w signal area with minimum or no enhancement.

*Encephalitis by Cytomegalovirus* is rare in adults except for immunodepressed individuals like HIV-affected; congenital or neonatal infections are more frequent (Striano et al. 2007).

Although CNS involvement typically takes the form of a meningoencephalitis or ventriculitis, it can also present as myelitis, polyradiculitis, and retinitis (Aiken 2010). CMV involves the gray matter and ventricular ependyma to a greater degree than the white matter; the most characteristic imaging finding is the presence of thin subependymal T2/FLAIR hyperintensity and contrast enhancement (Aiken 2010). Ventriculitis may be associated with an enhancement of the ependymal surface.

*Enteroviral encephalitis* (coxsackie-, echo-, and poliovirus) accounts for 10–20% of all viral encephalitis and is mostly pediatric infections. The clinical picture is nonspecific, and the prognosis is usually benign.

It may involve the brainstem, substantia nigra, nucleus dentatus, and the anterior horn of the spinal cord (Lee 2016); a correlation with the clinical suspicion is fundamental for the diagnosis. *Rabies virus encephalitis* results from the bite of infected dogs; rarely, the virus can penetrate from an infected wound or may be iatrogenic or following an organ transplant (Awasthi et al. 2001a, b).

Apart a classic form of presentation, the remaining 20% of cases causes a paralytic encephalitis. Reported cases, limited by its fatal prognosis, show T2-w hyperintense areas involving gray matter, especially the hippocampus, basal ganglia, and thalamus (Laothamatas et al. 2003). As the disease progresses, the areas of swelling and petechiae increase with enhancement after iv contrast medium injection.

In the paralytic form, the spinal cord involvement is more pronounced.

The *Japanese virus* is a flavivirus mainly spreading from Southeast Asia, whose reservoir is represented by domestic pigs and wild birds, while the carrier is the mosquito (Shibani and Garga 2012). This form of encephalitis has a severe clinical onset with fever, headache, and stiffness, progressing toward a meningoencephalitic state with nuchal rigidity, cachexia, hemiparesis, and convulsions.

While CT is almost always negative, MRI can demonstrate the presence of edema in the affected regions (hypointense on T1-w, hyperintense on T2-w images); in GRE/SWI, patchy blooming may be appreciated (Kumar et al. 1997; Prakash et al. 2004).

*HIV encephalitis* is a progressive neurodegenerative disease resulting from direct infection of CNS mononuclear cells and microglial cells. Among the various causes, besides those linked to the HIV infection, overinfections from opportunistic pathogens, alterations of the immune system, and complications related to the therapy are reported (Antinori et al. 2007; Navia et al. 1986a, b).

Patients present a subcortical dementia and cognitive and behavioral deficits (AIDS dementia complex).

MRI more often shows a diffuse form of leukoencephalopathy, with diffuse cerebral atrophy and symmetric T2 hyperintensity in the periventricular and deep white matter. There is no mass effect or contrast enhancement (Aiken 2010).

*JC virus encephalitis* is a secondary manifestation of infection in immunosuppressed patients (HIV-infected, long-standing hematological disorders, or immunosuppressed patients after organ transplantation) with the clinical findings of progressive multifocal leukoencephalopathy (PML) (Bag et al. 2010).

PML is a progressive demyelinating disease caused by a DNA papovavirus and the John Cunningham virus (JC virus), which directly infects the oligodendrocytes.

The clinical presentation is characterized by altered state of consciousness, motor deficit, ataxia, and visual deficit; PCR testing of the CSF for the JC virus allows the diagnosis with approximately 96% specificity, but the neuroradiologic findings are particularly useful.

MRI, more accurate than CT, demonstrates an asymmetric involvement of the subcortical and peri-ventricular white matter, predominantly in the parieto-occipital regions (Sarbu et al. 2016; Garrels et al. 1996). The lesions are hyperintense on T2-w and particularly hypointense on T1-w images, usually with no enhancement or mass effect. Reduced diffusion has been described in the early phases of the disease at the leading edge of active demyelination and may be a poor prognostic sign indicating a phase of disease progression (Fig. 21) (Aiken 2010).

Atypical patterns can occur, including faint peripheral enhancement, mass effect, and even focal hemorrhage. Contrast enhancement may represent a positive development, as an inflammatory reaction and elimination of the JC virus, but it can also be seen with immune reconstitution syndrome (IRIS) exacerbating PML (Aiken 2010; Sahraian et al. 2012).

### 2.4.3 Fungal Encephalitis

*Aspergillus encephalitis* is the most common fungal encephalitis and can occur by hematogenous diffusion from remote infections. It is prevalent in people with immunodeficiency, such as HIV-positive, patients with prolonged use of corticosteroids, neutrophil deficiency, and transplant recipients (Müller et al. 2007). As clinical and laboratory features do not always confirm the diagnosis, neuroimaging plays a key role (DeLone et al. 1999).

Imaging features depend on the evolution of the pathology and immunologic status of the patient (Tempkin et al. 2006; Almutairi et al. 2009; Marzolf et al. 2016). The angioinvasivity nature of the fungus explains the presence of cortical and subcortical septic infarctions. In severely immunocompromised patients, the lesions appear as poorly defined areas of CT hypodensity or MRI T2 hyperintensity, without significant mass effect, surrounding edema, or enhancement owing to the lack of a host immune response; hemorrhage may be associated with the infarct. In more immunocompetent patients, subtle peripheral or ring enhancement may be seen with surrounding vasogenic edema.

Invasive rhinosinusitis with intracranial extension has high morbidity and mortality (DeLone et al. 1999), associated with multiple brain abscesses and cerebral infarction; sometimes lesions may appear as a granulomatous mass (Azarpira et al. 2008; Siddiqui et al. 2006).

*Cryptococcus encephalitis* is the second most common among opportunistic CNS infections.

The etiologic agent is cryptococcus neoformans; clinically, it causes meningitis or meningoencephalitis, headache, convulsions, or blurred vision due to an increase in intracranial pressure.

Imaging findings may be very variable (Fig. 18). One of the most common imaging findings is hydrocephalus, because of the tendency of the disease to spread along perivascular spaces and to create cryptococcal pseudocysts in the midbrain and the basal ganglia (Takasu et al. 1991; Miszkiel et al. 1996; Awasthi et al. 2001a, b; Smith et al. 2008).

## 2.5 Cerebritis and Brain Abscesses

Cerebritis is defined as an area of poorly defined acute inflammation in the brain with increased

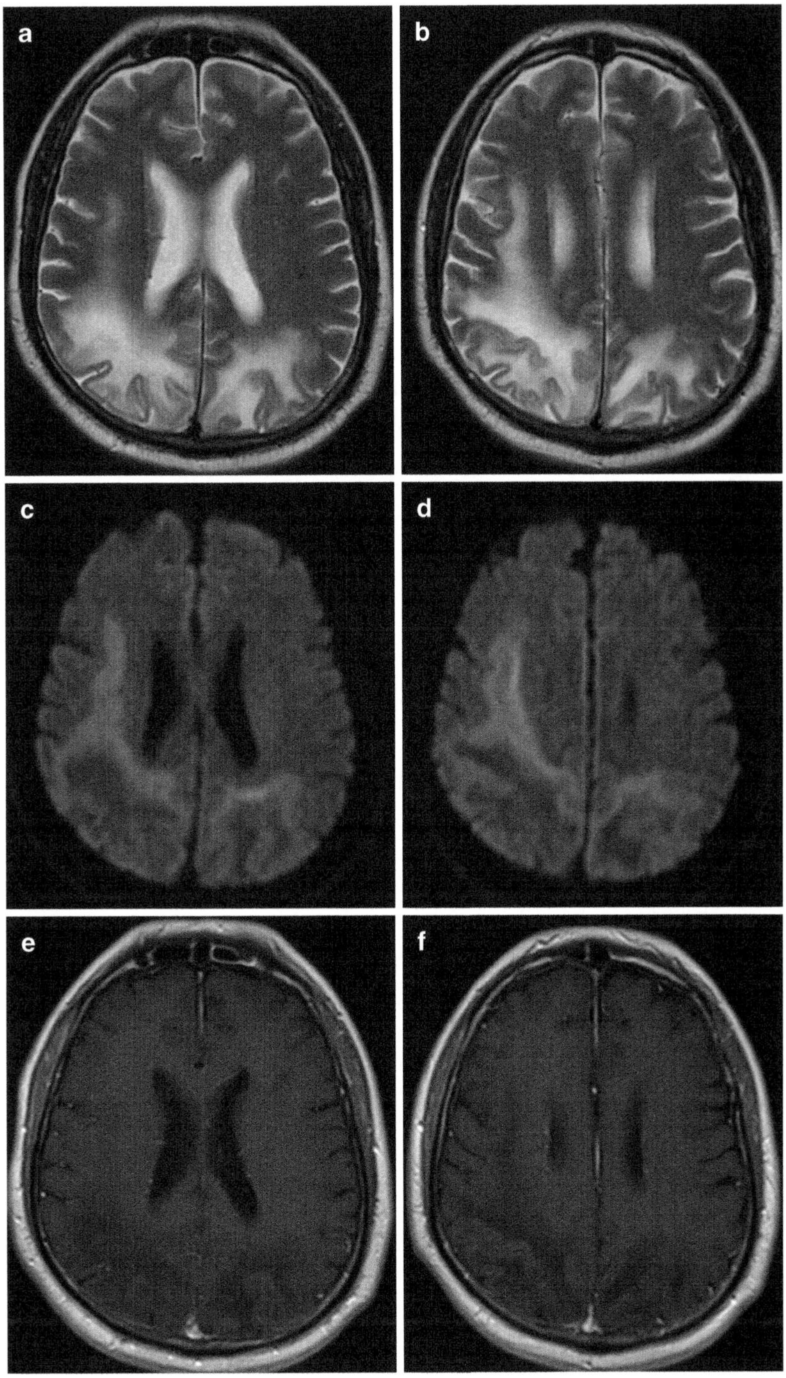


**Fig. 21** Progressive multifocal leukoencephalopathy. (**a** and **b**) T2-w axial sections: presence of extensive hyperintense lesions involving asymmetrically the right frontoparietal and the left parietal white matter, with cortical swelling and mild mass effect on right lateral ventricle. (**c** and **d**) DWI axial sections: Both the lesions show restricted diffusion at the leading edge of active demyelination. (**e** and **f**) T1-w axial sections after intravenous contrast medium injection: The lesions appear particularly hypointense on T1-w images, with no enhancement

permeability of the local blood vessels, possibly resulting from a variety of etiological factors, including pyogenic infection, and leading if untreated to brain abscess formation (Rath et al. 2012). Cerebral abscess is a localized CNS infection, formed by a central necrotic area surrounded by an external wall (collagen, granulation tissue, macrophages, gliosis).

Abscesses account for 1–2% of brain occupying space lesions in Western countries and

8% in developing countries. They are frequent in adults, while involving young patients (<15 years) in only 15–30% of the cases (Vajro et al. 2009).

Pyogenic brain abscesses are not common, accounting for one third of all the cerebral abscesses. They are caused by cerebral dissemination of bacteria coming from neighboring infections (sinusitis, otitis, mastoiditis) or by hematogenous spread of a remote infection (sepsis); in approximately 40% of cases, the primary site of infection remains unknown. Other causes of cerebral bacterial dissemination in CNS are craniofacial trauma, meningitis, and iatrogenic infections.

The evolution of pyogenic infection in the brain consists of four stages (Britt and Enzmann 1983; Muccio et al. 2014):

- early cerebritis (first stage, from the first to the third day), characterized by an inflammatory response with predominance of polymorphonuclear leukocytes;
- late cerebritis (second stage, from the fourth to the ninth day), in which the immune response is mediated by lymphocytes and macrophages, characterized by central necrosis formation with peripheral neoangiogenesis (with no blood–brain barrier) and presence of fibroblasts;
- early encapsulation (third stage, from the tenth to the 13th day), with the formation of surrounding peripheral wall with central necrosis;
- late capsule stage (fourth stage, from the 14th day), characterized by a mature encapsulated brain abscess with a wide central necrotic area.

Clinical features are different according to the site of the abscess. Diagnosis is challenging, and imaging has a primary role in differentiating brain abscesses from other lesions that can have similar clinical spectrum.

CT demonstrates early cerebritis as an area of ill-defined low attenuation (Fig. 22a) with a variable pattern of contrast enhancement (ranging from no to nodular or ring-like enhancement). The enhancement pattern is unchanged or progresses on delayed images obtained at 30–60 min after contrast administration (Rath et al. 2012). The late cerebritis phase shows persistent poorly defined low-attenuation edema, associated with post-contrast images with a thick ring-like or nodular enhancement that is stable or increases on delayed images (Rath et al. 2012). In both the early and late capsule stages, the pus-containing core appears as a round or ovoid area of low attenuation with a sometimes faintly visible surrounding capsule ring; following contrast administration, there is a ring enhancement that decays on delayed images corresponding to the granulation tissue of the capsule (Rath et al. 2012)

MR is the imaging modality of choice for diagnosis and follow-up of brain abscesses (Haimes et al. 1989). The early cerebritis stage is characterized by a nonspecific poorly defined area, hyperintense on T2-w, and is isointense to mildly hypointense on T1-w images, with ill-defined enhancement (Rath et al. 2012).

A mature brain abscess appears as a round/oval-shaped mass with a central area of suppurative necrosis (hypointense to the cerebral white matter on T1-w and variably hyperintense on T2-w images) and a complete peripheral capsule (typically hypointense on T2-w and hyperintense on T1-w images) (Fig. 22a and b). The short T1 and T2 of the rim seem to be due, respectively, to the presence of collagen fibers and to macrophages releasing free radicals with a paramagnetic effect; after intravenous injection of contrast medium, it shows a typical peripheral thin and regular "ring enhancement" (Fig. 22e).

The peripheral contrast enhancement can be stronger in the portion of the abscess closest to the gray matter, because of the stronger inflammatory reaction due to the bigger vascularization of the gray matter.

The surrounding vasogenic edema appears hypointense on T1-w and hyperintense on T2-w images; the presence of a satellite abscess (closely associated with a primary abscess) that gives a polylobate appearance to the mass is also possible.

DWI gives a critical support in the diagnosis of cerebral abscesses (Castillo 1999; Guo et al. 2001; Reddy et al. 2006), which appear typically

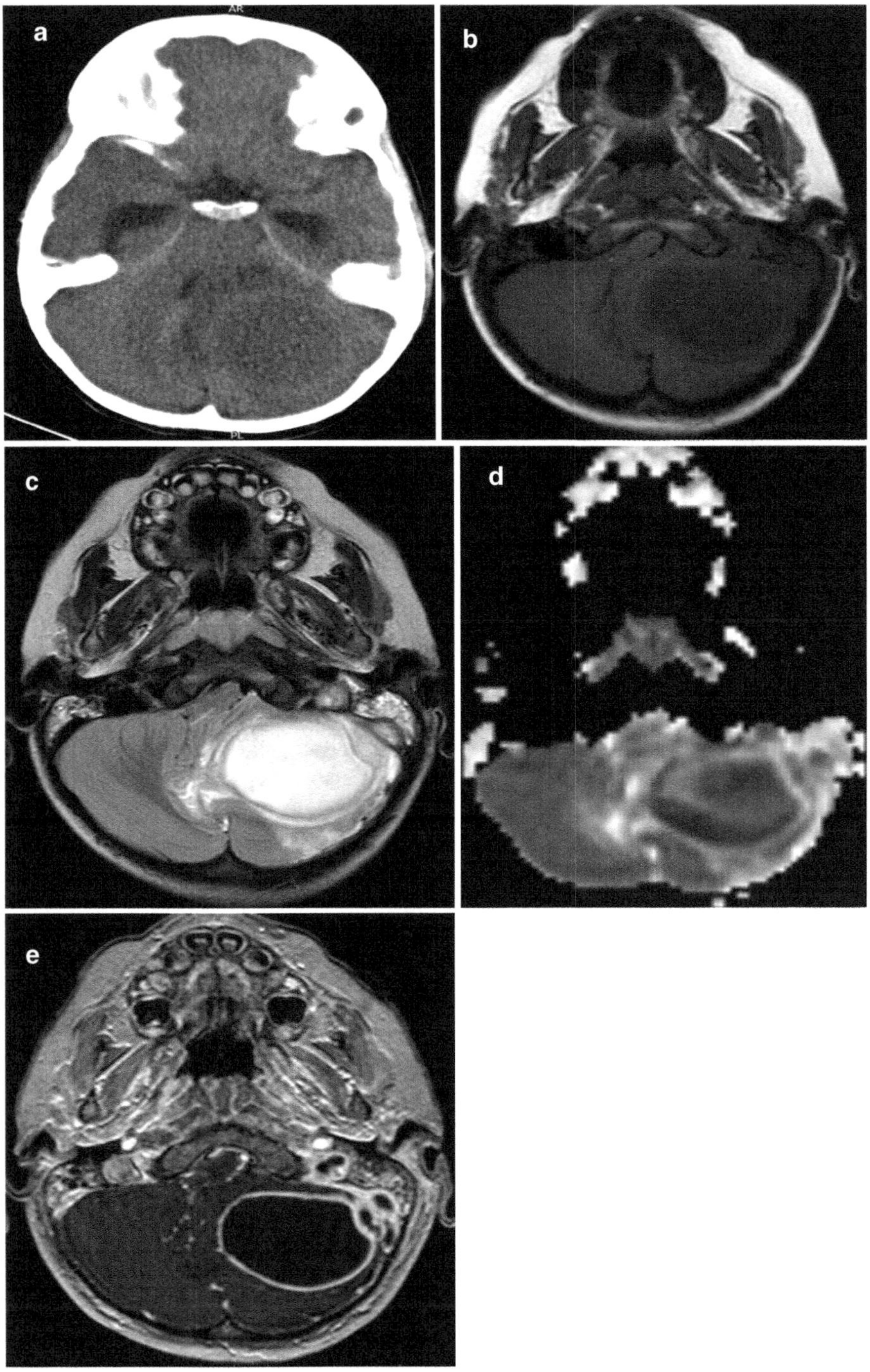


**Fig. 22** Cerebellar abscess. (**a**) CT scan. Presence of a left cerebellar hypodense mass, surrounded by edema, compressing e displacing the fourth ventricle; note temporal horn dilation. (**b** and **c**) T1 and T2-w axial sections; (**d**) ADC map axial section; (**e**) T1-w axial section after intravenous contrast medium injection. Presence of an oval-shaped mass with a central T1 hypointense, T2 hyperintense area of suppurative necrosis with restricted diffusion and a T2 hypointense peripheral capsule, showing a peripheral and regular "ring enhancement"; note also the mastoid air cells and tympanic cavity filled with a mass of soft tissue (by chronic otitis media) associated with transverse-sigmoid-jugular thrombophlebitis (arrows)

hyperintense, with low values on ADC maps (reported in the literature between 0.28 and 0.73 × $10^{-3}$ $mm^2/s$) because of the water restriction in the central necrotic area containing proteins and bacterial and cellular debris (Fig. 22d). However, the different concentration of bacteria and white cells, the different kinds of bacteria involved, and the immune response of the host can lead to a wider range of ADC values in the central necrotic area.

DWI is also useful to improve the diagnosis of an intraventricular rupture of a pyogenic abscess, with the purulent fluid appearing hyperintense in DWI with low values on the ADC maps in comparison with cerebrospinal fluid.

DWI may also be useful in the follow-up during treatment. The progressive increase in ADC values could be an earlier index of medical response to antibiotics earlier than the size reduction in the lesion and/or the presence of a gap in the peripheral rim enhancement; on the other hand, the persistence of low ADC values over time would be due to an ineffective therapy, and the recurrence of low ADC values suggests recurrence of active disease.

MR spectroscopy (1H-MRS) typically shows peaks corresponding to lipids (0.8–1.2 ppm), lactate (1.3 ppm), and amino acids (0.9 ppm) within the central necrotic area of pyogenic abscesses shows, without peaks corresponding to normal spectrum of nervous tissue (such as *N*-acetyl-aspartate and choline). Moreover, it is possible to find peaks of alanine (1.5 ppm), acetate (1.9 ppm), and succinate (2.4 ppm). The presence of lactate, acetate, and succinate is probably related to bacterial glycolysis and fermentation (Luthra et al. 2007).

Perfusion-w imaging shows different cerebral blood values related to the stage of the capsule: In early stage, the vascularization is higher than in the late stage in which the fibroblasts are dominant (Holmes et al. 2004; Muccio et al. 2014).

The differential diagnosis between pyogenic abscesses and other kinds of abscesses with a "ring-like" enhancement is not always possible with MRI only.

*Tuberculoma* is the localized form of CNS infection with Mycobacterium tuberculosis, more common in HIV-infected patients. It occurs at the corticomedullary junction, more common infratentorially in children and supratentorially in adults (Aiken 2010). MRI typically shows a hypointense T2 peripheral rim and a "ring-like" contrast enhancement after injection of gadolinium (Muccio et al. 2014). The center of the lesion shows iso/hypointensity on T1-w images and variable T2 signal related to the presence of caseous or liquefactive necrosis (Muccio et al. 2014): A dark T2 signal is thought to be caused by free radicals, and the solid caseation signal is attributed to cellular density (Jinkins et al. 1995; Garcia-Monco 1999; Bernaerts et al. 2003). Tubercular abscess is rare, more commonly in immunocompromised patients, and it appears similar to pyogenic abscess at MRI (Bernaerts et al. 2003).

*Cerebral toxoplasmosis* derives etiologically by toxoplasma gondii, causing a frank encephalitis and representing the main cause of brain abscess in HIV-positive patients. Fortunately, the number of cases has declined significantly because of the advent of highly active antiretroviral therapy (HAART). There is also a congenital form that occurs during transplacental passage during the third trimester of gestation.

The symptomatology is usually blurred, but when neurological symptoms appear in immunosuppressed patients it is always necessary to suspect toxoplasma encephalitis.

Cerebral toxoplasmosis consists itself of multiple lesions mainly to the basal ganglia, thalamus, and corticomedullary junction. CT can demonstrate hypodensity of the involved region and a "ring" enhancement around the lesion after contrast injection (Navia et al. 1986a, b); the lesions frequently calcify after treatment. MRI demonstrates multiple lesions in different stages of evolution, typically located in the subcortical and periventricular white matter, in the basal ganglia and thalami (rarely in cerebellum). The lesions are generally hypointense on T1-w images, while the T2 signal characteristics can be variable, ranging from hyperintense to isointense or even hypointense (Brightbill et al. 1996). The presence of an eccentric area of contrast enhancement ("eccentric target sign") is a typical feature of cerebral toxoplasmosis; the "concentric target sign" is a recently described MRI sign on T2-weighted imaging, and probably more specific, which consists of concentric alternating zones of hypo- and hyperintensities (Mahadevan et al. 2013; Roche et al. 2018). An imaging finding highly suggestive is the "asymmetric target sign," consisting of a small eccentric nodule of enhancement along the enhancing wall, thought to represent in folding of the cyst wall (Ramsey and Geremia 1988). DWI can be useful for differential diagnosis, since the center of the toxoplasma abscess has a hypo/isointense signal in DWI with ADC values higher than in pyogenic abscesses (Muccio et al. 2014).

## References


Adriani KS, Brouwer MC, van de Beek D (2015) Risk factors for community-acquired bacterial meningitis in adults. Neth J Med 73(2):53–60

Aiken AH (2010) Central Nervous System Infection. Neuroradiol Emerg Neuroimaging Clin N Am 20:557–580. In Gean AD (Ed)

Almutairi BM, Nguyen TB, Jansen GH, Asseri AH et al (2009) Invasive aspergillosis of the brain: radiologic-pathologic correlation. Radiographics 29(2):375–379

Antinori A, Arendt G, Becker JT et al (2007) Updated research nosology for HIV-associated neurocognitive disorders. Neurology 69(18):1789–1799

Awasthi M, Parmar H, Patankar T et al (2001a) Imaging findings in rabies encephalitis. AJNR Am J Neuroradiol 22(4):677–680

Awasthi M, Patankar T, Shah P et al (2001b) Cerebral cryptococcosis: atypical appearances on CT. Br J Radiol 74(877):83–85

Azarpira N, Esfandiari M, Bagheri MH et al (2008) Cerebral aspergillosis presenting as a mass lesion. Braz J Infect Dis 12(4):349–351

Bach F, Larsen BH, Rohde K et al (1990) Metastatic spinal cord compression. Occurrence, symptoms, clinical presentations and prognosis in 398 patients with spinal cord compression. Acta Neurochir 107(1–2):37–43

Bag AK, Curé JK, Chapman PR et al (2010) JC virus infection of the brain. AJNR Am J Neuroradiol 31(9):1564–1576

Baldwin KJ, Zivković SA, Lieberman FS (2012) Neurologic emergencies in patients who have cancer: diagnosis and management. Neurol Clin 30(1):101–128

Bang OY, Seok JM, Kim SG et al (2011) Ischemic stroke and cancer: stroke severely impacts cancer patients, while cancer increases the number of strokes. J Clin Neurol 7:53–59

Barkovich AJ, Atlas SW (1988) Magnetic resonance imaging of intracranial hemorrhage. Radiol Clin N Am 26:801–820

Battipaglia G, Avilia S, Morelli E et al (2012) Posterior reversible encephalopathy syndrome (PRES) during induction chemotherapy for acute myeloblastic leukemia (AML). Ann Hematol 91(8):1327–1328

Bernaerts A, Vanhoenacker FM, Parizel PM et al (2003) Tuberculosis of the central nervous system: overview of neuroradiological findings. Eur Radiol 13(8):1876–1890

Bognar L, Borgulya G, Benke P et al (2003) Analysis of CSF shunting procedure requirement in children with posterior fossa tumors. Childs Nerv Syst 19: 332–336

Brandsma D, Stalpers L, Taal W et al (2008) Clinical features, mechanisms, and management of pseudoprogression in malignant gliomas. Lancet Oncol 9:453–461

Brightbill TC, Post MJ, Hensley GT et al (1996) MR of toxoplasma encephalitis: signal characteristics on T2-weighted images and pathologic correlation. J Comput Assist Tomogr 20(3):417–422

Britt RH, Enzmann DR (1983) Clinical stages of human brain abscesses on serial CT scans after contrast infusion. Computerized tomographic, neuropathological, and clinical correlations. J Neurosurg 59(6):972–989

Brophy GM, Bell R, Claassen J et al (2012) Guidelines for the evaluation and management of status epilepticus. Neurocrit Care 17:3–23

Bulakbasi N, Kocaoglu M (2008) Central nervous system infections of herpesvirus family. Neuroimaging Clin N Am 18(1):53–84

Cakirer S, Başak M, Mutlu A et al (2002) MR imaging in epilepsy that is refractory to medical therapy. Eur Radiol 12(3):549–558

Caranci F, Tedeschi E, Ugga L et al (2018) Magnetic resonance imaging correlates of benign and malignant alterations of the spinal bone marrow. Acta Biomed 89:18–33

Castillo M (1999) Imaging brain abscesses with diffusion-weighted and other sequences. AJNR Am J Neuroradiol 20(7):1193–1194

Chamberlain MC (1997) Carcinomatous meningitis. Arch Neurol 54(1):16–17

Chamberlain M, Soffietti R, Raizer J et al (2014) Leptomeningeal metastasis: a response assessment in neuro-oncology critical review of endpoints and response criteria of published randomized clinical trials. Neuro-Oncology 16:1176–1185

Chi D, Behin A, Delattre J-Y (2008) Neurologic complications of radiation therapy. In: Schiff D, Kesari S, Wen PY (eds) Cancer neurology in clinical practice. Humana Press, New Jersey, pp 259–286

Cicala D, Briganti F, Casale L et al (2013) Atraumatic vertebral compression fractures: differential diagnosis between benign osteoporotic and malignant fractures by MRI. Musculoskelet Surg 97(Suppl 2):S169–S179
Clarke JL, Perez HR, Jacks LM et al (2010) Leptomeningeal metastases in the MRI era. Neurology 74:1449–1454
Coburn MW, Rodriguez FJ (1998) Cerebral herniations. Appl Radiol 27(5):10–16
Cook AM, Lau TN, Tomlinson MJ et al (1998) Magnetic resonance imaging of the whole spine in suspected malignant spinal cord compression: impact on management. Clin Oncol (R Coll Radiol) 10(1):39–43
Crocker M, Anthantharanjit R, Jones TL et al (2011) An extended role for CT in the emergency diagnosis of malignant spinal cord compression. Clin Radiol 66(10):922–927
D'Amico A, Briganti F, Caranci F et al (2003) MR study of CNS injury caused by chemotherapy and radiotherapy in childhood. Riv Neuroradiol 16(3):439–444
Damek DM (2010) Cerebral edema, altered mental status, seizures, acute stroke, leptomeningeal metastases, and paraneoplastic syndrome. Hematol Oncol Clin North Am 24(3):515–535
De Divitiis O, Elefante A (2012) Cervical spinal brucellosis: A diagnostic and surgical challenge. World Neurosurg 78(3–4):257–259
De la Fuente MI, DeAngelis LM (2014) The role of ventriculoperitoneal shunting in patients with supratentorial glioma. Ann Clin Transl Neurol 1:45–48
DeLone DR, Goldstein RA, Petermann G et al (1999) Disseminated aspergillosis involving the brain: distribution and imaging characteristics. AJNR Am J Neuroradiol 20(9):1597–1604
Destian S, Sze G, Krol G et al (1989) MR imaging of hemorrhagic intracranial neoplasms. AJR Am J Roentgenol 152:137–144
Elefante A, Tortora F, Volpe A et al (2003) Proposed protocol for neuroradiological study in the follow-up of CNS tumours in childhood. Riv Neuroradiol 16(3):471–475
Elefante A, Peca C, Del Basso De Caro ML et al (2012) Symptomatic spinal cord metastasis from cerebral oligodendroglioma. Neurol Sci 33(3):609–613
Elefante A, Caranci F, Del Basso De Caro ML et al (2013) Paravertebral high cervical chordoma: a case report. Neuroradiol J 26(2):227–232
Enting RH (2005) Leptomeningeal neoplasia: epidemiology, clinical presentation, CSF analysis and diagnostic imaging. Cancer Treat Res 125:17–30
Fewel ME, Thompson BG, Hoff JT (2003) Spontaneous intracerebral hemorrhage: a review. Neurosurg Focus 15:E1
Fischer M, Schmutzhard E (2017) Posterior reversible encephalopathy syndrome. J Neurol 264(8):1608–1616
Forsyth PA, Posner JB (1993) Headaches in patients with brain tumors: a study of 111 patients. Neurology 43(9):1678–1683
Garcia-Monco JC (1999) Central nervous system tuberculosis. Neurol Clin 17(4):737–759
Garrels K, Kucharczyk W, Wortzman G et al (1996) Progressive multifocal leukoencephalopathy: clinical and MR response to treatment. AJNR Am J Neuroradiol 17(3):597–600
Giglio P, Gilbert MR (2003) Cerebral radiation necrosis. Neurologist 9:180–188
Giglio P, Gilbert MR (2010) Neurologic complications of cancer and its treatment. Curr Oncol Rep 12(1):50–59
Glass JP, Melamed M, Chernik NL et al (1979) Malignant cells in cerebrospinal fluid (CSF): the meaning of a positive CSF cytology. Neurology 29(10):1369–1375
Gower DJ, Baker AL, Bell WO, Ball MR (1987) Contraindications to lumbar puncture as defined by computed cranial tomography. J Neurol Neurosurg Psychiatry 50:1071–1074
Groves MD (2011) Leptomeningeal disease. Neurosurg Clin N Am 22:67–78. vii
Guo AC, Provenzale JM, Cruz LC Jr et al (2001) Cerebral abscesses: investigation using apparent diffusion coefficient maps. Neuroradiology 43(5):370–374
Haacke EM, Xu Y, Cheng YC et al (2004) Susceptibility weighted imaging (SWI). Magn Reson Med 52:612–618
Haimes AB, Zimmerman RD, Morgello S et al (1989) MR imaging of brain abscesses. AJR Am J Roentgenol 152(5):1073–1085
Hammack JE (2012) Spinal cord disease in patients with cancer. Continuum (Minneap Minn) 18:312–327
Holmes TM, Petrella JR, Provenzale JM (2004) Distinction between cerebral abscesses and high-grade neoplasms by dynamic susceptibility contrast perfusion MRI. AJR Am J Roentgenol 183(5):1247–1252
Iwama T, Ohkuma A, Miwa Y et al (1992) Brain tumors manifesting as intracranial hemorrhage. Neurol Med Chir (Tokyo) 32(3):130–135
Jinkins JR, Gupta R, Chang KH et al (1995) MR imaging of central nervous system tuberculosis. Radiol Clin N Am 33(4):771–786
Jo JT, Schiff D (2017) Management of neuro-oncologic emergencies. Handb Clin Neurol 141:715–741
Kaal EC, Vecht CJ (2004) The management of brain edema in brain tumors. Curr Opin Oncol 16(6):593–600
Katabathina VS, Restrepo CS, Betancourt Cuellar SL et al (2013) Imaging of oncologic emergencies: what every radiologist should know. Radiographics 33(6):1533–1553
Klein SL, Sanford RA, Muhlbauer MS (1991) Pediatric spinal epidural metastases. J Neurosurg 74:70–75
Kumar S, Misra UK, Kalita J et al (1997) MRI in Japanese encephalitis. Neuroradiology 39(3):180–184
Lacy J, Saadati H, Yu JB (2012) Complications of brain tumors and their treatment. Hematol Oncol Clin North 26(4):779–796
Laothamatas J, Hemachudha T, Mitrabhakdi E et al (2003) MR imaging in human rabies. AJNR Am J Neuroradiol 24(6):1102–1109
Law M (2009) Neurological complications. Cancer Imaging 9:S71–S74

Lee KY (2016) Enterovirus 71 infection and neurological complications. Korean J Pediatr 59(10):395–401
Li KC, Poon PY (1988) Sensitivity and specificity of MRI in detecting malignant spinal cord compression and in distinguishing malignant from benign compression fractures of vertebrae. Magn Reson Imaging 6(5):547–556
Li XL, Zhou FM, Shangguan SQ et al (2014) Application of computed tomography for differential diagnosis of glioma stoke and simple cerebral hemorrhage. Asian Pac J Cancer Prev 15(8):3425–3428
Lieu AS, Hwang SL, Howng SL et al (1999) Brain tumors with hemorrhage. J Formos Med Assoc 98(5):365–367
Lin AL, Avila EK (2017) Neurologic emergencies in the patients with cancer. J Intensive Care Med 32(2):99–115
Little JR, Dial B, Belanger G et al (1979) Brain hemorrhage from intracranial tumor. Stroke 10:283–288
Logan SA, MacMahon E (2008) Viral meningitis. BMJ (Clin Res Ed) 336(7634):36–40
Lote K, Stenwig AE, Skullerud K et al (1998) Prevalence and prognostic significance of epilepsy in patients with gliomas. Eur J Cancer 34:98–102
Lulla R, Andrew MS, Foy AB et al (2011) Emergencies in children and young adults with central nervous system tumors. Clin Pediatr Emerg Med 12(3):213–223
Luthra G, Parihar A, Nath K et al (2007) Comparative evaluation of fungal, tubercular, and pyogenic brain abscesses with conventional and diffusion MR imaging and proton MR spectroscopy. AJNR Am J Neuroradiol 28(7):1332–1338
Luyken C, Blumcke I, Fimmers R et al (2003) The spectrum of long-term epilepsy-associated tumors: long-term seizure and tumor outcome and neurosurgical aspects. Epilepsia 44:822–830
Mahadevan A, Ramalingaiah AH, Parthasarathy S et al (2013) Neuropathological correlate of the "concentric target sign" in MRI of HIV-associated cerebral toxoplasmosis. J Magn Reson Imaging 38(2):488–495
Mak KS, Lee LK, Mak RH et al (2011) Incidence and treatment patterns in hospitalizations for malignant spinal cord compression in the United States, 1998–2006. Int J Radiat Oncol Biol Phys 80:824–831
Marino R, Gasparotti R, Pinelli L et al (2006) Posttraumatic cerebral infarction in patients with moderate or severe head trauma. Neurology 67:1165–1171
Martel S, De Angelis F, Lapointe E et al (2014) Paraneoplastic neurologic syndromes: clinical presentation and management. Curr Probl Cancer 38:115–134
Marzolf G, Sabou M, Lannes B et al (2016) Magnetic resonance imaging of cerebral aspergillosis: imaging and pathological correlations. PLoS One 11(4):e0152475
Maschio M (2012) Brain tumor-related epilepsy. Curr Neuropharmacol 10:124–133
McCurdy MT, Shanholtz CB (2012) Oncologic emergencies. Crit Care Med 40(7):2212–2222
Miszkiel KA, Hallcraggs MA, Miller RF et al (1996) The spectrum of MRI findings in CNS cryptococcosis in AIDS. Clin Radiol 51(12):842–850
Muccio CF, Caranci F, D'Arco F et al (2014) Magnetic resonance features of pyogenic brain abscesses and differential diagnosis using morphological and functional imaging studies: a pictorial essay. J Neuroradiol 41(3):153–167
Müller NL, Franquet T, Lee KS et al (2007) Imaging of pulmonary infections. Lippincott Williams & Wilkins, Philadelphia
Nagel MA, Gilden D (2013) The challenging patient with varicella-zoster virus disease. Neurol Clin Pract 3:109–117
Nathoo N, Nadvi SS, van Dellen JR et al (1999) Intracranial subdural empyemas in the era of computed tomography: a review of 699 cases. Neurosurgery 44(3):529–535
Navi B, Segal AZ (2009) Cancer and stroke. In: Geyer JD, Gomez CR (eds) Stroke: a practical approach. Lippincott Williams & Wilkins, Philadelphia, pp 48–55
Navi B, Reichman JS, Berlin D et al (2010) Intracerebral and subarachnoid hemorrhage in patients with cancer. Neurology 74:494–501
Navia BA, Jordan BD, Price RW (1986a) The AIDS dementia complex: I. Clinical features. Ann Neurol 19(6):517–524
Navia BA, PetitoCK GJW et al (1986b) Cerebral toxoplasmosis complicating the acquired immune deficiency syndrome: clinical and neuropathological findings in 27 patients. Ann Neurol 19(3):224–238
Oberndorfer S, Schmal T, Lahrmann H et al (2002) The frequency of seizures in patients with primary brain tumors or cerebral metastases. An evaluation from the Ludwig Boltzmann Institute of Neuro-Oncology and the Department of Neurology, Kaiser Franz Josef Hospital, Vienna. Wien Klin Wochenschr 114(21–22):911–916
Odaka M, Yuki N, Hirata K (2001) Anti-GQ1b IgG antibody syndrome: clinical and immunological range. J Neurol Neurosurg Psychiatry 70(1):50–55
Ogiwara H, Nordli DR, DiPatri AJ et al (2010) Pediatric epileptogenic gangliogliomas: seizure outcome and surgical results. J Neurosurg Pediatr 5:271–276
Pagliano P, Caggiano C, Acione T et al (2017) Characteristics of meningitis following transsphenoidal endoscopic surgery: a case series and a systematic literature review. Infection 45(6):841–848
Passarin MG, Sava T, Furlanetto J et al (2015) Leptomeningeal metastasis from solid tumors: a diagnostic and therapeutic challenge. Neurol Sci 36:117–123
Pater K, Puskulluoglu M, Zygulska AL (2014) Oncological emergencies: increased intracranial pressure in solid tumor's metastatic brain disease. Przegl Lek 71:91–94
Prakash M, Kumar S, Gupta RK (2004) Diffusion-weighted MR imaging in Japanese encephalitis. J Comput Assist Tomogr 28(6):756–761
Pruitt AA (2003) Nervous system infections in patients with cancer. Neurol Clin 21:193–219

Ramsey RG, Geremia GK (1988) CNS complications of AIDS: CT and MR findings. AJR Am J Roentgenol 151(3):449–454

Rath TJ, Hughes M, Arabi M et al (2012) Imaging of cerebritis, encephalitis, and brain abscess. Neuroimaging Clin N Am 22(4):585–607

Reddy JS, Mishra AM, Behari S et al (2006) The role of diffusion-weighted imaging in the differential diagnosis of intracranial cystic mass lesions: a report of 147 lesions. Surg Neurol 66(3):246–250

Ricard D, Psimaras D, Soussain C et al (2012) Central nervous system complications of radiation therapy. In: Wen P, Schiff D, Lee EQ (eds) Neurologic complications of cancer therapy. Demos Medical, New York

Roche AD, Rowley D, Brett FM et al (2018) Concentric and eccentric target MRI signs in a case of HIV-associated cerebral toxoplasmosis. Case Rep Neurol Med 2018:9876514

Ryken TC, Aygun N, Morris J et al (2014) AANS/CNS joint guidelines committee. The role of imaging in the management of progressive glioblastoma: a systematic review and evidence-based clinical practice guideline. J Neuro-Oncol 118(3):435–460

Sahraian MA, Radue EW, Eshaghi A (2012) Progressive multifocal leukoencephalopathy: a review of the neuroimaging features and differential diagnosis. Eur J Neurol 19:1060–1069

Sarbu N, Shih RY, Jones RV et al (2016) White matter diseases with radiologic-pathologic correlation. Radiographics 36(5):1426–1447

Savage P, Sharkey R, Kua T et al (2014) Malignant spinal cord compression: NICE guidance, improvements and challenges. QJM 107(4):277–282

Schettino C, Caranci F, Lus G et al (2017) Diffuse glioblastoma resembling acute hemorrhagic leukoencephalitis. Quant Imaging Med Surg 7(5):592–597

Schiff D, Batchelor T, Wen PY (1998a) Neurologic emergencies in cancer patients. Neurol Clin 16(2):449–483

Schiff D, O'Neill BP, Wang CH et al (1998b) Neuroimaging and treatment implications of patients with multiple epidural spinal metastases. Cancer 83(8):1593–1601

Schrader B, Barth H, Lang EW et al (2000) Spontaneous intracranial haematomas caused by neoplasms. Acta Neurochir 9(142):979–985

Scott BJ (2015) Neuro-Oncologic emergencies. Semin Neurol 35(6):675–682

Shibani M, Garga UC (2012) Role of imaging in herpes and Japanese encephalitis–two cases and review of literature. J Indian Acad Clin Med 13(4):338–343

Siddiqui AA, Bashir SH, Ali Shah A et al (2006) Diagnostic MR imaging features of craniocerebral aspergillosis of sino-nasal origin in immunocompetent patients. Acta Neurochir 148(2):155–166

Singer MB, Atlas SW, Drayer BP (1998) Subarachnoid space disease: diagnosis with fluid-attenuated inversion recovery MR imaging and comparison with gadolinium-enhanced spin-echo MR imaging blinded reader study. Radiology 208(2):417–422

Smith AB, Smirniotopoulos JG, Rushing EJ (2008) From the archives of the AFIP: central nervous system infections associated with human immunodeficiency virus infection: radiologic-pathologic correlation. Radiographics 28(7):2033–2058

Soussain C, Ricard D, Fike JR et al (2009) CNS complications of radiotherapy and chemotherapy. Lancet 374:1639–1651

Spennato P, Chiaramonte C, Cicala D et al (2016) Acute triventricular hydrocephalus caused by choroid plexus cysts: a diagnostic and neurosurgical challenge. Neurosurg Focus 41(5):E9

Spinazze S, Caraceni A, Schrijvers D (2005) Epidural spinal cord compression. Crit Rev Oncol Hematol 56:397–406

Stevens RD, Huff JS, Duckworth J et al (2012) Emergency neurological life support: intracranial hypertension and herniation. Neurocrit Care 17(Suppl 1): S60–S65

Straathof CS, de Bruin HG, Dippel DW et al (1999) The diagnostic accuracy of magnetic resonance imaging and cerebrospinal fluid cytology in leptomeningeal metastasis. J Neurol 246(9):810–814

Striano P, Tortora F et al (2007) Periodic myoclonus due to cytomegalovirus encephalitis in a patient with good syndrome. Arch Neurol 64(2):277–279

Sun H, Nemecek AN (2010) Optimal management of malignant epidural spinal cord compression. Hematol Oncol Clin North Am 24(3):537–551

Sze G, Soletsky S, Bronen R et al (1989) MR imaging of the cranial meninges with emphasis on contrast enhancement and meningeal carcinomatosis. AJR Am J Roentgenol 153(5):1039–1049

Takasu A, Taneda M, Otuki H et al (1991) Gd-DTPA enhanced MR imaging of cryptococcal meningoencephalitis. Neuroradiology 33(5):443–446

Tempkin AD, Sobonya RE, Seeger JF et al (2006) Cerebral aspergillosis: radiologic and pathologic findings. Radiographics 26(4):1239–1242

Thawait SK, Kim J, Klufas RA et al (2013) Comparison of four prediction models to discriminate benign from malignant vertebral compression fractures according to MRI feature analysis. AJR Am J Roentgenol 200(3):493–502

Tortora F, Caranci F, Belfiore MP et al (2015) Brainstem variant of posterior reversible encephalopathy syndrome: a case report. Neuroradiol J 28(6):634–637

Ullrich NJ (2009) Neurologic sequelae of brain tumors in children. J Child Neurol 24:1446–1454

Ullrich NJ, Robertson R, Kinnamon DD et al (2007) Moyamoya following cranial irradiation for primary brain tumors in children. Neurology 68:932–938

Vajro P, Sokal EM, Maddaluno S et al (2009) Brain abscess due to Klebsiella pneumoniae in a liver-transplanted child. Transpl Infect Dis 11(4):341–345

Van Breemen MS, Wilms EB, Vecht CJ (2007) Epilepsy in patients with brain tumours: epidemiology, mechanisms, and management. Lancet Neurol 6:421–430

Vaswani AK, Nizamani WM, Ali M et al (2014) Diagnostic accuracy of contrast-enhanced FLAIR magnetic resonance imaging in diagnosis of meningitis correlated with CSF analysis. ISRN Radiol 2014:578986. 7 pages

Wakai S, Yamakawa K, Manaka S et al (1982) Spontaneous intracranial hemorrhage caused by brain tumor. Its incidence and clinical significance. Neurosurgery 10:437–444

Walker MT, Kapoor V (2007) Neuroimaging of parenchymal brain metastases. Cancer Treat Res 136:31–51

Wassertrom WR, Glass JP, Posner J (2006) Diagnosis and treatment of leptomeningeal metastases from solid tumors; experience with 90 patients. Cancer 49:759–772

White JB, Piepgras DG, Scheithauer BW et al (2008) Rate of spontaneous hemorrhage in histologically proven cases of pilocytic astrocytoma. J Neurosurg 108:223–226

Witham TF, Khavkin YA, Gallia GL et al (2006) Surgery insight: current management of epidural spinal cord compression from metastatic spine disease. Nat Clin Pract Neurol 2(2):87–94

Zimmerman RD, Russell EJ, Leeds NE et al (1980) CT in the early diagnosis of herpes simplex encephalitis. AJR Am J Roentgenol 134(1):61–66

# Toxic–Metabolic Encephalopathies

H. Urbach and S. Weidauer

## Contents



H. Urbach (✉)
Department of Neuroradiology, University Medical Center, Faculty of Medicine, University of Freiburg, Freiburg, Germany
e-mail: horst.urbach@uniklinik-freiburg.de

S. Weidauer
Department of Neuroradiology, University Medical Center, Frankfurt/Main, Germany

**Abstract**

A patient who presents with a toxic–metabolic encephalopathy syndrome is often confused, uncooperative, somnolent, or even comatose. If emergency laboratory investigations (glu-



M. Scaglione et al. (eds.), *Emergency Radiology of the Head and Spine*, Medical Radiology Diagnostic Imaging, https://doi.org/10.1007/978-3-030-91047-1_8

cose, sodium) or the clinical history (medication, hypertension, radiation therapy, intoxication) suggests a specific diagnosis, CT including CT angiography or better MRI is performed to confirm the suspected diagnosis, to display disease-related complications, and to rule out differential diagnoses. In many patients, however, MRI is fundamental to suggest a diagnosis or at least to target the diagnostic direction. There is no definite MRI protocol; however, it should at least include DWI, FLAIR, 3D-TOF, and SWI sequences. Toxic–metabolic encephalopathies often show a symmetric lesion pattern. Special attention should be targeted on the pons (central pontine myelinolysis), mammillary bodies (Wernicke encephalopathy), globi pallidi (CO intoxication, cocaine, methamphetamine, and other synthetic drugs abuse), cortex and deep gray matter sparing the thalami (hypoglycemic encephalopathy), and white matter (heroin and adulterants). Also, drug abuse is considered in younger and middle-aged persons with hemorrhagic and ischemic strokes—30 % of strokes in patients younger than 45 years of age are considered to be drug-related.

## 1 Introduction

An encephalopathy syndrome is defined as altered consciousness with change in cognition and/or with a perceptual disturbance developing over hours or days and that was not better accounted for by a pre-existing or evolving chronic dementia. Toxic–metabolic encephalopathies perfectly fulfill this definition but encompass a broad spectrum of diseases with nonspecific clinical presentations and often uncooperative, confused, or even comatose patients (Sutter and Kaplan 2015). If the metabolic derangement is suggested by emergency laboratory investigations (glucose, sodium) or the clinical history (medication, hypertension, radiation therapy, intoxication), CT including CT angiography or better MRI is performed to confirm the suspected diagnosis, to display disease-related complications, and to rule out differential diagnoses (Table 1). In many patients, however, MRI is fundamental to suggest a diagnosis or at least to target the diagnostic direction. This is especially true for patients receiving illicit drugs since they will typically deny drug abuse (Table 2). These rather younger

**Table 1** Toxic–metabolic encephalopathies suggested by laboratory investigations or clinical history

| | Diagnostic hint | MRI |
|---|---|---|
| Hypoglycemic encephalopathy | Blood glucose ↓ or ↑ | T2 (DWI) lesions of basal ganglia, hippocampi, and cortex with sparing of the thalami, white matter, and cerebellum orinternal capsule and hemispheric white matter injury |
| Hyperglycemic encephalopathy | Blood glucose ↑, HbA1c ↑ | Often normal, may show reduced cortical T2 signal |
| Central pontine myelinolysis (CPM)<br>Extrapontine myelinolysis | Rapid correction of low blood sodium | Round, oval, or batwing-shaped hyperintensity in central pons with peripheral rim and sparing of the pyramidal tracts (and nuclei pontis)<br>(additional) basal ganglia, thalami, and cerebral white matter involvement |
| Hepatic encephalopathy (HE) | Acute liver failure (liver cirrhosis, portosystemic shunt)—Chronic hepatic encephalopathy (CHE) | AHE: Normal or rather symmetrical cortical DWI restriction CHE: T1 hyperintense signal of the globi pallidi, substantia nigra, anterior midbrain, innominate substance |
| Carbon monoxide poisoning | Clinical history | Symmetrical lesions of the globi pallidi |
| SMART syndrome | Radiation therapy many years ago | Cortical DWI restriction, hyperperfusion (rCBV ↑), and enhancement not confined to a vascular territory |
| Cerebral fat embolism | Clinical worsening with confusion some days after a polytrauma with (long) bone fractures | Microbleeds (splenium) + starfield pattern on DWI (≈1–4 days), white matter changes (≈5–14 days) |

**Table 2** Toxic–metabolic encephalopathies in which MRI may give to make the diagnostic hint

| | Diagnostic hint | MRI |
|---|---|---|
| Wernicke encephalopathy | Alcoholic patient with altered consciousness, ocular dysfunction (double vision, nystagmus), and ataxia | Symmetric T2/FLAIR hyperintensity of the medial thalami and the periventricular region of the III ventricle. Contrast enhancement of the mammillary bodies |
| Subacute combined degeneration | Patient with sensory ataxia with loss of vibration sense, spasticity, hyperreflexia, and positive Babinski sign | T2 hyperintense lesion of the dorsal spinal cord columns with an inverted V configuration. Rarely, the lateral columns of the spinal cord are also affected.T2 hyperintense signal changes in the centrum semiovale, and optic nerve enhancement may occur |
| Mild encephalopathy with reversible splenium lesion (MERS) | Presurgical epilepsy evaluation with withdrawal of antiepileptic drugsinfection with fluid dysbalance | Non-space-occupying symmetric lesion within the splenium of the corpus callosum with diffusion restriction (MERS type 1). Additional structures as the subcortical white matter or the anterior corpus callosum (MERS type 2) |
| PRES | Eclampsia, chemotherapeutic agents, subacute extensive hypertension, thrombotic microangiopathies (TTP/HUS), sepsis | Typical PRES: Patchy to confluent, cortical, and subcortical vasogenic edema "beginning" in the parieto-occipital regionsatypical PRES: Frontal lobe, basal ganglia, brain stem, and cerebellar involvement |
| RCVS | Clinical history with unusual, recent, severe headaches of progressive or sudden onset with or without focal neurological deficit and/or seizures | Cerebral vasoconstriction with at least 2 narrowings per artery on 2 different arteries (catheter angiography = gold standard, MRA, CTA)<br>Disappearance of arterial abnormalities on control angiogram in 3 months |
| Heroin | Patient's "environment" | Chasing the dragon leukoencephalopathy: Symmetric T2/FLAIR hyperintensity of the predominantly periventricular cerebral and cerebellar white matter |
| Cocaine | Patient's "environment" | (Subarachnoid and/or intracerebral) hemorrhageischemic infarctsBilateral (enhancing) globus pallidus lesions |
| Synthetic drugs | Patient's "environment" | Similar to cocaine |
| Mitochondrial disorders | Depending on the mitochondrial disorder. For example, MELAS: Stroke-like episodes, migraine-like headaches, epileptic seizures | MELAS: Cortical/subcortical lesions not confined to a vascular territory. Cortical DWI restriction. Sometimes: Basal ganglia, pulvinar thalami, dentate nuclei calcifications |

patients often present with ischemic or hemorrhagic strokes: 30% of strokes in patients younger than 45 years of age are considered to be drug-related.

## 2 Imaging

Due to the nonspecific clinical presentations, the often non-cooperative patients may be studied with non-enhanced CT and CT angiography or better with MRI. However, there is no definite MRI protocol. The MRI protocol should at least include DWI, FLAIR, 3D-TOF, and SWI sequences. Thus, cytotoxic edema, vasogenic edema, arterial occlusions, or narrowing and parenchymal (micro)-bleedings are displayed. In many instances, rapid T2-weighed or FLAIR sequences are needed. A typical such sequence is the propeller (Periodically Rotated Overlapping ParallEL Lines with Enhanced Reconstruction, GE) (Pipe 1999), BLADE (Siemens), or MultiVane (Philips) sequence with which the k-space is sampled in rotating, radially oriented strips or blades. The center of the k-space which contributes most to the image contrast is oversampled, so that the signal-to-noise and contrast-to-noise ratios are high. Oversampling also provides redundant information, and the data for each new blade can be compared with the previous one. If the patient moves between blades, the data for the second blade can be corrected or even completely discarded. Due to oversampling of the k-space, susceptibility artifacts are also slightly reduced. We typically finish our MRI protocol with a 3D-MPRAGE sequence with fat saturation following contrast administration.

In the acute phase, MRI may detect acutely injured brain areas with vasogenic or cytotoxic edema, whereas in the chronic phase MRI shows sequelae with parenchymal defects. The type and severity of the toxic–metabolic defect and the age of the patient at which the defect gets clinically manifest determine the lesion pattern. In most cases, toxic–metabolic encephalopathies are characterized by a symmetric lesion pattern. Due to high metabolic demand, deep gray matter and the cerebral cortex are often involved. In contrast, myelin with its high lipid content is particularly vulnerable to lipophilic toxic substances and the white matter is involved in many toxic–metabolic encephalopathies (Valk and van der Knaap 1992).

In the following, we will focus on adult-onset toxic–metabolic encephalopathies since they represent the major diagnostic challenge in those patients who often present in a confused and unresponsive state.

## 3 Diseases

### 3.1 Hypoglycemic Encephalopathy

Pathogenesis: Low serum glucose (<50 mg/dl), e.g., in diabetic patients on insulin therapy.

Clinical presentation: Coma, depressed level of consciousness, may be preceded by seizures.

MRI: Transient DWI and T2 lesions of basal ganglia, hippocampi, and cortex with sparing of the thalami and cerebellum. The lesions may show restricted diffusion. Lack of thalamic involvement is in favor of hypoglycemia and against hypoxic–ischemic encephalopathy (Fig. 1).

In another imaging pattern with a better prognosis, the deep white matter shows a symmetric hyperintensity involving the internal capsule, corona radiata, and splenium on T2-weighted images (Lo et al. 2006; Johkura et al. 2012).

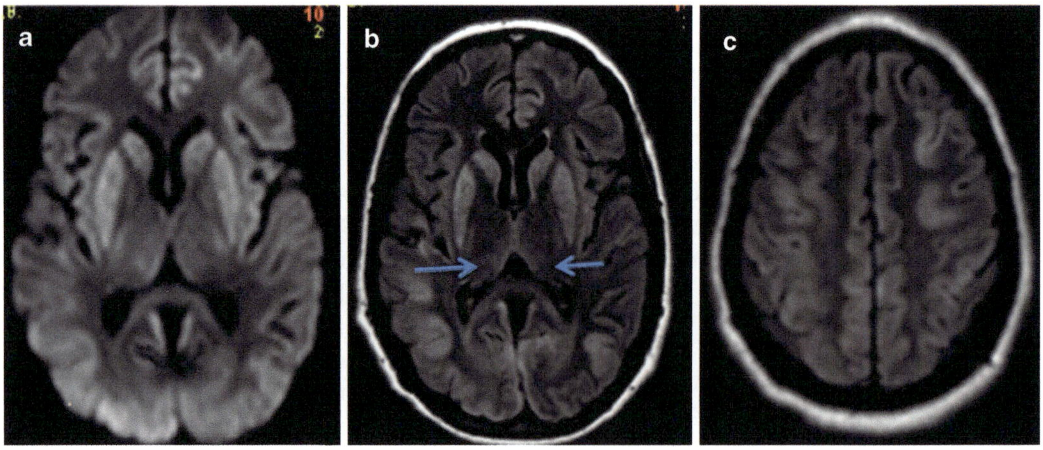


**Fig. 1** MRI 6 weeks after a 30-year-old woman presented with hypoglycemic coma. There is profound vasogenic edema of the basal ganglia (**a**, **b**) and the cortex (**c**), and the thalami are spared (**b**: arrows)

### 3.2 Hyperglycemic Encephalopathy (Non-Ketotic Hyperglycemia)

Pathogenesis: Non-ketotic hyperglycemia is a relatively common complication of diabetes mellitus type 2, especially in patients above 50 years of age.

Clinical presentation: The severity can vary from asymptomatic (for months, even years) to severely symptomatic patients (hyperosmolar coma and sometimes even death).

MRI: Often normal. Rarely and in close temporal relationship to seizures restricted diffusion reflecting cytotoxic edema on DWI and/or transient subcortical T2-weighted and FLAIR hypointensity predominantly in the posterior brain regions (Raghavendra et al. 2007). Unilateral striatal hyperintensity is another hint for non-ketotic hyperglycemia (Chu et al. 2002) (Fig. 2).

### 3.3 Osmotic Myelinolysis (Central Pontine Myelinolysis, Extrapontine Myelinolysis)

Definition: Myelinolysis in the center of the pons (central pontine myelinolysis). Extrapontine structures are involved in 50% of patients; however, extrapontine myelinolysis also may be seen in isolation. The term osmotic demyelination syndrome is used to encompass both entities.

Pathogenesis: Intramyelinic splitting, vacuolization, and rupture of myelin sheaths, presumably due to osmotic effects in the setting of correction of sodium levels (sodium level increases by more than 12 mmol/L/day). Often in alcoholic or malnourished patients. Also, uncorrected hyponatremia is considered as cause of confusion in, e.g., exercise-associated hyponatremia (EAH) among marathon runner (Noakes et al. 1985; Almond et al. 2005) or postoperative states (e.g., transurethral resection syndrome (TUR) due to the absorption of large volumes of non-electrolyte solutions (McGowan-Smyth et al. 2016).

Clinical manifestations: It varies from minimal symptoms to a complete locked-in syndrome, coma, or death.

MRI: It is centrally located T2-weighted and FLAIR-hyperintense pons lesion with relative sparing of the pyramidal tracts and a peripheral rim (Fig. 3). Sites of extrapontine myelinolysis include the basal ganglia, thalami, and cerebral white matter and, less commonly, the peripheral cortex, hippocampi, and lateral geniculate bodies (Fig. 4). DWI with cytotoxic edema (ADC ↓) is considered the earliest and most sensitive sequence but may be present only within the first days of the disease (Fig. 3).

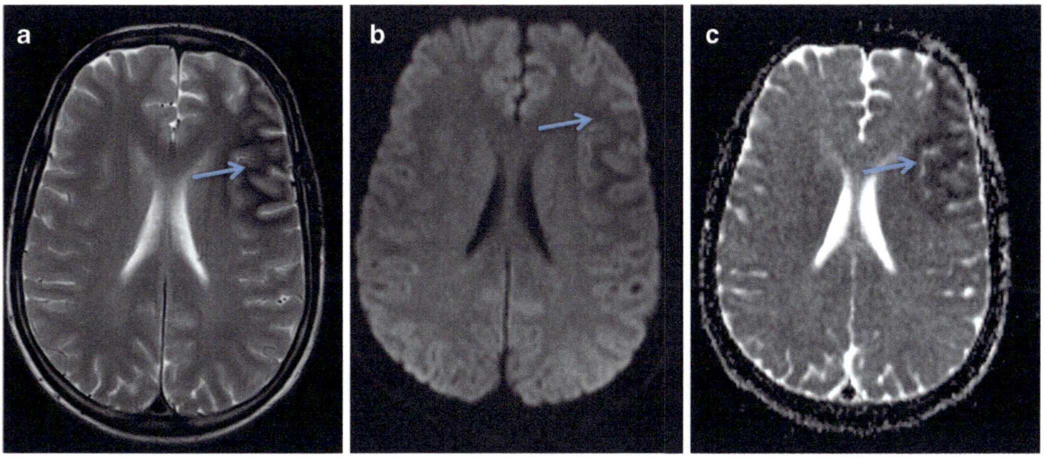


**Fig. 2** A 18-year-old man presented with somnolence and dysphasia. Blood sugar was 600 mg/dl. MRI showed signal changes in the left lateral frontal lobe: The cortical T2 hypointensity (**a**) without cytotoxic edema (**b**, **c**) is suggestive of non-ketotic hyperglycemia associated with epileptic seizures

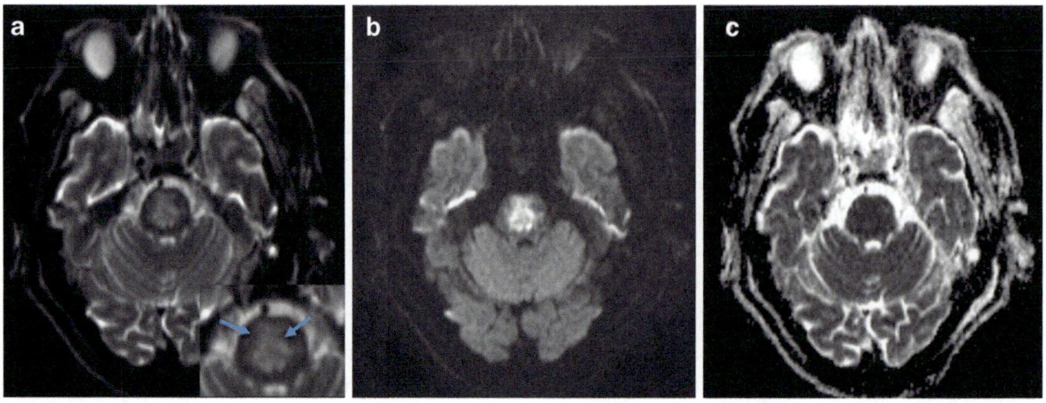


**Fig. 3** Central pontine myelinolysis in the pons with restricted diffusion (**b**: DWI, **c**: ADC map). The T2-weighted image shows a rather horizontal orientation, a peripheral rim (**a**), and sparing of the pyramidal tracts in the cerebral peduncles (**a**: inlay: arrows)

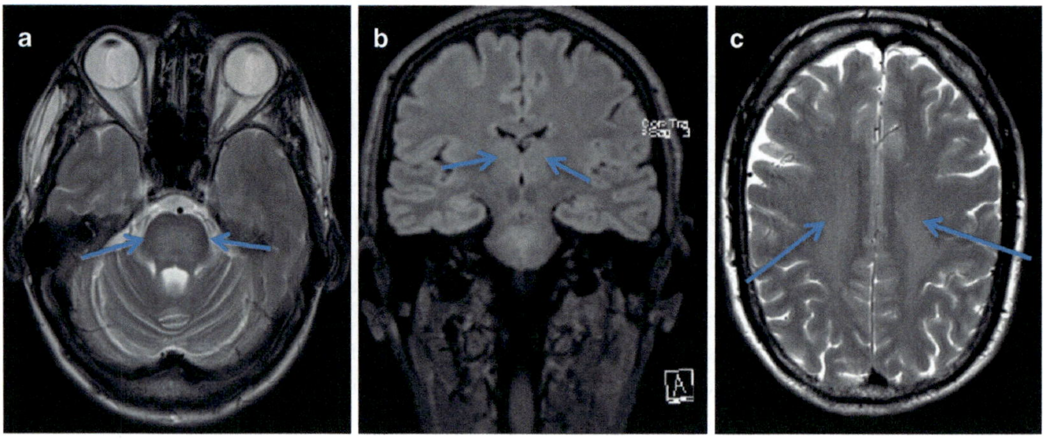


**Fig. 4** Pontine and extrapontine myelinolysis (osmotic myelinolysis) in a 46-year-old man with confusion. In addition to the symmetric signal changes in the pons (**a**: arrows), the thalami (**b**: arrows) and the supratentorial white matter (**c**: arrows) are involved

## 3.4 Hepatic Encephalopathy (HE)

Definition: Neurological and psychiatric abnormalities occurring in patients with liver dysfunction.

Pathogenesis: Brain overload with toxic substances such as ammonia and manganese and dysbalance between inhibitory and excitatory neurotransmitters (e.g., liver failure inactivates the glutamate transporter in astrocytes) (Rovira et al. 2008).

Clinical presentation: Broad spectrum ranging from subtle cognitive deficits to severe coma, rigidity, disorders of speech production, tremor, choreoathetoid movements, hyper- or hyporeflexia, and transient focal symptoms.

HE can be classified into three main groups on the basis of the duration and characteristics of the clinical manifestations (Ferenci et al. 2002): episodic, chronic, and minimal.

Episodic HE is characterized by the subacute development of a confusional state and neurologic abnormalities in patients with severe liver failure and/or portosystemic shunt surgery. Chronic HE either as relapsing or persistent chronic HE includes subtle abnormalities such as extrapyramidal signs and mild cognitive impairment or more severe abnormalities such as dementia, myelopathy, parkinsonism, ataxia, and tremor (Burkhard et al. 2003). Minimal HE patients are patients with liver cirrhosis or portal–systemic shunts with only subtle cognitive and neurologic deficits. However, for practical reasons it is easier to distinguish between acute hepatic encephalopathy and chronic hepatic encephalopathy.

MRI: In patients with acute HE, MRI may be normal. However, in patients with severe liver failure, it may show extended, rather symmetrical cortical DWI restrictions, that preferentially involve the insular cortices and relatively spare the perirolandic and occipital cortices. MRI in chronic HE shows T1 hyperintense lesions of the globi pallidi, substantia nigra, anterior midbrain, innominate substance, and less common the pituitary gland (Fig. 5).

## 3.5 Wernicke Encephalopathy

Pathogenesis: Acute neurologic disorder resulting from thiamine (vitamin B1) deficiency.

Clinical presentation: Triad with altered consciousness, ocular dysfunction (double vision, nystagmus), and ataxia (16–38% of patients).

MRI: Typical findings are symmetric T2/FLAIR hyperintensity of the medial thalami and the periventricular region of the III ventricle (80%) (Fig. 6), of the periaqueductal area (59%), mammillary bodies (45%), tectal plate (36%), and periventricular gray matter anteriorly to the IV ventricle (7%). Atypical findings are signal intensity alterations of the cerebellum, cerebellar vermis, cranial nerve nuclei, red nuclei, dentate nuclei, caudate nuclei, splenium, and cerebral cortex. Contrast enhancement occurs in around 2/3 of patients involving the mammillary bodies (39%), tectal plate (20%), thalamus (20%), periaqueductal area (17%), and cranial nerves nuclei (2%). Contrast enhancement of the mammillary bodies may be the only MRI sign of the disease (7%) and is significantly associated with alcohol abuse. In contrast, selective involvement of the cranial nerve nuclei is an established characteristic of nonalcoholic Wernicke encephalopathy (Zuccoli et al. 2009). Contrast enhancement may be the cause of microbleeds within the mammillary bodies, which are better detectable on SWI than on T2-weighted fast spin-echo images (Hattingen et al. 2016) (Fig. 7).

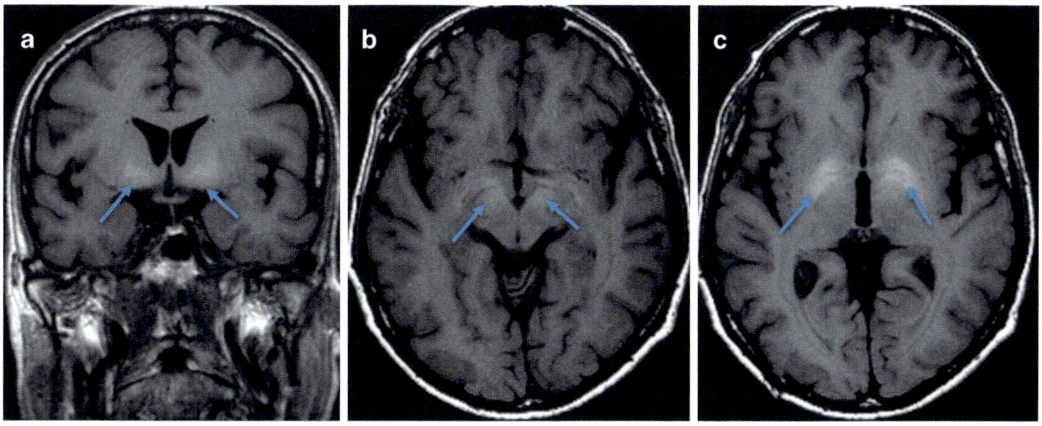


**Fig. 5** Coronal (**a**) and axial (**b**, **c**) T1-weighted SE images in a 71-year-old man with chronic HE show hyperintense lesions of the innominate substance (**a**: arrows), substantia nigra and anterior midbrain (B: arrows), and globi pallidi (**c**: arrows). T1 hyperintensity is considered to be due to manganese deposition

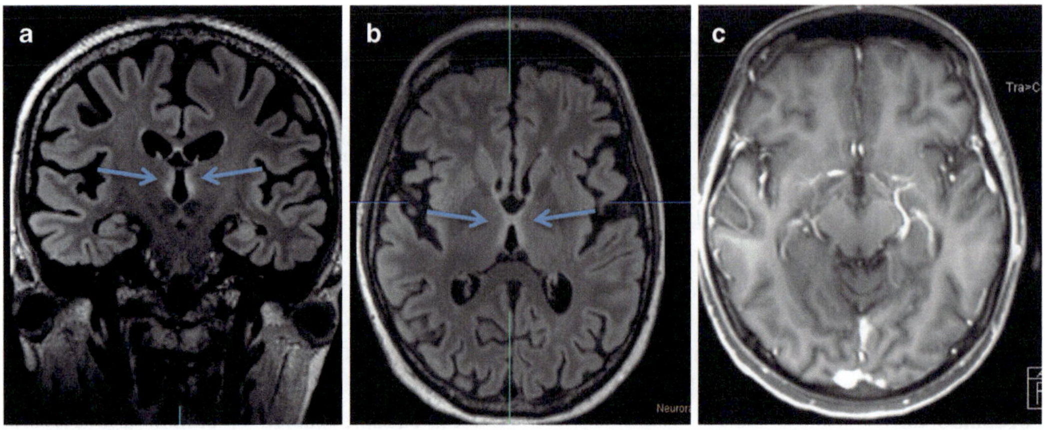

**Fig. 6** A 43-year-old man complained of blurred vision since 3 months. Three days ago, he suffered a sudden loss of visual acuity with central scotomas. He said to consume 2.5 L beer and 0.5 l wine/day. MRI shows Wernicke encephalopathy with a symmetric T2/FLAIR hyperintensity of the medial thalami and the periventricular region of the III ventricle (**a**, **b**: arrows), and the mammillary bodies do not enhance (**c**)

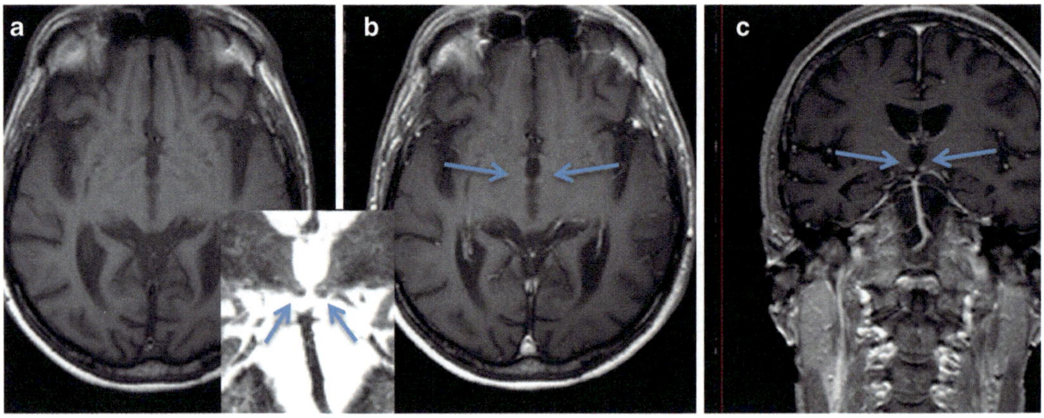

**Fig. 7** Wernicke encephalopathy in a 39-year-old alcoholic patient. MRI shows enhancing mammillary bodies (**b**, **c**: arrows). A coronal T2-weighted TSE image is compatible with hemorrhage within the mammillary bodies (**a**: inlay: arrows), and SWI was not performed

## 3.6 Carbon Monoxide Poisoning

Pathogenesis: Carbon monoxide is a colorless and odorless gas with a stronger affinity to the heme molecule than $O_2$.

Clinical presentation: Unresponsive patients with a "healthy" face color. CO is a major cause of suicidal deaths and accidental poisoning in Europe and North America.MRI: Usually bilateral and symmetric necrosis of the globi pallidi. Caudate, putamina, and cerebral white matter may also be affected. Patients with a good outcome have normal MRI or minimal involvement in the form of signal abnormalities in the globus pallidus. Patients with a poor outcome generally show more widespread involvement (Sharma et al. 2009) (Figs. 8 and 9).

## 3.7 SMART (Stroke-like Migraine Attacks after Radiation Therapy) Syndrome

Definition: Uncommon late complication (typically after many years) of cranial irradiation without evidence of residual or recurrent tumor (Kerklaan et al. 2011).

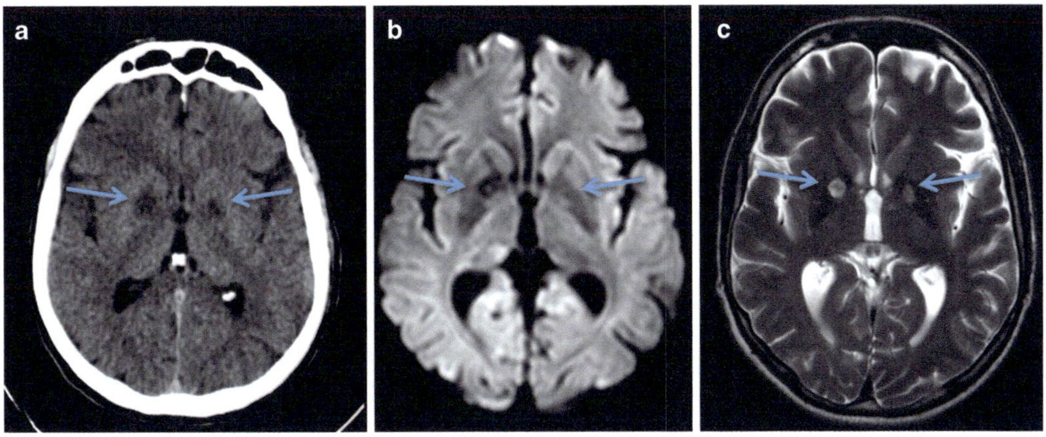


**Fig. 8** Carbon monoxide poisoning in a 53-year-old man attempting suicide. CT (**a**) and MRI (**b**: DWI, C: T2-w TSE) show selective involvement of the globi pallidi with the right side more severely injured (**a**–**c**: arrows)

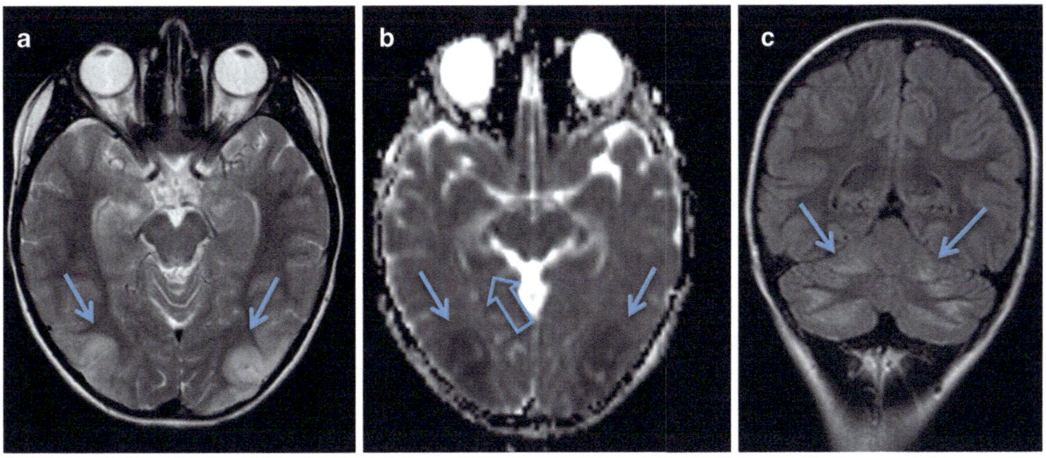


**Fig. 9** 15-year-old girl with flue gas poisoning from an apartment fire. MRI shows cytotoxic edema of the cerebellum (**c**: arrows), temporo-occipital cortex (**a**, **b**: arrows), and hippocampus on both sides. Basal ganglia including the globi pallidi are spared. This pattern likely results from the mixture of different gases (carbon dioxide, sulfur dioxide, carbon monoxide, cyanide, and others)

Pathogenesis: Post-radiation neuronal dysfunction with impairment of the trigeminovascular system or a lowered threshold for cortical spreading depression.

Clinical manifestations: The most striking clinical manifestations are migraine-like headaches (with or without aura) and focal seizures. Patients may also present with visuospatial deficits, aphasia, hemiparesis, confusion, and numbness (Black et al. 2006; Bradshaw et al. 2011).

MRI: Cytotoxic edema, contrast enhancement, and relative cerebral blood volume (rCBV) elevation of the (posterior parietal) cortex not confined to a vascular territory. Characteristic episodic nature of the deficits with spontaneous resolution over weeks (Fig. 10).

## 3.8 Subacute Combined Degeneration

Definition: Selective degeneration of the dorsal and sometimes the lateral spinal cord columns due to vitamin B12 deficiency, copper deficiency, zinc overload, genetically serum transcobalamin

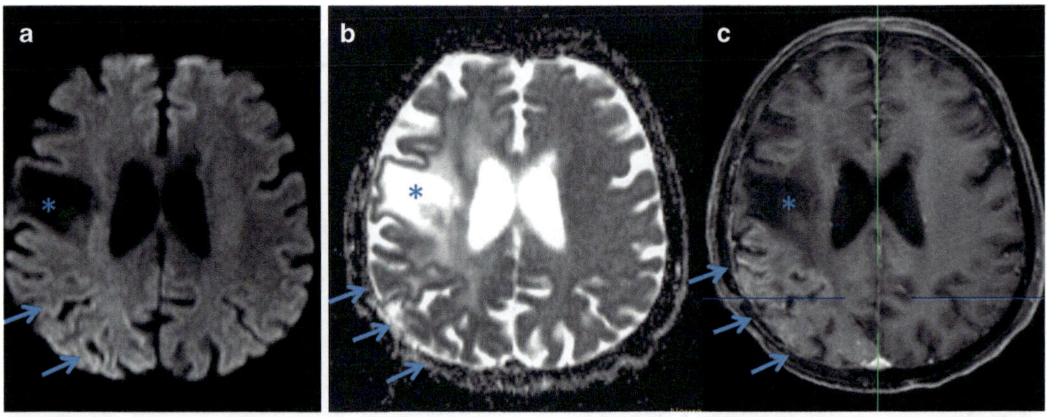


**Fig. 10** A 65-year-old woman who had radiation therapy following surgery of an oligodendroglioma 25 years ago (**a–c**: *) presented with headache, neglect, and left-sided epileptic seizures. MRI shows DWI restriction (**a**, **b**) and blood–brain barrier disruption (**c**) of the right-sided parietal cortex not confined to a vascular territory. Both disappeared on follow-up MRI 4 weeks later (not shown). Clinical complaints and temporal evolution fulfill criteria of a SMART syndrome

II deficiency, nitrous oxide ($N_2O$) abuse, and others.

Clinical presentation: The classic patient is an older woman who suffers from mild sensory ataxia with loss of vibration sense and spasticity, hyperreflexia, and positive Babinski sign. She has megaloblastic anemia and inadequate vitamin B12 intake from upper gastrointestinal surgery or immune-mediated with decreased availability of the intrinsic factor.

MRI: Longitudinal dorsal cord T2 signal increases with an "inverted V" on axial images (Fig. 11). The lateral spinal cord columns are less commonly affected (Fig. 11). There may be slight cord swelling and dorsal column enhancement. Low serum vitamin B12 level is also associated with (periventricular) white matter lesions (de Lau et al. 2009).

## 3.9 Cerebral Fat Embolism

Pathogenesis: Rare complication after long bone fractures (incidence 0.9–2.2%) or (cemented) hip arthroplasty (Parizel et al. 2001).

Clinical manifestations: Patients typically present with a triad of hypoxemia, neurological dysfunction, and petechial rash, commonly 12–72 h after trauma.

MRI: In the acute stage (1–4 days), released fat from bone marrow accumulates in the lungs; small vacuoles (diameter <5 μm) pass the capillaries and produce multiple cerebral emboli with a "starfield" pattern on DWI (Byrick et al. 1994). In the subacute stage (5–14 days), fat vacuoles are converted to free fatty acids that trigger a toxic reaction. A confluent cytotoxic edema in the periventricular and subcortical white matter may be followed by a vasogenic edema (Kuo et al. 2014). The late stage (>14 days) is characterized by atrophy and demyelination. Multiple petechial hemorrhages occur in all stages of the disease (Fig. 12).

## 3.10 Mild Encephalopathy with Reversible Splenium Lesion (MERS)

Definition: Rare but pathognomonic imaging finding likely caused by rapid reduction in antiepileptic drugs (AEDs). A common situation is AED withdrawal during presurgical work-up in order to provoke seizures. However, reversible splenium lesions are also found in patients with infections, chemotherapy, or other diseases affecting fluid balance systems.

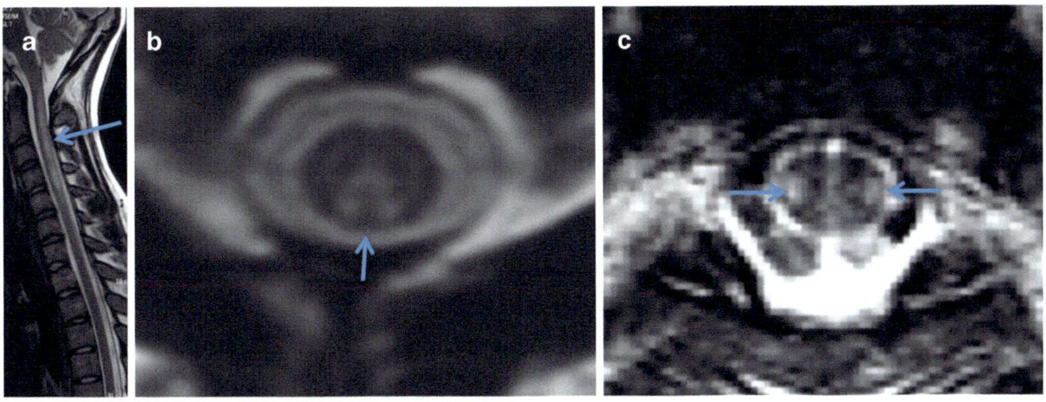


**Fig. 11** Sagittal (**a**) and axial (**b**) T2-weighted TSE images in a 40-year-old woman with loss of vibration sense, spasticity, and hyperreflexia. The T2 hyperintense lesion involves the posterior columns of the cervical spinal cord and has on axial images the shape of an inverted V (**b**: arrow). In another patient, the T2-weighted signal also involves the lateral columns including the lateral corticospinal tracts (**c**: arrows)

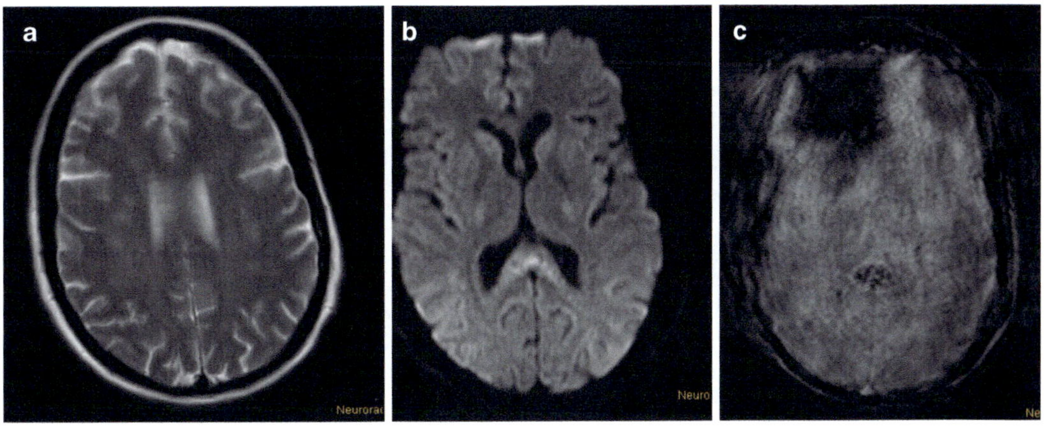


**Fig. 12** A 30-year-old initially awake polytrauma patient developed progressive vigilance loss after 3 days. MRI after 7 days show patchy and confluent T2 hyperintense signal changes within the centrum semiovale (**a**: arrows) and distinct DWI changes (**b**) and microbleeds (**c**) in the corpus callosum splenium

Clinical presentation: None related to the splenium lesion.

MRI: Non-space-occupying symmetric lesion in the center of the splenium with reduced diffusion. No contrast enhancement (MERS type 1). Complete or near-complete regression on follow-up MRI within 1–2 weeks (Nelles et al. 2006; Yuan et al. 2017). Additional structures such as the subcortical white matter or the anterior corpus callosum may also show symmetric lesions with restricted diffusion (MERS type 2) (Yuan et al. 2017) (Fig. 13).

## 3.11 Heroin

Pathogenesis: The highly lipophilic heroin easily penetrates the CNS and is converted into active morphine derivatives. Heroin is typically injected i.v., but in a heated form it may also be inhaled ("chasing the dragon"). Injected heroin leads to a central respiratory depression and hypoxic-ischemic leukoencephalopathy, while "chasing the dragon" is more toxic causing a spongiform leukoencephalopathy with intracytoplasmic vacuoles in the myelin sheaths and subsequent neuronal and glial degeneration. However, leukoencephalopa-

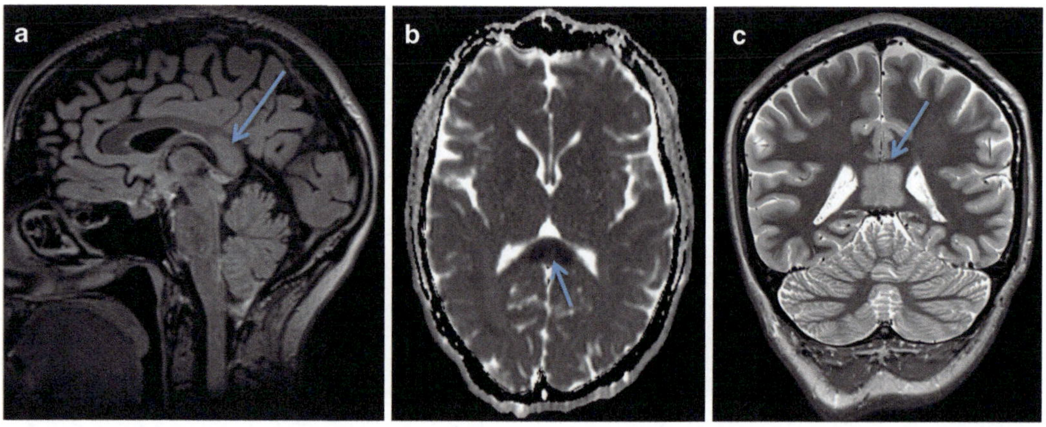


**Fig. 13** MERS type 1 in a 36-year-old presurgical epilepsy patient. The FLAIR (**a**: arrow)/T2 (**c**: arrow) hyperintense splenium lesion has a typical location and configuration and shows a distinct DWI reduction (**b**: arrow). It was incidentally detected and most likely due to the rapid withdrawal of antiepileptic drugs in order to provoke seizures for video EEG monitoring. The rapid withdrawal (most commonly of carbamazepine) causes fluid balance alterations. The lesion had disappeared on a MRI 4 months later (not shown)

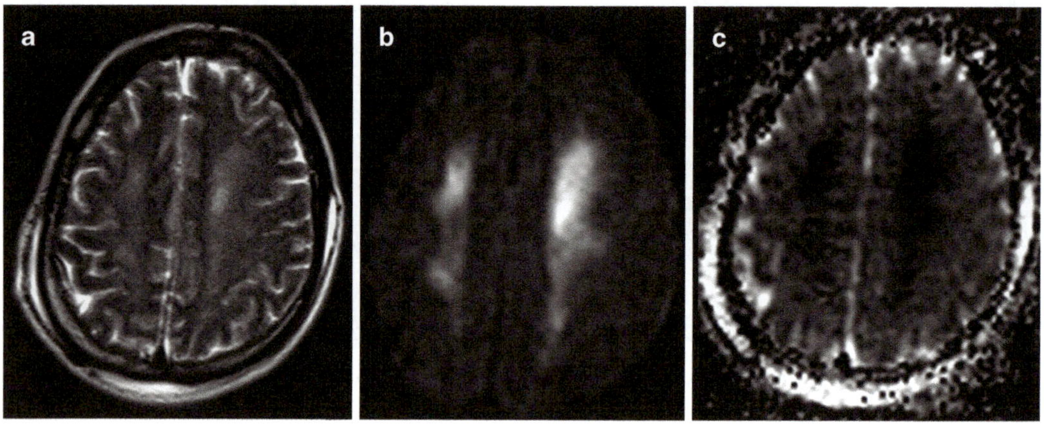


**Fig. 14** Spongiform encephalopathy with cytotoxic oedema of the supratentorial white matter (**a**: T2-weighted fast spin echo, **b**: DWI, **c**: ADC images) in a 28-year-old heroin abuser. As the cerebellum was not affected and heroin was not inhaled, the admixture of an adulterant such as levamisole possibly caused the leukoencephalopathy

thy cases without cerebellar involvement have been described and linked to the admixture of adulterants (Blasel et al. 2010) (Fig. 14).

Clinical manifestations: 3 clinical stages of "chasing the dragon" leukoencephalopathy. Stage 1 presents mostly cerebellar symptoms; stage 2 includes cerebellar and extrapyramidal symptoms, and stage 3 progresses to stretching spasms, akinetic, or hypotonic mutism (Bartlett and Mikulis 2005). High (23%) mortality rate.

MRI: Symmetric T2/FLAIR hyperintensity of the predominantly periventricular cerebral and cerebellar white matter sparing the dentate nuclei. Involvement of the posterior limb of the internal capsule and of the solitary tracts (Tamrazi and Almast 2012). The key to differentiate this type of leukoencephalopathy from other mimics is involvement of the cerebellum in a clinically non-hypertensive patient (Bartlett and Mikulis 2005). DWI shows restricted diffusion in the acute phase and elevated diffusion later on (Blasel et al. 2010).

## 3.12 Cocaine Encephalopathy

Pathogenesis: The short-lasting neurotoxic drug blocks the uptake of catecholamines and dopamine. It thus induces a severe vasoconstriction, for adulterants such as levamisole; also, white matter toxicity is discussed (Vosoughi and Schmidt 2015). In its most commonly used form, the highly lipid-soluble cocaine hydrochloride is ingested via mucosal membranes (sniffing, oral uptake). Crack, the alkaloidal form of cocaine hydrochloride, can also be smoked (Brown et al. 1992).

Clinical presentation: Cocaine leads to a short intense euphoria with feelings of elation, increased energy, and alertness. Complications are typically vascular with hemorrhages twice as common as ischemic strokes. However, for reasons that are not clearly understood, the alkaloidal form of the drug is associated with an equal frequency of ischemic and hemorrhagic events (Tamrazi and Almast 2012). Cocaine-induced cerebral hemorrhage includes both intraparenchymal and subarachnoid hemorrhage. Most cases of subarachnoid hemorrhage are secondary to aneurysm rupture, and approximately 40–50% of patients have underlying disease including aneurysms and arteriovenous malformations (Geibprasert et al. 2010). The causes for ischemic stroke include cocaine-induced vasoconstriction, vasculitis (due to unknown adulterants/impurities), vasospasm, and/or direct effects of cocaine on hemostasis. For example, cocaine enhances the responses of platelets to arachidonic acid, resulting in increased levels of thromboxane and increased platelet aggregation (Geibprasert et al. 2010).

MRI: Nasal septum necrosis, ischemic, and hemorrhagic complications, often involving the globi pallidi, white matter lesions, and less commonly confluent T2/FLAIR hyperintensities may be related to cocaine abuse. Infarctions often involve the subcortical white matter within the MCA territory (Fig. 15); however, they can be present anywhere in the brain (Geibprasert et al. 2010). The confluent T2/FLAIR hyperintensities in cocaine leukoencephalopathy spare the U fibers, have no restricted diffusion and no gadolinium enhancement (Vosoughi and Schmidt 2015), and resemble those of heroin-associated “chasing the dragon” leukoencephalopathy with the notable exception that the occipital predominance and cerebellar and brainstem involvement typical of heroin leukoencephalopathy are not seen (Bartlett and Mikulis 2005; Vosoughi and Schmidt 2015). Around 5–10% of cocaine abusers show ischemic, partially hemorrhagic lesions of the globi pallidi similar to those in CO poisoning or methamphetamine abuse (Alquist et al. 2012). These lesions often show a ring enhancement and are related to dopamine D3 receptor alterations (Kadi et al. 2014) (Fig. 16).

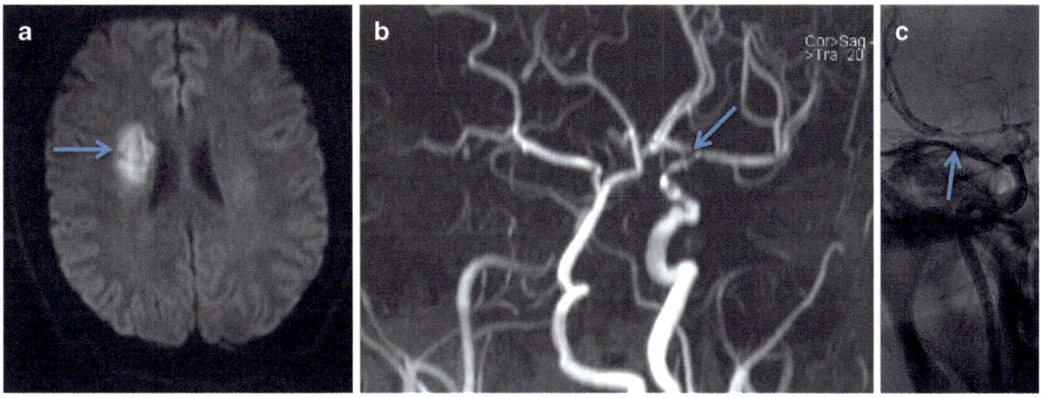


**Fig. 15** A 34-year-old man with cocaine abuse presented with progressive right hemispheric stroke. DWI showed a white matter infarct (**a**: arrow), and 3D-TOF-MRA right-sided carotid T occlusion and left-sided carotid T stenosis (**b**: arrow). Stent-retriever thrombectomy failed to re-open the right-sided occlusion (**c**: arrow)

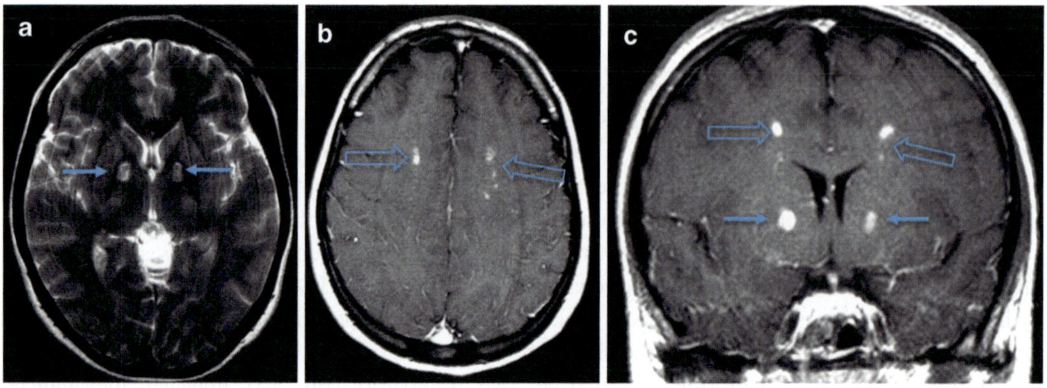


**Fig. 16** Cocaine-related ischemic lesions of the globi pallidi with some central hypointensity suggestive of hemorrhage (**a**: arrows). Note also the enhancement of the globi pallidi (**c**: arrows) and of lesions within the white matter (**b**, **c**: hollow arrows)

## 3.13 Synthetic Drugs

Definition: Synthetic drugs contain substances that are pharmacologically similar to those found in traditional illicit drugs (Creagh et al. 2018). The most well-known substances are synthetic marijuana (Spice K2), 3,4 methylenedioxymethamphetamine (MDMA, Ecstasy, Molly), N-methylamphetamine (Meth, Ice, Glass), and methadone (Saliva, Waver, Amidone).

Pathogenesis: Many of these substances share the same chemical properties and physiologic responses with the drugs they mimic but last longer and exaggerate the pathologic response in the brain. The methylamphetamine Ecstasy is primarily administered orally, and Meth is swallowed, smoked, snorted, or injected. These substances have similar effects as other amphetamines increasing the activity of dopamine, norepinephrine, and serotonin (Creagh et al. 2018). Methadone, which is usually swallowed or injected and used to manage pain and opioid addiction, is a synthetic narcotic with similar effects yet different chemical properties as morphine or heroin (Creagh et al. 2018).

Clinical presentation: Methamphetamine-associated hemorrhage is twice as common as ischemic stroke and particularly often in persons between 18 and 44 years. Both stroke types are more common in men than women, which may reflect the 3:1 ratio of use patterns in the general population and/or other risk factors for stroke in this age population. The route of administration differs notably: Ischemic stroke has a higher preponderance of inhalational use (ischemic stroke: oral: injection: inhalation ratio 1:1:4; hemorrhages: oral: injection: inhalation ratio 3:3:1) (Lappin et al. 2017).

Apart from stroke is headache, a predominant early presenting feature, together with hypertension vomiting, and seizures often developing over time (Lappin et al. 2017).

MRI: Amphetamines cause a long-lasting vasoconstriction and in long-term use have been found to decrease cortical gray matter volume and increase striatal volume. As in cocaine, ischemic complications show a spatial preponderance for the globus pallidus and occipital cortex, which is explained with the high serotonin receptor density in these areas (Reneman et al. 2001; Tamrazi and Almast 2012).

Methadone causes similar findings as heroin-associated “chasing the dragon” leukoencephalopathy with prominent involvement of the cerebellum. One plausible explanation is the high affinity of synthetic opioids for the mu-opioid receptors, which are more concentrated in the cerebellum and limbic system (Lucia et al. 1996; Xu et al. 2009; Salgado et al. 2010; Odia et al. 2010) (Fig. 17).

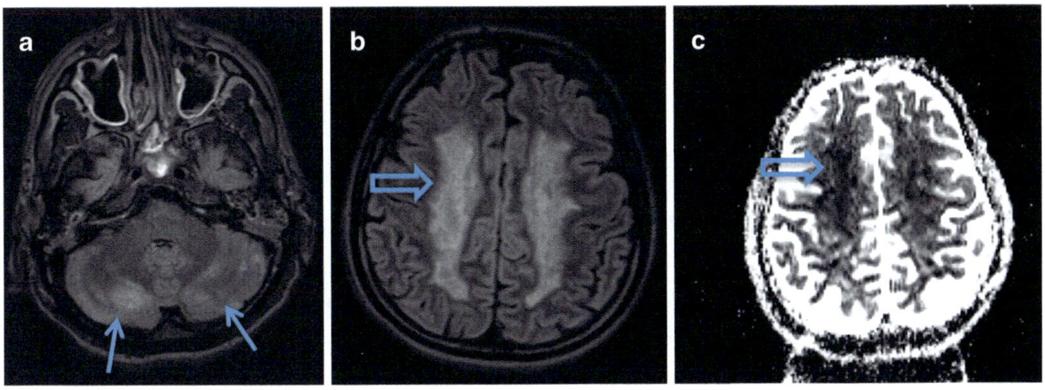


**Fig. 17** Cocaine and/or methadone leukoencephalopathy in a 40-year-old man admitted with somnolence progressing to coma. Cerebellar involvement (**a**: arrows) is in favor of opiate-related and/or levamisole leukoencephalopathy (resembling heroin-associated "chasing the dragon" leukoencephalopathy) and against cocaine leukoencephalopathy. The supratentorial white matter shows cytotoxic edema (**b**: FLAIR, **c**: ADC map: hollow arrow)

## 3.14 Posterior Reversible Encephalopathy Syndrome (PRES)

Definition: Clinico-neuroradiological syndrome characterized by insidious onset of headache, altered mental status, seizures, and others associated with posterior "leuko"encephalopathy on MRI.

Pathogenesis: Extremely elevated arterial blood pressure results in cerebral blood vessels autoregulatory failure and endothelial dysfunction with increased capillary permeability and vasogenic edema. Other common causes are cytotoxic agents causing direct endothelial toxicity (Hinchey et al. 1996) (Fig. 18) and thrombotic microangiopathies, often related to kidney diseases such as thrombocytic thrombocytopenic purpura (TTP)/hemolytic uremic syndrome (HUS).

Clinical presentation: The prototypic patient is the pregnant woman after 20 weeks of gestation with eclampsia. Chemotherapeutic agents such as cyclosporine or subacute extensive hypertension may also elicit PRES. MRI: Typical PRES: Nearly symmetrical, patchy to confluent, cortical, and subcortical vasogenic edema affecting the parieto-occipital regions, often in a watershed distribution.

Atypical PRES: Frontal lobe, basal ganglia, brain stem, and cerebellar involvement.

## 3.15 Thrombotic Thrombocytopenic Purpura (TTP)/Hemolytic Uremic Syndrome (HUS)

Definition: Triad of thrombocytopenia, hemolytic anemia, and acute renal failure. Pathogenesis: E. coli (0157:H7)-associated autoimmune disease-causing endothelial injury and microthrombi involving the kidneys and brain as well as bowel hemorrhage.

Clinical presentation: Seizures, variable neurological deficits, fever, lethargy, bloody diarrhea, low urine output, and others.

MRI: Multifocal peripheral hemorrhagic infarcts, PRES-like pattern.

## 3.16 Reversible Cerebral Vasoconstriction Syndrome (RCVS)

Definition and Pathogenesis: Transient disturbance of the cerebral vascular tone leading to potentially reversible vasoconstriction.

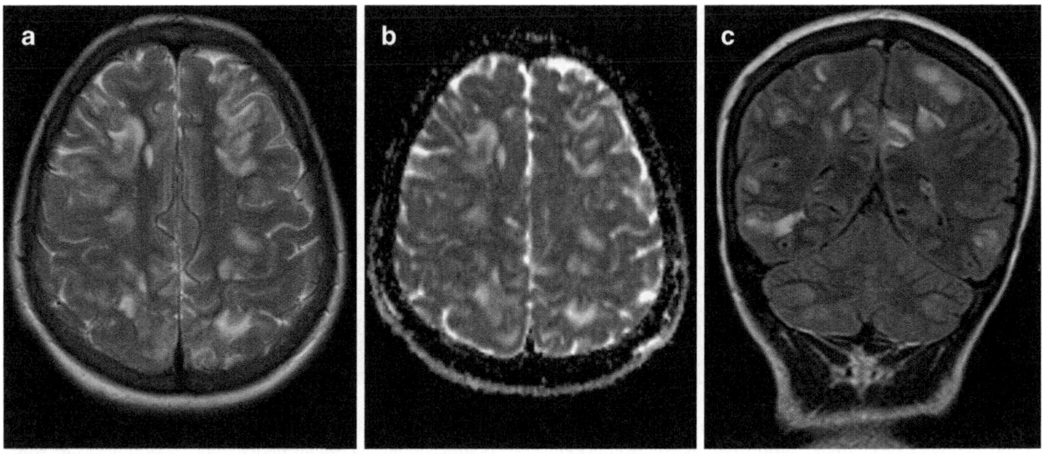


**Fig. 18** A 19-year-old woman presented with a seizure following autologous bone marrow transplantation 10 days ago. She had thrombocytopenia and leukopenia and uncontrolled hypertension. MRI shows typical PRES with symmetric vasogenic edema of the cortex and subcortical white matter (**a**, T2, **b**: ADC map, **c**: FLAIR) in vascular watershed zones. In typical PRES, the parieto-occipital regions, frontal lobes, temporal lobes, and cerebellum are affected with decreasing order

Recreational vasoactive drugs and post-partum period are typical triggers.

Clinical manifestations: Unusual, recent, severe headaches of progressive or sudden onset with or without focal neurological deficit and/or seizures (Ducros et al. 2010). 7% of acute headache patients, m:f = 1:2, hemorrhagic (convexity SAH 2/3, ICH 1/3) and ischemic complications in 7–54%, with hemorrhagic complications occurring in the first week and ischemic complications later. Up to 10% permanent disability can be associated with PRES (Miller et al. 2015a).

MRI: Cerebral vasoconstriction with at least 2 narrowings per artery on 2 different arteries (MRA, CTA, transfemoral angiography (most sensitive). Disappearance of arterial abnormalities on control angiogram in 3 months. The affected vessels show no wall enhancement on black-blood MRI (Mandell et al. 2012). Note: Cerebral vasoconstriction may not be visualized in up to one-third of patients with RCVS during the first week following symptom onset. It typically shows a centripetal pattern with the distal intracerebral arteries affected earlier than the proximal arteries. Ischemic infarcts often have a watershed territory pattern (Miller et al. 2015b) (Fig. 19).

## 3.17 Mitochondrial Disorders

Definition and Pathogenesis: Mitochondrial disorders are a group of disorders caused by dysfunctional mitochondria. They often affect the CNS due to its high energy needs. Clinical presentation: Most mitochondrial disorders occur in childhood and produce a wide range of symptoms including encephalopathy syndromes, strokes, epileptic seizures, neuropathy, dysarthria, ophthalmoparesis, and others (Finsterer and Zarrouk Mahjoub 2012).

MRI: The prototypic mitochondrial disorder is MELAS (mitochondrial encephalopathy with lactate acidosis and stroke-like episodes) characterized by multiple cortical and subcortical lesions not confined to a vascular territory. Typically, only the cortex shows DWI hyperintensity. Another common MELAS pattern is basal ganglia, pulvinar thalami, and dentate nuclei calcifications resembling those in Fahr's disease (Tschampa et al. 2013) (Fig. 20).

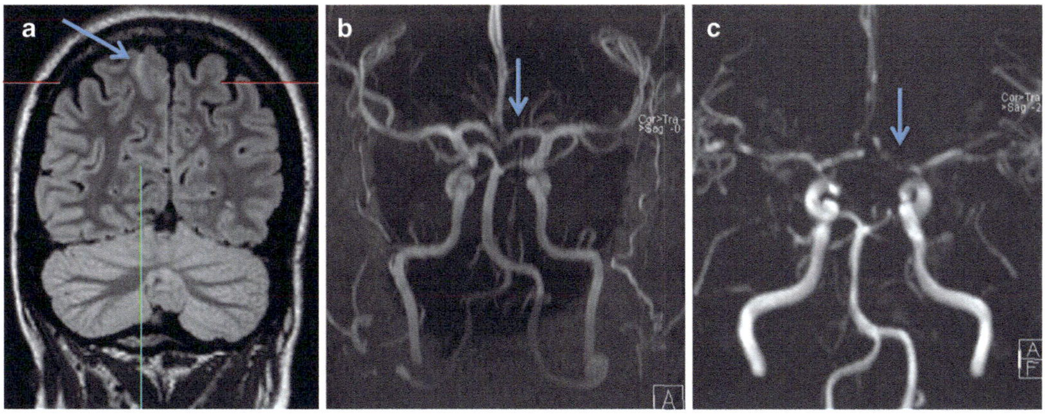


**Fig. 19** Reversible cerebral vasoconstriction syndrome (RCVS) in a 35-year-old woman who presented with repetitive right occipital headache attacks since 4 days. Coronal FLAIR MRI (**a**) shows right parietal sulcal subarachnoid effusion (**a**: arrow). Initial TOF-MRA (**b**) showed a discrete narrowing of the distal A1 segments (**a**: arrow), follow-up TOF-MRA 5 days later significant narrowing of both terminal ICA segments, of the left A1 (**c**: arrow), of both proximal A2 segmentation and the right MCA bifurcation

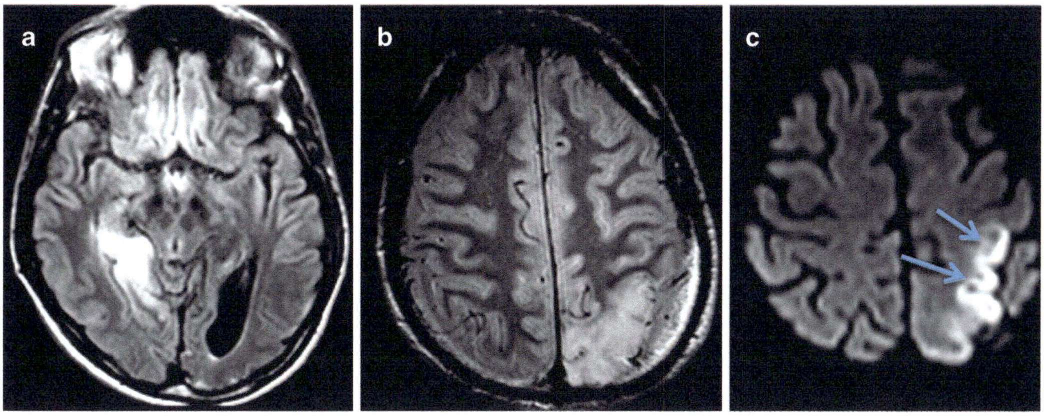


**Fig. 20** MELAS in a 42-year-old man with multiple stroke-like episodes and epileptic seizures. MRI shows an older right occipital infarct (**a**) and a subacute left parietal infarct (**b**, **c**). The left parietal infarct is not confined to a vascular territory, and the DWI hyperintensity only involves the cortex (**c**: arrows)

## References


Almond CS, Shin AY, Fortescue EB, Mannix RC, Wypij D, Binstadt BA, Duncan CN, Olson DP, Salerno AE, Newburger JW, Greenes DS (2005) Hyponatremia among runners in the Boston Marathon. N Engl J Med 352:15

Alquist CR, McGoey R, Bastian F, Newman W (2012) Bilateral globus pallidus lesions. J La State Med Soc 164:145–146

Bartlett E, Mikulis DJ (2005) Chasing "chasing the dragon" with MRI: leukoencephalopathy in drug abuse. Br J Radiol 78:997–1004

Black DF, Bartleson JD, Bell ML et al (2006) SMART: stroke-like migraine attacks after radiation therapy. Cephalalgia 26:1137–1142

Blasel S, Hattingen E, Adelmann M, Nichtweiß M, Zanella F, Weidauer S (2010) Toxic leukoencephalopathy after heroin abuse without heroin vapor inhalation. MR imaging and clinical features in three patients. Clin Neuroradiol 20(1):48–53

Bradshaw J, Chen L, Saling M et al (2011) Neurocognitive recovery in SMART syndrome: a case report. Cephalalgia 31:372–376

Brown E, Prager J, Lee HY, Ramsay RG (1992) CNS complications of cocaine abuse: prevalence, pathophysiology, and neuroradiology. AJR Am J Roentgenol 159:137–147

Burkhard PR, Delavelle J, Du Pasquier R, Spahr L (2003) Chronic parkinsonism associated with cirrhosis: a distinct subset of acquired hepatocerebral degeneration. Arch Neurol 60:521

Byrick RJ, Mullen JB, Mazer CD, Guest CB (1994) Transpulmonary systemic fat embolism. Studies in mongrel dogs after cemented arthroplasty. Am J Respir Crit Care Med 150:1416–1422

Chu K, Kang DW, Kim DE et al (2002) Diffusion-weighted and gradient echo magnetic resonance findings of hemichorea-hemiballismus associated with diabetic hyperglycemia: a hyperviscosity syndrome? Arch Neurol 59:448–452

Creagh S, Warden D, Latif MA, Paydar A (2018) The new classes of synthetic illicit drugs can significantly harm the brain: a neuro imaging perspective with full review of MRI findings. Clin Radiol Imaging J 2:000116

de Lau LM, Smith AD, Refsum H, Johnston C, Breteler MM (2009) Plasma vitamin B12 status and cerebral white-matter lesions. J Neurol Neurosurg Psychiatry 80:149–157

Ducros A, Fiedler U, Porcher R, Boukobza M, Stapf C, Bousser MG (2010) Hemorrhagic manifestations of reversible cerebral vasoconstriction syndrome: frequency, features, and risk factors. Stroke 41:2505–2511

Ferenci P, Lockwood A, Mullen K, Tarter R, Weissenborn K, Blei AT (2002) Hepatic encephalopathy: definition, nomenclature, diagnosis, and quantification—final report of the working party at the 11th world congresses of gastroenterology, Vienna, 1998. Hepatology 35:716–721

Finsterer J, Zarrouk Mahjoub S (2012) Epilepsy in mitochondrial disorders. Seizure 21:316–321

Geibprasert S, Gallucci M, Krings T (2010) Addictive illegal drugs: structural neuroimaging. AJNR Am J Neuroradiol 31(5):803–808

Hattingen E, Beyle A, Müller A, Klockgether T, Kornblum C (2016) Wernicke encephalopathy. SWI detects petechial hemorrhages in mammillary bodies in vivo. Neurology 87:1956–1957

Hinchey J, Chaves C, Appignani B, Breen J, Pao L, Wang A, Pessin MS, Lamy C, Mas JL, Caplan LR (1996) A reversible posterior leukoencephalopathy syndrome. N Engl J Med 334:494–500

Johkura K, Nakae Y, Kudo Y, Yoshida TN, Kuroiwa Y (2012) Early diffusion MR imaging findings and short-term outcome in comatose patients with hypoglycemia. AJNR Am J Neuroradiol 33:904–909

Kadi R, Rumy A, Statnik T, Cannie M, Mabiglia C, Divano L (2014) Bilateral lesions of the globus pallidus in a young woman. JBR-BTR 97: 118–120

Kerklaan JP, Nijeholt G, Wiggenraad RGJ, Berghuis B, Postma TJ, Taphoorn MJ (2011) SMART syndrome: a late reversible complication after radiation therapy for brain tumours. J Neurol 258:1098–1104

Kuo KH, Pan YJ, Lai YJ, Cheung WK, Chang FC, Jarosz J (2014) Dynamic MR imaging patterns of cerebral fat embolism: a systematic review with illustrative cases. Am J Neuroradiol 35:1052–1057

Lappin JM, Darke S, Farrell M (2017) Stroke and methamphetamine use in young adults: a review. J Neurol Neurosurg Psychiatry 88:1079–1091

Lo L, Tan AC, Umapathi T, Lim CC (2006) Diffusion-weighted MR imaging in early diagnosis and prognosis of hypoglycemia. AJNR Am J Neuroradiol 27:1222–1224

Lucia P, Pocek M, Passacantando A, Sebastiani ML, De Martinis C (1996) Multifocal leucoencephalopathy induced by levamisole. Lancet 348:1450

Mandell DM, Matouk CC, Farb RI, Krings T, Agid R, terBrugge K, Willinsky RA, Swartz RH, Silver FL, Mikulis DJ (2012) Vessel wall MRI to differentiate between reversible cerebral vasoconstriction syndrome and central nervous system vasculitis: preliminary results. Stroke 43:860–862

McGowan-Smyth S, Vasdev N, Gowrie-Mohan S (2016) Spinal anesthesia facilitates the early recognition of TUR syndrome. Curr Urol 9:57–61

Miller TR, Shivashankar R, Mossa-Basha M, Gandhi D (2015a) Reversible cerebral vasoconstriction syndrome, part 1: epidemiology, pathogenesis, and clinical course. AJNR Am J Neuroradiol 36:1392–1399

Miller TR, Shivashankar R, Mossa-Basha M, Gandhi D (2015b) Reversible cerebral vasoconstriction syndrome, part 2: diagnostic work-up, imaging evaluation, and differential diagnosis. AJNR Am J Neuroradiol 36:1580–1588

Nelles M, Bien CG, Kurthen M, von Falkenhausen M, Urbach H (2006) Transient splenium lesions in presurgical epilepsy patients: incidence and pathogenesis. Neuroradiology 48:443–448

Noakes TD, Goodwin N, Rayner BL, Branken T, Taylor RK (1985) Water intoxication: a possible complication during endurance exercise. Med Sci Sports Exerc 17:370–375

Odia M, Jinka M, Ziai WC (2010) Severe leukoencephalopathy following acute oxycodone intoxication. Neurocrit Care 13:93–97

Parizel PM, Demey HE, Veeckmans G, Verstreken F, Cras P, Jorens PG, De Schepper AM (2001) Early diagnosis of cerebral fat embolism syndrome by diffusion-weighted MRI (starfield pattern). Stroke 32:2942–2944

Pipe JG (1999) Motion correction with PROPELLER MRI: application to head motion and free-breathing cardiac imaging. Magn Reson Med 42:963–969

Raghavendra S, Ashalatha R, Sanjee V et al (2007) Focal neuronal loss, reversible subcortical focal T2 hypointensity in seizures with a nonketotic hyperglycemic hyperosmolar state. Neuroradiology 49:299–305

Reneman L, Majoie C, Habraken J, Gerard JG (2001) Effects of ecstasy (MDMA) on the brain in abstinent users: initial observations with diffusion and perfusion MR imaging. Radiology 220:611–617

Rovira A, Alonso J, Cordoba J (2008) MR imaging findings in hepatic encephalopathy. AJNR Am J Neuroradiol 29:1612–1621

Salgado RA, Jorens PG, Baar I, Cras P, Hans G, Parizel PM (2010) Methadone-induced toxic leukoencephalopathy: MR imaging and MR proton spectroscopy findings. AJNR Am J Neuroradiol 31:565–566

Sharma P, Eesa M, Scott JN (2009) Toxic and acquired metabolic encephalopathies: MRI appearance. Am J Roentgenol 193:879–886

Sutter R, Kaplan PW (2015) What to see when you are looking at confusion: a review of the neuroimaging of acute encephalopathy. J Neurol Neurosurg Psychiatry 86:446–59T3

Tamrazi B, Almast J (2012) Your brain on drugs: imaging of drug-related changes in the central nervous system. Radiographics 32:701

Tschampa HJ, Urbach H, Greschus S, Kuns WS, Kornblum C (2013) Neuroimaging characteristics in mitochondrial encephalopathies associated with the m.3243A>G MTTL1 mutation. J Neurol 260:1071–1080

Valk J, van der Knaap MS (1992) Toxic encephalopathy. AJNR Am J Neuroradiol 13:747–760

Vosoughi R, Schmidt BJ (2015) Multifocal leukoencephalopathy in cocaine users: a report of two cases and review of the literature. BMC Neurol 15:208

Xu N, Zhou W, Li S, Zhou G, Zhang N, Liang J (2009) Clinical and MRI characteristics of levamisole-induced leukoencephalopathy in 16 patients. J Neuroimaging 19:326–331

Yuan J, Yang S, Wang S, Qin W, Yang L, Hu W (2017) Mild encephalitis/encephalopathy with reversible splenial lesion (MERS) in adults-a case report and literature review. BMC Neurol 17:103

Zuccoli G, Santa Cruz D, Bertolini M, Rovira A, Gallucci M, Carollo C, Pipitone N (2009) MR imaging findings in 56 patients with Wernicke encephalopathy: nonalcoholics may differ from alcoholics. AJNR Am J Neuroradiol 30:171–176

# Herniation Syndromes

Merve Gürsoy and Cem Çalli

## Contents



## 1 Herniation Syndromes

The term "cerebral herniation" refers to a shift of a part of the brain from its normal anatomical location into an adjacent area. Cerebral herniation can stem from any infectious, ischemic, neoplastic, or traumatic cause that creates a mass effect in the brain. Extra-axial lesions (subdural hemorrhage, epidural hemorrhage, extra-axial brain tumor), focal brain lesions (primary/metastatic brain tumor, ischemic stroke, brain abscess, primary intracerebral hemorrhage), or diffuse brain lesions (traumatic brain injury, meningitis, encephalitis, subarachnoid hemorrhage) that cause increased intracranial pressure can be responsible for herniation syndromes (Stevens et al. 2015). Cerebral herniation should be rapidly diagnosed since it is among the neuroradiological emergencies that can result in death.

The cranium is a closed system that encompasses a constant total volume of the brain, cerebrospinal fluid (CSF), and blood. A volume increase in one of these is balanced with a volume reduction in others. This is called the Monro-Kellie doctrine (Mokri 2001). The brain has the

M. Gürsoy
Faculty of Medicine, Department of Radiology, Izmir Katip Celebi University, Izmir, Turkey

C. Çalli (✉)
Department of Radiology, Ege University Medical School, Izmir, Turkey



M. Scaglione et al. (eds.), *Emergency Radiology of the Head and Spine*,
Medical Radiology Diagnostic Imaging, https://doi.org/10.1007/978-3-030-91047-1_9

highest volume in the cranium, followed by CSF and blood, respectively. Since the volume of the brain cannot be changed, an increase in intracranial volume is balanced by a compensatory reduction in the volume of CSF or blood. However, if intracranial volume continues to increase and a reduction in blood or CSF volume is no longer possible, brain tissue becomes herniated.

There are various types of herniation and the clinical picture varies according to the type of herniation. The anatomical structure that is compressed as a result of herniation is responsible for the observed clinical signs. Pressure on the brain (corpus callosum, cingulate gyrus, midbrain, cerebral peduncles, inferior cerebellum, etc.), cranial nerves (oculomotor nerve), vascular structures (anterior and posterior cerebral artery, pericallosal artery, anterior choroidal arteries), or CSF drainage leads to signs associated with the compressed anatomical structure as well as hydrocephalus and ischemia/infarction in the watershed areas of the compressed arteries.

Brain herniations are mainly divided into two categories, i.e., intracranial and extracranial herniations. Moreover, intracranial herniations are classified as subfalcine, transtentorial, tonsillar, and transsphenoidal (transalar) herniations. Transtentorial herniations are also divided into two as ascending and descending transtentorial herniations. Descending herniations are classified as lateral and central, wherein lateral herniations are also divided into anterior (uncal) and posterior (parahippocampal) herniations (Nadgir and Yousem 2017; Riveros Gilardi et al. 2019) (Fig. 1). The classification of brain herniations is provided in Fig 2.

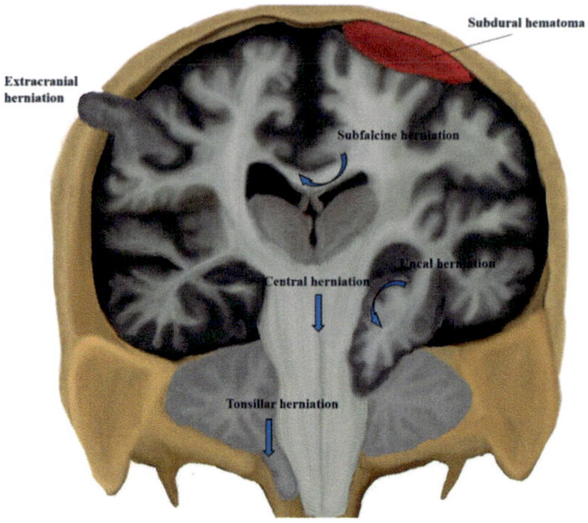


**Fig. 1** Coronal diagram demonstrates the different types of cerebral herniation

## 2 Neuroimaging of Herniation Syndromes

Since brain herniation syndromes are life-threatening emergencies, the priority should be to ensure airway patency, circulation, and ventilation in the patient. This is followed by noncontrast computed tomography (CT), i.e., the first imaging modality of choice in most of the neurologic emergencies. CT is especially preferred since it is available at many centers and it rapidly provides results. Both CT and magnetic resonance imaging (MRI) show the presence and type of herniation and the extent of herniated brain tissue with high sensitivity. However, MRI has a higher soft tissue resolution and shows anatomical details more precisely. MRI is superior in detecting small herniations and particularly herniations through the orbit, sella, and middle ear cavity in postoperative patients (Kaseff et al. 1992). MRI is superior to CT especially in determining whether the soft tissue density observed within the operation cavity on CT stems from herniated brain tissue or other pathologies in postoperative patients (Mosnier et al. 2000).

## 3 Anatomy

Herniation syndromes are classified based on the anatomical structure through which the brain tissue is herniated. The resulting clinical signs are closely associated with the compressed anatomical structure. Therefore, it is important to know the anatomical structures that are associated with herniation syndromes.

The cranial cavity is divided into several compartments by certain bony structures and dural reflections (Fig. 3). Dural reflections are formed by the dura mater, which covers the brain, folding into the cranial cavity to divide the cranium into

**Fig. 2** Types of brain herniations

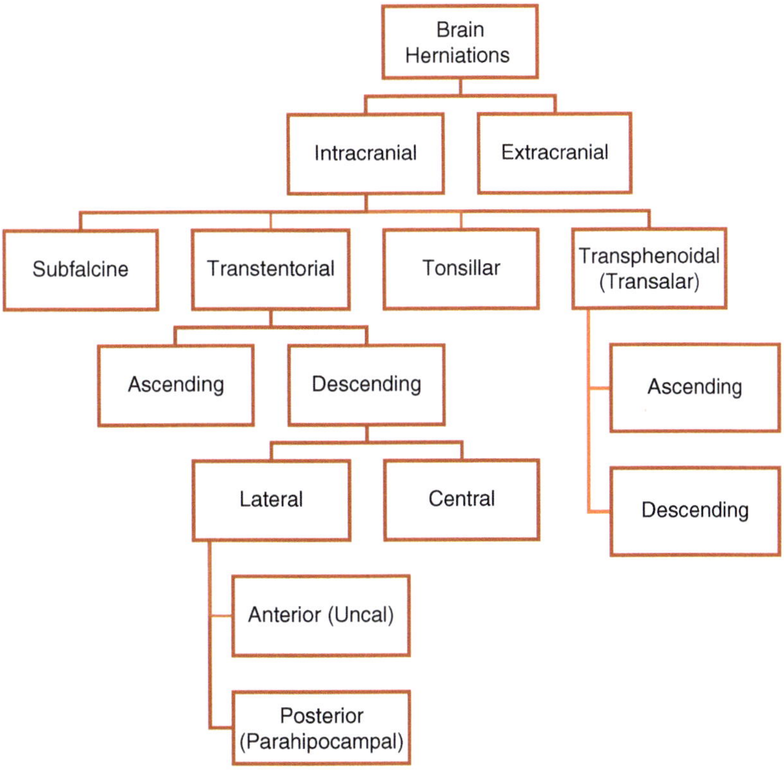


compartments. The most important dural reflections are falx cerebri, tentorium cerebelli, and falx cerebelli. Falx cerebri is tough with a fibrous membrane structure and lies in the anteroposterior direction. It is anchored to the crista galli of the ethmoid bone in the anterior and to the internal occipital protuberance of the occipital bone and superior surface of the tentorium cerebelli in the posterior aspect. It superiorly attaches to the inner table of the skull, and the lower edge of the falx cerebri is free. Corpus callosum is located right below the said free edge of the falx cerebri, whereas cingulate gyrus is located lateral to the free edge. Pericallosal sulcus is located between the corpus callosum and cingulate gyrus and the pericallosal artery (branch of the anterior cerebral artery) travels along this sulcus (Gray 1974). Falx cerebri divides the brain into two hemispheres, i.e., the right and left hemisphere. Moreover, the upper border of the falx cerebri contains the superior sagittal sinus, the lower free edge contains the inferior sagittal sinus, and the posteroinferior border that attaches to the tentorium cerebelli contains the straight sinus. Tentorium cerebelli is the second largest dural reflection after the falx cerebri. It lies in the transverse plane and divides the cranial cavity into two as the supratentorial and infratentorial compartments. The tentorium cerebelli is attached to the falx cerebri at its midline apex. Since this point is located more superiorly than the other parts, tentorium cerebelli is shaped like a tent. The base of the tentorium cerebelli is attached to the inner surface of the occipital bone and ends posteriorly at the internal occipital protuberance. It contains the transverse sinus in this area. In addition, the anterolateral margin attaches to the superior border of the petrous part of the temporal bone. This margin extends inferiorly to the tentorial incisura and attaches to the posterior clinoid process anteriorly. In this area, it contains the superior petrosal sinus.

The tentorium cerebelli has a notch called incisura cerebelli that provides communication between the supratentorial and infratentorial compartments. The midbrain and cerebral peduncles travel through the incisura. It is

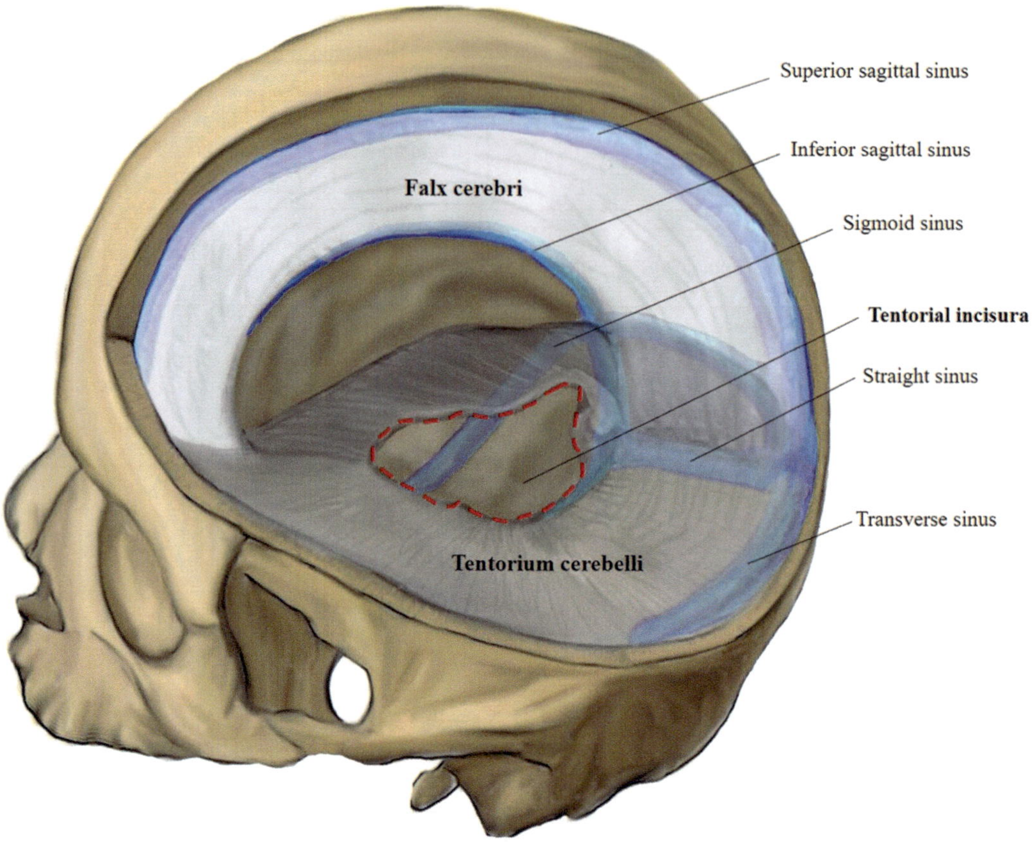


**Fig. 3** Drawing shows the main dural reflections, tentorial incisura, and dural venous sinuses

essential to know the anatomy associated with incisura, particularly for transtentorial herniations. The uncus and hippocampus slightly hang over the tentorium. The ambient cistern is closely associated with the free margin of the tentorium and contains the posterior cerebral arteries, anterior choroidal arteries, and internal cerebral veins. The third cranial nerve originates from the midbrain, crosses the interpeduncular cistern, and is located medial to the uncus.

# 4 Intracranial Herniations

## 4.1 Subfalcine Herniation

Subfalcine herniation is the most common type of intracranial herniations. In subfalcine herniation, the ipsilateral cingulate gyrus moves beneath the falx cerebri by pushing corpus callosum downwards due to a factor that causes supratentorial mass effect. If the pressure increase persists, the contralateral cingulate gyrus becomes compressed by herniated tissue. In the next stage, bilateral foramina of Monro would be compressed. Consequently, the contralateral lateral ventricle becomes dilated (the unilateral lateral ventricle is generally compressed due to a mass effect). The most important complication of subfalcine herniation is the compression of the pericallosal artery which is a branch of the anterior cerebral artery. An infarct can develop in the area from the cingulate gyrus, medial part of the superior frontal gyrus to the precuneus as a result of compression of the pericallosal artery, which is located between the corpus callosum and the cingulate gyrus. Edema caused by the infarct results in a further increased mass effect. Therefore, this vicious cycle may lead to a further enlarged herniation (Young 2011).

Subfalcine herniations are best evaluated with coronal MR images. In addition, axial MR and CT slices are used to measure the degree of midline shift. The degree of midline shift in the septum pellucidum is measured in millimeters from axial slices. The midline is represented by a line that connects the attachment points of the falx cerebri to the inner table of the skull anteriorly and posteriorly. A higher midline shift means poorer prognosis (Miller et al. 1977). It was shown that a septal shift more than 15 mm was associated with a poor prognosis (Ross et al. 1989). Another method that is less frequently used to determine midline shift is the measurement of the horizontal shift of the pineal gland. The degree of shift is correlated with the level of consciousness. Patients with a 0–3 mm shift are awake, whereas a shift of 3–4 mm causes drowsiness, a shift of 6–8.5 mm causes stupor and a shift of 8–13 mm causes coma (Ropper 1986).

## 4.2 Transtentorial Herniation

### 4.2.1 Descending Transtentorial Herniation

Descending transtentorial herniation (DTH) occurs as a result of the downward displacement of the brain through the tentorial incisura. It is the second most common type of herniation after subfalcine herniation. DTH constitutes great prognostic importance for the patient due to its potentially life-threatening outcomes.

Descending transtentorial herniation is divided into two categories as the lateral and central type. In addition, the lateral type is divided into two categories as the anterior and posterior type based on the herniated part of the medial temporal lobe. The uncus exhibits a downward displacement in the anterior type, and the parahippocampal gyrus exhibits a downward displacement in the posterior type through the tentorial incisura. On the other hand, central (bilateral) descending transtentorial herniation involves the diencephalon, midbrain, and pons. This type of herniation is generally observed with lateral herniation syndromes. Bilateral supratentorial masses, midline masses, or diffuse cerebral edema may lead to central type DTH.

In the anterior type, the uncus exhibits a downward displacement towards the ipsilateral crural cistern. Most DTHs initially begin with uncal herniation. In a later stage of herniation, posterior structures also become herniated due to the increased mass effect. The parahippocampal gyrus becomes herniated beneath the posterolateral part of the tentorial incisura in the posterior type. In more advanced posterior herniations, the fornical gyrus and the anterior part of the lingual gyrus can also become herniated. Anterior and posterior herniations occur as a result of herniation toward the ipsilateral crural cistern and lateral part of the quadrigeminal plate cistern, respectively. This leads to the rotation and compression of the brainstem. Whether the herniation is anterior or posterior depends on the localization of the space-occupying lesion as well as the width and shape of the tentorial incisura (Plant 1963).

#### 4.2.1.1 Lateral Herniation

Anterior (Uncal)

In the anterior type of DTH, the uncus exhibits a downward displacement from the free edge of the tentorial incisura. This is the most well-known type of herniation which can be easily detected by imaging modalities (CT and MRI) (Meyer 1920). The uncus is pushed inferiorly and medially and is displaced toward the lateral suprasellar cistern. In the early phase of herniation, the ipsilateral perimesencephalic cistern (interpeduncular, crural, ambient and quadrigeminal plate cistern) becomes enlarged and the contralateral side becomes compressed (Osborn 1977). Bilateral cisternal spaces become obliterated with the progression of herniation. There are studies showing that cisternal space obliteration is a poor prognostic factor. Moreover, the midbrain is compressed with the progression of herniation. The opposite cerebral peduncle is compressed against the contralateral tentorial edge. This leads to impaired integrity of the corticospinal tracts of the cerebral peduncle and motor deficit on the opposite side of the cerebral peduncle (same side as herniation). This hemiparesis on the same side as the mass is known as the Kernohan's notch phenomenon or false localizing sign (Collier 1904). Further compression of the midbrain causes damage to the reticular activating system and loss of consciousness. In this advanced stage of herniation, rupture is observed as a result of the tension in arterial structures located in the midbrain and pons. Small and multiple areas of bleeding in the midbrain and upper pons as a result of the rupture of the small penetrating branches of the basilar artery are called Duret's hemorrhages. These hemorrhages represent the most severe brainstem compression and dislocation, and generally result in coma and death.

The third cranial nerve and posterior cerebral artery are vulnerable to compression in anterior herniation due to their close anatomical location to the uncus. Due to the mentioned close anatomical location, the cardinal sign of uncal herniation is a blown pupil secondary to a compressed third cranial nerve. Another important complication of anterior DTH is occipital lobe infarction due to posterior cerebral artery compression. Patients develop homonymous hemianopsia as a result of occipital lobe infarct (Stovring 1977).

Pressure on the midbrain as a result of uncal herniation may cause the compression of the aqueduct of Sylvius, leading to increased intraventricular pressure. This may cause obstructive hydrocephalus. However, due to the mass effect of the supratentorial mass on the ipsilateral ventricle and the protective effect of the body of the sphenoid with the sella turcica and rigid posterior falx, dilatation is only observed in the contralateral temporal and occipital horns. The compression of the basal cisterns adjacent to the tentorial incisura due to herniated brain tissue also contributes to the impairment of cerebrospinal fluid (CSF) drainage.

#### Posterior (Parahippocampal)

In posterior DTH, the parahippocampal gyrus exhibits a downward displacement through the posterolateral part of the tentorial incisura. Posterior DTH is rarely isolated. Anterior (uncal) herniation is the initial event in most of the DTH cases and the herniation generally starts to involve the posterior structures with the progression of hernia. Unlike anterior herniation, the quadrigeminal plate and ambient cisterns are compressed; however, the lateral suprasellar cistern is generally preserved in the early phase of posterior DTH. As the hernia becomes enlarged, a wedge of necrosis, often accompanied by hemorrhage, occurs along the line of a groove in the parahippocampal gyrus (Mori et al. 1998). In the later stage, all cisternal spaces become obliterated and the midbrain becomes enlarged in the posterior-anterior plane and gets compressed and deformed (Blackwood and Corsellis 1976).

### 4.2.1.2 Central Herniation

Central herniation is observed in pathologies with diffuse involvement of the brain and in midline masses. It is characterized by a downward displacement of the diencephalon, midbrain, and pons through the tentorial incisura. Since masses rarely have midline localization, central herniation is generally accompanied by uncal and parahippocampal herniation.

Many secondary signs of central herniation can be easily detected with CT and MRI. These secondary signs include the obliteration of the cisternal spaces (the quadrigeminal and retrothalamic cisterns are totally effaced), caudal displacement of the basilar artery and pineal gland, rotation and deformity of the midbrain, an increase in sagittal diameter of the brainstem, posterior cerebral artery infarction, and inferoposterior displacement of the quadrigeminal plate (Hahn and Gurney 1985). While the compression of the cerebral aqueduct may lead to hydrocephalus, extremely small lateral ventricles can also be observed in pathologies that manifest with diffuse and severe brain edema. Ischemic lesions are observed in the occipital lobe and thalamus due to the compression of the posterior cerebral and thalamoperforating arteries. Third cranial nerve palsy and changes in consciousness can occur at the end of all these pathological processes, and even coma and death can be observed in the advanced stage of herniation. All these clinical signs reflect the order of diencephalic and brainstem dysfunction caused by herniation from the rostral to the caudal direction.

The incisural line was defined as a straight line from the anterior tuberculum sellae anteriorly to the inferior point of the confluence of the straight sinus, the great cerebral vein, and the inferior sagittal sinus posteriorly. Quantitative methods that employ the incisural line have been developed in order to measure the vertical downward displacement of the brainstem, which can be used to evaluate DTH. For instance, it was reported that a downward shift of 2 standard deviations (1.8 mm) of the proximal opening of the aqueduct (iter) could be used as an MRI criterion for DTH (in normal patients, the iter was 0.2 ± 0 0.8 mm below the incisural line) (Reich et al. 1993). However, since such measurements are challenging and time consuming in routine practice, qualitative evaluation of the downward shift is generally used more frequently.

### 4.2.2 Ascending Transtentorial Herniation

Ascending transtentorial herniation is an upward displacement of the cerebellum through the tentorial incisura due to any reason that creates a mass effect in the posterior fossa (Fig. 4). It generally occurs due to cerebellar masses; however, cerebellopontine angle tumors or masses located in the pons can also cause ascending transtentorial herniation. Another rarer cause of ascending transtentorial herniation is the sudden drop of intracranial pressure in patients who underwent shunt placement for hydrocephalus (Cuneo et al. 1979). Any mass effect in the posterior fossa may lead to ascending transtentorial herniation as well as tonsillar herniation through the foramen magnum. The width of the tentorial incisura and the vector direction of the mass effect (upwards or downwards) influence the type of herniation that will develop. Ascending transtentorial herniation is more possible in those with a wide tentorial incisura and an upward direction of mass effect.

As a result of ascending transtentorial herniation, the cerebellar vermis exhibits an upward displacement through the incisura. The midbrain and pons anteriorly shift to the clivus and become compressed. The inferior colliculus folds beneath the superior colliculus, and these two entities shift beneath the splenium of the corpus callosum. The fourth ventricle becomes distorted and obstructive hydrocephalus can be observed.

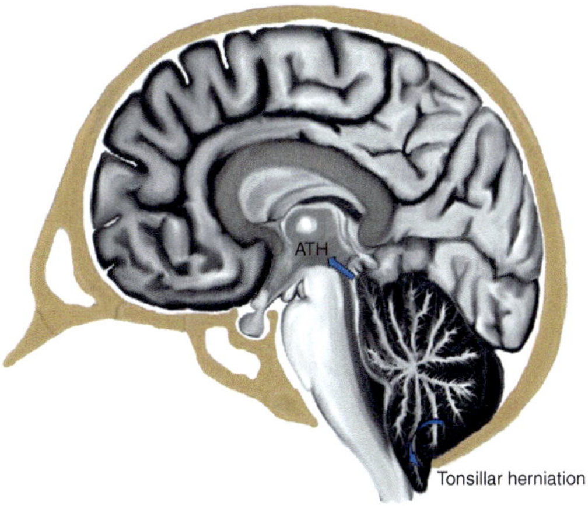


**Fig. 4** Sagittal diagram shows cerebellar tonsils extending below the foramen magnum (tonsillar herniation) and upward displacement of the cerebellum through the tentorial incisura (ATH). *ATH* ascending transtentorial herniation

The vein of Galen can be compressed in upward herniation since it runs at close proximity to the posterior tentorial incisura. This may lead to venous hemorrhagic infarction in the diencephalon and the adjacent white matter. Concerning the arteries, the superior cerebellar artery can be compressed against the tentorium, which may cause an infarct in the part of the cerebellar hemispheres located inferior to the tentorium (Sunderland 1958).

## 4.3 Tonsillar Herniation

Herniation types other than tonsillar herniation (transtentorial, subfalcine) are named after the dural margins at which intercompartmental displacement occurs. On the other hand, tonsillar herniation is named after the herniated brain tissue and described as the downward displacement of the cerebellar tonsils toward the cervical spinal canal along the foramen magnum

(Fig. 4). The most frequent cause of tonsillar herniation is infratentorial masses. However, in addition to causing tonsillar herniation, an infratentorial mass may also lead to ascending transtentorial herniation. Herniation is directed toward the foramen magnum if tentorial incisura is narrow and the vector direction of the mass effect is downward. Although supratentorial masses more frequently cause DTH, enlargement of herniation pushes the cerebellar tonsils downward through the foramen magnum. In support of this, previous studies also showed that nearly half of the patients with DTH also had tonsillar herniation (Reich et al. 1993).

Drawing a straight line from the inferior tip of the clivus to the posterior tip of the foramen magnum on sagittal MR images, a cerebellar tonsil location down to 3 mm inferior to this line is considered normal. A downward tonsillar displacement of 3–5 mm is considered borderline and 5 mm is considered pathological (Aboulezz et al. 1985). Other imaging findings associated with tonsillar herniation are anterior displacement of the brainstem and loss of CSF spaces around the brainstem. Sagittal MRI images are highly beneficial in showing all these changes. Beam hardening artifacts in the posterior fossa and partial volume averaging effects may complicate the evaluation of tonsillar herniation with CT.

Changes in consciousness that are generally observed in DTH and indicate upper brainstem compression are not expected in tonsillar herniation. A patient with tonsillar herniation is generally conscious. However, sudden death can be seen due to the involvement of cardiac and respiratory systems as a result of medulla compression (Howell 1959). Moreover, the compression of the posterior inferior cerebellar artery may lead to a cerebellar infarct and aqueduct compression, leading to hydrocephalus.

### 4.4 Transsphenoidal (Transalar) Herniation

Transsphenoidal herniation is rare and not as well-known as the other types of herniation. There are two types of transsphenoidal herniation, i.e., descending and ascending. In the descending type, the posterior frontal lobe is displaced toward the middle cranial fossa over the sphenoid wing. It occurs as a result of a mass effect in the anterior cranial fossa. Herniation may lead to the compression of the middle cerebral artery against the sphenoid wing, and infarction can be observed in the watershed areas of the middle cerebral artery. In the ascending type, the anterior temporal lobe is displaced toward anterior cranial fossa over the sphenoid wing. It occurs due to a mass effect in the middle cranial fossa. The supraclinoid internal carotid artery may be compressed against the anterior clinoid process and an infarct can be seen in the watershed areas of the anterior and middle cerebral arteries (Laine et al. 1995).

## 5 Extracranial Herniations

Extracranial herniations are the rarest form of all acquired herniations. They usually occur after surgery or trauma due to the herniation of swollen brain tissue through a defective area in the calvarium.

Decompressive craniectomy is a surgical procedure that is performed on patients with increased intracranial pressure. It reduces the intracranial pressure, thereby preventing the development of intracranial herniation and its complications. However, the surgical procedure also involves some complications. In patients with a small craniectomy defect, brain tissue can be herniated, protruding through the defect. In that case, brain parenchyma can be squeezed especially in the margins of the defect and lead to ischemia. Another undesired effect of decompressive craniectomy is that the brain tissue that is not protected by the calvarium becomes susceptible to infections. Another complication of decompressive craniectomy is paradoxical herniation which is rare but fatal. Paradoxical herniation is observed in patients who have a large craniectomy defect and who later undergo CSF drainage. This leads to a significant drop in intracranial pressure, which becomes lower than atmospheric pressure. The mentioned pressure difference causes subfalcine, transtentorial, or tonsillar herniation (Sinclair and Scoffings 2010). Clinical manifestations observed in patients include loss of consciousness, autonomic instability, focal neurologic deficits, pupillary changes, and signs of brainstem release (Chughtai et al. 2019).

Extracranial herniations can be demonstrated with high accuracy both with CT and MRI. However, MRI has a higher soft tissue resolution and is more superior in showing congenital extracranial herniations such as encephalocele.

## 6 Intracranial Hypotension

Intracranial hypotension typically occurs due to a CSF-venous fistula or CSF leak that is caused by a dural defect. As previously explained, the volume of the intracranial structures (brain, CSF and blood) is constant according to the Monro-Kellie doctrine. Therefore, a decrease in the volume of one component is compensated by an increase in the volume of another. A decrease in the volume of intracranial CSF is balanced by an increase in blood volume. This is visualized as smooth diffuse dural (pachymeningeal) enhancement and dural sinus engorgement on MR images, and these are the most common signs encountered in patients with intracranial hypotension (Amrhein and Kranz 2019).

Intracranial hypotension is among the causes of brain herniations and may cause central transtentorial herniation and/or tonsillar herniation. Intracranial hypotension should be suspected particularly in patients who have a herniation that is not proportional to the mass effect. Another sign of intracranial hypotension is bilateral subdural effusion. Although it is thought that herniations can develop secondary to the mass effect of subdural collections, the extent of displacement is generally not proportional to the mass effect caused by these collections (Chan et al. 2019). Patients with severe herniation frequently require blood patch or surgical repair of the dural defect, since an affected reticular formation in the brainstem can lead to coma and death.

**Acknowledgments** The authors thank Istemihan Coban, MD, for the illustrations.

## References


Aboulezz AO, Sartor K, Geyer CA et al (1985) Position of cerebellar tonsils in the normal population and in patients with Chiari malformation: a quanitative approach with MR imaging. J Comput Assist Tomogr 9:1033–1036

Amrhein TJ, Kranz PG (2019) Spontaneous intracranial hypotension: imaging in diagnosis and treatment. Radiol Clin N Am 57:439–451

Blackwood W, Corsellis JAN (1976) Greenfield's neuropathology, 3rd edn. Edward Arnold/Year Book, Chicago

Chan SM, Chodakiewitz YG, Maya MM, Schievink WI, Moser FG (2019) Intracranial hypotension and cerebrospinal fluid leak. Neuroimaging Clin N Am 29:213–226

Chughtai KA, Nemer OP, Kessler AT, Bhatt AA (2019) Post-operative complications of craniotomy and craniectomy. Emerg Radiol 26:99–107

Collier J (1904) The false localizing signs of intracranial tumors. Brain 27:490–508

Cuneo RA, Caronna JJ, Pitts L et al (1979) Upward transtentorial herniation. Seven cases and a literature review. Arch Neurol 36:618–623

Gray H (1974) In: Warwick R, Williams PL (eds) Gray's anatomy. Running Press, Philadelphia, pp 512–523

Hahn F, Gurney J (1985) CT signs of central descending transtentorial herniation. AJNR Am J Neuroradiol 6:844–845

Howell DA (1959) Upper brainstem compression and foraminal impaction with intracranial space-occupying lesions and brainstem swelling. Brain 82:525–551

Kaseff LG, Seidenwurm DJ, Nieberding PH et al (1992) Magnetic resonance imaging of brain herniation into the middle ear. Am J Otol 13:74–77

Laine FJ, Shedden AI, Dunn MM, Ghatak NR (1995) Acquired intracranial herniations: MR imaging findings. AJR Am J Roentgenol 165:967–973

Meyer A (1920) Herniation of the brain. Arch Neurol 4:387–400

Miller JD, Becker DP, Ward JD et al (1977) Significance of intracranial hypertension in severe head injury. J Neurosurg 47:503–516

Mokri B (2001) The Monro-Kellie hypothesis: applications in CSF volume depletion. Neurology 56:1746–1748

Mori K, Ishimaru S, Maeda M (1998) Uncoparahippocampectomy for direct surgical treatment of downward transtentorial herniation. Acta Neurochir 140:1239–1244

Mosnier I, Fiky LE, Shahidi A, Sterkers O (2000) Brain herniation and chronic otitis media: diagnosis and surgical management. Clin Otolaryngol Allied Sci 25:385–391

Nadgir R, Yousem DM (2017) Head trauma. In: Thrall JH (ed) Neuroradiology: the requisites, 4th edn. Elsevier, Philadelphia, PA, pp 150–173
Osborn AG (1977) Diagnosis of descending transtentorial herniation by cranial computed tomography. Radiology 123:93–96
Plant HF (1963) Size of tentorial incisura related to cerebral herniation. Acta Radiol Diagn 1:916–928
Reich JB, Sierra J, Camp W et al (1993) Magnetic resonance imaging: measurements and clinical changes accompanying transtentorial and foramen magnum brain herniation. Ann Neurol 33:159–170
Riveros Gilardi B, Muñoz López JI, Hernández Villegas AC et al (2019) Types of cerebral herniation and their imaging features. Radiographics 39:1598–1610
Ropper AH (1986) Lateral displacement of the brain and level of consciousness in patients with an acute hemispheral mass. N Engl J Med 314:953–958
Ross DA, Walter OL, Ross AM et al (1989) Brain shift, level of consciousness and restoration of consciousness in patients with acute intracranial hematoma. J Neurosurg 71:498–502
Sinclair AG, Scoffings DJ (2010) Imaging of the postoperative cranium. Radiographics 30:461–482
Stevens RD, Shoykhet M, Cadena R (2015) Emergency neurological life support: intracranial hypertension and herniation. Neurocrit Care 23(Suppl 2):S76–S82
Stovring J (1977) Descending tentorial herniation: findings on computed tomography. Neuroradiology 14:101–105
Sunderland S (1958) The tentorial notch and complications produced by herniations of the brain through that aperture. Br J Surg 455:422–438
Young GB (2011) Impaired consciousness and herniation syndromes. Neurol Clin 29:765–772

# Basic Neuro-Interventional Spine Procedures

Mario Muto, Giuseppe Leone, Roberto Izzo, Elisa Capone, Adrian Kastler, Gianluigi Guarnieri, and Francesco Briganti

## Contents



M. Muto (✉) · R. Izzo · E. Capone · G. Guarnieri
Neuroradiology Department, Cardarelli Hospital, Naples, Italy

G. Leone · F. Briganti
Unit of Interventional Neuroradiology, Department of Advanced Biomedical Sciences, Federico II University of Naples, Naples, Italy
e-mail: frabriga@unina.it

A. Kastler
Diagnostic and Interventional Neuroradiology Unit, Grenoble University Hospital, La Tronche, France

**Abstract**

Interventional spine procedures represent a well-known alternative to conservative management and highly debated surgical procedures in the management and relief of spinal pain.

Basic Neuro-Interventional Spine Procedures allow minimally invasive treatment for both degenerative and tumor conditions, such as spine metastasis, osteoid osteoma, vertebral hemangioma, aneurysmal bone cyst, and osteoblastoma.



M. Scaglione et al. (eds.), *Emergency Radiology of the Head and Spine*, Medical Radiology Diagnostic Imaging, https://doi.org/10.1007/978-3-030-91047-1_10

Diagnostic imaging, both MRI—T1w, T2w, and STIR sequences—and CT, is of main importance for understanding underlying condition and planning the best therapeutic approach. Epidural steroid injection in the care of radiculopathy, oxygen-ozone therapy for the treatment of herniated disk, and percutaneous vertebroplasty in the management of vertebral body compression fracture are only few of the most used and widely accepted techniques in the setting of neuro-interventional spine interventions.

In this chapter, we review the basic of anatomy and pathophysiology of spinal pain and then the current practice on neuro-interventional spinal interventions, including indications, contraindications, and complication and discuss the most used techniques in the clinical practice.

## Abbreviations

| | |
|---|---|
| ABC | Aneurysmal bone cyst |
| CNS | Central nervous system |
| CT | Computed tomography |
| DRG | Dorsal root ganglion |
| ESI | Epidural steroid injection |
| FJ | Facet joints |
| G6PD | Glucose-6-phosphate-dehydrogenase |
| GABA | Gamma-aminobutyric acid |
| Gd | Gadolinium |
| HIZs | High-intensity zones |
| IL | Interleukin |
| LBP | Low back pain |
| MMPs | Metalloproteinases |
| MRI | Magnetic resonance imaging |
| NGF | Nerve growth factor |
| NMDA | *N*-methyl-D-aspartate |
| NO | Nitric oxide |
| NOS | Nitric oxide synthase |
| O.O. | Osteoid osteoma |
| O2-O3 | Oxygen-Ozone |
| OB | Osteoblastoma |
| PGs | Prostaglandines |
| PMMA | Polymethylmetachrylate |
| PNS | Peripheral nervous systems |
| RF | Radiofrequency |
| SP | Substance P |
| SP | Substance P |
| TNF | Tumor necrosis factor |
| VBF | Vertebra body fracture |
| VP | Vertebroplasty |
| WDRNs | Wide dynamic range neurons |

## 1 Introduction

The concept of spine pain has bothered spine specialist since the origin of humanity, and pain management still remains an every-day struggle for healthcare. Among painful syndromes, spinal disorders and back pain represent the most frequent painful condition (Vos et al. 2017) and therefore represent the most expensive disease in industrialized countries (Wenig et al. 2009). Among the therapeutic options available in the management of patients suffering from spine pain, interventional spine procedures represent a valuable alternative to conservative management and highly debated surgical procedures. Owing to the access to high-quality imaging modalities, interventional radiologists are in the best position to perform spinal procedures. Galibert and Deramont (Galibert et al. 1987), a French neurosurgeon and neuroradiologist, were the first to perform a percutaneous vertebroplasty in a spinal hemangioma in the middle 1980s. Since then, a variety of spinal procedure have been developed and scientifically validated in the field of spinal disorder management. The object of this chapter is to describe the main therapeutic mini-invasive approaches in spine pain management, in the fields of both benign pain (degenerative pain disease) and malignant pain (primary and secondary tumors).

## 2 Pathophysiology of Spine Pain

Spinal pain, and in particular low back pain (LBP), is extremely common and represents a major cause of disability. Evaluating spinal pain, excluding few cases (about 1%) of subjects having underlying pathologies such as tumors or infection/inflammatory disease, the most important step is the identification of the exact source of the pain, which is often unexplained. This can be difficult in account to complex neuroanatomy of the spine. In fact, while somatic sensitive fibers travelling in the spinal nerves account for the well-localized pain, just as in radicular pain, the autonomic afferents coming from sympathetic sensitive fibers of paravertebral ganglia and chain (Hirsch et al. 1963) are responsible for the referred pain, just as in discogenic pain, that is diffuse, deep, and not well discriminated. Localized pain distributes in a well-defined cutaneous dermatome, while referred pain is perceived in the somatome area, which includes all tissues originating embriologically from the same somite. Any injury involving the disks, ligaments, and bones of the spine causes pain through tissue inflammation and production of a cascade of mediators such as prostaglandines (PGs), bradykinin, serotonin, histamine, excitatory amino acids, nitric oxide (NO), nerve growth factor (NGF), and hydrogen ions, all of which directly activate afferents and/or sensitize nociceptors (Dubner and Hargreaves 1989).

Fibers transmitting painful stimuli include C-type, unmyelinated (responsible for longlasting pain); A-delta, myelinated (accounting for fast, sharp pain); and A-gamma, the smallest myelinated fibers. A-beta fibers are normally proprioceptive, but can eventually produce nociceptive neuro-transmitters. Peripheral nociceptors can be specific (thermal, mechanical, chemical) or polymodal, also called "wide dynamic range neurons" (WDRNs) because they can respond to all stimuli. A major cause of non-specific lumbar pain is considered the disk disruption, being responsible for discogenic pain.

In healthy disks, free nerve endings are present only in the outermost few millimeters of the annulus, where tensile stresses overcome compressive loads, but they can grow in the degenerated disks favored from intranuclear pressure reduction, even penetrating the nucleus and producing substance P (SP).

On the other hand, healthy nociceptors of the external annulus may be stimulated to undergo abnormal stimulation secondary to instability or if peripheral tears expose them to effects of chemical mediators coming from the nucleus.

**Radicular pain** is due to radicular compression and/or inflammation caused in the majority of the cases by disk herniation and/or canal stenosis, through two different and complementary ways:

1. Mechanical (i.e., by direct compression of the nerve or dorsal root ganglion, DRG, or indirect compression on perineural vessels).
2. Inflammatory (i.e., by autoimmune cellular responses mounted if the disk is no longer segregated by the annulus and, so, is recognized as "non-self" by the immune system) and biochemical (through the action of mediators expressed by disk itself, such as phospholypase A2, PGE2, IL-6, and MMPs). That's why a protruding disk even without root compression can generate pain by releasing inflammatory mediators near the nerve root. Normally, inflammatory cells and mediators are absent in healthy disks and are more abundant in non-contained herniations than in contained ones.

In zygoapophysial joints, it is known that capsule, synovial membranes and subcondral bone facet joints are richly innervated, so representing a direct sources of pain. The facet joints receive double innervation (somatic and autonomic) so that facet pain can be local or distantly referred with possible overlapping among different levels. Degeneration—arthrosis or arthritis—of the facet joints is a frequent cause of radicular pain due to the compression of nerve roots in the lateral recesses and in the foramina due to hypertrophic and ostephytic remodeling subluxation, joint effusion with capsular tension, and synovial cysts.

Whatever is the origin, LBP can be classified as "acute" (lasting <4 weeks), "subacute" (5–12 weeks), and "chronic" (>12 week). Whereas acute forms generally resolve spontaneously, chronic pain is much more difficult to threat and resolves only in <5–10% of cases (Dunn and Croft 2004).

In acute pain, signals reaching the dorsal horns of the spinal cord have the same intensity as those travelling in neo-paleo-spinothalamic tracts and a descending countersignal coming from supraspinal centers dissolves and extinguishes arriving painful inputs (eudynia) (Moskowitz 2008).

The complex processes of central and peripheral sensitivization may influence the conversion of acute chronic pain, transforming a symptom into a disease through complex neuroplastic mutation occurring in the central nervous system (CNS) and peripherally in dorsal ganglia.

Sensitivization or hypersensitivity consists in a decrease in the threshold of neuron activation, increased response to stimuli, and even spontaneous neuronal firing.

The continuous stimulation from peripheral nociceptors can lead the spinal cord to reach a "hyper-excitable" state with a "wind-up" response through the properties of the WDRNs: neurons that do not normally transmit pain begin to do so. At the same time, others neurons activate even without stimuli, causing hyperalgesia and allodynia. The "wind-up" response involves the action of a lot of neurotransmitters. The unrelenting stimulation of the neurons in the dorsal horn promotes excessive release of substance P (SP) and glutammate from the presynaptic nerve endings of the peripheral primary-order neurons. The long-term depolarization of postsynaptic membranes of nociceptive-specific and also WDRNs removes the block normally exerted by magnetic ions upon *N*-methyl-D-aspartate (NMDA) receptors.

The binding of glutammate to NMDA receptors and its hyperactivation account for cellular influx of calcium which, in turn, activates nitric oxide synthase (NOS) resulting in the production of NO. NO diffuses across synapses and stimulates the presynaptic release of increasing amounts of SP and glutammate, creating a dangerous vicious cycle. At the same time, activation of NMDA receptors induces the production and membrane placement of new receptors. Intracellular calcium also promotes the breakdown of prostanoids to arachidonic acid, resulting in CNS inflammation. Just as in acute pain, the brain sends descending countersignal, but now the results are quite ineffective.

Gamma-aminobutyric acid (GABA), the major inhibitory neurotransmitter, loses its efficacy in front of excessive release of glutamate in central and peripheral nervous systems (PNS).

Although a constant input is needed to initiate the wind-up response, very little or any is needed to maintain it, perpetuating a positive feedback with minimal—or absent—peripheral stimuli.

In a healthy condition, peripheral discal nociceptors have a high threshold of activation and do not respond to physiological joint motion, pressure, stretching, or muscolar contraction. Inflammatory sensitization reduces the threshold for the activation of discal mechanoreceptors so that disk loading within the physiological range may cause pain.

In degenerating disk, in response to abnormal loads, chondrocytes proliferate and replace proteoglycan with abnormal types of collagen, upregulate MMPs which degrade the nucleus and annulus matrix, and promote macrophage infiltration which, in turn, produces multiple inflammatory mediators (bradykinin, IL-1, NO, TNF-a, phospholipase A2, and NGF) (Haro et al. 1996).

Inflammatory mediators can directly activate nocicepetors (bradykinin, serotonin, excitatory amino acids) and sensitize them by lowering the thresholds for firing and, by increasing the firing rates and finally recruiting new receptors, broadening the area of perception. Inflammatory sensitization of discal nociceptors may also arise from nerve fibrils accompanying the ingrowth of granulation tissue into the annular tears that, together with fluid collections, can be detected on magnetic resonance imaging (MRI) as high-intensity zones (HIZs). The granulation tissue seems to be a healing reaction to the annular injury, and the local inflammation it produces can stimulate the nociceptors generating pain from the fissures. Disks that are simply aging will not be painful because they do not have tears nor granulation tissue along with nerve fibrils (Peng et al. 2006).

The degeneration and disruption of disk are very often flanked by endplate changes, classified by Modic et al. into three stage, among which type I is commonly associated to painful instability.

Knowledge of the central and peripheral mechanism of pain is the fundamental to prevent the conversion of acute spinal pain in a chronic disease. Because of this possible evolution, it is very important to start the therapy as soon as possible taking care of both the symptom and its causes, and, if pain does not resolve, employ more aggressive treatment.

## 3 Mini-invasive Treatment for Degenerative Spine Disease

Degenerative spine disease may be a source of multiple back pain syndromes. Interventional radiologists should therefore be able to locate the origin of the pain described by the patient in order to offer the best possible interventional management, consistent with the affected spinal anatomical segment. Unfortunately, literature reports a poor radio-clinical correlation in the setting of degenerative disease. This requires, from the interventional radiologist, very careful image analysis to detect a possible source of pain. However, images are not the only subject of interest of the interventional radiologist, and both the patient and its clinical presentation should be the center of attention leading to a therapeutic decision.

### 3.1 Epidural Steroid Injection (ESI)

Epidural injection of corticosteroids is one of the most commonly used interventions in managing chronic spinal pain especially in case of associated radiculopathy (McLain et al. 2005). Indeed, radiculopathy is considered to be caused by inflammatory injury to the nerve roots in the condition of neural foraminal stenosis or herniated intervertebral disk (Saal et al. 1990). The principle of epidural steroid injection is to inject localized steroids immediately around the target nerve roots, thereby decreasing the inflammation of affected nerve roots and reducing the pain.

#### 3.1.1 Indications

Herniated disk with radiculopathy and spinal canal/foraminal stenosis are the two main indications for ESI. These conditions may affect the cervical, thoracic, or lumbar spine; and ESI may be performed at each of these levels. ESI must be reserved to failure of first-line conservative management including pharmacological, physical, and cognitive-behavioral therapy. Other indications may also be discussed, such as anterior facet joint cyst with radiculopathy, pain from post-laminectomy syndrome, post-herpetic pain (thoracic level), or post-traumatic pain syndromes (Fritz et al. 2007).

#### 3.1.2 Contraindications

Usual contraindications include known hypersensitivity to injected agents, local or systemic infection, bleeding diathesis, congestive heart failure, and uncontrolled diabetes mellitus. A history of surgery at the level of the puncture is not an absolute contraindication. Conditions in which the procedure will be performed depend on the national recommendations and guidelines (see side effects below). Also, patients with motor deficit are not adequate candidates for ESI and should be referred to surgical management.

#### 3.1.3 Imaging

Prior to any ESI, a CT or MRI should be performed. It is indeed mandatory to eliminate all of the red flags in spinal pain prior to performing an ESI. Also, precise assessment of spinal pathology correlated to clinical findings will help locate the level of the ESI and the type of ESI to perform (see above) and will evidently positively influence the outcome of the procedure. It is very important to keep in mind that because the source of back pain may be difficult to locate, correlation between clinical and radiological remains the key to a successful procedure.

#### 3.1.4 Technique

Epidural steroid injection may be achieved by several approaches (Fritz et al. 2007). The best technique is yet to be demonstrated, and debate remains over which one should be preferred, as the approach chosen depends on several factors: pain generator location, patients' anatomical presentation. Whatever the technique used, procedure should be performed under sterile conditions and with imaging guidance (fluoroscopy, CT scan, and MRI). The needle used may vary (20 Gauge or 22 Gauge) and the injection of contrast media is mandatory prior to steroid injection, in order to confirm the absence of vascular puncture.

*Transforminal Epidural Steroid Injection*: The needle is placed in immediate contact with the foraminal fatty space. The steroid is injected in the foraminal space directly. This approach should be reserved to foraminal or extraforaminal herniated disks or foraminal stenosis. There have been more cases of spinal cord infarct with this approach than with the above-described approaches.

*Interlaminar Epidural Steroid Injection*: This is a posterior approach. The goal is to target the posterior epidural space through the yellow ligament and via the interlaminar space. The approach can be paramedian, thereby targeting the posterior lateral epidural space or median, thereby targeting the posterior epidural space. This approach is preferred in case of posteriorly situated herniated disk and spinal canal stenosis.

### 3.1.5 Results

The evidence for ESIs in patients who have lumbar or cervical radiculopathy includes many small randomized controlled trials and a number of systematic reviews (Manchikanti et al. 2015a; b; Manchikanti et al. 2016). The heterogeneity of the technique performed, the multiplicity of the level injected, and the variety of the pathological conditions make it very difficult to obtain a high level of evidence, especially regarding long-term outcome. However, the evidence for ESI in radiculopathy is good with many trials and reviews reporting >50% pain relief lasting for several months. ESI may easily be repeated and therefore improve mid- to long-term outcome. Not more than 3 ESI may be performed per year.

The evidence for ESI in spinal stenosis is fair for short-term pain relief.

### 3.1.6 Side Effects

Risks associated with needle placement or with the injection of therapeutic substances include infection, bleeding (epidural hematoma), nerve injury, transient numbness or weakness, contrast reaction (allergy), steroid systemic side effects, and vaso-vagal syncope.

Several serious complications after ESI, including spinal cord and brain embolic infarctions, have been reported (Racoosin et al. 2015; MacMahon et al. 2009) and are subject to an ongoing debate whether or not ESI should continue to be performed by physicians (Manchikanti et al. 2014; Rathmell et al. 2015). There is no doubt that these procedures provide pain relief and remain the only conservative management options in case of LBP with radiculopathy able to avoid surgery. However, accurate information should be given to patients and informed consent on the risks should be obtained from them prior to any ESI.

In order to prevent these risks, careful attention should be brought to setting in which ESI is performed. Strict sterile conditions are mandatory to avoid infection. To avoid hemorrhagic complications, antiplatelet and anticoagulant therapy should be stopped, and coagulopathy disorders should be investigated. In order to avoid possible risk of intravascular injection and possible medullar infarct by steroid embolization of radiculomedullar arteries, the following steps should be followed:

Dexamethasone should be preferred in case of transforaminal approach and history of spine surgery. Small diameter needles (<22 Gauge) should be avoided.

Aspiration should be performed to exclude vascular puncture prior to steroid injection.

## 3.2 Disk Treatment

### 3.2.1 Indications

Interventional disk treatment is a second- to third-line management of radicular pain secondary to disk herniation. In these cases, only the lumbar region has been reported to be accessible to percutaneous disk management. Disk management may only be performed in patients presenting radicular pain rather than low back pain, with a history of failed conservative management and a good clinical/radiological correlation as shown by clinical and radiological data. In some specific cases, disk treatment may only be proposed in cases of the failure of ESI. This is particularly the case for mechanical decompression.

### 3.2.2 Contraindications

Usual contraindications include allergy to the injected drugs, local or systemic infection, bleeding disorder, patients with motor deficits or cauda equine syndrome, neoplasm, pregnancy, glucose-6-phosphate-dehydrogenase (G6PD) deficiency (only for oxygen-ozone treatment), hyperthyroidism, severe anemia, and recent myocardial infarction. Calcified herniated disk is not accessible to percutaneous disk management. Specific to mechanical decompression: uncontained disk herniation. Loss of discal height greater than 50% and dehydrated disk on T2 imaging are specific contraindications for all the types of decompressive technique such as coablation and decompressor.

### 3.2.3 Imaging

A detailed CT or MRI of the affected lumbar spine segment should be performed and compared to the clinical findings. Radiological screening must demonstrate disk herniation with radicular irritation and rule out other possible causes of radiculopathy. In that sense, MRI may appear superior to CT scan in evaluating the radiculopathy secondary to the disk herniation as well as disk hydration status. However, CT is a better imaging means to rule out calcified herniated disk.

### 3.2.4 Technique

#### 3.2.4.1 Oxygen-Ozone Therapy

Oxygen-Ozone ($O_2$-$O_3$) is a strongly anti-oxidant gas with antiseptic, immuno-modulating, analgesic, and anti-inflammatory properties (Giurazza et al. 2017). $O_2$-$O_3$ therapy may be administered directly into the disk in the form of $O_2$-$O_3$ mixture at non-toxic concentrations. Disk access is performed extra pedicular foraminal approach using a 19 or 22 Gauge needle until centrally situated in the disk: the ideal needle position is considered to be at the junction between the posterior and the middle third of the disk. Gas mixture [1–3 ml: 2% $O_2$-$O_3$ (30–40 μg/ml) in 98% $O_2$] is then injected into the disk. Another 10 mL of mixture is injected into the foramen at needle retrieval, along with steroid injection (Fig. 1).

#### 3.2.4.2 Mechanical Decompression

Several devices have been commercialized throughout the past decade, but the principle remains common: to perform a percutaneous debulking of the herniated disk and to relieve the pressure on the radicular nerve. The procedure may be performed under either CT or fluroroscopy. The best indications are median paramedian contained herniated disk.

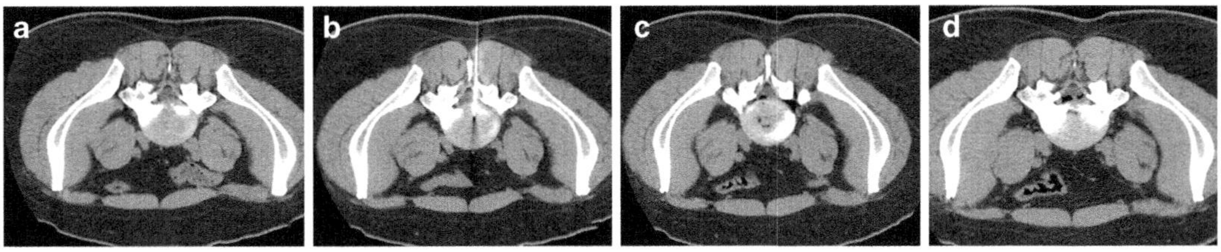


**Fig. 1** (**a**) Patient in the prone position; right paramedian lateral herniated disk with thecal compression. (**b**) Under CT guidance with a transligament approach, the disk at the L5-S1 level is reached. (**c**, **d**) The gas mixture $O_2$-$O_3$ is injected in the amount of 3 mL in the disk and 7 mL in epidural space with good distribution inside and outside the disk

### 3.2.5 Results

In the appropriate clinical/imaging context, intradiscal injection of $O_2$-$O_3$ has a reported success rate that reaches 90% at short-term follow-up (6 months) and a 75–82% success rate at long-term follow-up (12 months) with no major or minor side effects (Giurazza et al. 2017).

Results of mechanical decompression are debated in the literature and level of evidence is not sufficient to date. However, the most recent studies report a very good outcome in cases of lateral foraminal and extraforaminal herniated disk with a 6-month postoperative success rate of 79% in lateralized herniated disks ($\geq$70% decrease in pain), and 50% in case of posteromedian herniated disk (Amoretti et al. 2012).

### 3.2.6 Complications

The overall complication rates of these intradiscal therapies are very low (Giurazza et al. 2017; Amoretti et al. 2012). Diskitis may be one of the most feared complications; however, with the antiseptic properties of ozone, only one reported case exists in the literature (Vanni et al. 2016).

## 3.3 Facet Treatment

### 3.3.1 Indication

Facet joint procedures will be performed in case of (Manchikanti et al. 2001) facet joint syndrome, which typically includes the following clinical symptoms:

- Posterior LBP.
- Increased at palpation, extension, and trunk rotation.
- Inferior limb pain radiation is possible, in the buttock the posterior aspect of the thigh and in some cases even below the knee, referred to as "pseudo-sciatica."

### 3.3.2 Contraindication

Apart from the basic contraindication for any spine procedure (infection, hemorrhagic condition), there is no specific contraindications to performing facet procedures.

### 3.3.3 Imaging

Patients must benefit from at least a CT or an MR scan, in order to rule out other causes of back pain. Careful attention will then be brought to facet degeneration changes. Facet joint syndrome may be present in patients suffering from facet degenerative disease, with classical osteoarthritis signs. One of the most specific signs which should be detected is bone edema situated in the pediculo-articular area. This will require an MRI with T2 STIR sequences. However, in some cases, no pathological signs are detected at radiological screening.

### 3.3.4 Technique

#### 3.3.4.1 Facet Joint Injection

Facet joint (FJ) injections are a crucial step in facet joint disease management, as facet therapeutic injections present a double interest, both diagnostic and therapeutic. Indeed, because diagnosis of facet joint syndrome is not always reliable when based only on clinical and radiological data, it has been suggested that FJ injection be performed to confirm diagnosis.

The site of injection (intra articular, pericapsular, or medial branch block) should be determined depending on the objective of the FJ injection. European guidelines do not recommend the use of intraarticular steroids in the management of chronic LBP. In case of FJ injection to select patient for denervation, the International Spine Intervention Society has recommended that the FJ block be performed at the medial branch. The adjunction of steroids may be performed and this specific point remains a debate in the literature.

#### 3.3.4.2 Facet Joint Denervation

The ideal candidate for FJ denervation is a patient who underwent medial branch infiltration with significant pain relief after failure of conservative management. Due to the dual nerve supply of a given FJ, electrodes or cryoprobes should be placed at two subsequent levels. Nerve fibers can be destroyed either by physical means, heat (radiofrequency—RF) or cold (cryoneurolysis), or by chemical means (alcohol/phenol).

#### 3.3.4.3 Facet Screwing

Trans-facets screwing is an emerging technique which is possible to perform percutaneously under CT and fluoroscopic guidance.

### 3.3.5 Results

Here again, due to the heterogeneity of the approaches and the variety of the possible facet joint pain, results in the literature are mixed in facet joint management (Manchikanti et al. 2015a; b; Cohen and Raja 2007). However, due to the presence of inflammatory mediators into and around degenerative FJ, short to intermediate pain relief should occur after steroid injections (several months). Facet joint denervation however provides long-term results with a mean efficacy duration of 12 months in 60–70% of patients.

### 3.3.6 Complications

Common complications of FJ procedures include: hemorrhagic, infectious complications, vasovagal syncope, and steroid-related complications if administered. Other complications specific to denervation technique include motor nerve lesioning neuritis and muscle atrophy.

These complications can easily be avoided by using imaging guidance and motor stimulation prior to denervation.

## 3.4 Spine Spacer

### 3.4.1 Indications

The ideal interspinous spacer indication is focal (1 level) spinal canal stenosis with the visualization of posterior ligamentum flavuum bulking into the canal.

### 3.4.2 Contraindications

- Multilevel canal stenosis.
- Fracture of the spinous processes.
- Neurological deficit.

### 3.4.3 Imaging

Both MR and CT are required pre-procedures in order to asses both osseous and soft tissue components of the spinal canal stenosis. Careful attention must be brought to assessing the posterior spinous processes which will receive the spacer device. Also, baseline imaging is mandatory for follow-up after the procedure.

### 3.4.4 Technique

Target of interspinous spacer will be planned on CT images, which is definitively needed for this procedure. The approach will be lateral, in order to access the interspinous space perpendicular to the processes. The patient is therefore placed in supine position. The procedure begins with the insertion of a spinal needle for local anesthesia. Then, the dilation of the path is performed and the spacer is inserted through a large coaxial needle with the tip in place in the interspinous space.

Some authors advocate performing adjunct spinous process cementoplasty to prevent possible fracture while deploying the spacer device; this technique remains confidential and will need further assessment.

### 3.4.5 Results

There is a lack of studies assessing the results of such device in the literature today. Only a few centers perform such procedures, but the results are very promising. As always, the successful outcome mainly depends on the indication, which is made on both clinical and radiological data.

### 3.4.6 Complications

Cases of spinous process fracture have been reported along with device malpositioning.

## 3.5 Vertebroplasty (VP)

### 3.5.1 Indications

Percutaneous vertebroplasty has become a widely performed and accepted treatment of porotic vertebral body compression fracture (VBF), less frequently for spine metastasis, primary benign tumors, or spine traumatic fractures. Mechanism of action is the stabilization of the microfractures involved in the pathogenesis of spinal pain (Muto et al. 2016). The most common indication for VP is acute or subacute VBF in both osteoporotic and traumatic settings. A very strong debate still exists about the treatment of osteoporotic fractures as some authors report that there is little added value of VP in case of VBF compared with conservative treatments (Comstock et al. 2013; Kroon et al. 2014), while others report the usefulness of VP in this setting (Mathis et al. 1998; Gangi et al. 2003; Muto et al. 2015). Two randomized controlled trials in 2009 suggested also placebo effects of those treatments, but many biases are present in the study as inclusion/exclusion criteria, cross-over of the treated/untreated patients, and imaging technique (Buchbinder et al. 2009; Kallmes et al. 2009). Another technique became very popular and correspond to vertebral augmentation techniques in which vertebral height restoration is obtain by balloon (kyphoplasty), or by metallic implant (vertebral stenting, spine jack), mostly indicate for the treatment of vertebral trauma. In this case, vertebral kyphosis reduction to restore vertebral body height is the goal associated to vertebral consolidation. Indications of this method are highly kyphotic vertebral bodies, particularly in the thoraco-lumbar junction (T8-L2).

### 3.5.2 Contraindications

Absolute contraindications include uncorrectable coagulopathy, active local or systemic infection, and allergy to polymethylmetachrylate (PMMA). Absence of pain or improvement under conservative treatment may also be viewed as contraindications; however, VP and vertebral augmentation techniques may be discussed in cases of high kyphotic vertebral angle. Posterior wall disruption is not an absolute contraindication; however, neurological deficits or instable fracture involving the posterior arch of burst instable fractures may require surgical management.

### 3.5.3 Imaging

Osteoporotic VBF requires an MR examination to assess the acute nature of the fracture and the number and levels of these fractures. Hypointensity in the vertebral body on T1WI and hyperintensity on T2 STIR images allow targeting the accurate vertebral levels.

In the acute trauma setting, a CT is also mandatory in order to rule out posterior wall involvement and posterior arch fractures.

### 3.5.4 Technique

Two steps may be differentiated in VP: needle placement and cement injection. Needle placement may be performed under CT guidance, fluoroscopic (mono or bi plane) guidance, or cone beam CT guidance. Injection of the cement however should be performed under direct fluoroscopic visualization. Therefore, if the needle is placed under CT guidance, adjunct C-Arm fluoroscopic control should be available for cement injection. Visualization of the cement diffusion is advised in order to avoid cement leakage. The setting of VP is the same whatever the imaging guidance modality used (Figs. 2 and 3).

Strict sterile conditions are required; local, general anesthesia or conscious sedation may be used, depending on operator and patient's preference. Uni- or bilateral approach is possible, and trans- or lateropedicular routes may be used. Several levels can be treated at the same time. The quantity of injected cement is not fixed and depends on several factors (level of the VBF, type of cement, cement distribution, etc.).

### 3.5.5 Results

Several factors should be considered when evaluating the impact of VP in the setting of VBF.

When considering pain improvement after VP, many observational studies have shown VP to be effective and safe for the treatment of osteoporotic (Yang et al. 2016) and acute traumatic VBF (Knavel et al. 2009). However, the improvement of pain may not be the only benefit of VP, as it is well known that presence of pain influences disability and patient discomfort and, in elderly patients, may lead to bed rest complications. Many observational studies support these results (McKiernan et al. 2004; Rapan et al. 2017). The same is applicable in the trauma setting; unpublished results of the VOLCANO study showed that, when comparing VP and bracing in the acute setting of nonosteoporotic fractures, although pain improvement was higher immediately after VP compared with bracing, the effect of improvement of pain decreased in the 6-month follow-up period. However, the improvement in functional disability was evidently higher the entire follow-up period and therefore led to shorter work stoppages and less bed rest complications (Kastler et al. 2013).

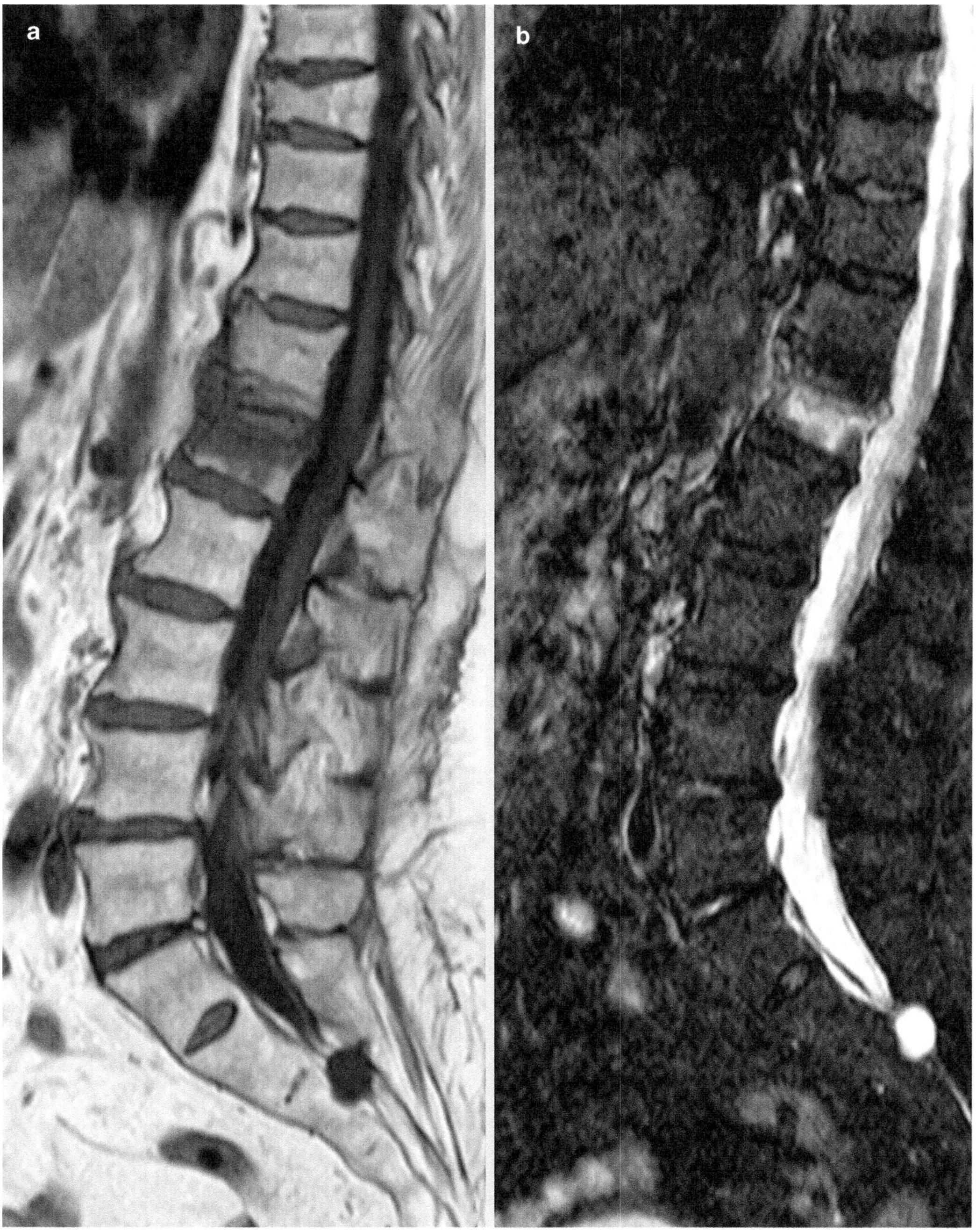


**Fig. 2** (**a**) Sagittal T1-weighted MRI shows a vertebral porotic fracture at the L1 level with hypointense signal. (**b**) Sagittal STIR MRI shows the hyperintense signal due to bone-marrow edema. (**c**) Unipeducolar approach for VP at the L1 level. (**d**, **e**) Preventive VP at the D12 and L2 levels

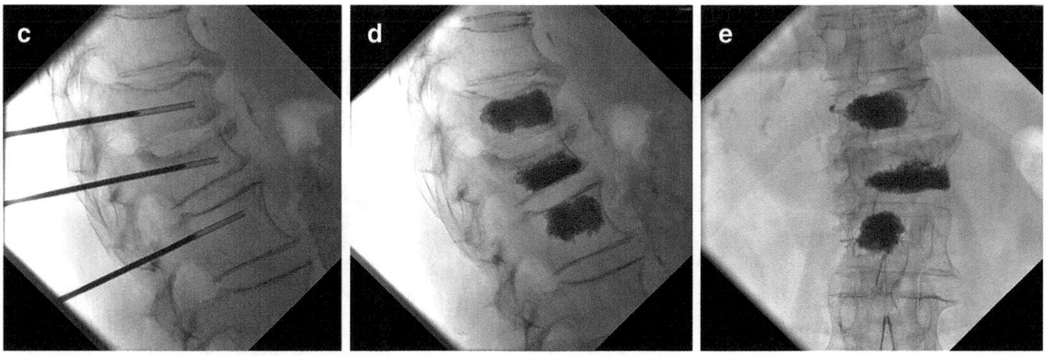


**Fig. 2** (continued)

### 3.5.6 Complications

The overall complication rate following VP is very low, between 1% and 5% depending on the studies and the type of pathology (Hochmuth et al. 2006; McGraw et al. 2003). Apart from complications which may occur in any spinal procedure (infection, bleeding, needle misplacement), specific complications of VP essentially include cement leakages. Most of the reported leakages are asymptomatic (intradiscal, anterior, or lateral cement leakages). However, the most feared complications during VP are spinal canal leakage and pulmonary embolism. These complications are exceptional, and highly diminished by the use of realtime fluoroscopic monitoring, improvement of cement viscosity slow cement injection. A debate exists on the impact of VP on future spinal fractures. It has been shown that VP does not influence the occurrence of secondary fractures, through many reports.

## 4 Percutaneous Treatment of Primary and Secondary Tumors

### 4.1 Introduction

Primary spine tumors are quite frequent and they include multiple lesions that can be classified into benign (hemangioma, aneurysmal bone cyst, osteochondroma, osteoblastoma, eosinophilic granuloma, hemangiopericitoma, giant cell tumor) or malignant being solitary (chordoma, chondrosarcoma, Ewing sarcoma, plasmacytoma) or multiple (multiple myeloma, lymphoma, leukemia).

A second classification distinguish tumors based on tissue origin dividing primary spine tumors in osteogenic, condrogenic, fibrogenic, vascular, emo-lymphatic, and notochordal.

The most common primary malignant tumors is multiple myeloma (9.8% of all cases) followed by chordoma (8.5% of all cases) while the most common primary benign spine tumor is certainly vertebral hemangioma (28.1% of all cases) followed by giant cell tumor (15.7% of all cases), osteoblastoma (4.4% of all cases), and aneurysmal bone cyst (1%) (Zhou et al. 2017; Zileli et al. 2013).

Spine metastases are the most frequent malignant bone lesions. Breast, lung, prostate cancers represent the most common primary tumors causing bone metastasis involving different portions of the metamer, with often untreatable pain and oncologic instability. A majority of them (Constans et al. 1983) have osteolytic features (70.9%), while the 21.1% are mixed and only the 8.0% have an osteoblastic pattern.

The management of primary or secondary vertebral lesion must be multidisciplinary and multiple treatment options (Ha et al. 2015; Lim et al. 2009) are available for neoplastic patients depending on primary tumor, biological markers, disease stage, and risk of recurrence.

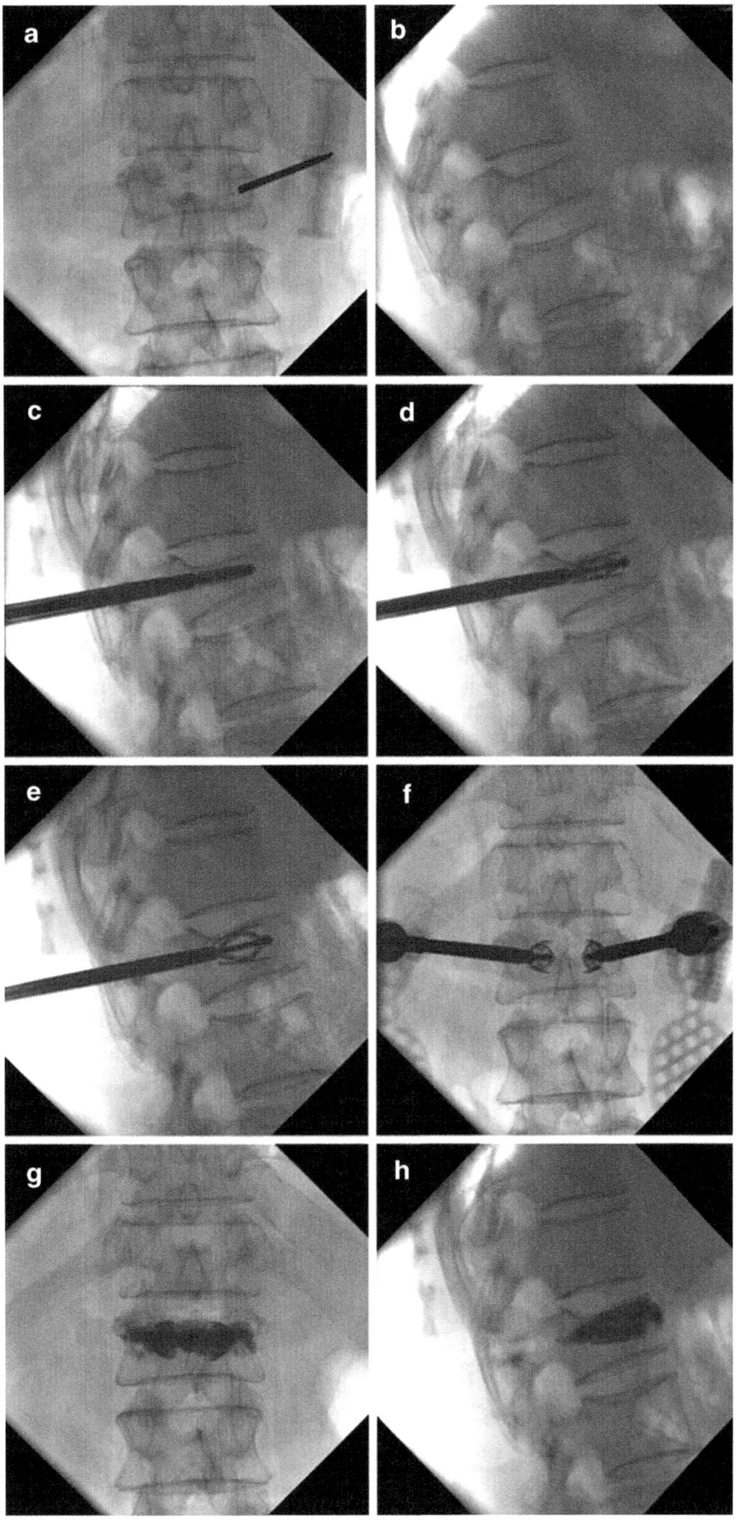


**Fig. 3** (**a**, **b**) Recent traumatic fracture at the L1 level with superior endplate fracture. (**c**, **d**) Percutaneous bilateral approach with spine jack positioning to create a cavity and to restore vertebral height. (**e**, **f**) X-ray control after opening spine jack. (**g**, **h**) Final control after cement injection with vertebral height restoration

## 4.2 Mini-invasive Treatment of Spine Metastasis

The choice of the treatment depends on multiple factors such as clinical symptoms, the age of patient, tumor nature, biological marker, and disease diffusion. The best treatment must be established on each patient with a combination of different options: surgery, radiation therapy, chemotherapy, hormono-therapy, radio-metabolic therapy, medical therapy with biphosfonates, endovascular embolization (for renal cell cancer or thyroid cancer), RF-cryoablation, or mini-invasive approach by vertebroplasty (VP).

Prevention of vertebral collapse (Taneichi et al. 1997) plays a significant role in maintaining or improving the patient quality of life, and it can be obtained only by surgery or percutaneous techniques.

VP is a mini-invasive procedure consisting in the injection of cement into vertebral body affected by tumor by trans-peduncolar, para-peduncolar, or trans-somatic approach under fluoroscopy or CT control obtaining pain relief and vertebral stabilization effect.

It is necessary to add also RF ablation or cryo-ablation to obtain an antineoplastic effect (Fig. 4).

RF ablation and VP are indicated in patients affected by pain resistant to conventional treatment without neurological deficit and without spinal cord compression, without or with vertebral compression fracture.

Secondary osteolytic or mixed malignant lesions can be treated with good outcome increasing the quality life of patients leading to those three targets.

Only in cases of pathologic fractures in patients with osteoblastic lesions, a VP can be suggested.

MRI with T2WI-STIR sequence for bone marrow abnormality detection is mandatory to check the treatment and the number of vertebral bodies to treat; in fact in only 12% of cases there is the involvement of one metamer. Gadolinium (Gd) injection can be performed to better understand epidural or paravertebral tumor extension. CT is also recommended to evaluate better bony structure.

The antineoplastic effect is obtained by using RF ablation device before cement injection. Osteolytic lesions in the absence of symptomatic spinal cord or roots compression can be treated without any major complications.

Patients with spinal cord compression or associated local infection (osteomyelitis, discitis, or epidural abscess) and coagulative disorders are absolute RF-VP contraindication to percutaneous treatment.

## 4.3 Osteoid Osteoma (O.O)

O.O. is a benign bone abnormality which occurs usually in adolescent male patients between 10 and 20 years of age, involving the spine only in 1% of the cases more often at lumbar level. The lesion is characterized by a lytic nidus surrounded by a sclerotic rim that can be of different size and it is composed of well-organized trabecular bone with vascular fibrous connective stroma.

Pain is the most important symptom, very often resistant to medical therapy influencing the quality of life, especially night time relief with aspirin oral therapy.

Spontaneous evolution is really rare, medical treatment is ineffective, surgical en bloc resection or mini-invasive percutaneous procedure (Klass et al. 2009) with RF ablation is the suggested treatment option.

RF ablation (Liberman et al. 2010) is performed under CT guidance in order to obtain a thermal necrosis of the lesion thanks to RF probe placed into the lesion with pain relief effect and sclerotic effect (Fig. 5).

## 4.4 Vertebral Hemangioma

Vertebral hemangioma is the most common spine tumor with a frequency of 12% in adults, and it is, in the majority of the cases, completely asymptomatic.

By contrary, symptomatic and/or aggressive vertebral hemangiomas can be treated by the percutaneous approach obtaining pain and stabilization effect.

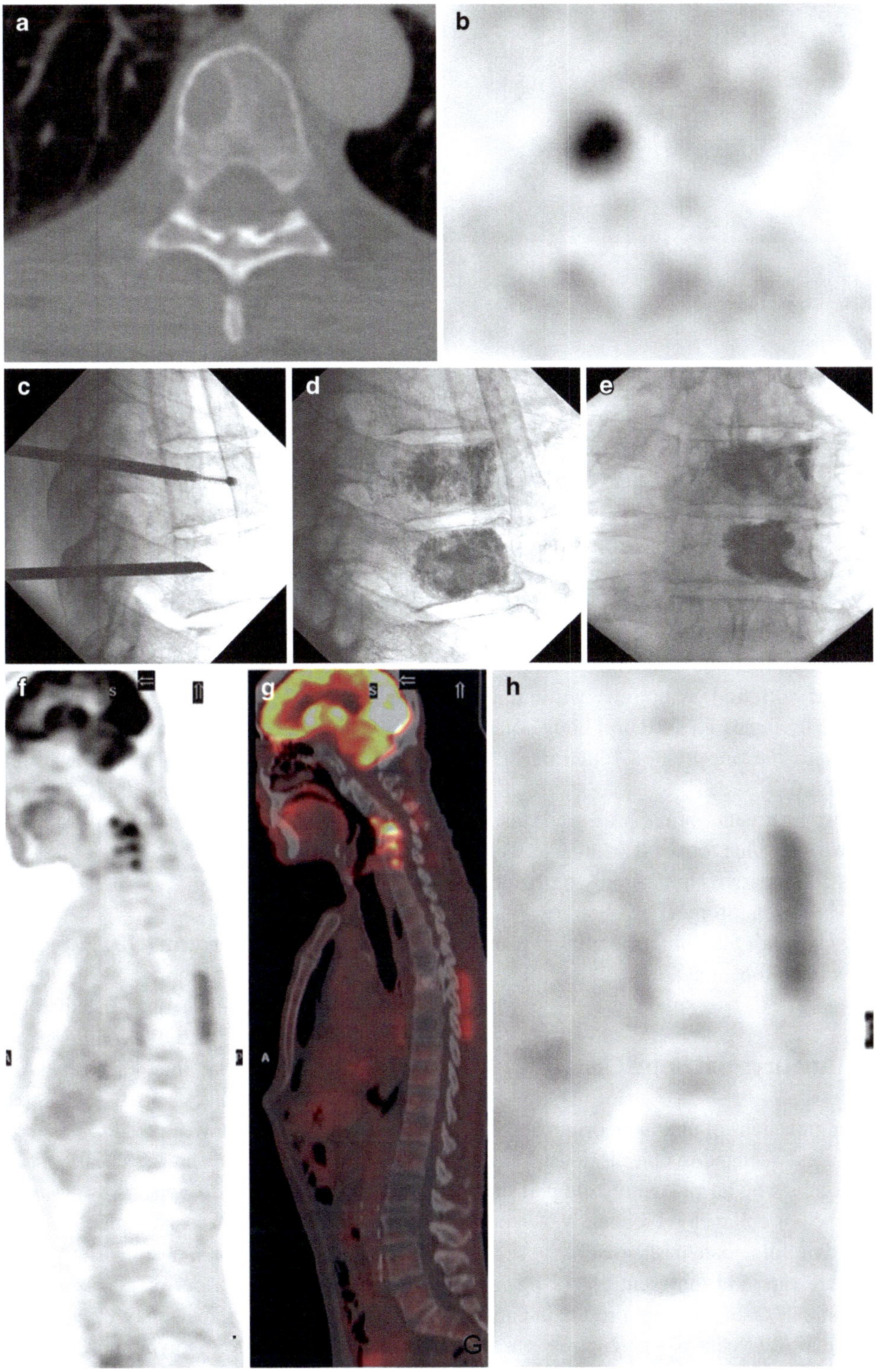


**Fig. 4** (**a**, **b**) Patient with primary breast cancer and lytic lesion in the right half of T6 vertebra with positive PET correlation. (**c**–**e**) Percutaneous treatment of the radiofrequency at T6 level and VP to T6 and T7 levels. (**f**–**h**) PET-TC follow-up at 3 months shows disappearance of the uptake at T6 lesion with the evidence of other lesions at cervical region

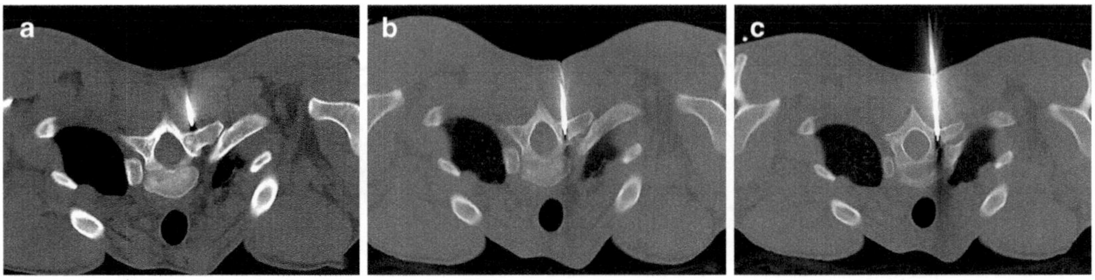


**Fig. 5** (**a**–**c**) Under CT guidance, working cannula and radiofrequency needle are positioned for the treatment of right T2 pedicle osteoid osteoma

Multiple lesions are frequent up to 25–30% of the cases, especially at thoracic level.

They are characterized by capillar venous cavernoma with a mature vascular space between bone stroma and fatty tissue.

Patients affected by symptomatic and aggressive vertebral hemangioma even with epidural extension can benefit from VP as a valuable, mini-invasive, and quick method that allows a complete and enduring resolution of the painful vertebral symptoms without findings of the fracture of a vertebral body adjacent or distant to the one treated (Guarnieri et al. 2009) (Fig. 6).

Another treatment option is the endovascular approach with glue or ONIX in acute phase before decompressive laminectomy or the percutaneous injection of pure alcohol to obtain a venous sclerosis obtaining an epidural vascular reduction (Cianfoni et al. 2014).

## 4.5 Aneurysmal Bone Cyst (ABC)

ABC benign lesions of unknown origin and up to 30–50% are associated to other lesions. They are vascularized cystic lesions with solid part due to the presence of collagene. Frequently it is possible to find multiloculate cyst.

They are rare and represent 1% of primitive bone tumors. 80% of ABC are present in patients younger than 20 years old as contrary to giant cell tumors with mild prevalence in female (Zileli et al. 2013).

20% of ABC have spine location, mostly located at cervical and thoracic level.

Patients can be suffered by pain and acute spinal cord compression.

The pattern is characterized by lytic lesion with thinning of cortical layer with internal septa with multiple blood levels visible at MR and CT imaging.

Treatment options are:

- Surgery with frequent risk of recurrence.
- Vascular embolization with glue injection or alcohol injection.
- VP using a bioactive material injected into aneurysmal bone cyst at spinal level producing an immediate pain relief with stabilization effect and bone formation thanks to its action of osteoconduction.

## 4.6 Osteoblastoma (OB)

OB is a rare, benign bone tumor usually observed in young populations, and this condition involves the spine in up to one-third of cases (Arrigoni et al. 2017). It involves spinal segment in the 4.4% of all cases. They can lead to pain resistant to medical treatment (Zhou et al. 2017).

On CT imaging, OB appears as an expansion of bone with lytic lesion and with cortical expansion demarcated by the thin shell of bone. Sometimes, multiple foci of matrix mineralization or extensive sclerosis may be observed. On T1W MRI, the lesion is hypointense and mixed signal on T2W due to variable matrix mineralization and it enhances after intravenous Gd administration. Rarely, tumor may be aggressive with bone destruction, breaking the cortex, wide zone

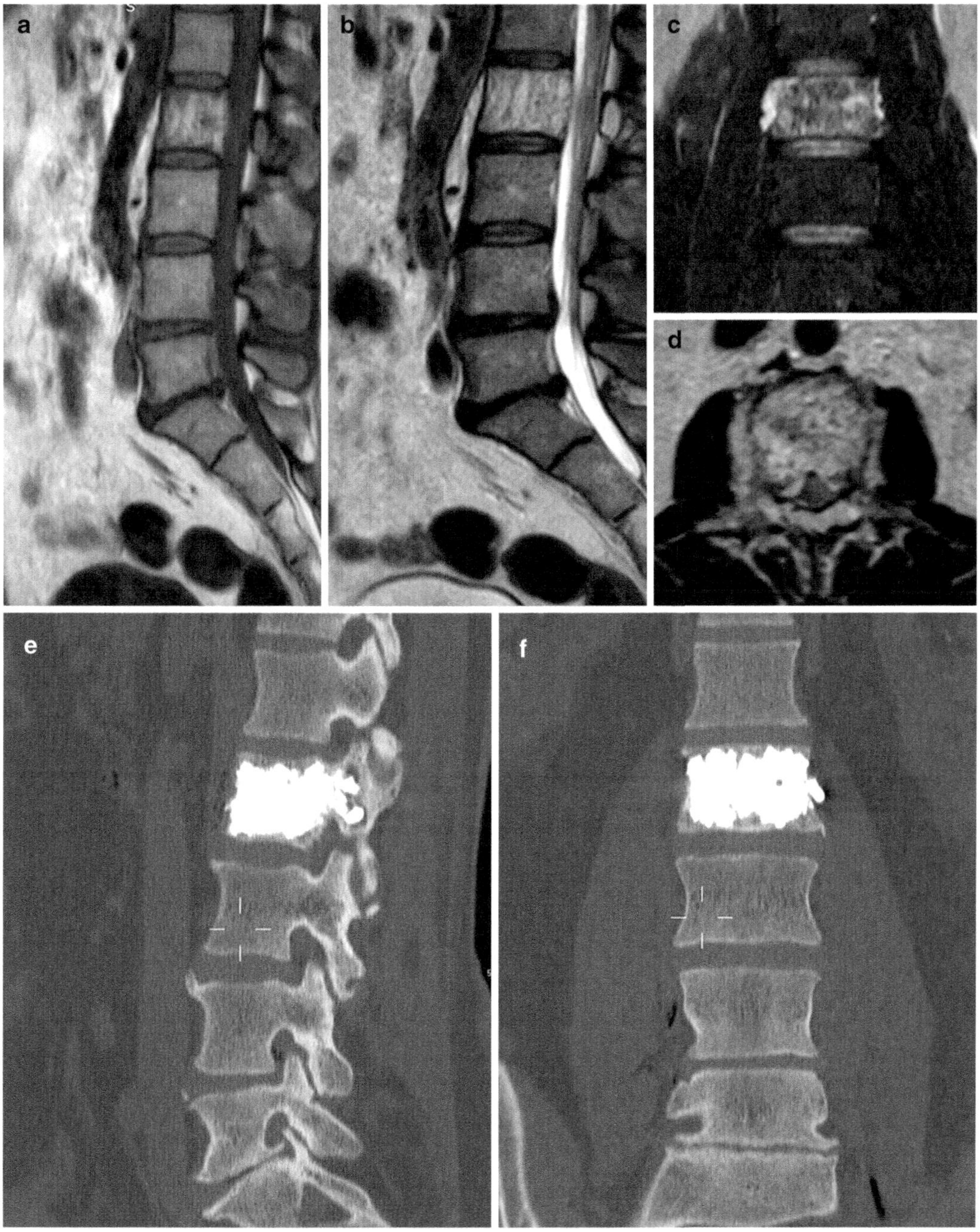


**Fig. 6** (**a–d**) MRI shows aggressive osteoangioma at L2 level with disomogeneal signal intensity in T1-weighted and T2-wieghted imaging and epidural extension more evident on the right side. (**e, f**) Complete filling of the vertebral aggressive hemangioma by bilateral peducolar approach with associated peducolar filling

of transition, characteristic perilesional edema in bone and soft tissue extending beyond the lesion resulting in flare phenomenon (Patnaik et al. 2016).

Curettage with marginal excision or wide en bloc resection is a treatment option, although surgery can lead to instability of the spine, requiring additional interventions to stabilize the segments involved, and can cause the precocious onset of arthrosis or other degenerative diseases (Galgano et al. 2016).

The minimally invasive procedure of spinal OB using RF ablation under CT guidance is an option treatment with low rate of complications achieving a complete success in terms of pain relief (Arrigoni et al. 2017).

## 5 Conclusions

Mini-invasive percutaneous treatment with vertebroplasty with or without radiofrequency ablation association is a safe treatment in patients affected by primary or secondary vertebral tumor with good outcome and low complication rate increasing the quality life of patients.

## References


Amoretti N et al (2012) Percutaneous discectomy on lumbar radiculopathy related to disk herniation: why under CT guidance? An open study of 100 consecutive patients. Eur J Radiol 81(6):1259–1264

Arrigoni F, Barile A, Zugaro L, Fascetti E, Zappia M, Brunese L (2017) Masciocchi C CT guided radiofrequency ablation of spinal osteoblastoma: treatment and long-term follow-up. Int J Hyperth 9:1–7

Buchbinder R, Osborne RH, Ebeling PR, Wark JD, Mitchell P, Wriedt C, Graves S, Staples MP, Murphy B (2009) A randomized trial of vertebroplasty for painful osteoporotic vertebral fractures. N Engl J Med 361(6):557–568

Cianfoni A, Massari F, Dani G, Lena JR, Rumboldt Z, Vandergrift W (2014) Percutaneous ethanol embolization and cement augmentation of aggressive vertebral hemangiomas at two adjacent vertebral levels. J Neuroradiol. 41(4):269–267

Cohen SP, Raja SN (2007) Pathogenesis, diagnosis, and treatment of lumbar zygapophysial (facet) joint pain. Anesthesiology 106(3):591–614

Comstock BA et al (2013) Investigational vertebroplasty safety and efficacy trial (INVEST): patient-reported outcomes through 1 year. Radiology 269(1):224–231

Constans JP, de Divitiis E, Donzelli R, Spaziante R, Meder JF, Haye C (1983) Spinal metastases with neurological manifestations. Review of 600 cases. J Neurosurg 59(1):111–118

Dubner R, Hargreaves KM (1989) The neurobiology of pain and its modulation. Clin J Pain S2:S1–S6

Dunn KM, Croft PR (2004) Epidemiology of natural history of low back pain. Eur Med Phys 40:9–13

Fritz J et al (2007) Management of chronic low back pain: rationales, principles, and targets of imaging-guided spinal injections. Radiographics 27(6):1751–1771

Galgano MA, Goulart CR, Iwenofu H, Chin LS, Lavelle W, Mendel E (2016) Osteoblastomas of the spine: a comprehensive review. Neurosurg Focus 41(2):E4

Galibert P et al (1987) Preliminary note on the treatment of vertebral angioma by percutaneous acrylic vertebroplasty. Neurochirurgie 33(2):166–168

Gangi A et al (2003) Percutaneous vertebroplasty: indications, technique, and results. Radiographics 23(2):e10

Giurazza F et al (2017) Intradiscal O2O3: rationale, injection technique, short- and long-term outcomes for the treatment of low back pain due to disc herniation. Can Assoc Radiol J 68(2):171–177

Guarnieri G, Ambrosanio G, Vassallo P, Pezzullo MG, Galasso R, Lavanga A, Izzo R (2009) Muto M Vertebroplasty as treatment of aggressive and symptomatic vertebral hemangiomas: up to 4 years of follow-up. Neuroradiology 51(7):471–476

Ha KY, Min CK, Seo JY et al (2015) Bone cement augmentation procedures for spinal pathologic fractures by multiple myeloma. J Korean Med Sci 30(1):88–94

Haro H, Shinomiya K, Komori H et al (1996) Upregulated expression of chemokines in herniated nucleus pulposus resorption. Spine 21:1647–1652

Hirsch C, Ingelmark B-E, Miller M (1963) The anatomical basis for low back pain: studies on the presence of sensory nerve endings in ligamentous, capsular and intervertebral disc structures in the human lumbar spine. Acta Orthop Scand 33:1–17

Hochmuth K et al (2006) Percutaneous vertebroplasty in the therapy of osteoporotic vertebral compression fractures: a critical review. Eur Radiol 16(5):998–1004

Kallmes DF, Comstock BA, Heagerty PJ, Turner JA, Wilson DJ, Diamond TH, Edwards R, Gray LA, Stout L, Owen S, Hollingworth W, Ghdoke B, Annesley-Williams DJ, Ralston SH, Jarvik JG (2009) A randomized trial of vertebroplasty for osteoporotic spinal fractures. N Engl J Med 361(6):569–579

Kastler A, Huguonnet E, Jean B, Gabrillargues J, Pereira B, Chabert E, Coste A, Claise B, Achim V, Khalil T, Sinardet D, Coll G, Irthum B, Chazal J (2013) Efficacy of vertebroplasty for non osteoporotic spinal compression fractures. The VOLCANO study: vertebroplasty vs. conservative treatment in acute non osteoporotic vertebral fractures. R.S.o.N. America, Editor. Chicago

Klass D et al (2009) CT guided RF ablation of spinal OO with Concomitant perineural and epidural irrigation for neuroprotection. Eur Radiol 19(9):2238–2243

Knavel EM, Thielen KR, Kallmes DF (2009) Vertebroplasty for the treatment of traumatic non-osteoporotic compression fractures. AJNR Am J Neuroradiol 30(2):323–327

Kroon F et al (2014) Two-year results of a randomized placebo-controlled trial of vertebroplasty for acute osteoporotic vertebral fractures. J Bone Miner Res 29(6):1346–1355

Liberman B, Gerniak A, Eshed I, Chechick A, Weiss I, Shabshin N (2010) Percutaneous CT guided radio-

frequency ablation of osteoid osteoma and osteoblastoma. Harefuah 149(8):494–497. 552
Lim BS, Chang UK, Youn SM (2009) Clinical outcomes after percutaneous vertebroplasty for pathologic compression fractures in osteolytic metastatic spinal disease. J Korean Neurosurg Soc 45(6):369–374
MacMahon PJ, Eustace SJ, Kavanagh EC (2009) Injectable corticosteroid and local anesthetic preparations: a review for radiologists. Radiology 252(3):647–661
Manchikanti L et al (2001) Evaluation of the relative contributions of various structures in chronic low back pain. Pain Physician 4(4):308–316
Manchikanti L et al (2014) Epidural steroid warning controversy still dogging FDA. Pain Physician 17(4):E451–E474
Manchikanti L et al (2015a) Efficacy of epidural injections in the treatment of lumbar central spinal stenosis: a systematic review. Anesth Pain Med 5(1):e23139
Manchikanti L et al (2015b) A systematic review and best evidence synthesis of the effectiveness of therapeutic facet joint interventions in managing chronic spinal pain. Pain Physician 18(4):E535–E582
Manchikanti L et al (2016) Epidural injections for lumbar radiculopathy and spinal stenosis: a comparative systematic review and meta-analysis. Pain Physician 19(3):E365–E410
Mathis JM, Petri M, Naff N (1998) Percutaneous vertebroplasty treatment of steroid-induced osteoporotic compression fractures. Arthritis Rheum 41(1):171–175
McGraw JK et al (2003) Society of Interventional Radiology quality improvement guidelines for percutaneous vertebroplasty. J Vasc Interv Radiol 14(7):827–831
McKiernan F, Faciszewski T, Jensen R (2004) Quality of life following vertebroplasty. J Bone Joint Surg Am 86-A(12):2600–2606
McLain RF, Kapural L, Mekhail NA (2005) Epidural steroid therapy for back and leg pain: mechanisms of action and efficacy. Spine J 5(2):191–201
Moskowitz MH (2008) Central influences of pain. In: Slipman CW, Derby R, Simeone FA et al (eds) Interventional spine. An algorithmic approach. Saunders Elsevier, Philadelphia, pp 39–52
Muto M et al (2015) Assisted techniques for vertebral cementoplasty: why should we do it? Eur J Radiol 84(5):783–788
Muto M et al (2016) What's new in vertebral cementoplasty? Br J Radiol 89(1059):20150337
Patnaik S, Jyotsnarani Y, Uppin SG, Susarla R (2016) Imaging features of primary tumors of the spine: a pictorial essay. Indian J Radiol Imaging 26(2):279–289
Peng B, Hou S, Wu W et al (2006) The pathogenesis and clinical significance of a high-intensity zone (HIZ) of lumbar intervertebral disc on MR imaging in the patient with discogenic low back pain. Eur Spine J 15:583–558
Racoosin JA et al (2015) Serious neurologic events after epidural glucocorticoid injection – The FDA's risk assessment. N Engl J Med 373(24):2299–2301
Rapan S et al (2017) Quality of Life in Patients Following Vertebroplasty. Open Access Maced J Med Sci 5(1):42–47
Rathmell JP et al (2015) Safeguards to prevent neurologic complications after epidural steroid injections: consensus opinions from a multidisciplinary working group and national organizations. Anesthesiology 122(5):974–984
Saal JS et al (1990) High levels of inflammatory phospholipase A2 activity in lumbar disc herniations. Spine (Phila Pa 1976) 15(7):674–678
Taneichi H, Kaneda K, Takeda N et al (1997) Risk factors and probability of vertebral body collapse in metastases of the thoracic and lumbar spine. Spine 22:239–245
Vanni D et al (2016) Intraforaminal ozone therapy and particular side effects: preliminary results and early warning. Acta Neurochir 158(5):991–993
Vos T, GBD 2016 Disease and Injury Incidence and Prevalence et al (2017) Global, regional, and national incidence, prevalence, and years lived with disability for 328 diseases and injuries for 195 countries, 1990–2016: a systematic analysis for the Global Burden of Disease Study 2016. Lancet 390(10100):1211–1259
Wenig CM et al (2009) Costs of back pain in Germany. Eur J Pain 13(3):280–286
Yang EZ et al (2016) Percutaneous vertebroplasty versus conservative treatment in aged patients with acute osteoporotic vertebral compression fractures: a prospective randomized controlled clinical study. Spine (Phila Pa 1976) 41(8):653–660
Zhou Z, Wang X, Wu Z, Huang W, Xiao J (2017) Epidemiological characteristics of primary spinal osseous tumors in Eastern China. World J Surg Oncol 15(1):73
Zileli M et al (2013) ABC of the spine. Eur Spine J 22(3):593–601

# Part III

# Spine: Traumatic Emergent Injuries
(M. Scaglione, IT, J. Spraat & E. Dick, UK)

# Introduction: Traumatic Spinal Cord and Spine Injury. Stability and Instability Concepts

Alfredo Bucciero

## Contents



Spinal traumas are injuries resulting from extrinsic insults inflicted on the vertebral column (vertebrae, intervertebral articulations, ligaments) and/or structures contained in the vertebral canal (spinal cord, nerve roots). They are caused by road, work or sport accidents, violences, or falls. The mechanism of injury can be direct or indirect: direct mechanism is due to contact forces secondary to impact of the spine, whereas indirect mechanism is due to non-contact forces secondary to exaggerated movements of the spine.

*Injuries to the vertebral column* are determined by impact, compression, tension, shear, bending, rotation/torsion, or combined forces and depend on the resistance at the failure of the vertebral column structures

A. Bucciero (✉)
Department of Neurosurgery, Pinetagrande, Castel Volturno, Italy

**According Frank and Frank (2016):**

- Tensile failure load (kg) is 102 for cervical vertebrale, 147 for upper thoracic vertebrae, 298 for lower thoracic vertebrae, 409 for lumbar vertebrae, 88 for cervical discs, 118 for upper thoracic discs, 244 for lower thoracic discs, and 325 for lumbar discs.
- Compression failure load (kg) is 305 for cervical vertebrae, 308 for upper thoracic vertebrae, 345 for middle thoracic vertebrae, 458 for lower thoracic vertebrae, 505 for lumbar vertebrae, 320 for cervical discs, 450 for upper thoracic discs, 1150 for lower thoracic discs, and 1500 for lumbar discs.
- Torsional failure moment (kg × cm) is 49 for upper thoracic vertebrae, 90 for middle thoracic vertebrae, 239 for lower thoracic vertebrae, 214 for lumbar vertebrae, 31 for cervical discs, 84 for upper thoracic discs, 167 for middle thoracic discs, 265 for lower thoracic discs, and 440 for lumbar discs.



M. Scaglione et al. (eds.), *Emergency Radiology of the Head and Spine*,
Medical Radiology Diagnostic Imaging, https://doi.org/10.1007/978-3-030-91047-1_11

According to Myklebust et al. (1988), tensile forces at failure (N) is 233 for anterior atlantooccipital membrane, 83 for posterior atlantooccipital membrane, 214 for apical ligament, 357 for alar ligament, 436 for vertical cruciate ligment, 76 for tectorial membrane, from 47 (C2–C3, C3–C4) to 676 (L3–L4) for anterior longitudinal ligament, from 38 (L3–L4) to 160 (L2–L3) for posterior longitudinal ligament, from 63 (Th2–Th3) to 429 (L1–L2) for joint capsule, from 56 (C4–C5) to 334 (L4–L5) for ligamentum flavum, from 24 (Th9–Th10) to 185 (L1–L2) for interspinous ligament, and from 92 (Th5–Th6) to 750 (L3–L4) for sospraspinous ligament.

## 1 Injuries Can Be Stable or Unstable

*Spinal stability* is the capacity of the vertebrae to remain cohesive and to preserve the normal displacement in all physiological body movements (AAOS, 1985). It is ensured by a stabilizing system consisting of a passive subsystem, a neural subsystem, and an active subsystem (Panjabi 1992a, b). The passive subsystem includes vertebrae, intervertebral articulations (intersomatic joints, facet joints), ligaments, and the passive mechanical properties of the muscles. It sends a continuous flow of information about position, motion, and loads from the vertebral column to the neural subsystem. The neural subsystem includes the central nervous system and somatic nervous system. It receives proprioceptive information from the passive subsystem, determines specific requirements for spinal stability, and sends motor stimuli to the active subsystem. The active subsystem includes all muscles and tendons surrounding the vertebral column. It receives motor stimuli from the neural subsystem and generates forces required for an appropriate and coordinate muscular activity. Stability of the spine thus obtained is necessary to allow movements between body parts, to carry loads, and to protect the spinal cord and nerve roots (Panjabi 1992a, b).

*Spinal instability* is the loss of stability of vertebral column in such a way that there are displacements of vertebrae beyond their normal physiological limits (Louis 1993). Vertebral displacements indicative of spinal instability differ relative to the involved region of the vertebral column. According to White and Panjabi (1990) they correspond to:

For the upper cervical spine

- Axial rotation C0–C1 to one side >8°.
- C0–C1 translation >1 mm.
- Overhang C1–C2 (right + left) >7 mm.
- Axial rotation C1–C2 to one side >45°.
- C1–C2 translation at the atlantodental interval >3 mm.

For the subaxial cervical spine

- Sagittal plane translation >3.5 mm or 20%.
- Sagittal plane rotation >20%.
- Sagittal plane angulation >11°.

For the thoracic spine

- Sagittal plane translation >2.5 mm.
- Sagittal plane angulation >5°.

For the lumbosacral spine

- Sagittal plane translation >4.5 mm or 15%.
- Sagittal plane rotation at L1–2, L2–3 or L3–4 >15°.
- Sagittal plane rotation at L4–5 >20°.
- Sagittal plane rotation at L5-S1 >25°.

Spinal instability is caused by segmental vertebral column injuries resulting in loss of spinal stiffness, increased neutral zone of the intervertebral motion, and alterated ratio between translation and rotation at any phase of intervertebral movement (Bogduk 2005).

Spinal stiffness is the ability of the spine to resist by force to a deformation (Kurutz 2010).

The entire range of the physiological intervertebral motion (range of motion or ROM) may be divided into two parts: neutral zone (NZ) and elastic zone (EZ). The NZ (measured from the neutral position up to the beginning of the EZ) is the part within which the spinal motion is produced with a minimal internal resistance, whereas the EZ (measured from the end of the NZ up to the physiological limit of the intervertebral motion) is the part within which the spinal motion is produced against a significant internal resistance (Panjabi 1992a, b).

The values of both stiffness and NZ (as well as of the EZ) vary relative to the spinal levels and movements.

According to White and Panjabi (1990) and Ferguson (2008):

- Cervical spine stiffness is 1317 N/mm in compression and 33 N/mm in lateral shear.
- Thoracic spine stiffnes is 1250 N/mm in compression, 900 N/mm in anterior shear, and 100 N/mm in lateral shear.
- Lumbar spine stiffness in 667 N/mm in compression, 145 N/mm in anterior shear, 143 N/mm in posterior shear, and 6.9 Nm/degree in torsion,

According to White and Panjabi (1990) and Sis et al. (2016), mean values (degree) of NZ and EZ are as follows:

- At C0–C1, the NZ is 1.1 in flexion, 1.1 in extension, 1.5 in lateral binding, and 1.6 in rotation; the EZ is 2.4 in flexion, 19.9 in extension, 4.0 in lateral bending, and 5.6 in rotation.
- At C1–C2, the NZ is 3.2 in flexion, 3.2 in extension, 1.2 in lateral binding, and 29.6 in rotation; the EZ is 8.3 in flexion, 7.7 in extension, 5.5 in lateral bending, and 9.3 in rotation.
- At C3–C7, the NZ is 10.7 in flexion, 3.6 in extension, 9.3 in lateral binding, and 5.8 in rotation; the EZ is 6.9 in flexion, 3.5 in extension, 4.3 in lateral bending, and 9.2 in rotation.
- At Th1–Th12, the NZ ranges from 0.96 (Th4–Th8) to 2.85 (Th1–Th4) in flexion/extension, from 2.90 (Th4–Th9) to 3.35 (Th8–Th12) in lateral bending, and from 1.68 (Th4–Th8) to 2.66 (Th1–Th4) in rotation; the EZ ranges from 2.09 (Th4–Th8) to 4.76 (Th1–Th4) in flexion/extension, from 1.24 (Th1–Th4) to 5.31 (Th8–Th12) in lateral bending, and from 3.59 (Th4–Th8) to 5.58 (Th8–Th12) in rotation.
- At L1–L5, the NZ is 1.5 in flexion, 1.5 in extension, 1.6 in lateral bending, and 0.7 in rotation; the EZ is 6.1 in flexion, 2.3 in extension, 5.0 in lateral bending, and 1.7 in rotation.
- At L5-S1, the NZ is 3.0 in flexion, 3.0 in extension, 1.8 in lateral bending, and 0.4 in rotation; the EZ is 7.0 in flexion, 4.8 in extension, 3.7 in lateral bending, and 1.0 in rotation.

All movements exhibited by the spine involve a combination of vertebral translation and rotation. The ratio of range of translation $\Sigma(dT)_i$ to range of rotation $\Sigma(d\theta)_i$ for each of motion *(I)* is called *instability factor (IF)*: $IF = \Sigma(dT)_i/\Sigma(d\theta)_i$. The normal value of the IF is 25.5 ± 8.7 mm/rad (Weiler et al. 1990), and values beyond the upper two SD range are expression of spinal instability (Bogduk 2005).

In the upper cervical spine, segmental vertebral column injuries causing instability include injuries to the transverse atlantal ligament with or without involvement of the alar and apical ligaments, and injuries to the capsular joints (atlanto-occipital joints, atlantoaxial joints) (Riascos et al. 2015). In the subaxial spine, segmental vertebral column injuries causing instability may be distinguished into anatomical structural injuries and anatomical column injuries (Oxland et al. 1991). Anatomical structural injuries consist of injuries to the vertebral column structures. They include injuries to the interspinous/supraspinous ligaments and ligamentum flavum (flexion instability), injuries to the anterior longitudinal ligament and pedicle (extension instability), injuries to the anterior disc-end-plate and capsular ligament (axial rotation instability), and injuries to the posterior disc-end-plate (lateral bending instability). Anatomical column injuries consist of injuries to the complex of the vertebral column structures at any level of the subaxial spine. They include injuries affecting at least two contiguous columns of the Denis' three column system (1983).

By using the Denis' three column system, we may divide the spine from C3 to S1 into three vertical parallel columns: anterior, middle, and posterior. Anterior column includes the anterior longitudinal ligament, the anterior two-thirds of the vertebral body, and the anterior two-thirds of the intervertebral disc. Middle column includes the posterior one-third of the vertebral body, the posterior one-third of the intervertebral disc, and the posterior longitudinal ligament. Posterior column includes the neural arch and interconnecting ligaments.

Spinal instability can be a cause of spinal cord and/or nerve root compression, spinal deformity, and spinal pain. White and Panjabi (1990) defined *clinical instability* as the loss of the spine's ability to maintain its patterns of displacement under physiologic loads so there is no initial or additional neurologic deficit, no major deformity, and no incapacitating pain. They also proposed a specific point system in which a score of five or more points indicates a clinically unstable spine.

According to White and Panjabi (1990), the criteria for the diagnosis of clinical instability vary relative to the spinal levels.

1. Subaxial Cervical Spine
   (a) Anterior elements destroyed or unable to function = 2 points,
   (b) Posterior elements destroyed or unable to function = 2 points.
   (c) Positive stretch test = 2 points.
   (d) Radiographic criteria = 4 points (flexion-extension X-ray: sagittal plane translation >3.5 mm or 20% = 2 points; sagittal plane rotation >20° = 2 points. Resting X-ray: sagittal plane displacement >3.5 mm or 20% = 2 points; relative sagittal plane angulation >11° = 2 points).
   (e) Developmentally narrow spinal canal (sagittal diameter <13 mm or Pavlov's ratio <0.8) = 1 point.
   (f) Abnormal disc narrowing = 1 point.
   (g) Spinal cord damage = 2 points.
   (h) Nerve root damage 1 point.
   (i) Dangerous loading anticipated = 1 point.
2. Thoracic and Thoracolumbar Spine
   (a) Anterior elements destroyed or unable to function = 2 points.
   (b) Posterior elements destroyed or unable to function = 2 points.
   (c) Disruptions of costovertebral articulations = 1 point.
   (d) Radiographic criteria = 4 points (sagittal plane displacement >2.5 mm = 2 points; relative sagittal plane angulation >5° = 2 points).
   (e) Spinal cord or cauda equina damage = 2 points.
   (f) Dangerous loading anticipated = 1 point.
3. Lumbar Spine
   (a) Anterior elements destroyed or unable to function = 2 points.
   (b) Posterior elements destroyed or unable to function = 2 points.
   (c) Radiographic criteria = 4 points (flexion-extension X-ray: sagittal plane translation > 4.5 mm or 15% = 2 points; sagittal plane rotation >15° at L1–L2, L2–L3, or L3–L4; > 20° at L4–L5; >25° at L5-S1 = 2 points. Resting X-ray: sagittal plane displacement >4.5 mm or 15% = 2 points; relative sagittal plane angulation >22° = 2 points).
   (d) Cauda equina damage = 3 points.
   (e) Dangerous loading anticipated = 1 point.

*Injuries to the vertebral canal content* are determined by impact with transient or persistent compression, as well as by flexion, hyperextension, flexion-rotation, and extension-rotation. Mechanical injury (primary injury) to the spinal cord and/or nerve roots triggers then a chain of events extending the damage to the nervous tissue (secondary injury). The secondary mechanism of spinal cord injury includes neurogenic shock, vascular insults, excitotoxicity, calcium-mediated injury, fluid-electrolyte disturbance, immunologic injury, apoptosis, disturbances in mitochondrion function, activation of μ and δ opioid receptors, and increase in acetylcholine and 5-hydroxytryptamine levels (Dumont et al. 2001). In turn, the secondary mechanism of nerve root injury includes increase in intraneural pressure, decrease in intraneural blood flow, hypoxia with tissue acidosis, accumulation of sodium channels, release of cytokines (TFN-α, IL-1, IL-6), increased expression of hyperpolarization-activated cyclic nucleotide-gated (HCN) channels, activation of acid-sensing ion channels 3 (ASIC3), and protease-activated protein receptor 2 (PAR) (Lin et al. 2014).

## 2 Pathology

Lesions characterizing spinal traumas may be distinguished into vertebral column changes, extradural, subdural, and subarachnoid hematomas, meningeal tears, spinal cord changes, and nerve root changes.

1. Vertebral column changes may be classified as follows (AO Spine 2018):
   (a) *Upper Cervical Spine.*
      - Occipital condyle and craniocervical junction.
        - Type A. isolated bony injury (condyle).
        - Type B. non-displaced ligamentous injury (craniocervical).
        - Type C. any injury with displacement.
      - C1 ring and C1–2 joint.
        - Type A. isolated bony only (arch).
        - Type B. ligamentous injury (transverse atlantal ligament).
        - Type C. atlantoaxial instability/translation in any plane.
      - C2 and C2–3 joint.
        - Type A. bony injury only without ligamentous, tension band, discal injury.
        - Type B. tension band/ligamentous injury with or without bony injury.
        - Type C. any injury that leads to vertebral body translation in any derectional plane.

Upper cervical spine injuries may be also divided into:

1. *Occipital condyle fractures*
   (a) Anderson-Montesano classification (1988)
      - Type I: comminuted fracture without displaced fractures into the foramen magnum.
      - Type II: skull base fracture radiating into the occipital condyle.
      - Type III: avulsion fracture of the occipital condyle.

   (b) Tuli classification (1997)
      - Type I: nondisplaced fracture.
      - Type IIA: displaced fracture with no ligamentous instability.
      - Type IIB: displaced fracture with ligamentous instability.
2. Atlas fractures
   (a) Gehweiler classification (1980).
      - Type I: isolated fracture of the anterior arch.
      - Type II: isolated, usually bilateral, fracture of the posterior arch.
      - Type III: fracture of the anterior and posterior arch.
      - IIIa: transverse atlantal ligament intact.
      - IIIb: transverse atlantal ligament damaged.
      - Type IV: isolated simple or burst fracture of the lateral mass.
      - Type V: isolated fracture of the transverse process.

   (b) Lendells and Van Peterghem classification (1988).
      - Type I: fracture confined to a single arch that does not cross the equator of the atlas; each arch can be involved.
      - Type II: fracture involving both arches that crosses the equator of atlas; two or more fragment mat be present.
      - Type III: a lateral mass fracture that extends into one arch only.

        *Jefferson fracture* is a burst fracture of atlas described as a four-part fracture involving bilaterally the anterior and posterio.r arches.
3. Atlantooccipital dissociation
   (a) Traynelis classification (1986).
      - Type I: ventral dislocation of the occiput with respect to C1 anterior arch.
      - Type II: longitudinal distraction of the occiput from C1.
      - Type III: dorsal dislocation of the occiput with respect to C1.

4. Transverse atlantal ligament injury
   (a) Dickman classification (1996).
      - Type I: disruption of the substance of the transverse ligament.
      - Type II: fracture and avulsion involving the tubercle for the insertion of the transverse ligament on the C1 lateral mass.
5. Odontoid fractures
   (a) Anderson-D'Alonzo classification (1974):
      - Type I: fracture of the tip of the odontoid peg.
      - Type II: fracture running through the base of the odontoid peg.
      - Type III: fracture involving the base of the odontoid peg and running through the body of the axis.

      Grauer et al. (2005) divided Anderson-D'Alonzo type II fractures into: Type A (fracture with minimal or no displacement or comminution), Type B (displaced fracture extending antero-superior to posteroinferiorly or transverse fracture), and Type C (fracture extending from anteroinferior to posterosuperior direction or fracture with significant comminution).
6. Axis body fractures
   (a) Benzel classification (1994)
      - Type I: coronally oriented fracture.
      - Type II: sagittally oriented fracture.
      - Type III: horizontal rostral fracture (=Anderson-D'Alonzo type III fracture).
7. Fujimura classification (1996)
   (a) Avulsion fracture.
   (b) Transverse fracture.
   (c) Burst fracture.
   (d) Sagittal fracture.
8. Hangman's fractures
   (a) Effendi classification (1981)
      - Type I: isolated hairline fracture of ring of axis with minimal displacement of the body of C2. The fracture may involve any part of the ring of the axis and may extend anteriorly into the body of C2. The fracture line is then oblique, involving usually one or rarely both posteroinferior corners of the body. The disc space below the axis is normal and stable.
      - Type II: displacement of anterior fragment, with an abnormal disc below axis. The body of the axis may be displaced in extension, flexion, or obvious forward listhesis.
      - Type III: displacement of the anterior fragment with the body of the axis in the flexed position; but in addition, the facet joints at C2–3 are dislocated and locked. Type III lesion must be suspected when the body of the axis is in a position of flexion; it has not been seen when it is in a position of extension or of forward listless.
9. Francis classification (1981)
   (a) Type I: displaced <3.5 mm, angulated <11°.
   (b) Type II: displaced <3.5 mm, angulated >11°.
   (c) Type III: displaced between 3.5 mm and 1/2 vertebral width, angulated <11°.
   (d) Type IV: displaced between 3.5 mm and 1/2 vertebral width, angulated >11°.
   (e) Type V: any disc disruption.
10. Levine and Edwards classification (1985)
   (a) Type I: hairline fracture, < 3 mm anterolisthesis, no angulation.
   (b) Type II: significant angulation, dislocation > 3 mm.
   (c) Type IIa: significant angulation, no translation ("hinging" of the anterior longitudinal ligament).
   (d) Type III: uni- or bilateral locked facet joint.

## 2.1 Subaxial Cervical Spine

*Type A. compression injuries*

A0. minor, nonstructural fractures: no bony injury or minor injury such as an isolated lamina fracture or spinous process fracture.

A1. wedge-compression: compression fracture involving a single endplate without the involvement of the posterior wall of the vertebral body.

A2. split: coronal split or pincer fracture involving both endplates without the involvement of the posterior wall of the vertebral body.

A3. incomplete burst: burst fracture involving a single endplate with the involvement of the posterior vertebral wall.

A4. complete burst: burst fracture or sagittal split involving both endplates.

*Type B. tension band injuries*

B1. posterior tension band injury (bony): physical separation through fractured bony structures only.

B2. posterior tension band injury (bony capsuloligamentous, ligamentous): complete disruption of the posterior capsuloligamentous or bony capsuloligamentous structures together with a vertebral body, disk, and/or facet injury.

B3. anterior tension band injury: physical disruption or separation of the anterior structures (bone/disk) with tethering of the posterior elements.

*Type C. translation injuries*

C. translational injury in any axis-displacement or translational of one vertebral body relative to another in any direction.

*Type F. facet injuries*

F1. nondisplaced facet fracture: with fragment <1 cm in height, <40% of lateral mass.

F2. facet fracture with potential for instability: with fragment >1 cm, > than 40% lateral mass, or displaced.

F3. floating lateral mass.

F4. pathologic subluxation or perched/ dislocated facet.

BL. bilateral injuries.

## 2.2 Thoracolumbar Spine

*Type A. compression injuries*

A0. minor, nonstructural fractures: fractures, which do not compromise the structural integrity of the spinal column such as transverse process or spinous process fractures.

A1. wedge-compression: fracture of a single endplate without the involvement of the posterior wall of the vertebral body.

A2. split: fracture of both endplates without the involvement of the posterior wall of the vertebral body.

A3. incomplete burst: fracture with any involvement of the posterior wall; only a single endplate fractured. Vertical fracture of the lamina is usually present and does not constitute a tension band failure.

A4. complete burst: fracture with any involvement of the posterior wall and both endplates. Vertical fracture of the lamina is usually present and does not constitute a tension band failure.

*Type B. distraction injuries*

B1. transosseous tension band disruption. Chance fracture: monosegmental pure osseous failure of the posterior tension band.

B2. posterior tension band disruption: bony and/or ligamentary failure of the posterior tension band together with a Type A fracture.

B3. hyperextension: injury through the disc or vertebral body leading to a hyperextended position of the spinal column. Commonly seen in ankylotic disorders. Anterior structures, especially the anterior longitudinal ligament, are ruptured but there is a posterior hinge preventing further displacement.

*Type C. translation injuries*

C. displacement or dislocation: there are no subtypes because various configurations are possible due to dissociation/dislocation. Can be combined with subtypes of A or B.

1. Extradural, subdural, and subarachnoid hematomas are collections of blood due to rupture of spinal extra-axial vessels.
2. Meningeal tears affect the dura mater with or without the involvement of the arachnoid mater. They can cause cerebrospinal fluid leakage or pseudomeningocele (with or without arachnoidal lining).
3. Spinal cord changes include edema, contusion, hemorrhage, and laceration/transection. According to Rowland et al. (2008), spinal cord injury phases may be distinguished as follows:
   - Primary immediate phase (≤2 h): primary mechanical injury, traumatic severing of

axons, gray matter hemorrhage, hemorrhagic necrosis, microglial activation.
- Early acute phase (≤48 h): vasogenic and cytoxic edema, continued hemorrhage and necrosis, neutrophil invasion, peak blood-brain barrier permeability, early demyelination (oligodendrocyte death), neuronal death, axonal swelling.
- Secondary subacute phase (≤14 days): macrophage infiltration, initiation of astroglial scar (reactive astrocytosis), blood-brain barrier repair, and resolution of edema.
- Intermediate phase (≤6 months): continued formation of glial scar, cyst formation, lesion stabilization.
- Chronic/late phase (≥6 months): prolonged Wallerian degeneration, persistence of spared, demyelinated axons, potential structural and functional plasticity of spared spinal cord tissue.

4. Nerve root changes include edema, contusion, laceration, and transection/avulsion

## 3 Clinical Presentations

Spinal traumas can be amyelic or myelic. Amyelic traumas manifest with mechanical pain and disability, whereas myelic traumas manifest with medullary and/or radicular syndromes. Medullary syndromes include transverse cord syndrome, central cord syndrome, anterior cord syndrome, Brown-Sequard syndrome, posterior cord syndrome, and conus medullaris syndrome. According to the International Standards of Neurological Classification of Spinal Cord Injury (ISNCSCI), published by the American Spinal Injury Association (ASIA), sensory and motor deficits due to spinal cord injury may be graded as follows (Kirshblum et al. 2011):

- A = Complete. No motor and sensory function is preserved in the sacral segment S4–S5.
- B = Sensory incomplete. Sensory but no motor function is preserved below the neurological level and includes the sacral segment S4–S5, and no motor function is preserved more than three levels below the motor level on either side of the body.
- C = Motor incomplete. Motor function is preserved below the neurological level, and more than half of key muscle functions below the single neurological level of injury have a muscle grade less than 3.
- D = Motor incomplete. Motor function is preserved below the neurological level, and at least half (half or more) of key muscle functions below the neurological level of injury have a muscle grade >3.
- E = Normal. If sensation and motor function as tested with the ISNCSCI are graded as normal in all segments, and the patient had prior deficits, then the Asia Impairment Scale (AIS) grade is E.

Spinal cord injury without radiographic abnormality (SCIWORA) is a syndrome characterized by clinical symptoms of traumatic myelopathy with no radiographic or computed tomographic features of spinal fracture or instability (Pang and Wilberger Jr. 1982). According to magnetic resonance imaging patterns, it may be distinguished into the following types (Boese and Lechler 2013):

- Type I: no detectable abnormalities.
- Type IIa: extraneural abnormalities (disc protrusion or herniation, flavum bulging, spondylosis, ossification of the posterior longitudinal ligament, prevertebral soft tissue swelling, ligamentous abnormalities).
- Type IIb: intraneural abnormalities (edema, hemorrhage, contusion, partial or complete transection).
- Type III: extraneural and intraneural abnormalities.

Radicular syndromes can be uni- or multisegmental, as well as uni- or bilateral. They also include cauda equina syndrome.

## 4 Treatment

Spinal traumas may be treated conservatively or by surgery.

According to AO Surgery Reference (2018):

1. The following injuries require conservative treatment:
   (a) Upper cervical spine injuries
      - Occipital condyle fractures.
      - Gehweiler type I, II, IIIa, and V fractures.
      - Gehweiler type IV fracture with minimal displacement.
      - Reducible acute C1–C2 rotatory subluxation.
      - Anderson-D'Alonzo type I fracture.
      - Anderson-D'Alonzo type II fracture.
      - Anderson-D'Alonzo type III fracture without or with minimal displacement.
      - C2 body fractures without or with minimal displacement.
      - Effendi type I fracture.
      - Effendi type II fracture without or with minimal displacement.
      - Effendi type III fracture without or with minimal displacement.

   (b) Subaxial cervical spine injuries
      A0 and A1 fractures.
      A2, A3, and A4 undisplaced fractures.
      B1 minor fractures.

   (c) Thoracolumbar spine injuries
      A0 and A1 fractures.
      A2, A3, and A4 stable fractures.
2. The following injuries require surgical treatment
   (a) Upper cervical spine injuries
      - Ooccipital condyle fractures (> 8° axial rotation to one side and > 1 mm C0–C1 translation, neurological compromise).
      - Atlantooccipital dissociation.
      - Gehweiler type IIIb fracture.
      - Gehweiler type IV fracture with severe displacement.
      - C1–C2 rotatory subluxation.
      - C1–C2 dislocation.
      - Anderson-D'Alonzo type II fracture.
        - With transverse fracture of the neck of the odontoid process.
        - With associated C1–C2 instability.
        - With fracture line running from anterior caudal to posterior cranial, severe comminution, transdental luxation, or associated C1 injury
      - Anderson-D'Alonzo type III fracture.
        - With sufficient bone stock in the C2 body to secure a stable construct.
        - With displacement and associated C2 injuries
      - C2 body fracture.
        - With dislocation.
        - With the involvement of C1–C2 or C2–C3 segments.
        - With traumatic spondylolisthesis
      - Effendi type II fracture with severe displacement.
      - Effendi type III fracture with severe displacement.

   (b) Subaxial Cervical Spine Injuries
      - A1 fracture.
        - With severe wedging.
        - With neurological compromise
      - A2, A3, and A4 fractures.
        - With displacement.
        - With neurological compromise
      - B1 fracture.
        - With excessive posterior bony gap.
        - With neurological compromise
      - B2, B3, and C fractures.

   (c) Thoracolumbar Spine Injuries
      - A1 fracture with severe wedging and local kyphosis.
      - A2, A3, or A4 unstable fractures with or without neurological compromise.
      - B1, B2, B3, and C fractures.

According to Joaquim and Patel (2014), the following treatment algorithm may help in therapeutic decision-making process for upper cervical spine injuries:

1. In the presence of ligamentous injury (abnormal misalignment, outside the normative ranges of alignment, perched/locked facet joints, increase atlantodens interval >3.5 mm), surgery is indicated.
2. In the absence of ligamentous injury, it is necessary to check the fracture morphology:
   - Occipital condyle and atlas fractures require initial conservative management with cervical orthosis.
   - Axis fractures require initial conservative management, considering surgical treatment in case of:
     - Fracture in the base of the odontoid process in: patients >50 years old, fracture with displacement greater than 5 mm or severe comminution in the dens base.
     - Fracture that does not heal after conservative management or does not achieve a good cervical alignment.

According to the Spine Trauma Study Group (STSG), the following region-specific scoring systems may help in therapeutic decision-making process for subaxial spine injuries:

*Subaxial Injury Classification System (SLIC) and Injury Severity Score* (Patel et al. 2008).

1. Injury morphology.
   - No abnormality: 0 points.
   - Compression: 1 point.
   - Burst: +1 point.
   - Distraction: 2 points.
   - Translation: 3 points.
2. Integrity of the discoligamentous complex.
   - Intact: 0 points.
   - Indeterminate: 1 pont.
   - Disrupted: 2 points.
3. Neurologic status.
   - Intact: 0 points.
   - Nerve root injury: 1 point.
   - Complete: 2 points.
   - Incomplete: 3 points.
   - Persistent cord compression: +1 point.

Treatment suggestion:

- Score ≤3: non-operative treatment.
- Score of 4: consider for operative or non-operative treatment.
- Score ≥5: operative treatment.

*Thoracolumbar Injury Classification and Severity Score (TLICS)* (Lee et al. 2005).

1. Injury morphology
   (a) Compression
   - Compression fracture: 1 point.
   - Burst fracture: 2 points.

   (b) Translation/rotation: 3 points.
   (c) Distraction: 4 points.
2. Posterior ligamentous complex integrity.
   (a) Intact: 0 points.
   (b) Suspected injury or indeterminate: 2 points.
   (c) Injured: 3 points.
3. Neurologic involvement.
   (a) Intact: 0 points.
   (b) Nerve root: 2 points.
   (c) Cord/conus medullaris (incomplete): 3 points.
   (d) Cord/conus medullaris (complete): 2 points.
   (e) Cauda equina: 3 points.
   Treatment suggestion:
   (a) Score ≤3: non-operative treatment.
   (b) Score of 4: consider for operative or non-operative treatment.
   (c) Score ≥5: operative treatment.

## References

Anderson LD, D'Alonzo RT (1974) Fractures of the odontoid process of the axis. J Bone Joint Surg Am 56:1663–1674

Anderson PA, Montesano PX (1988) Morphology and treatment of occipital condyle fractures. Spine 13:731–736

AO Spine Injury Classification Systems (2018) (https://aospine.aofoundation.org/Structure/education/online-education/surgery-reference/Pages/surgery-reference.aspx)

AO Spine Surgery Reference (2018) (https://aospine.aofoundation.org/Structure/education/online-education/surgery-reference/Pages/surgery-reference.aspx)

Benzel EC, Hart BL, Ball PA et al (1994) Fractures of the C-2 vertebral body. J Neurosurg 81:206–212
Boese CK, Lechler P (2013) Spinal cord injury without radiologic abnormalities in adults: a systematic review. J Trauma Acute Care Surg 75:320–330
Bogduk N (2005) Clinical anatomy of the lumbar spine and sacrum, 4th edn. Elsevier, Amsterdam
Denis F (1983) The three column spine and its significance in the classification of acute thoracolumbar spinal injuries. Spine 8:817–831
Dickman CA, Greene KA, Sonntag VK (1996) Injuries involving the transverse atlantal ligament: classification and treatment guidelines based upon experience with 39 injuries. Neurosurgery 38:44–50
Dumont RJ, Okonkwo DO, Verma S et al (2001) Acute spinal cord injury, part I: pathophysiologic mechanisms. Clin Neuropharmacol 24:254–264
Effendi B, Roy D, Dussault RG et al (1981) Fracture of the ring of the axis. A classification based on the analysis of 131 cases. J Bone Surg Br 63: 319–327
Ferguson S (2008) Biomechanics of the spine. In: Boos N, Aebi M (eds) Spinal disorders. Fundamentals of diagnosis and treatment. Springer, Cham
Francis WR, Fielding JW, Hawkins RJ et al (1981) Traumatic spondylolisthesis of the axis. J Bone Joint Surg Br 63-B(3):313–318
Franck H, Franck D (2016) Forensic biomechanics and human injury: criminal and civil applications – an engineering approach. CRC Press, Taylor & Francis Group, Boca Raton
Fujimura Y, Nishi Y, Kobayashi K (1996) Classification and treatment of axis body fractures. J Orthop Trauma 10:536–540
Gehweiler JA, Osborne RL, Becker RF (1980) The radiology of vertebral trauma. Saunders, Philadelphia
Grauer JN, Shafi B, Hilibrand AS et al (2005) Proposal of a modified, treatment-oriented classification of odontoid fractures. Spine J 5:123–129
Joaquim AF, Patel AA (2014) Subaxial cervical spine trauma: evaluation and surgical decision-making. Global Spine J 4:63–70
Kirshblum SC, Burns SP, Biering-Sorensen F et al (2011) International standards for neurological classification of spinal cord injury (Revised 2011). J Spinal Cord Med 34:535–546
Kurutz M (2010) Finite element modeling of the human lumbar spine. In: Moratal D (ed) Finite element analysis. InTech, London
Lee JY, Vaccaro AR, Lim MR et al (2005) Thoracolumbar injury classification and severity score: a new paradigm for the treatment of thoracolumbar spine trauma. J Orthop Sci 10:671–675
Lendells CD, Van Peteghem PK (1988) Fractures of the atlas: classification, treatment and morbidity. Spine 13:450–452
Levine AM, Edwards CC (1985) The management of the traumatic spondylolisthesis of the axis. J Bone Joint Surg Am 67:217–226
Lin JH, Chiang YH, Chen CC (2014) Lumbar radiculopathy and its neurobiological basis. World J Anesthesiol 3:162–173
Louis R (1993) Spinal stability and instability as sefined by the Louis three-column spine concept. In: RNN H, PC MC, JPC F, Winston H (eds) Spinal instability. Contemporary perspectives in neurosurgery. Springer, Cham
Myklebust JB, Pintar F, Yoganandan N et al (1988) Tensile strength of spinal ligaments. Spine 13:526–531
Pang D, Wilberger JE Jr (1982) Spinal cord injury without radiographic abnormalities in children. J Neurosurg 57:114–129
Panjabi MM (1992a) The stabilizing system of the spine. Part 1. Function, dysfunction, adaptation, and enhancement. J Spinal Disord 5:389–390
Panjabi MM (1992b) The stabilizing system of the spine. Part 2. Neutral zone and instability hypothesis. J Spinal Disord 5:390–397
Patel AA, Dailey A, Brodke DS et al (2008) Subaxial cervical spine trauma classification: the Subaxial Injury classification system and case examples. Neurosurg Focus 25:E8
Riascos R, Bonfante E, Cotes C et al (2015) Imaging of atlanto-occipital and atlantoaxial traumatic injuries: what the radiologist needs to know. Radiographics 35:2121–2134
Rowland JW, Hawryluk GWJ, Kwon B et al (2008) Current status of acute spinal cord injury pathophysiology and emerging therapies: promise on the horizon. Neurosurg Focus 25:E2
Sis HL, Mannen EM, Wong BM et al (2016) Effect of follower load on motion and stiffness of the human thoracic spine with intact rub cage. J Biomech 49:3252–3259
Traynelis VC, Marano GD, Dunker RO, Kaufman HH (1986) Traumatic atlanto-occipital dislocation. Case report. J Neurosurg 65:863–870
Tuli S, Tator CH, Fehlilngs MG, Mackay M (1997) Occipital condyle fractures. Neurosurgery 41:368–376. discussion 376-377
Weiler PJ, King GJ, Gertzbein SD (1990) Analysis of sagittal plane instability of the lumbar spine in vivo. Spine 15:13000–11306
White AA, Panjabi MM (eds) (1990) Clinical biomechanics of the spine, 2nd edn. JB Lippincott, Philadelphia

# Traumatic Emergent Injuries: Cranio-Cervical Junction

Antonia Sorbo, Filomena Pezzullo, Roberto Picascia, Alessandra Perillo, Naail Alzuhir, Francesca Iacobellis, and Mariano Scaglione

## Contents



A. Sorbo · F. Pezzullo
Department of Radiology, Pineta Grande Hospital, Castel Volturno (CE), Italy

R. Picascia · A. Perillo
Department of Radiology, University of Campania L. Vanvitelli, Naples, Italy

N. Alzuhir
Department of Radiology, Sunderland Royal Hospital, NHS, Sunderland, UK

F. Iacobellis
Department of Radiology, AORN A. Cardarelli Hospital, Naples, Italy

M. Scaglione (✉)
Department of Medical, Surgical and Experimental Sciences, University of Sassari, Sassari, Italy

Department of Radiology, Pineta Grande Hospital, Castel Volturno, Italy

Department of Radiology, James Cook University Hospital/Teesside University, Middlesbrough, UK
e-mail: mscaglione@uniss.it


M. Scaglione et al. (eds.), *Emergency Radiology of the Head and Spine*, Medical Radiology Diagnostic Imaging, https://doi.org/10.1007/978-3-030-91047-1_12

**Abstract**

The cranio-cervical junction area is a very special and complex region of the spine. Junctional traumatic injuries are common in clinical practice and are mostly due to blunt trauma. In adults it more frequently involves the lower cervical spine, whereas in children the atlanto-axial region is more prone to injuries. Vertebral trauma may cause temporary or permanent disability that may be seen immediately after the traumatic event or, at a distance, as a result of mechanical instability. Traumatic injuries may involve the bone, the ligamentous system, and the spinal cord. Plain film of the cervical spine could be the first imaging examination requested in patients with suspected cervical trauma; however, it has low diagnostic performance, especially in patients with C-spine collar. Multidetector computed tomography represents the imaging technique of choice in emergency settings to evaluate the bone injuries. Magnetic resonance is indicated for the identification of the ligamentous and spinal cord injuries and for the preoperative assessment of the unstable cervical spine. Diagnostic pitfalls are related with technical and anatomical factors; the knowledge of these factors is important to avoid misdiagnosis. In this chapter, the relevant literature concerning all of these topics is finally summarized.

## Abbreviation

| | |
|---|---|
| CCJ | Cranio-cervical junction |
| CVJ | Craniovertebral junction |
| CT | Computed tomography |
| MR | Magnetic resonance |
| MDCT | Multidetector computed tomography |
| MPR | Multiplanar reform |
| OCFs | Occipital condyles fractures |
| TAL | Transverse atlantal ligament |
| OCD | Occipitocervical dissociation |
| SCI | Spinal cord injury |
| EDH | Extradural hemorrhage |

## 1 Introduction

The cranio-cervical (or craniovertebral) junction (CCJ or CVJ) area is a very special, intricate, and complex region of the spine.

This functional unit is constituted by bony segments connected via a complex ligamentous system whose vulnerability to injury may compromise the structural integrity of the cranio-cervical junction.

A comprehensive and detailed knowledge of this anatomical region is the key not only for an adequate surgical management of the disorders affecting this area but also to avoid complications.

The CCJ is the transition from the head to the spine; and it carries unique anatomical, biomechanical, and functional properties (Brotis et al. 2015).

It is composed of three bone elements: the first and second cervical vertebrae (also known as atlas and axis, respectively), and the occiput, in conjunction with a ligamentous complex, structured to perform its unique role of providing stability and mobility of the cervical spine.

The end-result is a magnificent interplay between motion and stability. The occipital condyles form the cranial end of the CCJ and articulate with the atlas or C1 vertebra at the atlanto-occipital joint. The latter is mainly responsible for flexion and extension movements. Similarly, atlas meets the axis vertebra (C2) at the atlanto-axial joint. This joint is responsible for most of the CCJ rotation (Brotis et al. 2015).

Junctional traumatic injuries are common in clinical practice. In fact, about half of all cervical fractures occur in this area (Fine et al. 1979).

Blunt trauma represents the most frequent mechanism of injury in modern countries.

Blunt trauma resulting injuries essentially depends on changes in pressure and shear forces produced by three main mechanisms: (1) direct-impact, (2) compression, and (3) rapid acceleration/deceleration injuries. Combined compression and deceleration (airbag/seat belt injuries) cause spinal trauma most frequently (Romano et al. 2017).

Approximately 10–30% of all spinal trauma results in spinal cord injury (Fine et al. 1979), which is considered a major source of morbidity and mortality, particularly in young people (Hu et al. 1996).

Clinical examination of upper cervical spine trauma can be considered a diagnostic challenge, since many neurological scenarios are possible, and the patient may often have an associated head trauma that may alter the level of consciousness and complicate examination.

The diagnosis of CCJ lesions in traumatized patients is a complex task and often involves multiple steps where radiologic imaging plays a central role.

In the setting of blunt trauma to the cranio-cervical junction, imaging plays a major role in the management and prognosis of these injuries. The acute imaging evaluation of what are usually high-energy mechanisms of injury typically involves an initial computed tomography (CT) assessment and, frequently, subsequent emergency magnetic resonance imaging (MR) assessment.

Injuries involving the upper cervical spine may be distinguished in: injuries affecting mainly bone structures (Menezes and Traynelis 2008) and predominantly ligamentous injury (Hadley 2002). Thus basing on the principle that bone injuries may heal with conservative treatment, whereas ligamentous injury would not heal properly, leading to an unstable spine.

The current imaging recommendations in the trauma scenario include an initial CT evaluation followed by MR, in case of significant bony injury or when a ligamentous injury is suspected (Sundgren et al. 2007).

In this chapter, the relevant literature concerning this issue, particularly focusing on "rare" CCJ traumatic events, is summarized.

## 2 Imaging Approach

CCJ injuries are observed, predominantly, as a result of motor-vehicle accidents, falls from heights, and sports; and thus, young men are more affected. Another age peak is seen in the elderly who have preexisting degenerative vertebral disease.

Even though plain films of the cervical spine are often the first imaging examination requested in patients with suspected cervical trauma, its low diagnostic performances, especially in patients with C-spine collar, and the wider availability of multidetector computed tomography (MDCT) have changed this algorithm (Tins and Cessar-Pullicino 2004; Frankel et al. 1994; Stiell et al. 2001).

Vertebral trauma is responsible for temporary or permanent disability that may be seen immediately after the traumatic event or, at a distance, as a result of mechanical instability.

MDCT imaging best depicts the biomechanical parameters that have caused specific injuries and thus helps to provide rapid and stable therapy decisions (Schueller et al. 2015a).

In addition to the diagnosis of bony lesions, MDCT scan allows an accurate assessment of the stability/instability of the injury, which leads to the timing of surgical treatment, although the issue is still controversial in the literature (Parizel et al. 2010).

The radiologist must be able to recognize vertebral fractures, to classify according to the different patterns of fracture (compression, distraction, rotation), to drive the continuation of the diagnostic plan, and to indicate the use of MRI to rule out or characterize spinal cord injury (Schueller et al. 2015b).

The concept of stability is extremely important for the choice of therapy and is based on the "three-column model" by Denis: the anterior column consists in the anterior longitudinal ligament and the anterior two-thirds of the vertebral body, the middle column is the posterior one-third of the vertebral body including the anulus fibrosus and posterior longitudinal ligament, and the posterior column, which includes all structures posterior to the posterior longitudinal ligament (Schueller et al. 2015a).

The availability of fast, cost-effective imaging methods with high sensitivity and specificity in the detection of any potentially unstable injury that may cause or exacerbate neurologic deficits makes MDCT the imaging modality of choice for the evaluation of patients with acute traumatic injury of the CCJ and of the cervical spine (Diaz Jr. et al. 2005). An appropriately thin-section axial source data-set of 0.75 mm is recommended to obtain adequate MPR (ideally, 2 mm or less).

For the diagnosis of spinal lesions, axial images and sagittal reconstructions are necessary. Because of the curvatures of the vertebral column in the sagittal plane, the coronal images are not optimal and rarely provide additional information. However, sagittal and coronal reconstructions are recommended for a complete examination.

To obtain good quality sagittal and coronal MPR, a slice thickness of 1.0/1.5 mm and a reconstruction interval of 1.5 mm are suggested, both in the unenhanced and enhanced MDCT scans.

MDCT is fast, reduces motion artifacts, reduces partial volume effects, reduces image noise, and provides better i.v. contrast material opacification of blood vessels, enhancement of parenchymal organs, and high-quality MPR and isotropic visualization, which increase the diagnostic power of this imaging modality, to the benefit of traumatized emergency patients.

Since sagittal and coronal references are considered standard in the CT of the spine, they must therefore be included in the study protocol. In some cases of spine fracture, 3D surface renderings can provide additional information in diagnostic interpretation and surgical planning (Bensch et al. 2012).

If axial images and sagittal reformulations of sufficient quality are available, in most cases it is possible to confirm or rule out unstable lesions by distinguishing the direct and indirect signs of pathology.

The bone lesion presents as cortical defects with sharp non-sclerotic edges and fracture lines that extend into the bone. The degree of destruction of the vertebra varies from mild-to-severe comminution.

The evident malposition of the joints or vertebrae is a precise sign of injury and should be considered as such until proven otherwise, even in the absence of bone defects. Three-dimensional surface renderings can help to clarify whether a joint is in a physiological or pathological position.

If only soft tissue structures such as the intervertebral discs and the ligamentous complex are involved, the dislocation of the vertebral bodies indicates instability. Furthermore, the widening of the facet joint spaces is a sign of soft tissue injury and may involve instability. There are normal variations, but they are rarely limited to a single disk or joint.

Enlargement and/or angulation of 1 or more isolated intervertebral spaces also suggests lesions. A fracture or rupture of soft tissue structures is usually accompanied by an adjacent hemorrhage, which looks like a soft tissue vertebral column. Most lesion patterns show a preference for the segments of the spine that are biomechanically more susceptible to each specific type of injury (Bensch et al. 2004).

MR is indicated for the identification the ligamentous injuries and the treatment planning of the unstable cervical spine, for the direct evaluation of the spinal cord if its traumatic involvement is suspected, and in patients who cannot be clinically evaluated for more than 48 h due to altered level of consciousness (Como et al. 2009).

## 3 Bone Injuries

### 3.1 Occipital Condyle Fractures

Occipital condyle fractures (OCFs) are relatively unusual, occurring nearly universally in the setting of high-energy blunt trauma (Anderson and Montesano 1988; Aulino et al. 2005).

Often difficult to identify based on plain radiographs alone, OCFs are now diagnosed more frequently due to the widespread use of MDCT in the standard trauma evaluation (Bloom et al. 1997; Wasserberg and Bartlett 1995).

Occipital condyle fractures have typically been associated with lower cranial nerve palsies, particularly hypoglossal nerve injury.

Anderson and Montesano first classified OCFs based on the vector of force precipitating the injury according to this classification system:

- *Type I* injuries result from axial loading, and the fractured condyle is comminuted with minimal or no displacement; generally stable lesions.
- *Type II* fractures result from direct trauma to the skull and occur in conjunction with basilar skull fractures: these injuries are usually stable, with some potential degree of instability if the condyle is separated from *the cranium* (Fig. 1).
- *Type III* injuries are avulsion fractures that occur from lateral flexion or rotatory forces with resultant pulling by the alar ligament; these injuries can be potentially unstable, especially if a bilateral lesion is present, lead-

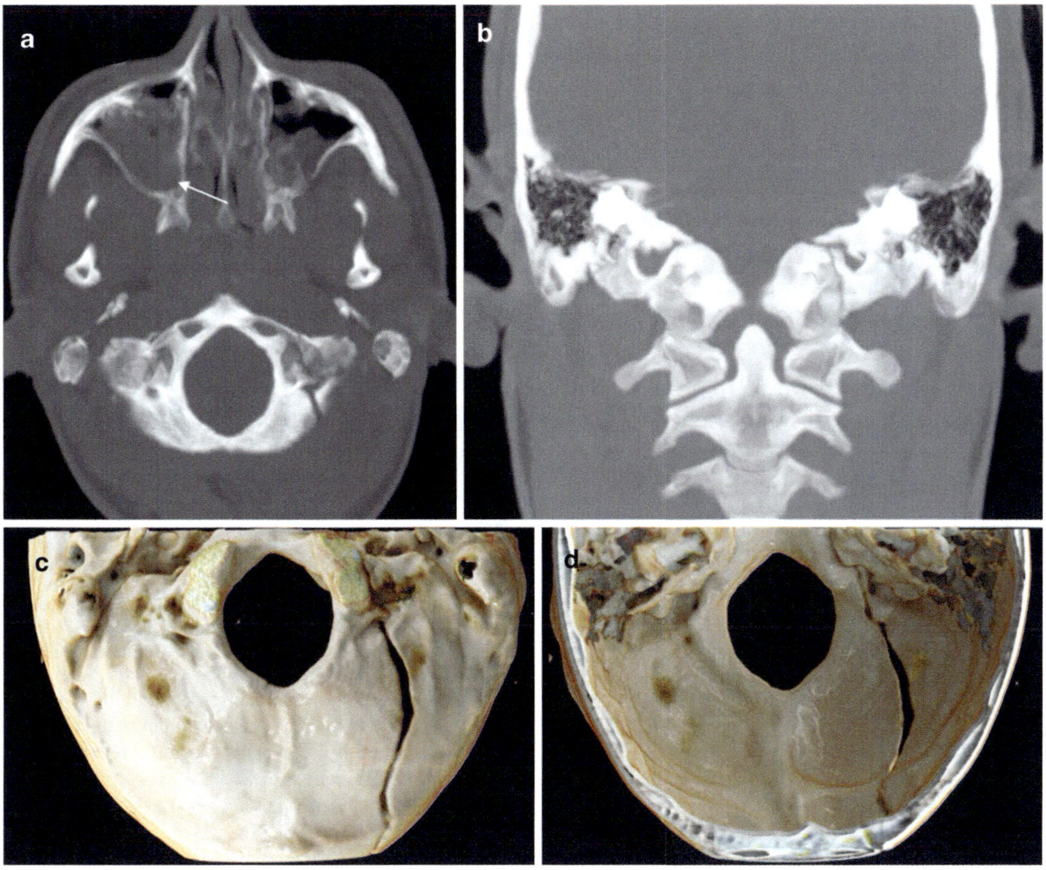


**Fig. 1** A 17-year-old male was admitted to the Emergency Department after a head blunt trauma. Axial (**a**), coronal (**b**) MIP and 3D reconstruction (**c**, **d**) images show a fracture of the occipital bone extending to the left condyle (type II fracture sec. Anderson and Montesano, type I sec. Tuli). There is also a bilateral haemosinus (arrow). This fracture can be associated with lower cranial nerve palsies, particularly hypoglossal nerve injury

ing to atlanto-occipital dissociation, implying ligamentous injury.

Tuli et al. (Tuli et al. 1997) proposed a classification oriented to the treatment and based on the presence of fragment displacement, stability of the atlanto-occipital and atlantoaxial joints, and MR imaging evidence of ligamentous injury. The classification divides OCFs into 2 major categories:

- *Type 1*: without displacement of fragments.
- *Type 2*: with displacement of fragments.

Displaced OCFs were further subdivided into those fractures without radiographic evidence of instability of the occipitoatlantoaxial joint complex (Type 2a) and those demonstrating radiographic evidence of instability (Type 2b).

In the Tuli classification, OCFs types I and II of Anderson and Montesano classification are grouped together as Tuli type 1, as they have the same treatment. Tuli type 2A fractures may require a rigid collar, whereas type 2B lesions require surgical intervention (Tuli et al. 1997; Caroli et al. 2005).

## 3.2 Atlas Fractures

Atlas fractures may be difficult to diagnose. Classically, patients with C1 fractures present with pain in the upper neck and a history of trauma to the top of the head such as in shallow diving or in automobile collision (Garrett et al. 2010).

Once identified, atlas fractures can be classified by the fracture pattern.

Jefferson in 1920 described 4 types of atlas fractures:

- *Type 1:* fractures involving the posterior arch only.
- *Type 2:* anterior arch only.
- *Type 3:* both arches involved.
- *Type 4:* lateral mass fracture.

Similarly, Gehweiler in 1976 proposed a five-tired classification of the C1 vertebra:

- *Type I:* fracture of the anterior arch.
- *Type II:* fracture of the posterior arch.
- *Type III:* combination fractures of anterior and posterior arches.
- *Type IV:* lateral mass fractures.
- *Type V:* fracture of the transverse process.

Landels and Van Peteghem in 1988 reduced the injury patterns in three:

- *Type I:* fractures involving a single arch (Figs. 2, 3, and 4).
- *Type II:* fractures involving both anterior and posterior arches (Fig. 5).
- *Type III:* representing lateral mass fractures.

Levin and Edwards (Bellabarba et al. 2006) in 1991 classified C1 fractures in the following five groups:

- *Type I:* posterior arch fracture (Fig. 2).
- *Type II:* burst fracture.
- *Type III:* anterior arch fracture (Fig. 3).
- *Type IV:* transverse process fracture.
- *Type V:* lateral mass fracture.

No classification scheme from the above has been tested for validity and reliability, and none guides treatment or prognosis.

C1 fractures are a complex group of upper cervical injuries, and diagnosis and treatment thereof require a holistic approach. The context of any concurrent spinal trauma in addition to patients' overall health (e.g., obesity, myelopathy, ability to comply with treatment, osteoporosis) will dictate treatment methods. According to the latest recommendations, the treatment of isolated C1 fracture is independent from the specific injury pattern. The majority of these injuries can be treated with nonoperative immobilization and a hard cervical collar or a halo-vest; certain fracture characteristics will require surgical fixation or fusion. The coexistence of a simultaneous transverse atlantal ligament rupture (TAL) or a long-term local instability requires cranio-cervical fixation (Ryken et al. 2013).

The surgeon must be aware of the fracture patterns that require more extensive stabilization and follow patients closely for signs of instability and deformity after nonoperative management (Mead et al. 2016).

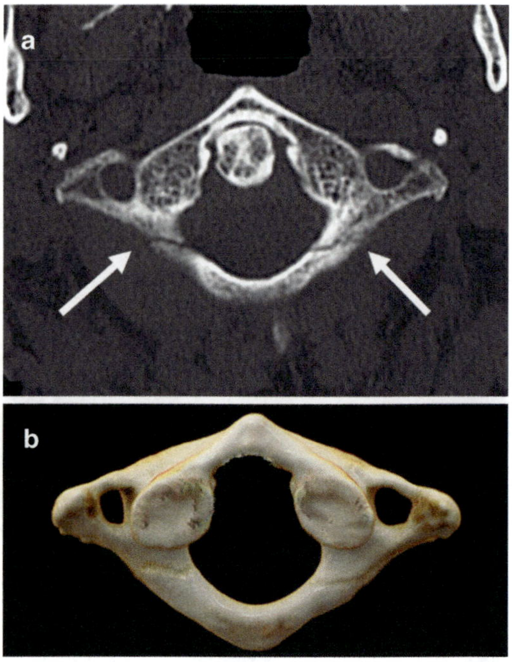


**Fig. 2** An 88-year-old man was admitted to the Emergency Department after a head blunt trauma due to a car collision. Axial CT (**a**) and image 3D reconstruction (**b**) show linear fracture (arrows) of the posterior arc of the atlas (type I both sec. Landels and sec. Levin and Edwards)

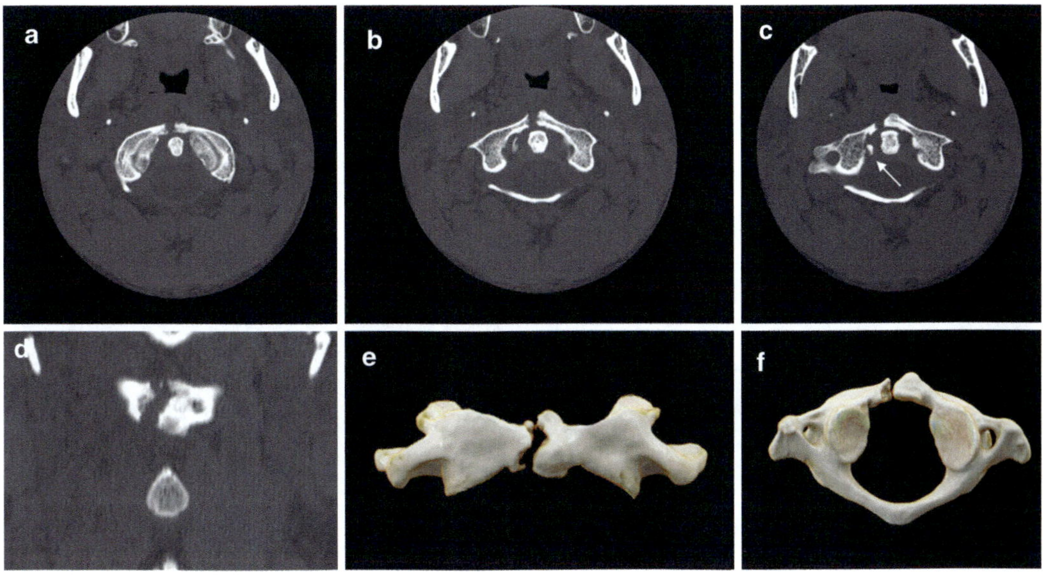


**Fig. 3** A 54-year-old man admitted to the Emergency Department with a history of car accident. Axial (**a–c**) and coronal (**d**) CT images show a fracture of the anterior arch of the atlas (type I sec. Landels, and type III sec. Levin and Edwards), and partial avulsion of the right tubercle for the insertion of the transverse ligament on the C1 lateral mass (**c**, arrow) (type II sec. Dickman and Sonntag) (**b**, **c** not visible on 3D reconstruction). 3D reconstruction images give an overall assessment of atlas injuries (**e**, **f**). Coexistence of a simultaneous transverse atlantal ligament rupture (TAL) requires cranio-cervical fixation

## 3.3 Axis Fractures

Andersons and D'Alonzo classified it into three categories:

- *Type I:* apical dens fracture.
- *Type II:* fracture through the base of the dens.
- *Type III:* with the fracture line into the C2 body (Figs. 6 and 7).

Type II Anderson's and D'Alonzo's odontoid fractures have been further subclassified by Roy-Camille according to the inclination of the fracture line into subtype 1 (forward), subtype 2 (backwards), subtype 3 (horizontal), and subtype 4 (fracture with rotation or English policeman's hat) (Brotis et al. 2015).

Of the three fracture patterns described, Type 1, the least common, involves an obliquely oriented fracture through the distal third of the odontoid, typically distal to the level of the transverse cruciate ligament. These fractures are often secondary to an avulsion injury involving the apical ligament and in, the absence of other ligamentous disruption, are stable injuries. Type 2, the most common of the three, involves a horizontal fracture through the neck (or base) of the odontoid at its intersection with the C2 body. Of the three types, these are noted to have the highest non-union rate with non-operative treatment. Type 3 fractures are, in fact, C2 vertebral body fractures wherein the fracture line extends into one or both of the superior articulating processes, toward the C1–2 joint. These fractures demonstrate a high rate of union with non-operative treatment (Jefferson and Harrop 2017).

Pars interarticularis fractures are best seen on transverse and parasagittal CT images. They are often asymmetric and are considered atypical when the fracture extends into the posterior vertebral body. Atypical fracture patterns are actually quite common and may involve the transverse foramen, placing the vertebral artery at risk for injury (Al-Mahfoudh et al. 2016).

### 3.3.1 Hangman's Fractures

Also named as traumatic spondylolisthesis of C2, Hangman's fracture refers to bilateral pars interarticularis fractures, which bear similarities to

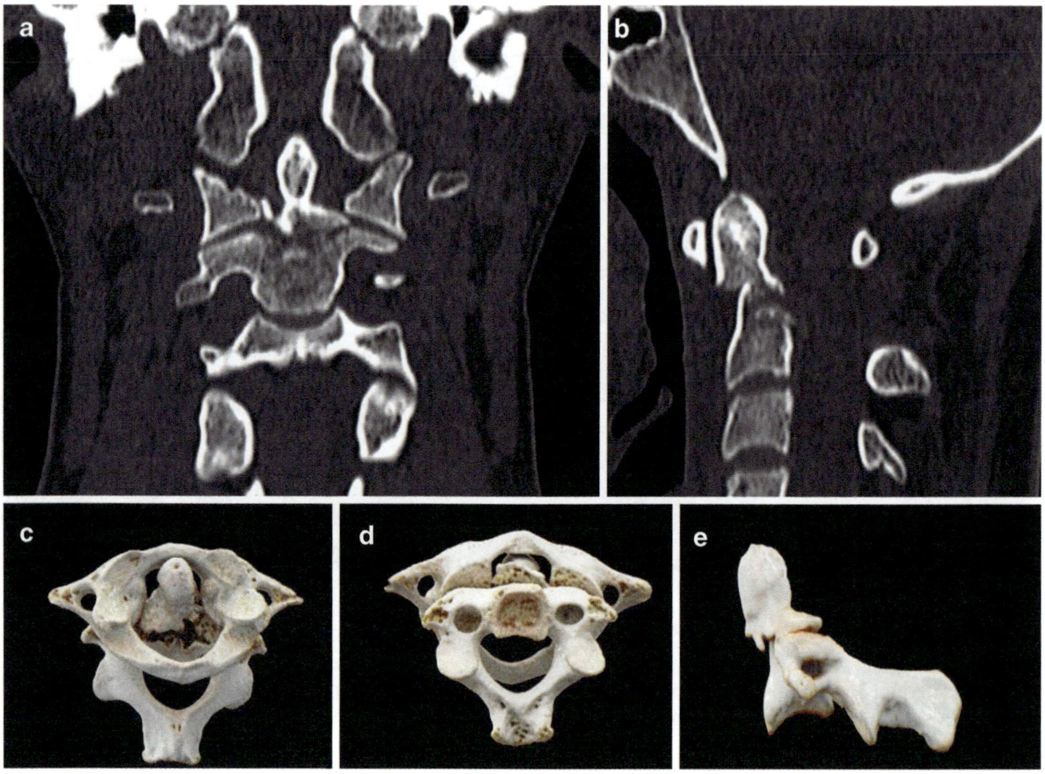


**Fig. 4** A 20-year-old woman after a motorbike accident. Coronal (**a**), sagittal (**b**), and 3D reconstruction (**c–e**) images show a fracture through the odontoid and into the lateral masses of C2 (type III sec. Anderson's and D'Alonzo's classification) with slight posterior dislocation of C2

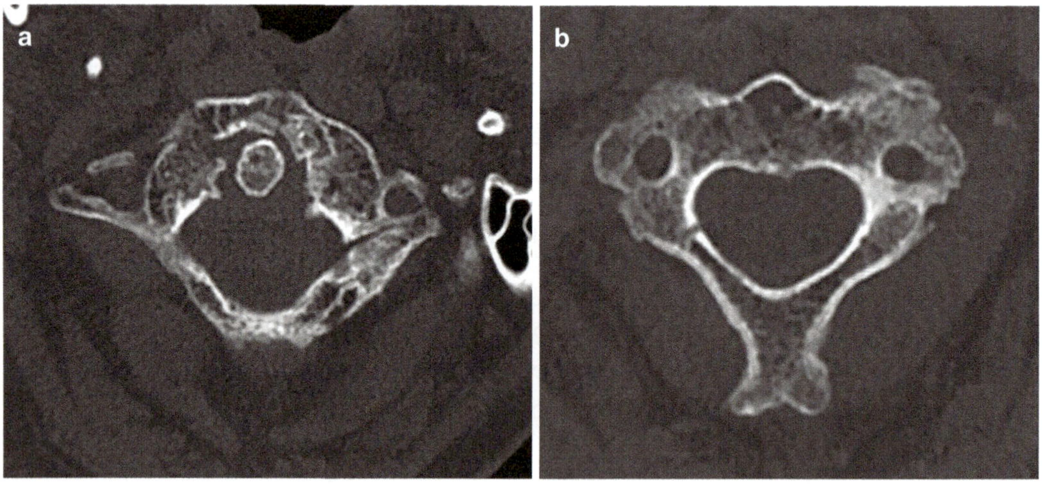


**Fig. 5** A 72-year-old woman after a fall from ladder. Axial CT scans (**a, b**) show a fracture of anterior and posterior arches of the atlas (**a**) (type II sec. Landels, and type II sec. Levin and Edwards), and posterior arch of the axis (**b**)

findings seen in persons who have undergone judicial hanging. Most of these fractures result from falls and motor vehicle crashes and reflect a variety of injury mechanisms.

The most widely used classification for traumatic spondylolisthesis is the system devised by Effendi and modified by Levine and Edwards, as outlined in the following subsections:

- *Type 1 fractures* – Type 1 fractures are bilateral pars fractures without angulation or significant translation. These result from hyperextension and axial loading and are considered mechanically and neurologically stable.
- *Type 2 fractures* – Type 2 fractures include disruption of the C2–3 disk with anterior translation of the C2 body. These are the most common hangman's fracture type and result from hyper-extension with axial loading followed by hyperflexion. They are unstable and may produce a small posterior fracture fragment that can narrow the canal and cause spinal cord injury (Figs. 4 and 7).
- *Type 2A fractures* – Type 2A fractures are unstable flexion-distraction injuries with C2 angulation but without translation (Fig. 8).
- *Type 3 fractures* – Type 3 fractures are combined anterior translation and angulation with facet subluxation or frank dislocation. These are highly unstable injuries that result from hyperflexion and compression (Bernstein and Baxter 2012).

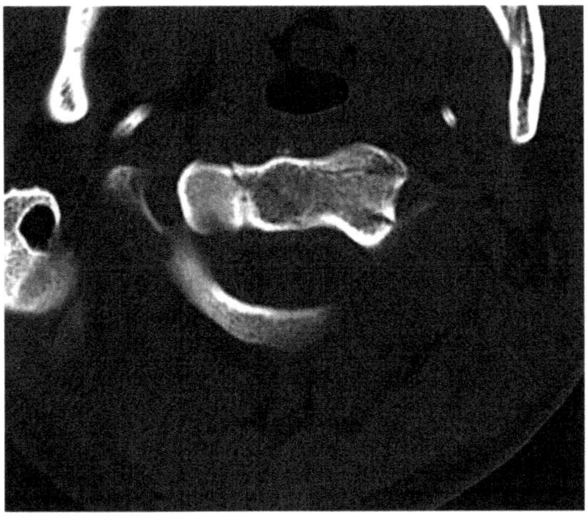

**Fig. 6** A 54-year-old polytrauma patient admitted to the Emergency Department after a car accident. Axial CT scan shows fracture through the odontoid process of C2 (type III sec. Anderson's and D'Alonzo's classification). She also had right femur and left wrist fractures

## 4 Ligamentous Injuries

The cranio-cervical junction is composed of two major joints: the atlanto-occipital joint and the atlanto-axial joint. These two joints are responsible for the majority of the movement available in the entire cervical spine and the anatomical

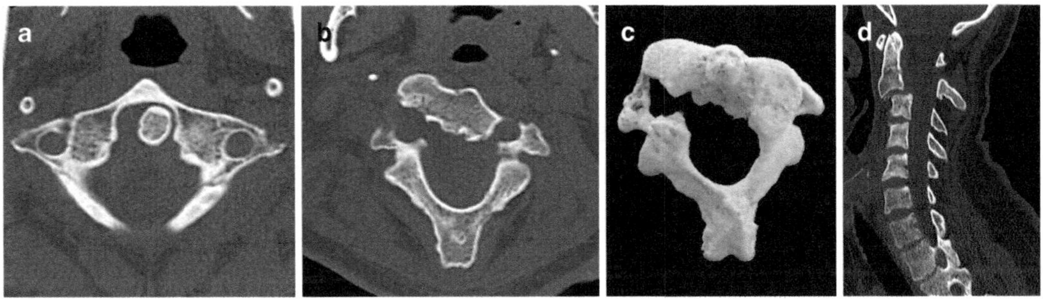


**Fig. 7** A 23-year-old male was admitted to the Emergency Department after a motor vehicle crash. CT in axial plane (**a**, **b**), 3D reconstruction (**c**), and CT in sagittal plane (**d**) showing a fracture of the posterior arc of the atlas (**a**) (type I both sec. Landels and sec. Levin and Edwards), detachment of bilateral pars interarticularis of C2 (**b**), and anterior translation of the C2 body (**d**) "Hangman fracture type II sec. Levine and Edwards". It is the most common type of Hangman's fracture and results from hyper-extension followed by hyperflexion. It is unstable and may produce a small posterior fracture fragment that can narrow the canal and cause spinal cord injury (**c**)

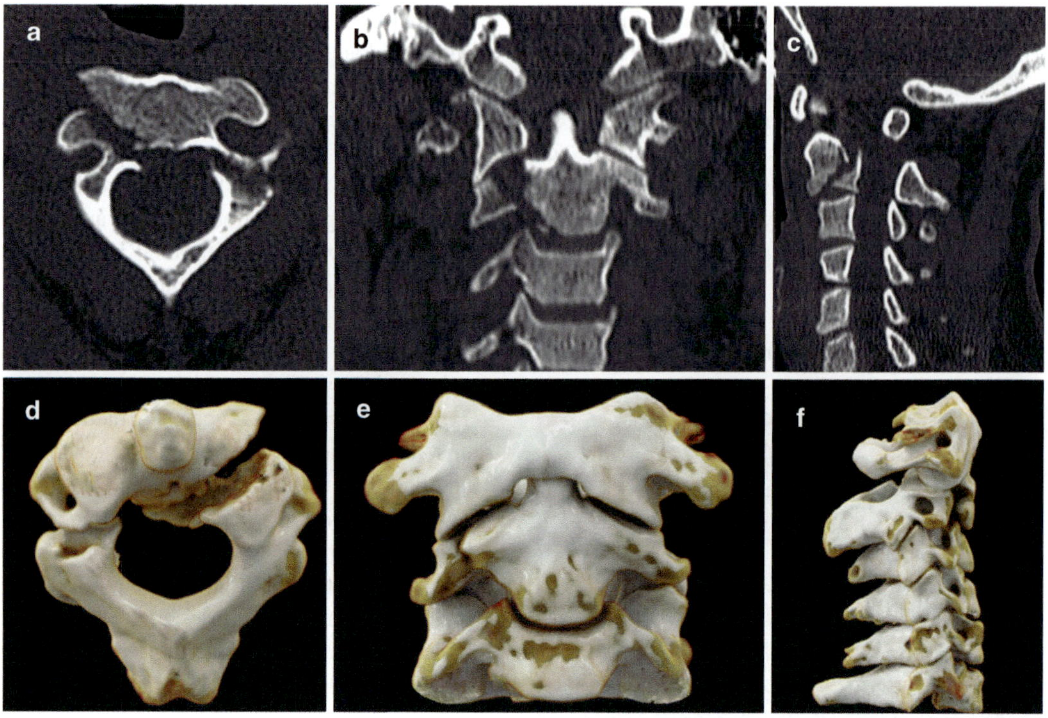


**Fig. 8** A 35-year-old male was admitted to the Emergency Department after a motor vehicle crash. Axial (**a**) and coronal (**b**) and sagittal (**c**) CT images and 3D reconstructions (**d–f**) showing detachment of bilateral pars interarticularis of C2, with a slight translation of the C2 body and an oblique line of fracture and angulation of the fragments (**c**). "Hangman fracture type IIa sec. Levine and Edwards." This is an unstable fracture

structure of each is based on different biomechanical principles. The mechanical properties of the atlanto-occipital joint are primarily determined by bony structures, whereas those of the atlanto-axial joint are primarily determined by ligamentous structures.

## 4.1 Occipitocervical Dislocation

Traumatic occipitocervical dissociation (OCD) represents a spectrum of often fatal injuries between the head and the atlas.

It results from ligamentous injury to the cranio-cervical junction and is associated with high mortality and significant neurologic morbidity.

The widespread availability of MDCT and the development of better diagnostic criteria allow a timely diagnosis and a good clinical outcome for this quite rare injuries, once considered fatal (Blackwood III 1908).

Up to 20% of patients with OCD may have only neck pain as symptom, with normal neurological examination at presentation (Horn et al. 2007; Mendenhall et al. 2015; Sweet et al. 2010). So, any patient involved in high-energy trauma should be suspected for OCD, irrespective of clinical findings, and appropriate precautionary measures should be taken until the diagnosis is ruled out.

Traynelis et al. (Traynelis et al. 1987) classified OCD patterns into three types according to the direction of dislocation of the occiput relative to the cervical spine:

- *Type I* OCD consists in anterior displacement of the occiput with respect to C1.
- *Type II* is primarily a longitudinal distraction with separation of the occiput from the atlas.
- *Type III* OCD exists when the occiput is posteriorly dislocated from C1.

Bellabarba et al. (Bellabarba et al. 2006) recently published a three-stage classification, also known as Harborview classification system more "clinically oriented." It considers the injury severity and quantifies the stability of the occipitocervical junction with the therapeutic implications. Stage I injury is defined as a stable minimally or nondisplaced cranio-cervical injury in which there is sufficient preservation of ligamentous integrity, thus allowing nonoperative treatment. Stage 2 injury includes partially or completely spontaneously reduced bilateral OCD involving minimal displacement (Harris lines within ≤2 mm beyond the upper limit of normal) in which a positive traction test confirms a complete loss of cranio-cervical ligamentous integrity, requiring internal fixation. Stage 3 injury refers to a highly unstable injury defined by gross cranio-cervical malalignment (Harris lines >2 mm beyond acceptable limits), requiring internal fixation (Bellabarba et al. 2006).

Although these represent a spectrum of cranio-cervical injury severity, we reserve the term "cranio-cervical dissociation" for Stage 2 and 3 injuries, where ligamentous instability is complete.

### 4.2 Transverse Atlantal Ligament Injury

The TAL has the role to retain the odontoid process against the anterior arch of atlas, preventing its backward dislocation that may compress or transect the rostral cervical spinal cord causing instantaneous death or severe neurological deficit (Riascos et al. 2015).

Dickman and Sonntag classified the TAL injury in two types:

- *Type I*, disruptions of the substance of the ligament, without an osseous component.
- *Type II*, fractures and avulsions involving the tubercle for the insertion of the transverse ligament on the C1 lateral mass (Type II injuries) (Fig. 3).

These two kinds of injuries have specific clinical characteristics leading to different treatment.

TAL lesions in avulsion (type II) present high rate of healing with conservative treatment (external immobilization), different from lesions of the substance of TAL (type I), in which the conservative treatment rarely lead to heal, being the early surgical internal fixation the best treatment in these cases.

## 5 Craniovertebral Junction Injuries in Children

Atlanto-axial region in children is more prone to injuries than in adults where lower cervical spine is involved more frequently.

The high cervical region in children has several well-described characteristics which predisposes it to injuries:

- Increased ligamentous laxity which allows excessive motion of the spine.
- More horizontally oriented facets that allow excess translational rotation in an antero-posterior.
- Less mature bone maturation (ossification).
- Higher fulcrum of cervical movement (C2-C3) (in adults at C5-C6).
- Higher inertia and torque forces associated with a large head/body mass ratio, which shifts fulcrum hip to up (Oppenlander et al. 2014; Joaquim and Alpesh 2011).

Fractures of the odontoid process of the axis account for 10–20% of all cervical spine fractures. Clinical evidence of acute cord injury for at least 1 day and evidence of acute cord injury, spinal cord or column injuries by imaging or electrophysiological studies.

In newborns, all upper cervical injuries usually are associated with cephalic presentation and the use of forceps for rotational maneuvers.

Combination fractures of C1-C2, as already mentioned, are relatively common (Calvy et al. 1987).

Vehicular trauma is the most common cause of upper cervical injuries (56%), followed by falls (17%), twice as frequent in young children. Athletic- and sports-related injuries (wrestling, football, diving, gymnastics, etc.) constitute 13% (more common in old children), whereas, penetrating injuries account for 4% of all spinal injuries. Odontoid epiphysiolysis is typically seen in children <7 years. The neurocentral synchondrosis, which may not fuse completely until the age of 7 years, represents a vulnerable site of injury in young children. Birth injuries are a known cause for SCI (spinal cord injury) in neonates (6%).

The craniovertebral junction which comprises the basi-occiput, atlas, axis, and their supporting ligaments constitutes the most complex and dynamic region of the cervical spine. The wide range of movements possible at this region makes it vulnerable to injury and instability.

Scott et al. (Scott et al. 1990) in a study on the treatment of atlanto-occipital instability in pediatric patients categorized the CVJ injuries in 4 broad categories:

- Atlantoaxial rotatory subluxation.
- Atlantoaxial ligamentous instability.
- Traumatic atlantoaxial fracture.
- Atlanto-occipital dislocation.

After receiving a child or adult with trauma, physical examination is important in aiding diagnosis; and in a patient with suspected spinal trauma, primary goal should be to achieve immobilization of the spine along with ensuring adequate airway, ventilation, and perfusion. Spinal immobilization prevents vertebral column and spinal cord from further injury during imaging or transportation to a specialized center. In children <8 years, head is relatively larger as compared to torso which forces the neck into a position of flexion when the head and torso are supine on a flat surface.

As children can suffer multiple-level injury, evaluation of entire spinal axis is essential The initial evaluation of C1-C2 injury begins with obtaining plain X-ray films (Shin et al. 2010).

Fracture or nondiagnostic findings on plain radiographs are further delineated by either thin section CT. All patients with neurological deficit undergo MR scans to exclude an acute surgical lesion like extradural hemorrhage (EDH) or herniated disc although the latter is extremely uncommon in children.

Management of spinal cord injuries is usually conservative in children as in adults. Halo vest provides superior immobilization in upper cervical and CCJ injuries and can be used in a child as young as 1 year of age with minimal difficulty (Kim et al. 2011). Custom molding brace has been used especially for lower cervical injuries.

Indications for early surgical intervention, i.e., within 2 weeks of injury, include:

1. Injuries that cannot be reduced and stabilized by external means.
2. Partial spinal cord injury with progressive neurological deficit.
3. EDH.
4. Herniated discs.

## 6 Pitfalls

Pitfalls in imaging refer to imaging findings which could be misinterpreted as pathology, when they may be a normal appearance or of a less significant etiology than originally thought. These may be related with uncorrected technique or to normal developmental anatomy and normal developmental variance.

### 6.1 Technical Factors

High-quality radiographs require careful patient positioning relative to the X-ray tube and appropriate exposure factors (kV and mAs). Underexposure can diminish bone detail, and overexposure can obscure soft tissue signs which could facilitate diagnosis and injury detection.

A rotated spine can result in loss of alignment of endplate margins and poor visibility of facet joints. In the cervical region, this can simulate facet joint subluxation. Rotation can lead to asymmetry in the odontoid lateral mass interval which could be misinterpreted as a sign of fracture of the atlas ring.

In the odontoid projection, if the mouth is not adequately opened, the incisor teeth may overlie the peg, mimicking a rare vertical fracture of the peg.

If there is too much or too little tilt of the X-ray tube through the open mouth, there is superimposition of the occiput or of the anterior arch of the atlas, respectively, on the base of the odontoid peg which can simulate a fracture, unless the arch of C1 is followed across and beyond the peg (Keller et al. 2015).

Movement artifacts may affect images especially in the traumatized spinal injury patient who may also have associated brain injury.

At CT, the presence of metalwork in the spine, e.g., previous surgery, can result in significant artifacts especially if instrumentation is made in stainless steel, whereas titanium results in rather less artifact. Imaging technique, such as slight angulation of the gantry and altered exposure factors, or the availability of new reconstruction software, may help to reduce the degree of artifact and improve interpretation. The use of ultrafine slice thickness, slice overlap, and appropriate windowing will facilitate high-resolution sagittal and coronal reconstructions, which will help to increase fracture detection and minimize the risk of missed fracture (Sugimoto et al. 2012).

## 6.2 Anatomical Factors

In the developing skeleton, the recognition of normal appearances at different stages of growth together with knowledge of normal variants is crucial to avoid pitfalls of interpretation in spinal injury.

In the immature skeleton, areas of lucency may be representative of cartilaginous development due to the expected sites of secondary ossification centers. Each vertebra typically ossifies from three primary ossification centers, one in each half of the vertebral neural arch and one in the body, termed the centrum. Ossification starts at different times in the vertebral arches and in the body. Generally, the vertebral arches unite between 1 and 3 years of age, while the centrum unites with the arches at the neurocentral synchondroses between 3 and 6 years of age. In the upper cervical spine, the centrum unites with the posterior neural arch at approximately the third year.

Exceptions to the above ossification process occur in the first and second cervical vertebrae.

The C1 vertebra ossifies from three centers. Initially, there is an ossification center for each lateral mass which gradually extends into the posterior arch, where the two usually fuse later than in other vertebrae at about the age of 3 or 4 years. Toward the end of the first year, a third center of ossification appears within the anterior arch and unites with the lateral masses between the ages of 6 and 8 years. Failure of fusion or congenital absence of any of these ossification centers may simulate a fracture, but awareness of the normal developmental process, the typical location, and the smooth margins at the defect site will help to avoid misinterpretation (Fesmire and Luten 1989).

The central pillar of the axis (C2) also develops from three segments, namely, the tip of the dens, the base of the dens, and the centrum. The basilar odontoid synchondrosis usually fuses between 3 and 6 years but may be delayed. This should not be mistaken for a fracture. The vestigial form may persist, being represented by a fine sclerotic line, and not to be misinterpreted as a fracture line, which would appear clearly lucent with an irregular margin (Fig. 9). Synchondroses tend to be symmetrical in location, occur at typical sites, and have smooth well-corticated margins.

Secondary centers of ossification (apophyses) occur at typical locations, as do accessory ossicles, and should not be confused with fracture fragments.

Typically, ossicles are corticated and usually have a smooth margin although occasionally they may have a very subtle marginal irregularity. The Bergman ossicle at the proximal tip of the odontoid peg is a developmental ossicle (the primor-

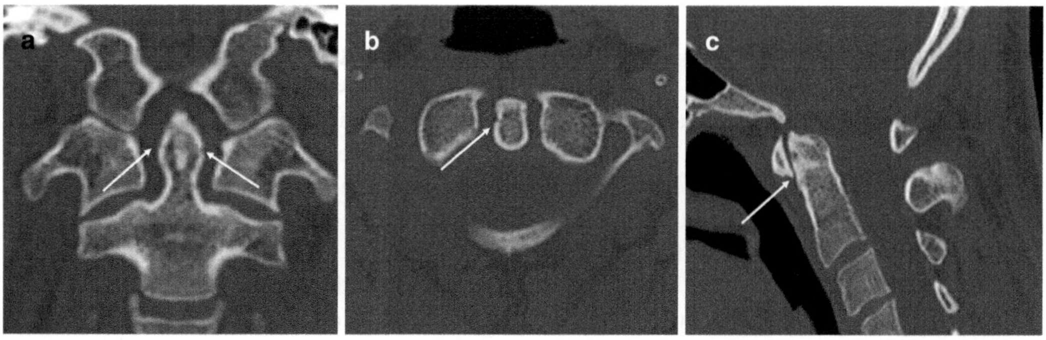


**Fig. 9** A 34-year-old man was admitted at the Emergency Department after a head blunt trauma. Coronal (**a**), axial (**b**), and sagittal (**c**) images show a discontinuity through the odontoid, which may mimic a fracture (arrows). Smooth corticated margin, opposed to the irregular margin of a fresh fracture, helps differentiate this normal finding from an injury

dial proatlas) and forms the tip of the dental axis. It is frequently located in a V-shaped vertical cleft at the apex of the dens and fuses between the ages of 2 and 12 years, but may remain as a separate ossicle and may not be confused with an avulsion injury (Macalister 1893).

The os odontoideum is not a true accessory ossicle but the result of multiple minor avulsion injuries in childhood. It should not be misdiagnosed as fracture and is correctly identified by the smooth corticated margins opposed to the irregular margins of a fresh facture with cortical break/disruption. The os odontoideum can be stable or unstable. The unstable os odontoideum is associated with abnormal movement which can be readily detected on flexion and extension radiographs, MR may identify secondary effects on the cord as focal atrophy and intrinsic cord signal change or fluid signal between the ossicle and its bone origin. These features are the results of chronic instability and are not related with acute event (Platzer et al. 2007).

Other potential pitfalls in the normally developed spine include prominent lucency of the posterior border of the vertebral body, at the site of the basivertebral venous plexus, and also venous channels within the vertebral body as seen on axial CT images which may simulate a fracture (Fig. 9). The typical Y configuration extending to the basivertebral venous plexus almost confirms the venous nature and excludes a fracture (Kohler and Zimmer 1993).

## 7 Conclusions

CCJ injuries may cause acute catastrophic neurologic deficits as well as chronic disability.

Although similar in the mechanism of injury, each lesion requires a specific treatment to optimize the patient outcome. Many injuries may be conservatively treated; others, however, require a more aggressive surgical approach.

Due to the rarity of some of the described injuries, general recommendations for the treatment are often difficult to establish.

As a general rule, ligamentous injuries should be considered unstable lesions requiring surgical treatment. Bony injuries in the majority of cases can be conservatively treated, reserving surgery for unstable patterns.

The instability and the presence of a neurological injury can guide surgical treatment, which often involves early stabilization and rehabilitation. However, in the literature many cases of unstable injuries associated with neurological deficit successfully non-operatively managed are described. Often the prolonged immobilization and the bed rest may be associated with side effects. In some of these cases, occult instability is noted with delayed dynamic imaging and requires late surgical intervention.

The speed and the accuracy of MDCT, both in acquiring data and in reformatting images, make it the most suitable diagnostic method in the total body evaluation of the polytrauma patient.

Actually, it allows promptly managing the patient, establishing if conservative or operative approach is needed (interventional or surgical). MR is intended as second-level examination for the evaluation of soft tissues and cord injuries.

The imaging evaluation of the spine can be challenging and there are many pitfalls to be avoided. Familiarity with normal radiological anatomy, awareness of technical factors which can lead to misinterpretation, and knowledge of normal ossification and normal variants will minimize the risk of over- or under-reporting radiological findings.

## References


Al-Mahfoudh R, Beagrie C, Woolley E et al (2016) Management of typical and atypical Hangman's fractures. Global Spine J 6(3):248–256. https://doi.org/10.1055/s-0035-1563404

Anderson PA, Montesano PX (1988) Morphology and treatment of occipital condyle fractures. Spine 13:731–736

Aulino JM, Tutt LK, Kaye JJ et al (2005) Occipital condyle fractures: clinical presentation and imaging findings in 76 patients. Emerg Radiol 11:342–347

Bellabarba C, Mirza SK, West GA et al (2006) Diagnosis and treatment of craniocervical dislocation in a series of 17 consecutive survivors during an 8-year period. J Neurosurg Spine 4:429–440

Bensch FV, Kiuru MJ, Koivikko MP et al (2004) Spine fractures in falling accidents: analysis of multidetector CT findings. Eur Radiol 14(4):618–624. Epub 2003 Oct 7

Bensch FV, Koivikko MP, Koskinen SK (2012) Multidetector computed tomography of spinal fractures. Semin Roentgenol 47(4):330–341. https://doi.org/10.1053/j.ro.2012.05.003

Bernstein MP, Baxter A (2012) Cervical spine trauma: pearls and pitfalls. Pitfalls in clinical imaging

Blackwood NJ III (1908) Atlo-occipital dislocation: a case of fracture of the atlas and axis, and forward dislocation of the occiput on the spinal column, life being maintained for thirty-four hours and forty minutes by artificial respiration, during which a laminectomy was performed upon the third cervical vertebra. Ann Surg 47:654–658

Bloom AI, Neeman Z, Slasky BS et al (1997) Fracture of the occipital condyles and associated craniocervical ligament injury: incidence, CT imaging and implications. Clin Radiol 52:198–202

Brotis AG, Paraskevi TM, Tsitsopoulos P et al (2015) An evidence-based approach towards the cranio-cervical junction injury classifications. Eur Spine J 24(5):931–939

Calvy TM, Segall HD, Gilles FH (1987) CT anatomy of the craniovertebral junction in infants and children. AJNR Am J Neuroradiol 8(3):489–494

Caroli E, Rocchi G, Orlando ER et al (2005) Occipital condyle fractures: report of five cases and literature review. Eur Spine J 14(5):487–492

Como JJ, Diaz JJ, Dunham CM, Chiu WC, Duane TM, Capella JM et al (2009) Practice management guidelines for identification of cervical spine injuries following trauma: update from eastern association for the surgery of trauma practice management guidelines committee. J Trauma 67(3):651–659

Diaz JJ Jr, Aulino JM, Collier B et al (2005) The early work-up for isolated ligamentous injury of the cervical spine: does computed tomography scan have a role? J Trauma 59:897–904

Fesmire FM, Luten RC (1989) The pediatric cervical spine: developmental anatomy and clinical aspects. J Emerg Med 7:133–142

Fine PR, Kuhemeir KV, DeVivo MJ et al (1979) Spinal cord injury: an epidemiologic perspective. Paraplegia 17:237–250

Frankel HL, Rozycki GS, Ochsner MG et al (1994) Indications of obtaining surveillance thoracic and lumbar spine radiographs. J Trauma 37:673–676

Garrett M, Consiglieri G, Kakarla UK et al (2010) Occipitoatlantal dislocation. Neurosurgery 66(3):48–55

Hadley MN (2002) Guidelines for management of acute cervical injuries, vol 50. Neurosurgery 50:S1–S6

Horn EM, Feiz-Erfan I, Lekovic GP et al (2007) Survivors of occipito-atlantal dislocation injuries: imaging and clinical correlates. J Neurosurg Spine 6:113–120

Hu R, Mustard CA, Burns C (1996) Epidemiology of incident spinal fractures in a complete population. Spine 21:492–499

Jefferson RW, Harrop JS (2017) Update on upper cervical spine injury classifications. Semin Spine Surg 29(1):9–13

Joaquim AF, Alpesh A (2011) Cranio-cervical traumatic injuries: evaluation and surgical decision making. Global Spine J 1(1):37–42

Keller S, Bieck K, Karul M et al (2015) Lateralized odontoid in plain film radiography: sign of fractures? A comparison study with MDCT. Rofo 187(9):801–807

Kim SK, Shin JJ, Kim TH et al (2011) Clinical outcomes of halo-vest immobilization and surgical fusion of odontoid fractures. J Korean Neurosurg 50(1):17–22

Kohler A, Zimmer EA (1993) Shoulder girdle and thorax. In: Schmidt S, Freyschmidt J, Kohler A (eds) Borderlands of normal and early pathologic findings in skeletal radiology, 4th edn. Thieme Medial Publishers, New York, pp 234–245

Macalister A (1893) Notes on the development and variations of the atlas. J Anat Physiol. 27:519–542

Mead LB, Millhouse PW, Krystal J et al (2016) C1 fractures: a review of diagnoses, management options, and outcomes. Curr Rev Musculoskelet Med 9(3):255–262
Mendenhall SK, Sivaganesan A, Mistry A et al (2015) Traumatic atlanto-occipital dislocation: comprehensive assessment of mortality, neurologic improvement, and patient-reported outcomes at a Level 1 trauma center over 15 years. Spine J 15:2385–2395
Menezes AH, Traynelis VC (2008) Anatomy and biomechanics of normal craniovertebral junction (a) and biomechanics of stabilization (b). Childs Nerv Syst 24:1091–1100
Oppenlander ME, Clark JC, Sonntag VK et al (2014) Pediatric craniovertebral junction trauma. Adv Tech Stand Neurosurg 40:333–353
Parizel PM, van der Zijden T, Gaudino S et al (2010) Trauma of the spine and spinal cord: imaging strategies. Eur Spine J 19(1):8–17
Platzer P, Jaindl M, Thalhammer G et al (2007) Cervical spine injuries in pediatric patients. J Trauma 62:389–396
Riascos R, Bonfante E, Cotes C et al (2015) Imaging of atlanto-occipital and atlantoaxial traumatic injuries: what the radiologist needs to know. Radiographics 35(7):2121–2134
Romano F, Iacobellis F, Guida F et al (2017) Traumatic injuries: mechanisms of lesions. In: Diagnostic imaging in polytrauma patients. Springer, Cham, pp 35–50
Ryken TC, Aarabi B, Dhall SS et al (2013) Management of isolated fractures of the atlas in adults. Neurosurgery 72(2):127–131
Schueller G, Scaglione M, Linsenmaier U et al (2015a) The key role of the radiologist in the management of polytrauma patients: indications for MDCT imaging in emergency radiology. Radiol Med 120(7):641–654
Schueller G, Scaglione M, Linsenmaier U et al (2015b) The key role of the radiologist in the management of polytrauma patients: indications for MDCT imaging in emergency radiology. Radiol Med 120(7):641–654. https://doi.org/10.1007/s11547-015-0500-x
Scott EW, Haid RW Jr, Peace D (1990) Type I fractures of the odontoid process: implications for atlanto-occipital instability. Case report. J Neurosurg 72(3):488–492
Shin JJ, Kim SJ, Kim TH et al (2010) Optimal use of the halo-vest orthosis for upper cervical spine injuries. Yosei Med J 51(5):648–652
Stiell IG, Wells GA, Vandemheen KL et al (2001) The Canadian C-spine rule for radiography in alert and stable trauma patients. JAMA 286:1841–1848
Sugimoto Y, Ito Y, Shiozaki Y, Shimokawa T, Mazaki T (2012) Motion induced artifact mimicking cervical dens fracture on the CT scan: a case report. Asian Spine J 6(3):216–218
Sundgren PC, Philipp M, Maly PV (2007) Spinal trauma. Neuroimaging Clin N Am 17:73–85
Sweet J, Ammerman J, Deshmukh V et al (2010) Cruciate paralysis secondary to traumatic atlanto-occipital dislocation. J Neurosurg Spine 12:19–21
Tins BJ, Cessar-Pullicino VN (2004) Imaging of acute cervical spine injuries: review and outlook. Clin Radiol 59:865–880
Traynelis VC, Marano GD, Dunker RO et al (1987) Traumatic atlanto-occipital dislocation. Case report. J Neurosurg 66(5):789
Tuli S, Tator CH, Fehlings MG (1997) Occipital condyle fractures. Neurosurgery 41:368–377
Wasserberg J, Bartlett RJ (1995) Occipital condyle fractures diagnosed by high-definition CT and coronal reconstructions. Neuroradiology 37:370–373

# Cervical Spine Injury

Gerd Schueller and Ulrich Linsenmaier

## Contents



**Abstract**

The assessment of cervical spine injury during the initial clinical evaluation is challenging as patients often present with a decreased level of consciousness according to concurrent head injuries or intensive care medication. Hence, the timely and accurate diagnosis is one of the key issues for emergency radiologists, representing a prerequisite for the initiation of a proper clinical management in cervical spine trauma. In particular, timely considering fractures as stable or instable and reporting existing and helping to avoid subsequent injury to the spinal cord define the crucial tasks. CT and MR imaging are the workhorses in the cervical spine injury workup. These modalities are essential in the comprehensive assessment of the patterns and the extent of an injury, and in providing a prediction of the patients' out-

G. Schueller (✉)
ERS Emergency Radiology Schueller,
Zug, Switzerland
e-mail: info@emergencyradiology.ch

U. Linsenmaier
Helios Kliniken Munich, Munich, Germany
e-mail: ulrich.linsenmaier@helios-kliniken.de



M. Scaglione et al. (eds.), *Emergency Radiology of the Head and Spine*,
Medical Radiology Diagnostic Imaging, https://doi.org/10.1007/978-3-030-91047-1_13

come. This chapter outlines the fundamental keys to the classifications, biomechanical considerations and the diagnosis of the subaxial cervical spine.

## 1 Introduction

The prevalence of cervical spine injury (CSI) is reported to be 1–14% of all trauma patients and represents a potentially devastating trauma with an associated in-hospital mortality as high as of 6% (Jain et al. 2015). The incidence of cerebral spine fracture is 12/100,000, being more common in males than in females (Clayton et al. 2012; Lowery et al. 2001; Sanchez et al. 2005). The highest incidence rate is reported to be among patients aged from 15 to 45 years, with a second peak in those aged from 65 to 80 years (Clayton et al. 2012; Leucht et al. 2009; Ryan and Henderson 1992). In these, pre-existing degenerative disease makes the cervical spine more prone to sustaining acute damage.

The cervical spine is most often injured in motor vehicle accidents, after falls from heights, and during sports activities (Roberge et al. 1988; Thompson et al. 2009). The incidence of CSI in the setting of head injury has been reported to range between 1.8 and 9% (Hills and Deane 1993; Mulligan et al. 2010; Yanar et al. 2007). Conversely, the incidence of moderate-to-severe head injuries in patients with CSI is reported to be between 18 and 40% (Michael et al. 1989; Mulligan et al. 2010). Cervical spine injuries occur in more than the half the cases in which these predicting factors come together: male under 45 years of age; alcohol consumption; motor vehicle accident with no seat belts fastened (Schueller 2010). In particular, CSI injury is frequently encountered in multiply and severely injured patients (Vaccaro et al. 2007).

Neurological deterioration ranging from incomplete spinal cord injury (SCI) and radiculopathy to complete SCI occurs in 12–50% of patients with cervical spine fractures (Kattail et al. 2009; O'Malley and Ross 1988; Sanchez et al. 2005).

The cranio-cervical junction (the segments C0 to C2) injuries account for about a third of cervical spine fractures. They are comprehensively described in the "Cranio-Cervical Junction" chapter of this book. In contrast, with a peak observed in the segments C5 to Th1, the subaxial cervical spine injuries account for two thirds of cervical vertebral fractures (Chilvers et al. 2017) and are subject to this chapter.

## 2 Classifications, Stability and Instability

Several spine stability concepts are reviewed in the "Introduction" section of Part III of this book. In order to comprehensively asses the subaxial cervical spine and to understand the variety of injury mechanisms and their radiological patterns, however, dedicated classification systems are also highlighted here. The ideal classification of the subaxial cervical spinal trauma does not yet exist, primarily because the implementation of morphological, biomechanical, and clinical parameters in a single nomenclature have been proven a difficult task. For radiologists and surgeons, only a few classifications of injury patterns have been shown to be useful enough to provide essential therapy decisions in daily practice.

Among the first classifications of the cervical spine trauma was the publication of Holdsworth (Holdsworth 1970), suggesting the concept of columns and their damage being responsible for instability. Holdsworth described anterior (vertebral body and disc) and posterior (facets, posterior ligaments) columns and six fracture types: anterior compression, fracture-dislocation, rotation-fracture dislocation, extension, burst, and shear fractures. From a clinical point of view, one of the drawbacks of the Holdsworth-classification was, due to a simplification of biomechanical processes, the characterization of burst fractures as stable injuries.

Magerl explained vertebral spine injury by a two columns model (Magerl et al. 1994). This classification was adopted by the Swiss-based *Arbeitsgemeinschaft für Osteosynthesefragen* (AO). It described three fundamental injury mechanisms, increasing in severity from A to C:

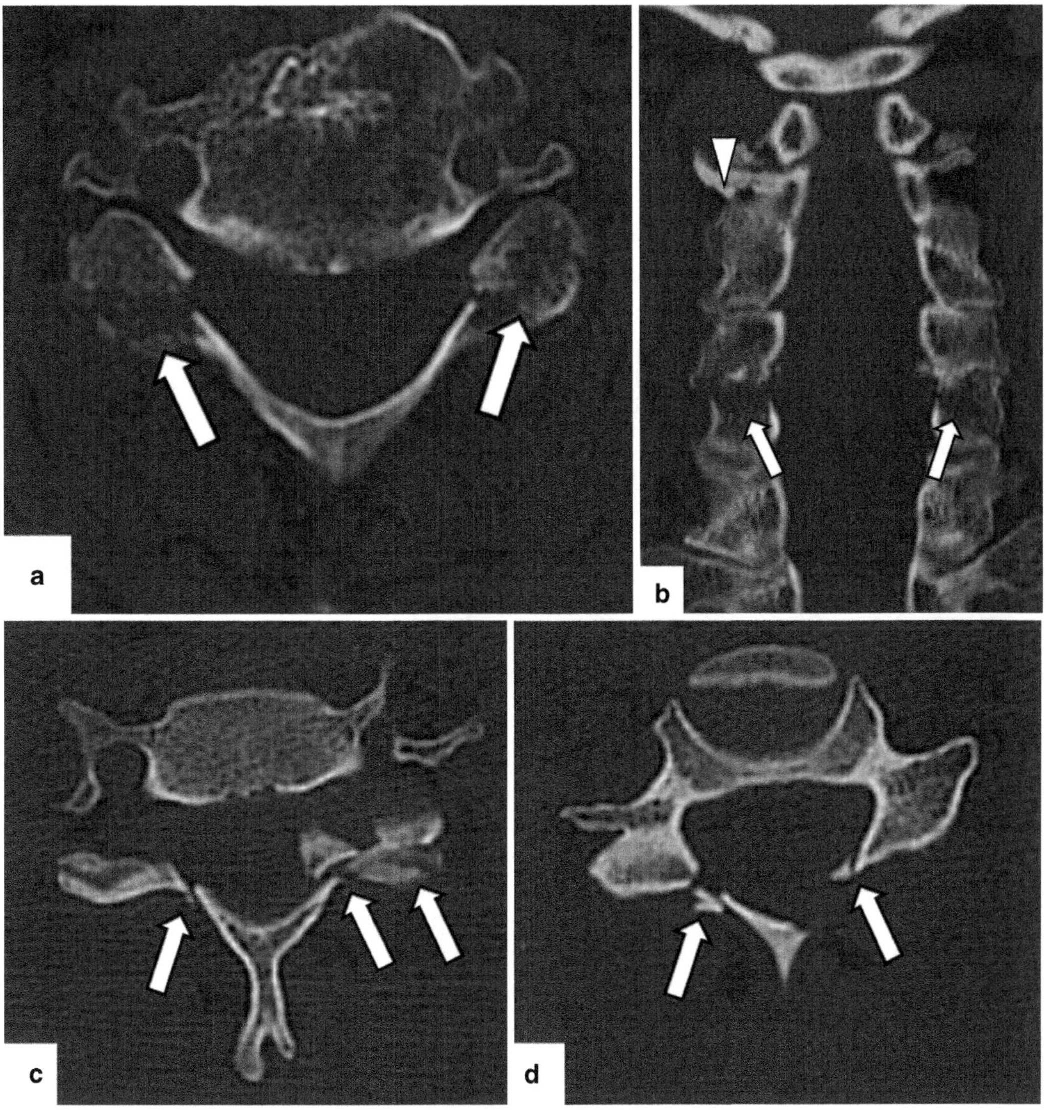


**Fig. 1** Fracture of the posterior vertebral elements (arrows) of C5 in a 69-year-old male (**a** and **b**) as well as a 33-year-old female (**c** and **d**) after motor vehicle accidents. In each patient, the anterior and middle columns are intact, suggesting stable injuries. Note: the non-displaced fracture of the right arch of C2 (arrowhead). NECT, axial (**a**, **c**, and **d**) and coronal (**b**) reconstructions

A = compression; B = distraction; C = rotation injuries. The intent of the Magerl classification was to classify thorcaolumbar vertebral trauma. However, in daily practise, it is used to classify the subaxial cervical trauma as well (Reinhold et al. 2006).

The three columns model is the one most frequently used to understand pathological response to an impact to the spine (Denis 1983; Denis 1984). The anterior column is composed of the anterior longitudinal ligament and the anterior two-thirds of the vertebral bodies, the cartilaginous endplates, and the intervertebral discs. The middle column is composed of the posterior third of these structures and of the posterior ligament. The posterior column contains all posterior osseous and ligamentous elements. If the anterior or the posterior column is disrupted, the other columns are supposed to provide sufficient stability to prevent spinal cord injury (Figs. 1 and 2). If

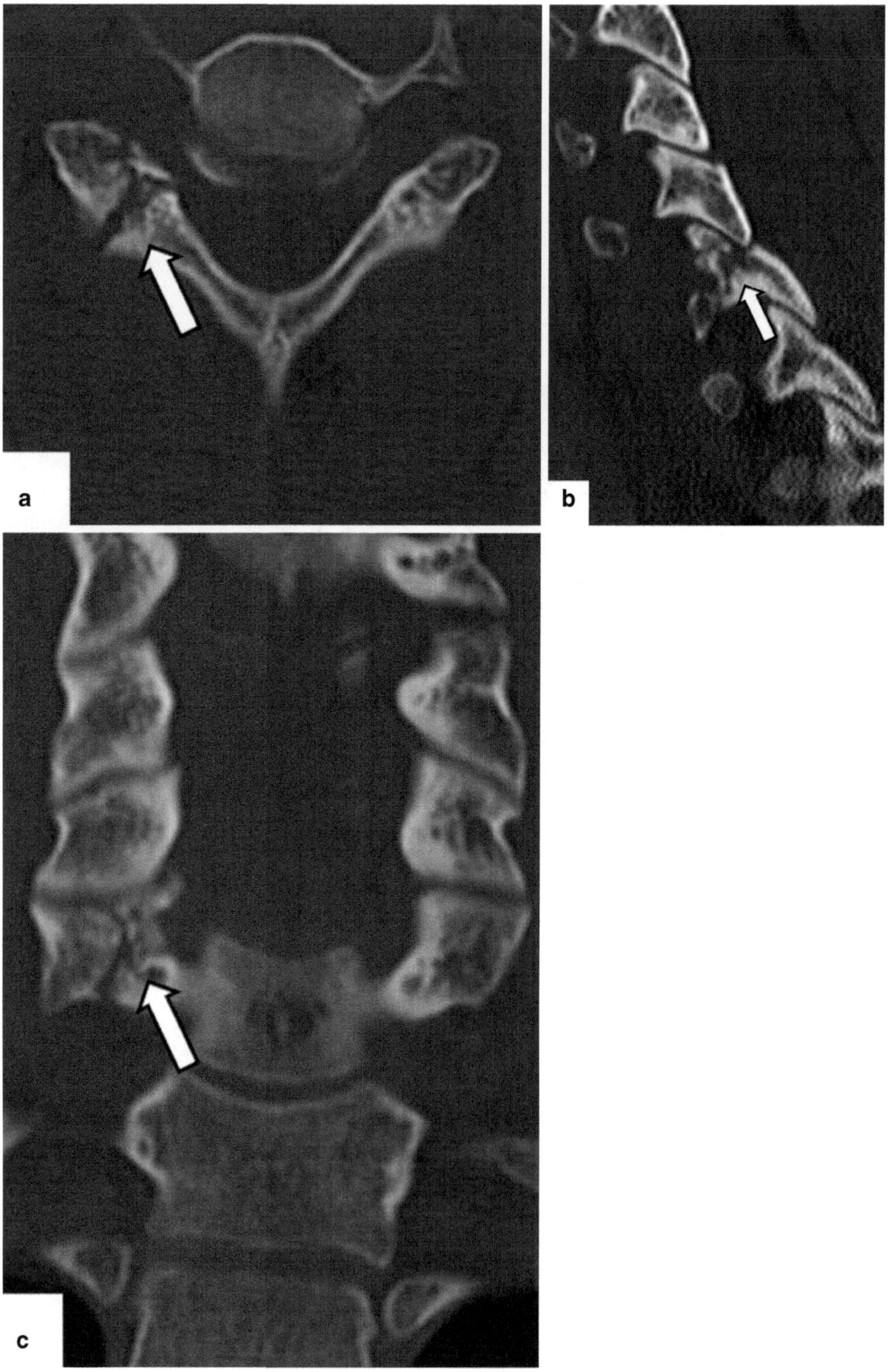


**Fig. 2** Fracture of the right posterior column (arrows) of C7 in a 31-year-old male after a blunt trauma. The right facet of C7 is comminuted. The anterior and middle columns are intact suggestive of a stable injury. NECT, axial (**a**), sagittal (**b**), and coronal (**c**) reconstructions

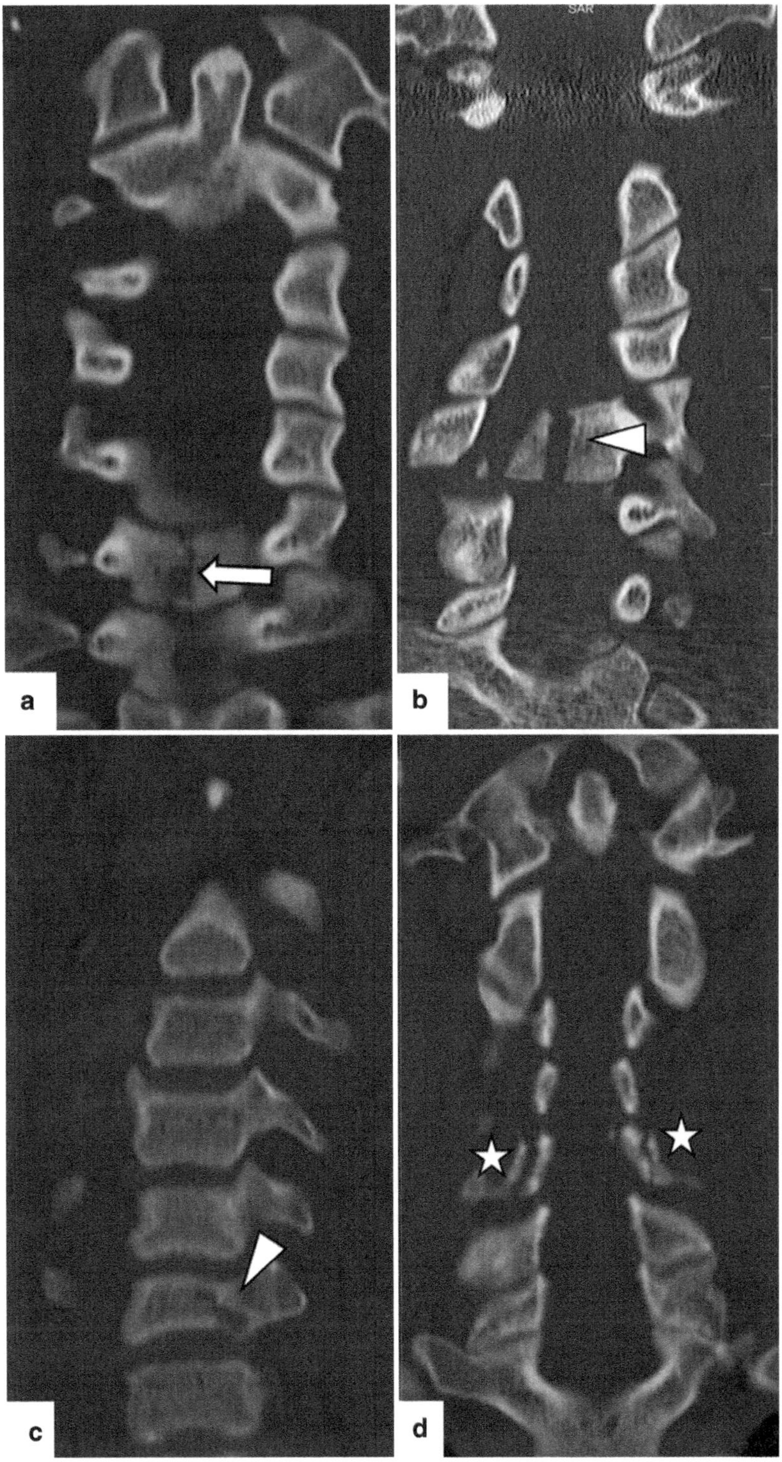


**Fig. 3** Instability of C6 in a 39-year-old male after a motor vehicle accident. The anterior (arrow), middle (arrowhead), and posterior (asterix) columns are fractured. NECT, coronal reconstructions (**a**-**d**)

two columns are disrupted, the spine is distracted as two separate units, resulting in instability (Fig. 3). In the Denis classification, four injury patterns were described: compression (anterior column); burst (anterior and middle columns); flexion-distraction (anterior and posterior columns; middle column is the centre of rotation); and fracture-dislocation (all columns).

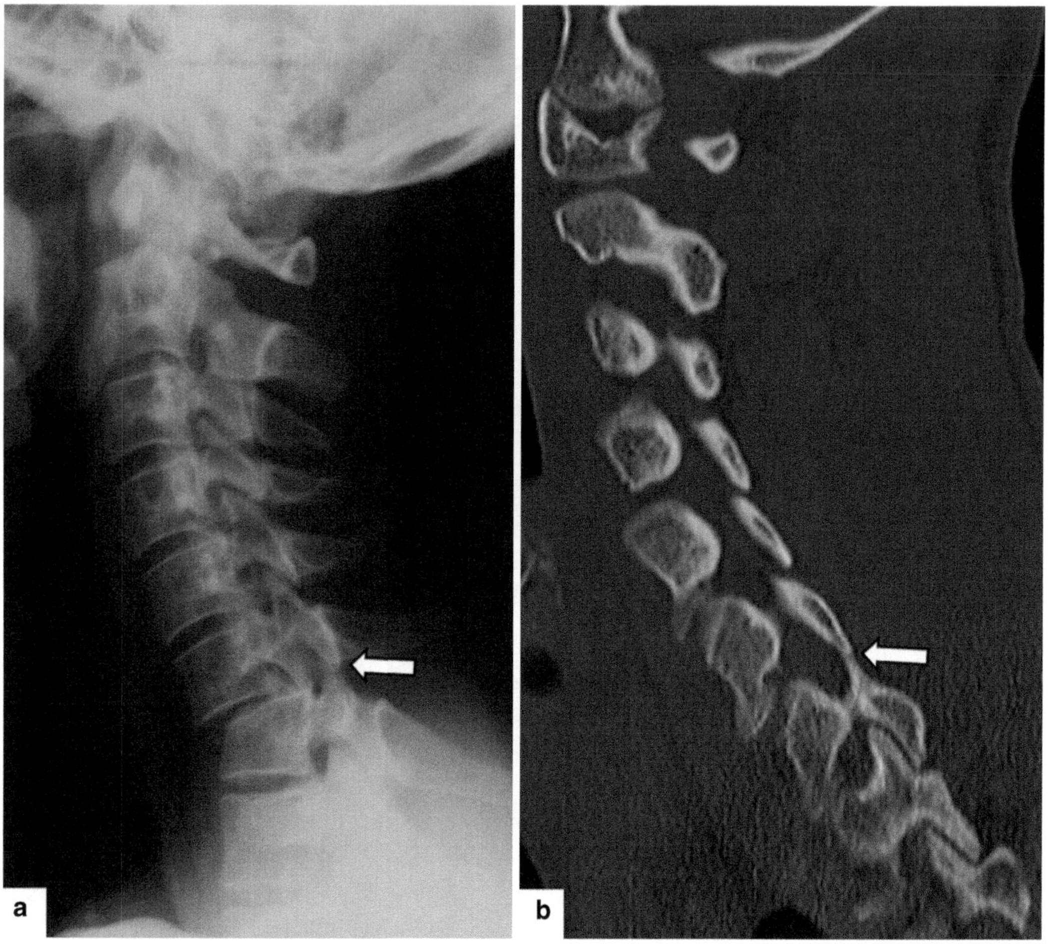

**Fig. 4** Facet joint luxation of the segments C6/C7. A jumped facet (arrows), anterior displacement of 25–50% and more than 11° of hyperkyphosis of the vertebra C6 in relation to C7. Lateral radiograph (**a**) and NECT sagittal reconstruction (**b**) of a 34-year-old female

White and Panjabi stated that specific injury mechanisms accordingly cause specific injury patterns due to the complexity of the specific mechanical force vectors, moments and positions (White 3rd et al. 1975). Among other findings of their biomechanical analyses, instability of the subaxial cervical spine includes more than 3.5 mm horizontal displacement of one vertebra in relation to an adjacent vertebra and more than 11° of rotation difference to that of either adjacent vertebra (Fig. 4).

Equally important biomarkers suggestive of subaxial cervical spine instability are summarized in Table 1. Among these relative imaging features are: a dislocation of a vertebral body

**Table 1** Biomarkers suggestive of subaxial cervical spine instability

| |
|---|
| >3.5 mm horizontal displacement of one vertebra in relation to an adjacent vertebra |
| >11° horizontal displacement of one vertebra in relation to an adjacent vertebra |
| Displaced vertebral body |
| Increased interlaminar and/or interspinous distance |
| Wide facet joints |
| Increased vertical and horizontal distance of the pedicles |
| Discontinuous posterior edge of a vertebral body |
| Spinal canal stenosis >50% |
| Reduction in the height of the anterior vertebral edge >50% |
| Inhomogenous spinolaminar line C2/C3 |

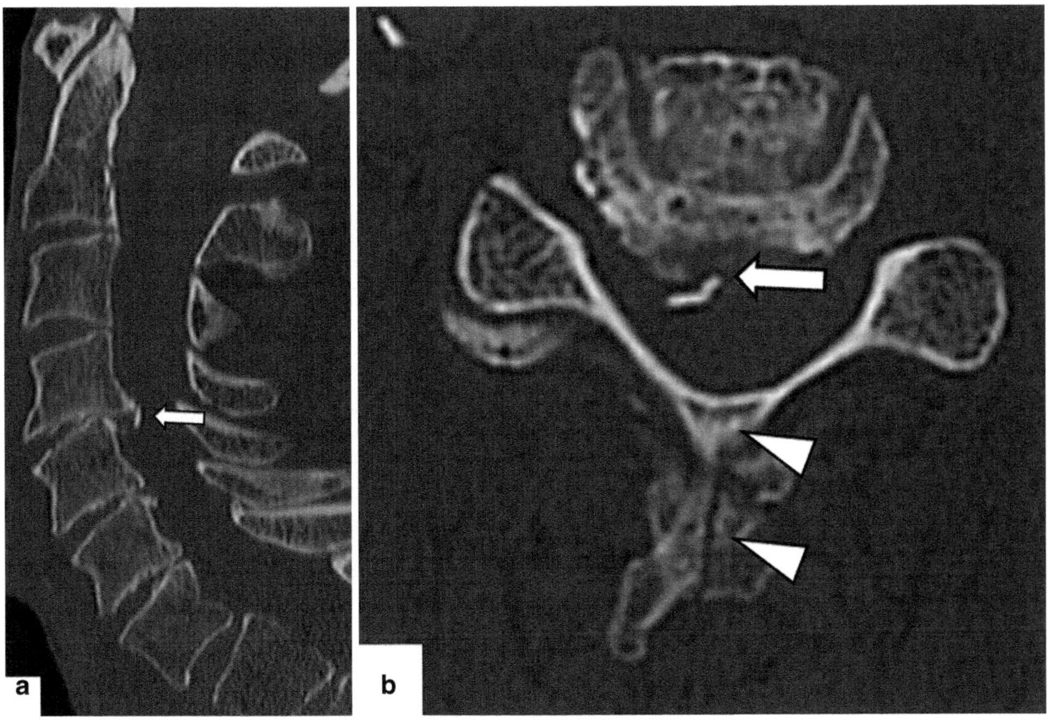


**Fig. 5** Unilateral luxation of the left facet joint C4/C5, fractures of the posterior vertebral body edge (arrows), the posterior arch as well as the spinous process (arrowheads) of C4. First-line radiography was suggestive for malalignment along the posterior vertebral body edges; however, fractures of the posterior vertebral elements were not seen (not shown). NECT in a 59-year-old male after a motor vehicle accident, coronal (**a**) and axial (**b**) reformations

(Fig. 5); an increased interlaminar and/or interspinous distance (Fig. 6); wide facet joints, indicating subluxation (Fig. 4); an increased vertical and horizontal distance of the pedicles (Fig. 7); and a discontinuous posterior edge of a vertebral body. From a clinical point of view, a minority of compression fractures, some burst fractures, most flexion-distraction fractures, and all fracture-dislocation injuries are instable injuries. From a radiologic point of view, however, the stability or instability of vertebral spine fractures is not unequivocally delineated in some cases, particularly in burst fractures. However, there is broad consensus about what constitutes stability, based on imaging features, including a spinal canal stenosis <50% in neurologically unremarkable patients as well as a reduction in the height of the anterior vertebral edge <50% (Willen et al. 1990).

When radiographs are used as a first-line examination in cervical spine trauma, one has to consider the tremendously high false-negative rate of radiography in CSI documented in literature; see Sect. 4.2. High-Risk Patients. However, in order to reveal information as scrunitely as possible from radiographs, these patterns are among normal cervical spine radiographical findings: the cervical vertebral bodies must fulfil a mild lordosis; the anterior and posterior edges of the vertebral bodies as well as the posterior laminar line (spinolaminar line) must parallel each other; the facets must align on lateral radiographs (additional oblique views may be considered helpful); AP view must show a homogenous line along the spinous processes; intervertebral height must be within normal range, according to the patient's age; prevertebral soft tissue on lateral views must be thin; however, in the paediatric population, it can measure up to 6 mm and even more in views taken in exspiration; in infants, on lateral views the spinolaminar line is a relevant marker to judge pseudoluxation of C2/

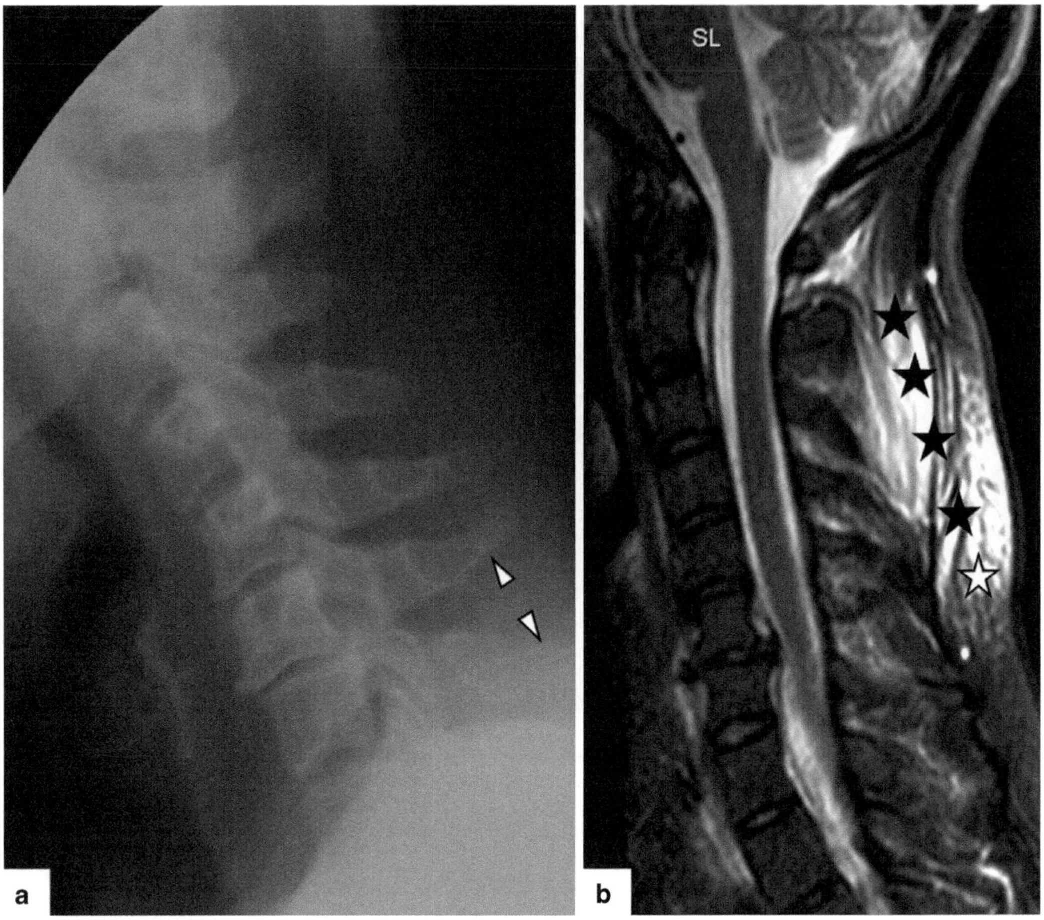


**Fig. 6** Hyperflexion injury in a 58-year-old male. Lateral radiograph (**a**) shows increased interlaminar and interspinous distances (arrowheads). Sagittal T2-weighted MR imaging (**b**) reveals a substantial paravertebral soft tissue hematoma along the segments C2 to C7 (asterices)

C3 from traumatic injury of the junction of the upper and lower cervical spine (Fig. 8).

The classification systems mentioned are based on the mechanism of injury extracted from plain radiographs or CT scans, ignoring the contribution of the ligaments to stability and the role of MR imaging in the assessment of subaxial cervical spine trauma (Martinez-Perez et al. 2014). Moreover, the neurological status may be the single most influential factor to discriminate conservative from surgical management. Hence, it was the Spine Trauma Study Group to develop the Subaxial Cervical Spine Injury Classification (SLIC) system (Vaccaro et al. 2007). This severity score is based on three components: fracture morphology, affection of the posterior ligamentous complex, and the neurological status, since these entities reflect independent determinants of prognosis and management. The total number of points is calculated for a subaxial cervical fracture or dislocation (see Table 2). Injuries with a SLIC score of 4 or less are considered manageable conservatively. Fractures with a score of 6 or more are usually surgically stabilized, whereas injuries with a score of 5 may be managed either with surgery or nonoperatively (Dvorak et al. 2007). Hence, although of being far from an ideal classification for cervical trauma, by building the system on injury patterns from less severe to more severe, the SLIC severity score helps to optimize the therapeutic decision-making process in cervical spine injuries.

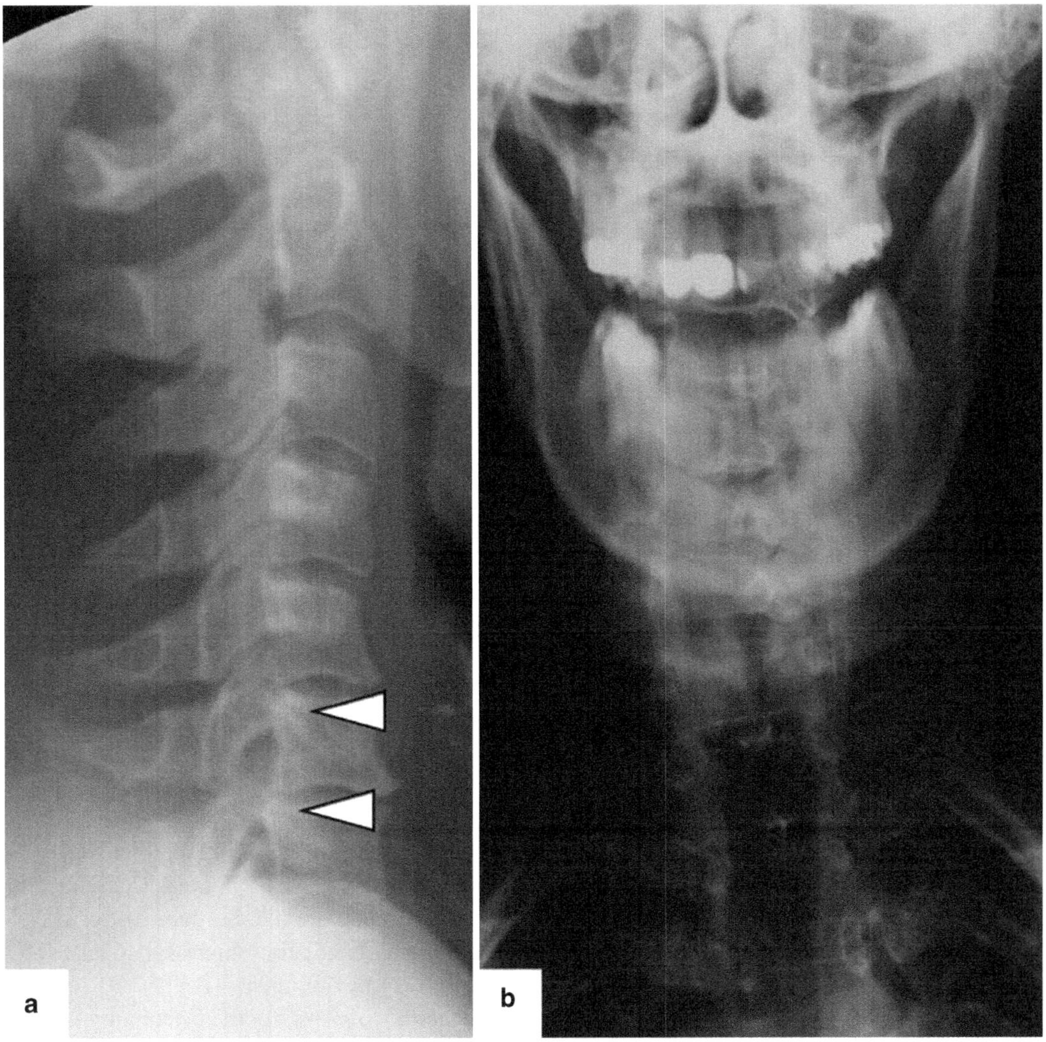


**Fig. 7** Lateral (**a**) and AP (**b**) radiographs in a 70-year-old female with severe pain in the lower neck after a blunt trauma. The increased horizontal distance of the pedicles (arrowheads) in (**a**) is suggestive of an acute intervertebral disc injury C6/C7; in these segments, pre-existing osteochondral degenerative disease is evident. AP radiography is technically and diagnostically insufficient in this patient

## 3 Injury Patterns

Subaxial CSI imaging reveals predictable, specific radiological patterns, regardless the level of an injury. Since there is a wide spectrum of stress factors responsible for each injury mechanism, it is the combination of all forces which results in the main traumatizing vector (Schueller and Schueller-Weidekamm 2014). The instantaneous axis of rotation of one vertebra to another reflects an important paradigm in the biomechanic considerations on the deformity of the vertebral spine, since, in relation to the instantaneous axis of rotation, the traumatizing vector causes different injuries. For example, the instantaneous axis of rotation of the segment C5/C6 is considered in the anterocentral portion of C5. If the traumatizing vector is effective anteriorly to this axis, then a flexion injury is the result. On the opposite, the vector being effective posteriorly leads to an extension trauma.

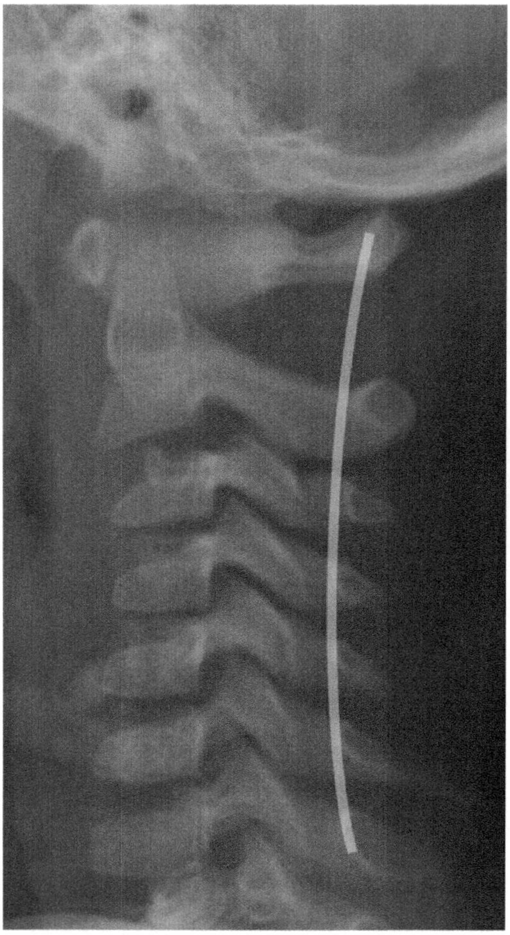

**Fig. 8** Pseudoluxation at C2/C3 in an infant. On the lateral radiograph, the normal alignment of the spinolaminar line (semi-transparent line) along all segments differentiates a normal from a trauma-induced appearance

## 3.1 Flexion

Hyperflexion disrupts the posterior ligaments, including the capsular ligaments, and angulates the vertebral body anteriorly (Fig. 9). Injuries are mechanically instable because of the disrupted ligaments, compromising the middle column. In addition, disc displacement may contribute to spinal cord and nerve root compression. The major radiologic features are the diminished height of the anterior edge of a vertebral body, the enhanced spaces between the spinous processes as well as widened or jumped facets. Even on radiographs, a focal kyphosis may be anticipated. The reason why the cervical spine is more often involved in traumatic injury to the facets than the thoracolumbar spine is that the cervical articular processes are smaller than the thoracolumbar ones and are distributed more horizontally with only little overlap of the articular surfaces, rendering them more prone to flexion as well as extension injuries. The segments C5 to C7 are mostly involved. However, in many cases, not only one segment is injured. Consequently, the entire spine should be thoroughly investigated for non-contiguous injury in patients with a proven hyperflexion injury (Fig. 9). CT imaging is suggested to search for the facet injuries, while T2-weighted and STIR MR imaging depicts the soft tissue and ligamentous trauma (Fig. 10) as well as CSI best (Fig. 11).

**Table 2** The subaxial injury classification and severity (SLIC) score (Vaccaro et al. 2007)

| Characteristics | | Points |
|---|---|---|
| Morphology | No abnormality | 0 |
| | Compression | 1 |
| | Burst | 2 |
| | Distraction | 3 |
| | Rotation/translation | 4 |
| Disco-ligamentous complex | Intact | 0 |
| | Indeterminate | 1 |
| | Disrupted | 2 |
| Neurological status | Intact | 0 |
| | Root injury | 1 |
| | Complete cord injury | 2 |
| | Incomplete cord injury | 3 |
| | Continuous compression with deficit | 1 |

If the traumatizing vector is weaker than described above and causes only a longitudinal pull on the anterior ligament, as a consequence, the anterior vertebral body bears most of the force. The result is a wedge compression fracture. The anterior column is injured, without disruption of the posterior elements (Denis 1984). These fractures are considered to be stable (Fig. 9). In the elderly, CT imaging also reveals injuries of the ossified anterior ligamentous and bony structures (Fig. 12).

When a flexion mechanism is combined with a severe axial compression at the cervical spine, flexion teardrop fractures occur. In some classifi-

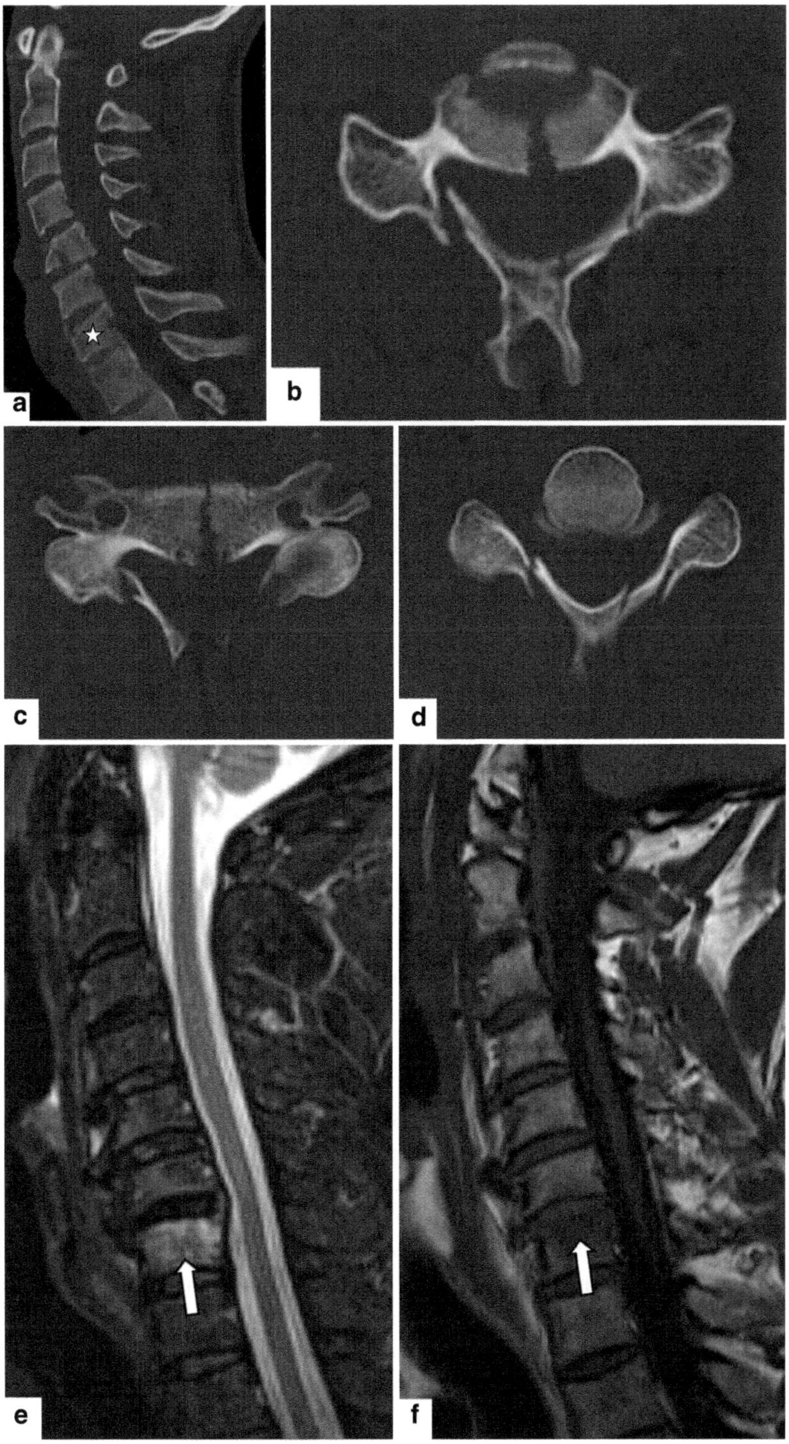


**Fig. 9** Instability of the segment C5 in a 28-year-old pedestrian struck by a motorbike. The vertebral body C5 is angulated anteriorly and its anterior edge is reduced in height. The hyperflexion injury has caused a disruption of all columns. Note: compression fracture of the vertebral body C7 (asterix in (**a**)) with intact middle and posterior columns as well in another patient (**e**, **f**), representing a stable fracture. Moderate bone marrow oedema is noted associated with the fractured vertebral body (arrows in **e**, **f**). NECT, sagittal (**a**) and axial (**b**–**d**) reconstructions; 1.5 Tesla sagittal T2 weighted (**e**) and T1 weighted (**f**) MR imaging

cations, these are described as a variant of burst fractures. They are typically caused by diving into shallow water or comparable accidents. The anterior longitudinal ligament is ruptured and the anteroinferior aspect of the vertebral body is fractured (Raniga et al. 2014). This fragment is displaced anteriorly and resembles a teardrop. CT imaging discriminates two fracture types: type I

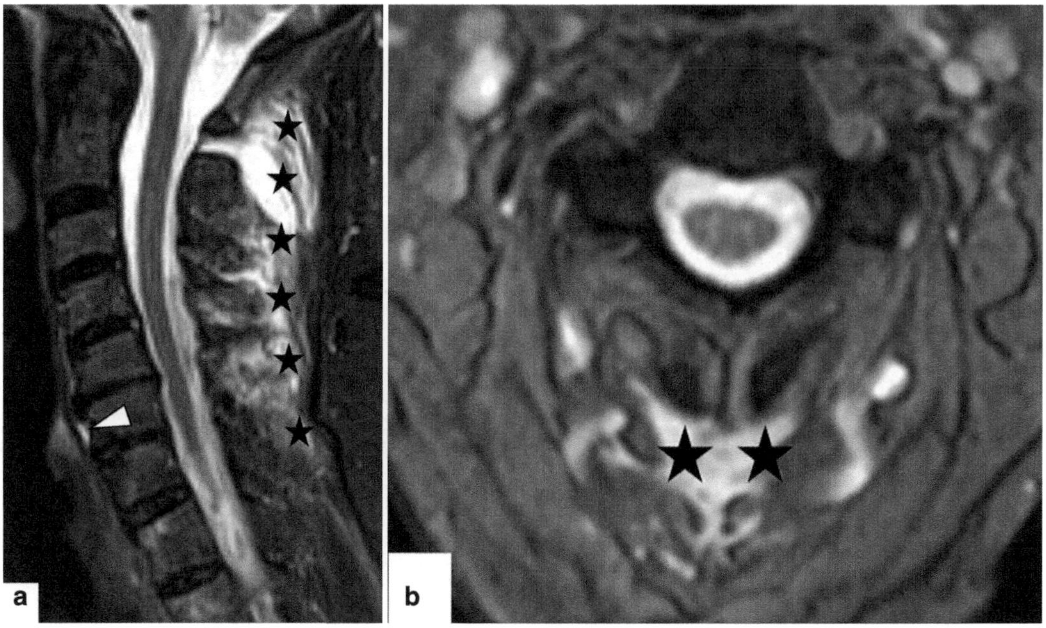


**Fig. 10** 61-year-old male having sustained a hyperflexion injury. Moderate bone bruise is noted in the vertebral bodies C7, Th1, and Th2 as well as a small anterior paravertebral hematoma of C5/C6 (arrowhead in (**a**)). Substantial soft tissue damage and posterior ligamentous sprain are evident ranging from C1 to C7 (asterices). 3.0 Tesla sagittal (**a**) and axial (**b**) T2-weighted MR imaging

includes the findings described above, whereas type II additionally shows the displacement of the posterior vertebral body edge, widened facet joints, and a widened interlaminar space as a sign of significant posterior ligamentous disruption (Fig. 13). Hence, the injury involves all three columns. It is highly instable and neurological compromise according to spinal cord injury is usually observed.

Hyperflexion injury should be discriminated from whiplash injury. In the latter, the sequelae of extension and flexion leads to the fracture of the laminae as well as the vertebral body of the involved segment (Fig. 14). More recent literature suggests that the combination of axial compression and excentrical rotation leads to an anterior disc distraction and a posterior facet joint compression (Bogduk and Yoganandan 2001). In clinical practise, however, isolated muscular and capsuloligamentous injuries are most often observed which are suitably seen with MR imaging (Fig. 15). In addition, MR angiography may be undertaken in order to exclude carotideal and vertebral artery injury. However, according to literature, the indication of cross-sectional imaging for whiplash injuries remains controversial, since therapeutically relevant alterations are seen in the minority of patients only (Ronnen et al. 1996).

## 3.2 Burst

Burst fractures occur when a severe compressive force is transmitted to the spine axially and a disc fractures into its adjacent lower vertebral body, causing a disruption of this vertebral body. This injury mechanism leads to the discontinuity of the anterior and middle columns. The posterior column has variable degrees of injury. Radiologically, fragments are seen that narrow the spinal canal and compress the myelon. At the cervical spine, burst fractures most often occur as injuries of the cranio-cervical junction, including Jefferson fractures (Han et al. 1976) and occipital condyle fractures.

In brief, the Jefferson fracture is a synonym for a fracture of the atlas ring (Fig. 16). An axially transmitted force displaces the masses later-

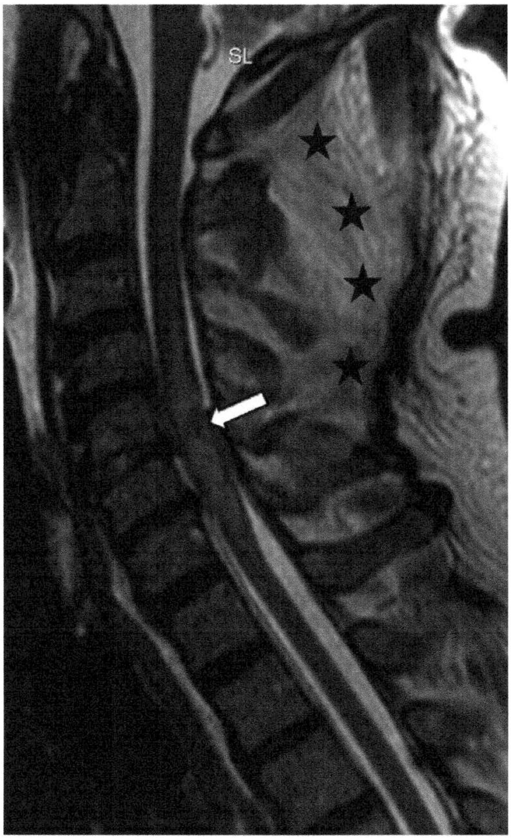


**Fig. 11** Type 3 spinal cord injury according to Kulkarni and Bondurant (Bondurant et al. 1990). There is a substantial high T2 cord signal from C4 to C7 in keeping with an oedema; in addition, small foci of low central signal are noted at C5/C6, representing haemorrhage (arrow). There is a large oedema in the posterior soft tissue, suggestive of a hyperflexion trauma mechanism (asterices). 3.0 Tesla sagittal T2-weighted MR imaging

ally and causes fractures of the anterior and posterior arches. The avulsion of the transverse ligament is the major cause of the Jefferson fracture's instability (Gehweiler et al. 1976). In general, fractures of the atlas were classified by Gehweiler into five types. Originally, a four-fragment fracture was described and is classified as a Gehweiler type III fracture. In daily practise, fractures with three fragments are also referred to as Jefferson fractures. Type I and II fractures are isolated lesions of the anterior or posterior arches, also referred to as nutcracker fractures, since they are a result of an anterior distraction and a posterior compression between the occipital condyles and the axis. Type IV and V fractures are isolated stable fractures of the lateral mass or of a transverse process, respectively. These fractures can lead to the dissection of the vertebral artery and are, in addition to all fractures involving the pedicles or the transverse processes, considered an indication for CT angiography of the supraaortic branches (Langner et al. 2008; Malhotra et al. 2007) (Fig. 17).

Until the event of multidetector CT imaging, occipital condyle fractures were probably underreported. The classification most widely accepted was described by Anderson and Montesano. It comprises three types: type I is an impaction fracture with or without a minor displacement (Fig. 18). Bilateral lesions may be considered instable. Type II is more extensive than type I, unilateral damage being considered a stable fracture (Fig. 19). A type III fracture is an avulsion fracture with a substantial medial fragment displacement into the foramen magnum (Anderson and Montesano 1988).

For a comprehensive description of these entities, refer to the "Cranio-Cervical Junction" chapter of this book.

## 3.3 Hyperextension

Due to forceful posterior displacement of the head, the traumatizing vector is effective dorsally in relation to the instantaneous axis of rotation (see above). Hence, a hyperextension mechanism occurs and leads to the distraction, i.e., elongation of the anterior column. This injury is defined as instable due to the disruption of the posterior column. At the anterior column, a bony disruption is frequently visible as well as widening of the intervertebral space and retrolisthesis of the upper vertebral body of the involved segments (Fig. 20). The injury pattern includes the malalignment of the posterior osseous and ligamentous structures at the level of the injury. Commonly, the interspinous alignment is disturbed and the laminae are fractured (Fig. 21). Typically, the mid and lower cervical spine is injured.

The pathognomonic findings are accompanied by severe soft tissue damage to the intervertebral

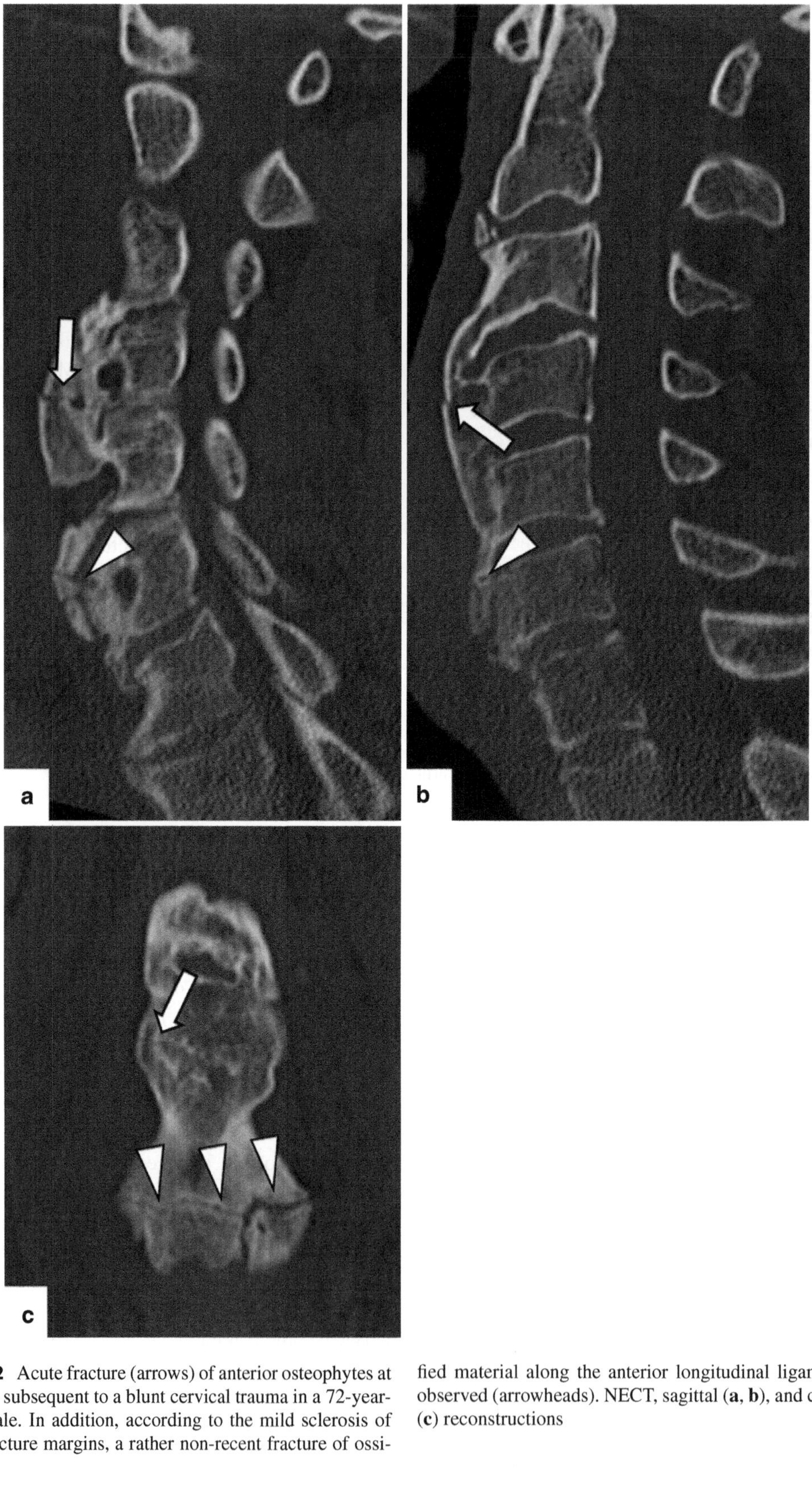


**Fig. 12** Acute fracture (arrows) of anterior osteophytes at C3/C4 subsequent to a blunt cervical trauma in a 72-year-old male. In addition, according to the mild sclerosis of the fracture margins, a rather non-recent fracture of ossified material along the anterior longitudinal ligament is observed (arrowheads). NECT, sagittal (**a**, **b**), and coronal (**c**) reconstructions

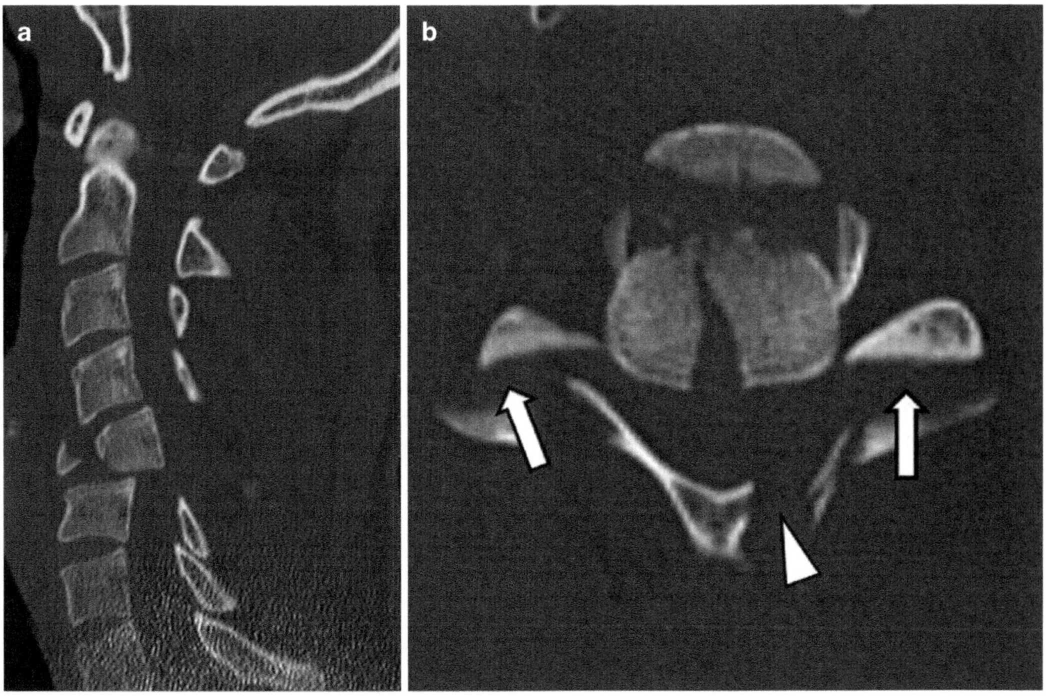


**Fig. 13** Teardrop fracture of C5 in a 33-year-old male after a motor vehicle accident. There is a displacement of the antero-inferior vertebral body (teardrop; arrow in **a**). The vertebral body is substantially displaced posteriorly (arrowheads in **a**), the laminae are fractured (arrowhead in b), the facet joints are subluxated (arrows in **b**), and, consequently, the interlaminar space is widened. A marked posterior soft tissue hematoma is noted (asterix). NECT, sagittal (**a**) and axial (**b**) reconstructions

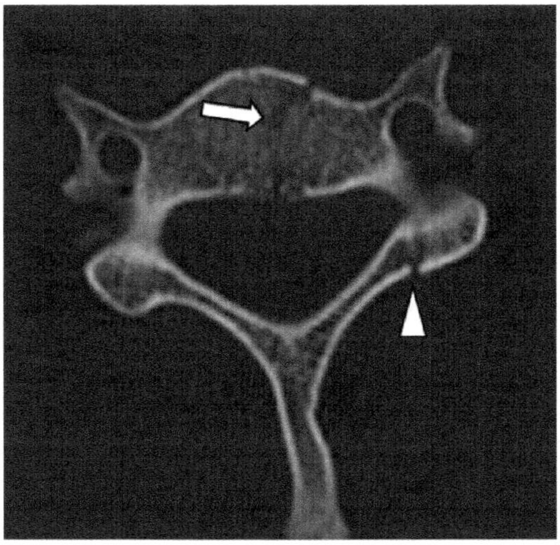

**Fig. 14** Whiplash injury after a motor vehicle accident in a 21-year-old female. Fractures of the vertebral body (arrow) and the left lamina (arrowhead) are noted. NECT, axial reformation

discs and to the posterior vertebral elements, suitably diagnosed by MR imaging (Fig. 20). Rarely, the deforming force to the anterior ligament leads to an associated avulsion fracture of the anterior vertebral body, which then is called teardrop. This pattern should not be confused with the teardrop fracture occurring with a hyperflexion mechanism (see above). CT is necessary for the detection of the posterior arch fractures. Vertebral artery involvement is discriminated by CT angiography. On MR imaging, non-displaced fractures of the posterior bony elements are rarely depicted. However, with T2-weighted and STIR images, the soft tissue damage as well as the cord injuries are unequivocally diagnosed. Rarely, relevant traumatic disc herniations are also seen. Hyperextension injuries should not be misinterpreted as Clay shoveler's fractures. This synonym stands for the avulsion fracture of spinous processes sustaining severe forces on the

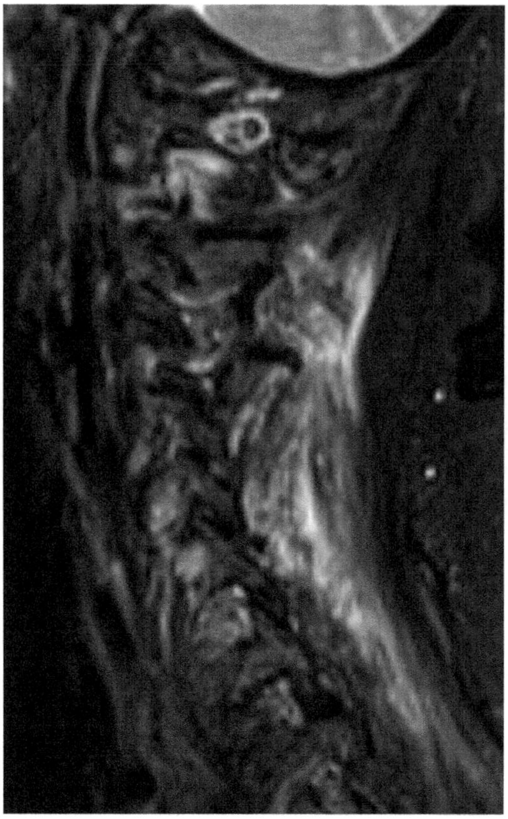

**Fig. 15** Acute posterior muscular and ligamentous oedema and haemorrhage from C2 to Th1, in keeping with a whiplash injury. Substantial bone bruise from C5 to C7 is noted; however, no fracture was observed on CT imaging (not shown). 3.0 Tesla sagittal STIR MR imaging

nuchal ligament, usually sparing the laminae (Figs. 22 and 23).

Occurring during motor vehicle accidents, at the level of the upper cervical spine, this injury mechanism causes the traumatic spondylolysis of the axis, i.e., Hangman's fracture (Effendi et al. 1981). The fracture involves the interarticulate parts bilaterally and/or the pedicles, the body, the facets as well as the transverse processes (Fig. 24). Also, the intervertebral disc C2/C3 is ruptured. For details, see the "Cranio-Cervical Junction" chapter of this book.

## 3.4 Fracture-Dislocation and Hyperflexion-Rotation

Fracture-dislocation is caused by severe shear and rotational forces. This type of injury was initially described as a disruption of the cervical spine with a rotatory subluxation of the anterior and posterior vertebral elements (Denis 1984). The injury pattern includes the vertebral disruption as well as unilateral or bilateral facet joint luxations (Fig. 25). On axial CT images, the malrotation of one vertebra to its neighbour is substantially better obtained than on radiographs. Perhaps oblique radiographs help to detect the injuries, if initial AP and lateral views are not normal; however, CT imaging providing thin section multidimensional reformations is necessary to make the diagnosis. "Naked" inferior facets are seen (Fig. 26), describing the absence of the superior facet of the neighbouring lower vertebral body and the lateral mass jumped anteriorly to its inferior neighbour (O'Callaghan et al. 1980).

The cervical vertebral facets have a more horizontal orientation than the thoracolumbar facets; hence, they are prone to subluxation subsequent to ligamentous trauma. A unilateral luxation is rather caused by the combination of rotation and flexion, whereas a bilateral luxation frequently occurs after rotation and compression (Palmieri et al. 2006). In unilateral trauma, the vertebral body is anteriorly displaced by about 25%. On the opposite, the bilateral luxation represents a highly instable condition. The horizontal vertebral body dislocation of the injured segment is at least 50% (Fig. 27). Another radiologically useful sign is the Reversed Hamburger bun sign (Daffner and Daffner 2002). It reflects a convex rather than a normal concave appearance of the articular surfaces (Fig. 28).

In addition, with facet joint trauma, uncovertebral displacement occurs as well. The uncinate processes create a postero-lateral frame for the cervical vertebrae C3 to C7. A rotational injury causes the displacement of the uncovertebral facets. In coronal images this resembles headphones put on asymmetrically and, accordingly, is referred to as Positive headphones sign (Palmieri et al. 2006).

Typically, the mid and lower cervical spine is involved in dislocation and rotation trauma. Unless the segment C7 is not affected, CT angiography should urgently be performed in order to exclude vertebral artery intramural hematoma, dissection, or occlusion (Fig. 29). MR imaging is

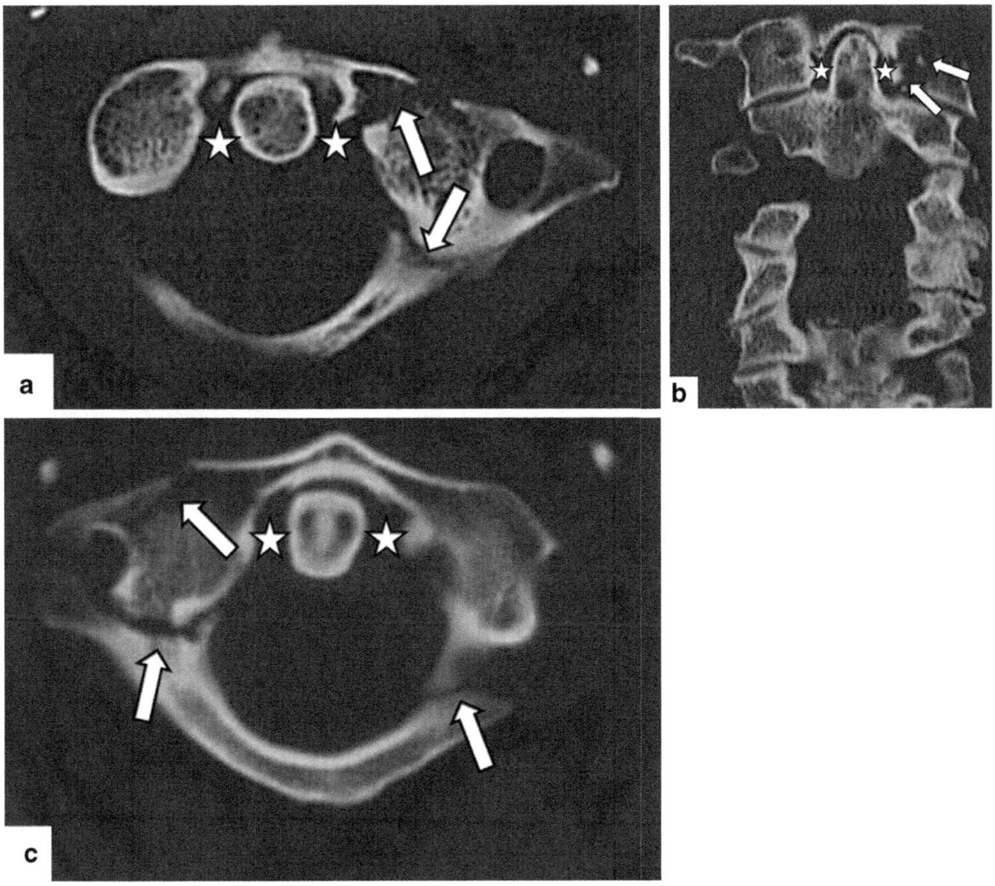


**Fig. 16** Fractures of the left anterior and posterior atlas ring in a 54-year-old male after a fall from height (**a**, **b**) and of the posterior arches on both sides in a 32-year-old patient after a motor vehicle accident (**c**), in keeping with Jefferson fractures (arrows). No relevant displacement of the dens axis, i.e., no evidence of instability, is noted (asterices). NECT, axial (**a**, **c**) and coronal (**b**) reconstructions

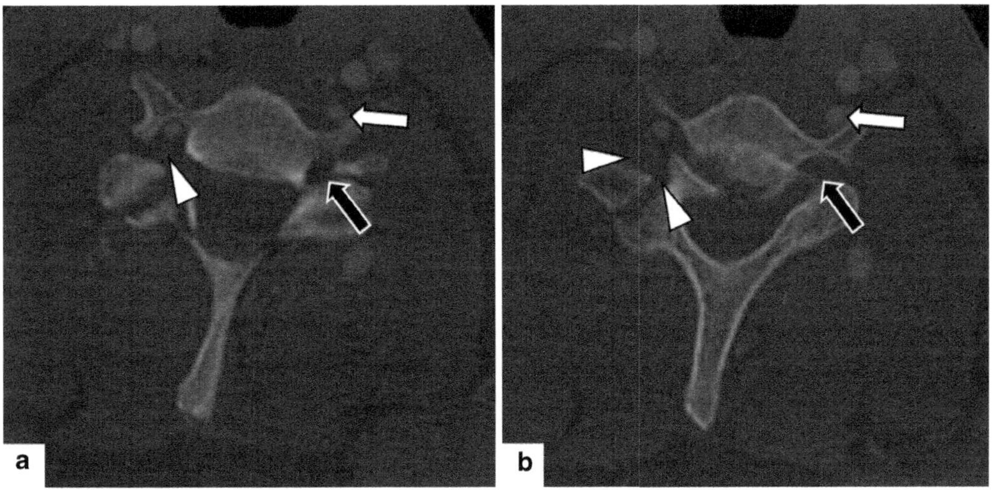


**Fig. 17** Fracture and mild displacement of the right pedicle of C6 in a 39-year-old male sustaining a motor vehicle accident. There is mild soft tissue swelling along the transverse foramen (arrowheads); however, no signs of a vascular injury were noted. As a variant, the left vertebral artery (white arrows) has not entered the vertebral artery canal (black arrows) at C6. CT angiography, axial reconstructions (**a**, **b**)

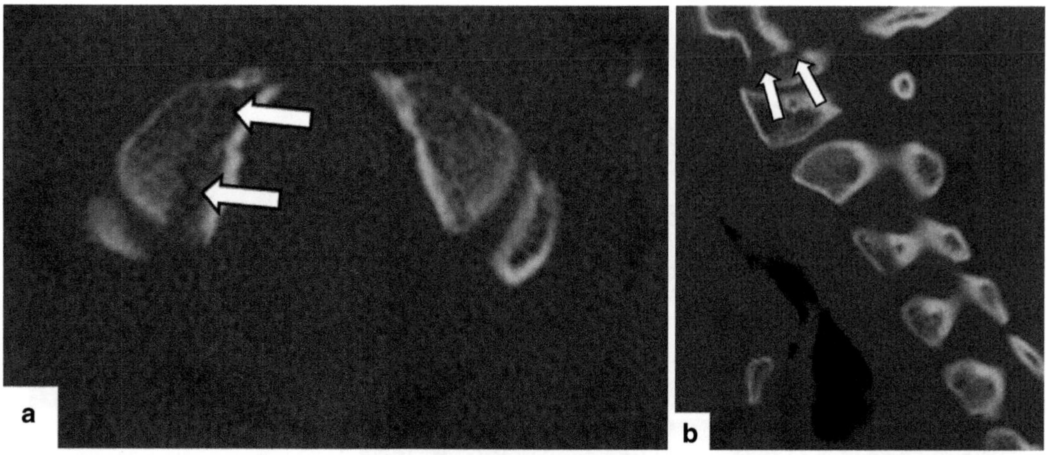


**Fig. 18** Right occipital condyle fracture in a 28-year-old male after diving into shallow water. A minor fracture displacement is noted (arrows). NECT, axial (**a**) and coronal (**b**) reconstructions

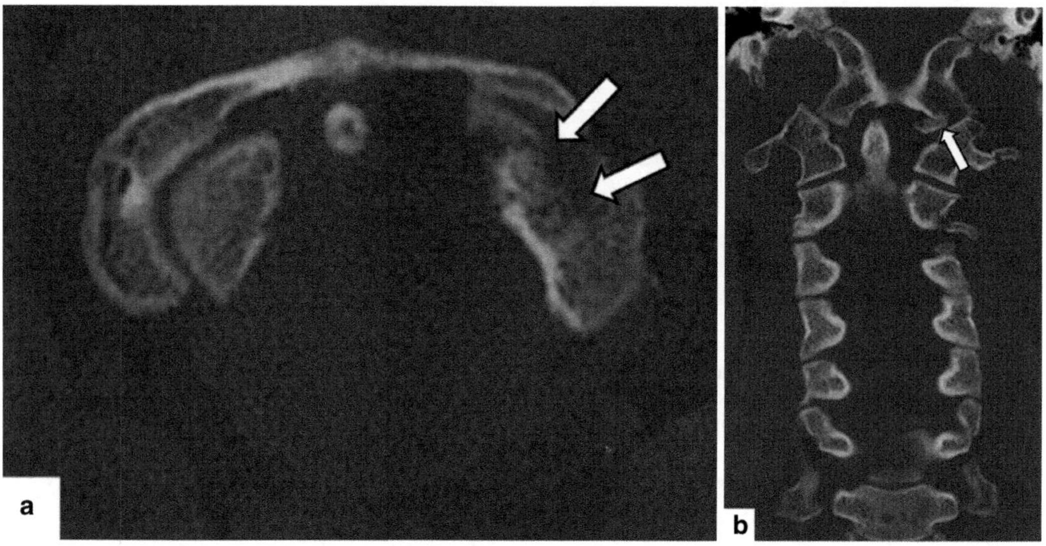


**Fig. 19** Unilateral occipital condyle fracture on the left in a 39-year-old female after an axial impact onto the head. NECT axial (**a**) and coronal (**b**) reconstructions show a pronounced displacement of the fragment (arrows)

considered a standard in the diagnosis of ligamentous, capsular, discal, and cord trauma in these patients, most often performed subsequent to the stabilization of the vertebral fractures.

## 3.5 Ligamentous Injury and Disc Herniation

The direct signs of ligamentous trauma include thinning and elevated T2 signal of ligaments (strain, grade 1), subtotal ligamentous disruption (partial tear, grade 2), and discontinuity (complete tear, grade 3) (Groves et al. 2005; Vaccaro et al. 2001).

The indirect signs include elevated signal on T2-weighted images and thickening of ligaments (Hawighorst et al. 2001), intraspinous and paravertebral hematoma, and bone bruise particularly along the vertebral body edges.

Traumatic disc herniations are noted in the minority of cases of blunt cervical trauma; how-

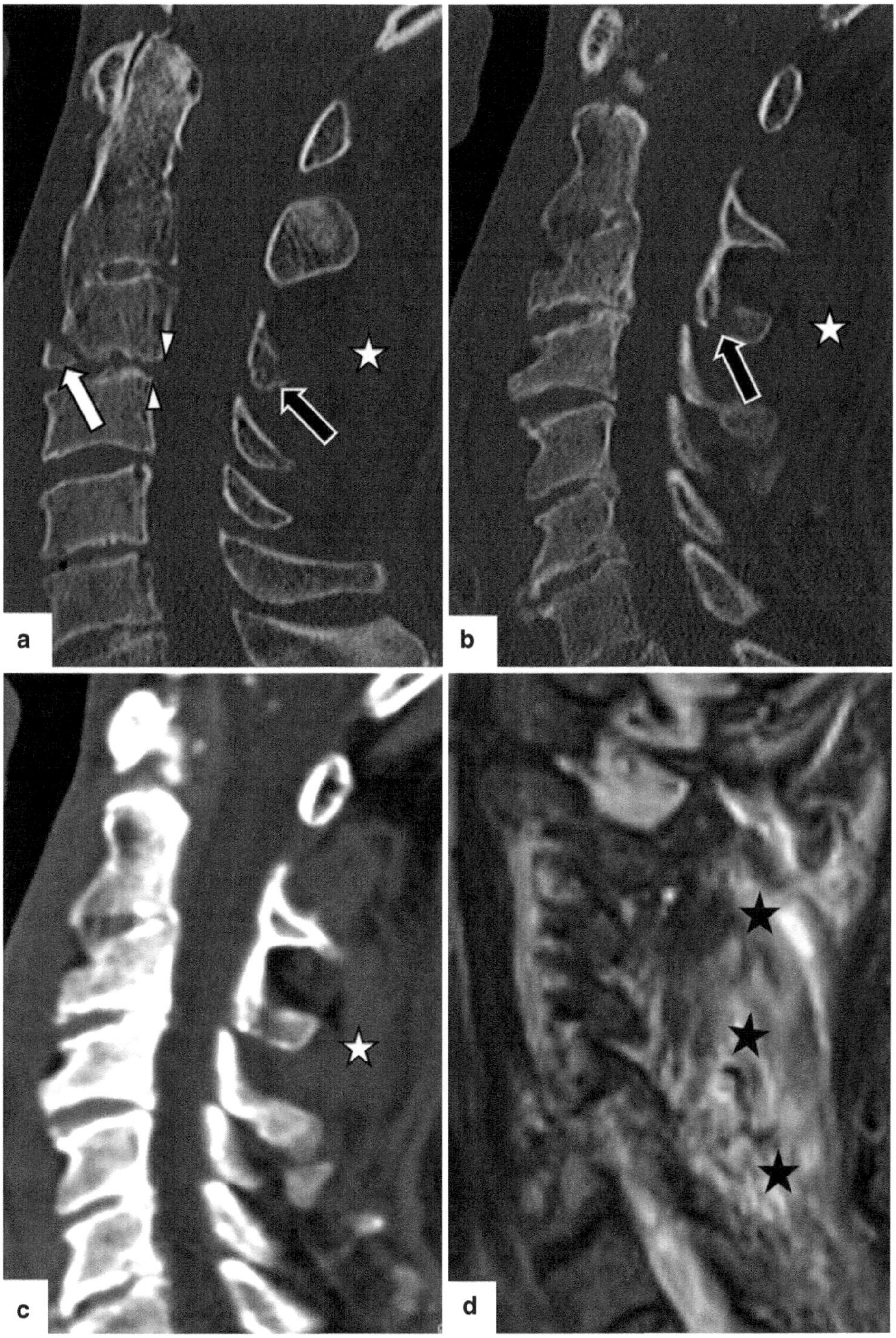


**Fig. 20** Hyperextension injury in a 68-year-old car driver. A fracture fragment of the anterior column is displaced (arrow). The vertebral body of C3 is mildly displaced posteriorly (arrowheads). The posterior column is fractured (black arrows), and a substantial posterior soft tissue hematoma is noted (asterices). NECT, coronal reconstructions in bone (**a**, **b**) and soft tissue (**c**) windows; 3.0 Tesla sagittal T2-weighted MR imaging (**d**)

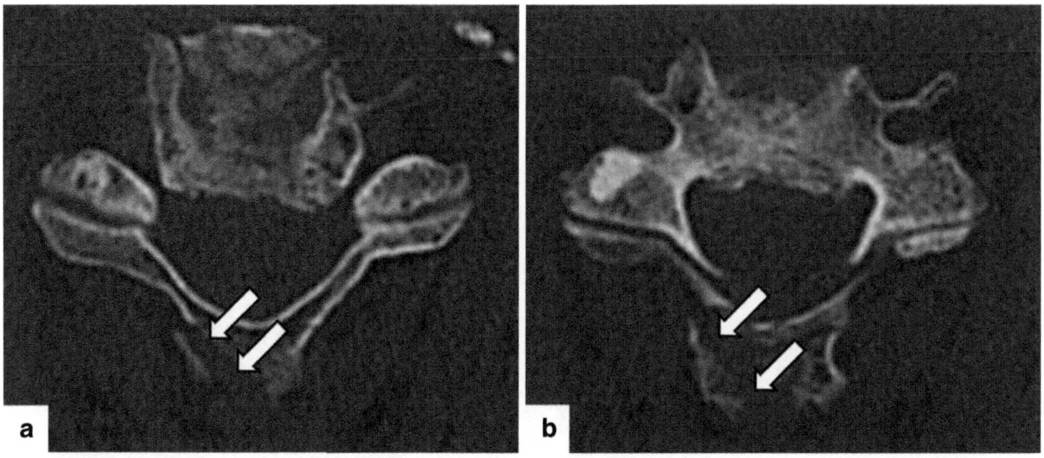


**Fig. 21** Same patient as in Fig. 20. Lamina fracture, extending to the spinous process (arrows) of C3, indicates a posterior column injury. NECT, axial reconstructions (**a**, **b**)

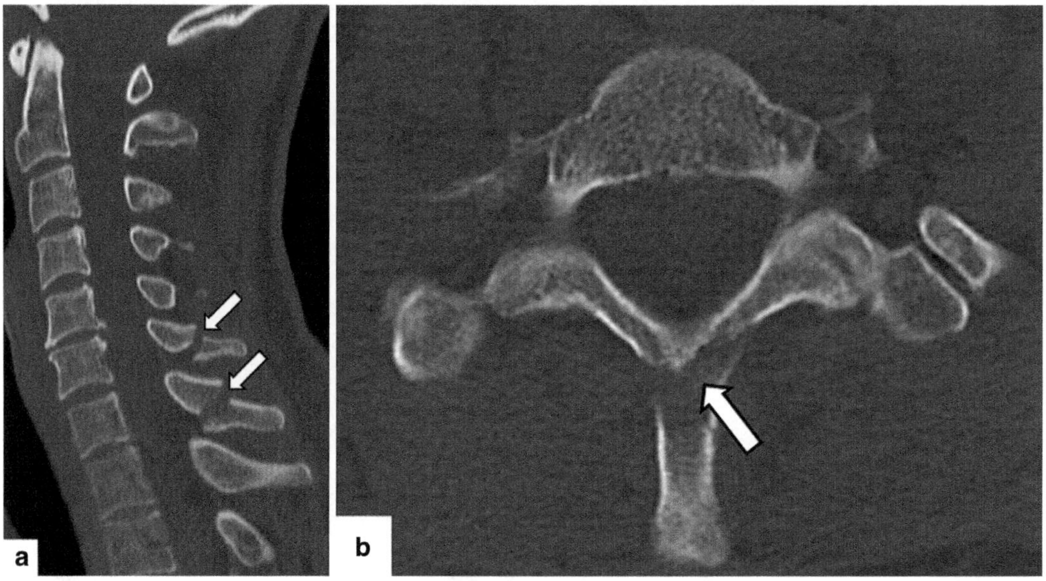


**Fig. 22** Clay shoveler's fracture of C6 and C7 in a 48-year-old male after garden work. Mildly displaced avulsion fractures (arrows) of the spinous processes are seen on NECT sagittal (**a**) and axial (**b**, C7 is shown) reconstructions. The laminae are intact

ever, in instable injuries, they are observed in almost half of the cases. Usually, a disc herniation is observed at the level of an injury or one level adjacent to it (Fig. 30). Its appearance resembles the herniation of disc material observed in non-traumatic cases. In the minority of patients, therapeutical decisions can be drawn from CT imaging. In some, dense material is observed effacing the spinal canal of the neuroforamina (Fig. 31). In fact, MR imaging is the key to the diagnosis; in particular T2-weighted images provide the relation of herniated disc material and the epidural space, the cord, and the nerve roots. With a rupture of the posterior longitudinal ligament, free fragments may be seen within the anterior epidural cerebrospinal fluid with no connection to the disc. In the elderly, preexisting disc pathology is not always unequivo-

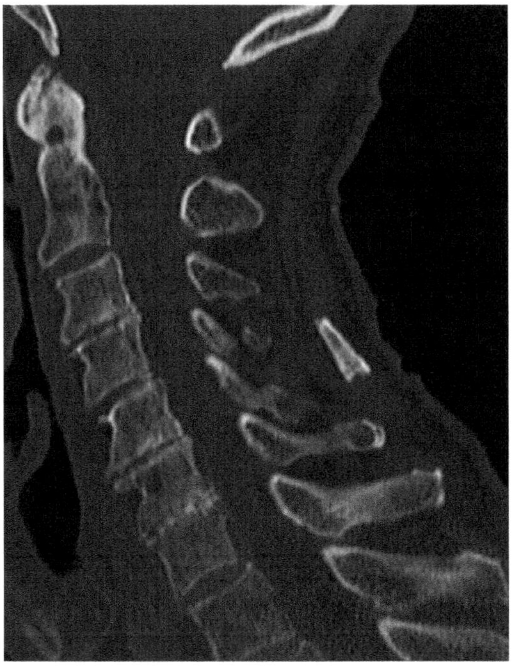

**Fig. 23** Sesamoid ossicles of the nuchal ligament must not be misinterpreted as posterior column fractures! NECT sagittal reconstruction shows a 14 mm calcification of the nuchal ligament

cally differentiated from an acute trauma. Particularly in these, ligamentous and soft tissue damage may lead to the diagnosis.

## 3.6 Spinal Cord Injury

The most common causes of spinal cord trauma are motor vehicle accidents, followed by falls. Male patients aged under 30 years are most often affected. The most common location of spinal cord injury is at the levels C4 to C6 (Schueller and Schueller-Weidekamm 2014). CT imaging solely provides a swollen and hyperdense cord as a sign of haemorrhagic transformation, but cannot be used to underline therapeutical considerations. MR imaging is well established for the detection of spinal cord injury. Predominantly, T1-weighted, STIR, and T2-weighted gradient echo sequences are used. Findings include cord swelling and high T2 signal representing oedema. Cord haemorrhage has a crucial impact on the patients´ outcome. Due to susceptibility effects, it is best visible as hypointense signal on T2-weighted gradient echo sequences. Acute trauma must be differentiated from chronic degenerative disease, including chronic disc herniation and osseous as well as discogenic spinal canal stenosis. In these patients, superimposed trauma usually results in cord oedema well visible on T2-weighted images (Hendey et al. 2002) (Fig. 32). Vice versa, chronic findings can be well distinguished from acute injuries by MR imaging (Fig. 33).

In infants, the spinal cord's high elasticity makes it prone to sustaining a trauma. However, trauma can occur without a radiological correlation, which is referred to as SCIWORA (Pang and Wilberger Jr 1982).

Generally accepted grading criteria have been developed and published by the American Spinal Injury Association (ASIA). According to the Frankel classification, the severity score has five grades, E being normal and A indicating a complete deficit with no motor or sensory functions below the level of the injury (Maynard Jr. et al. 1997).

From a radiological point of view, the publication of M. Kulkarni, F. Bondurant, and coworkers (Bondurant et al. 1990) is of good help in order to correlate MR imaging results with the patients´ clinical prognosis. The prognosis is dependent on the extent of the oedema and is deteriorated by haemorrhage. Type 1 of the Kulkarni and Bondurant classification contains cord haemorrhage evident as a T1 signal inhomogeneity and low T2 signal. It has a poor prognosis. Most commonly, type 2 injuries are noted. T2 signal is hyperintense, the cord is edematously swollen, and T1 signal is normal. It has the best prognosis. Type 3 is comparably rare; it includes peripheral high T2 signal and a low T2 signal in the centre (Fig. 11). T1-weighted images usually are without findings. It has a moderate prognosis. The poorest prognosis, as a matter of fact, is correlated with a spinal cord transsection. It is best depicted on T1-weighted images. Without the presence of transsection, the combination of the factors, patients older than 50 years and the location of spinal cord injury at the levels C4 to C6, has a markedly poor prognosis.

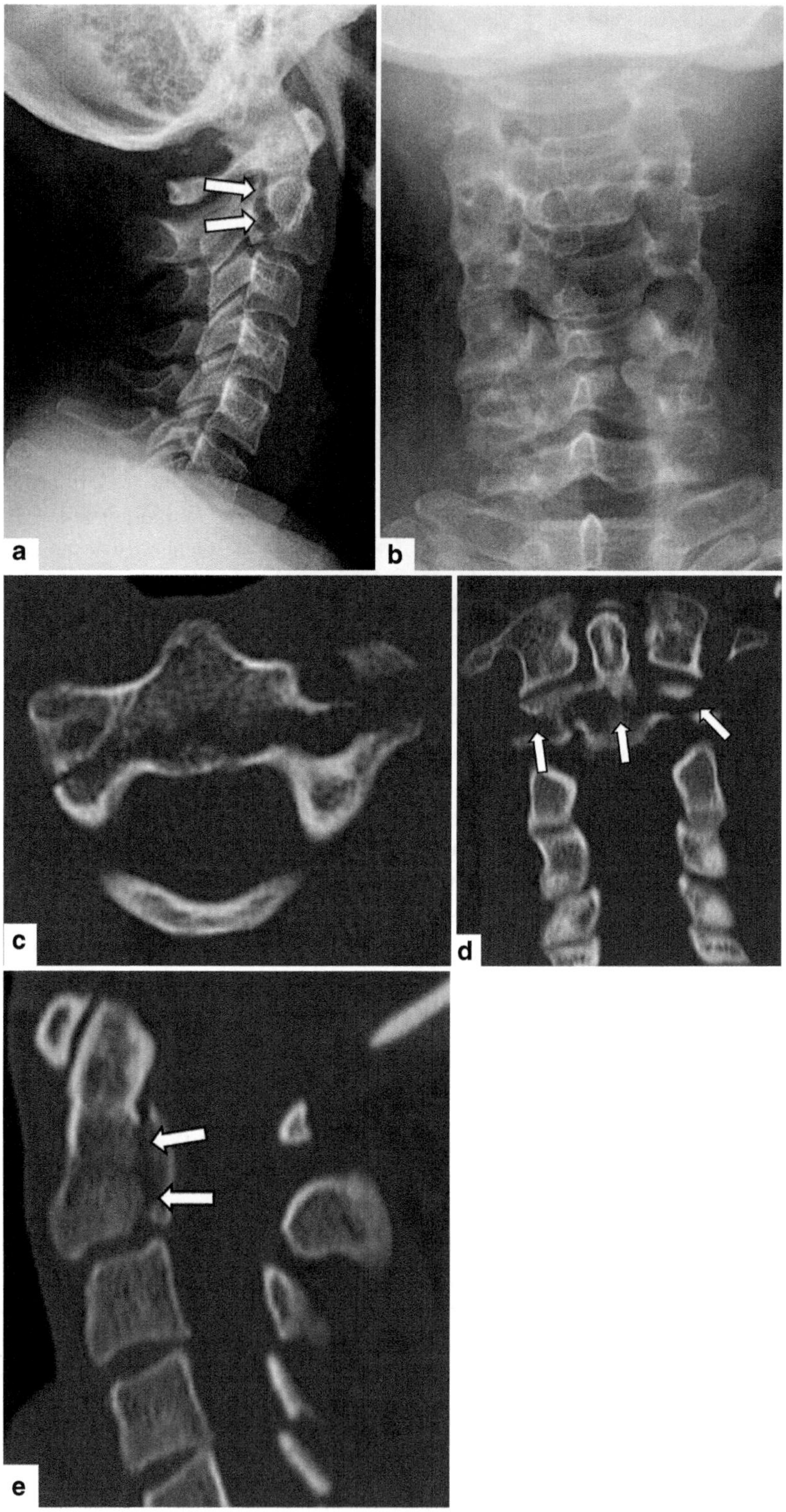


**Fig. 24** Hangman's fracture of C2. Bilateral fractures through the interarticulate parts and the pedicles (arrows) are noted on the lateral (**a**) radiograph as well as on axial (**c**), coronal (**d**), and sagittal (**e**) NECT reconstructions. AP radiograph (**b**) is inconclusive in this patient

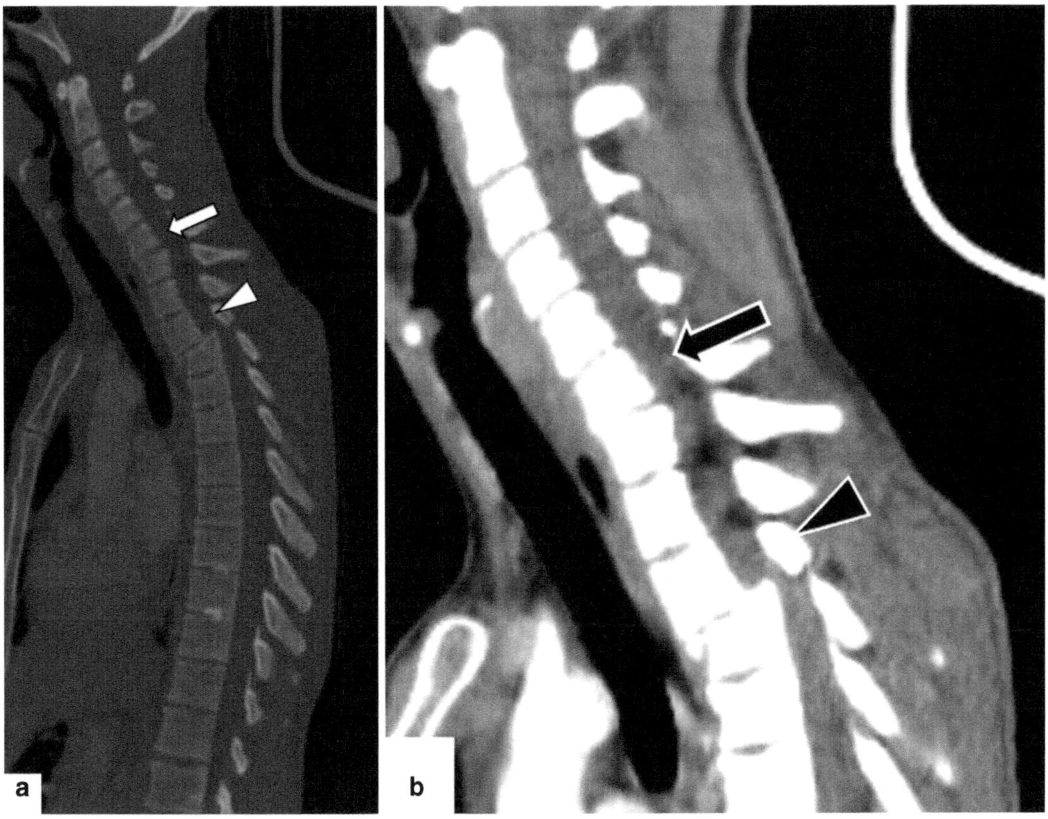


**Fig. 25** Multisegmental dislocations of the segments C6/C7 and Th2/Th3 in a 33-year-old car driver. Anterior displacement according to unilateral facet joint luxation of C6 (arrows) as well as bilateral facet joint luxation of Th2 (arrowheads) is noted. There is an absolute spinal canal stenosis Th2/Th3; the cord is substantially compressed. Sagittally reconstructed NECT in bone (**a**) and soft tissue (**b**) windows

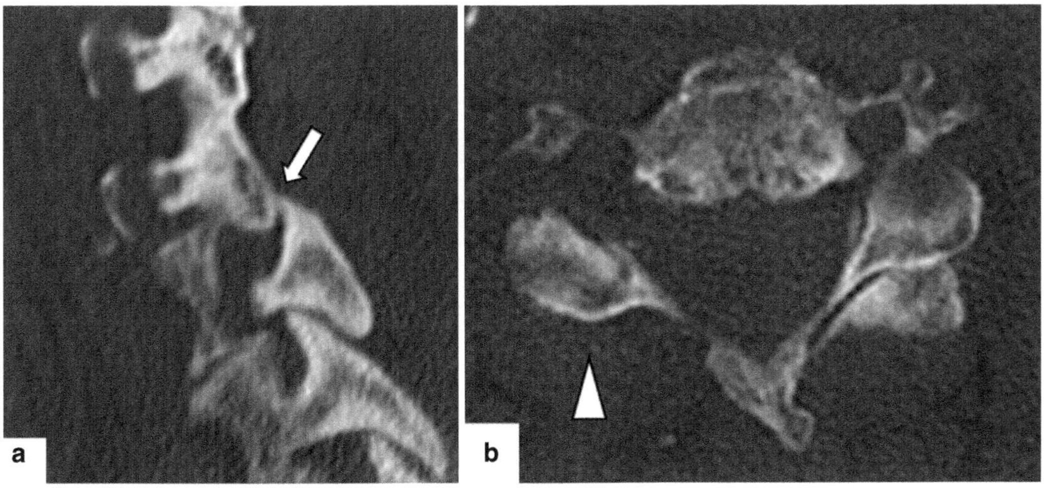


**Fig. 26** Unilateral luxation of C6 with a jumped facet on the right (arrow) and the naked facet sign (arrowhead). NECT, sagittal (**a**) and axial (**b**) reconstructions

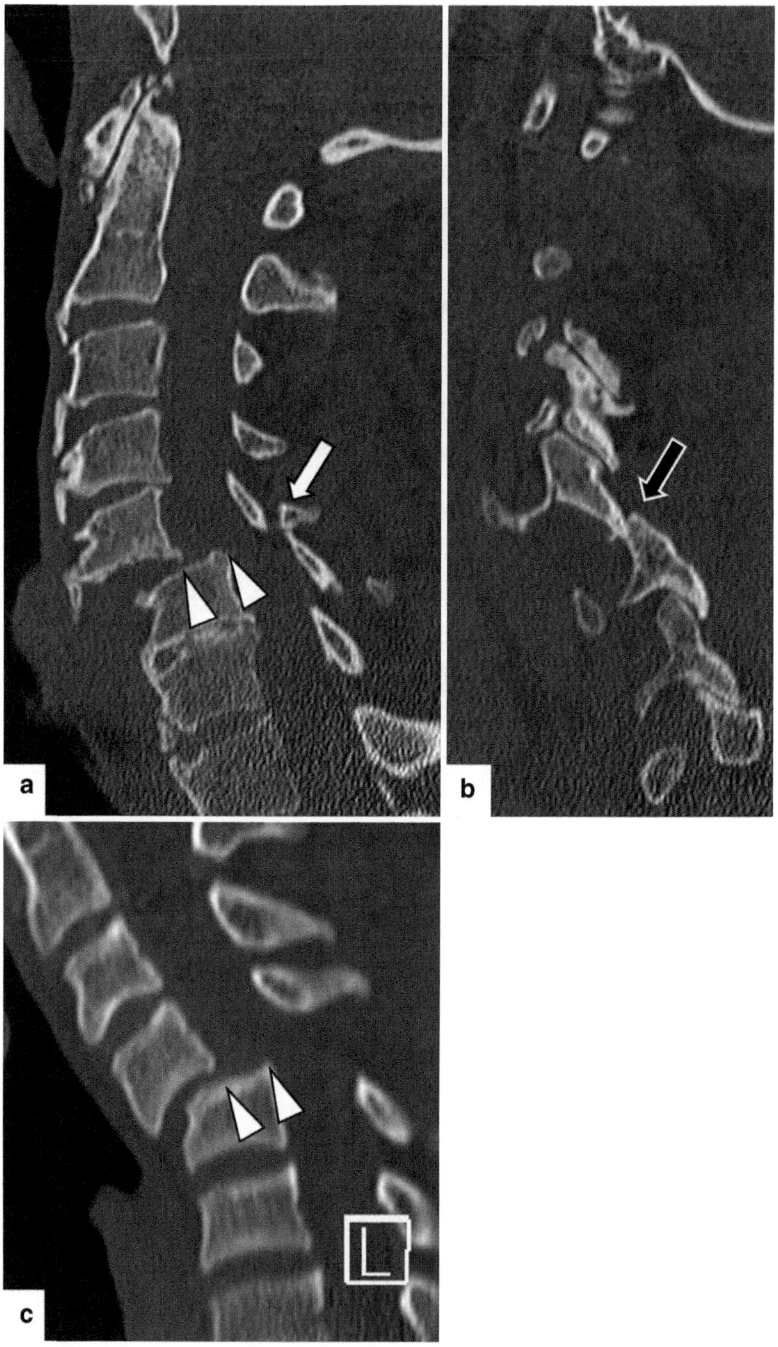


**Fig. 27** Bilateral facet joint luxations of C5/C6 (arrows) in an 81-year-old motor cycle driver (**a**, **b**) and of C4/C5 in a 29-year-old male (**c**) after jumping into shallow water. The horizontal displacement of the vertebral bodies of C6 (**a**) and of C4 (**c**) is about 50% each (arrowheads). In (**b**) the jumped facet (black arrow) on the left is shown. NECT, sagittal reconstructions

## 4 Imaging Modalities

On the one hand, a low threshold in the use of cross-sectional imaging is presumably associated with an increased detection of CSI. On the other hand, this strength must be thoroughly weighed against the shortcomings, including the costs of CT and MR imaging. In addition, concerns about the radiation exposure require a careful patient selection.

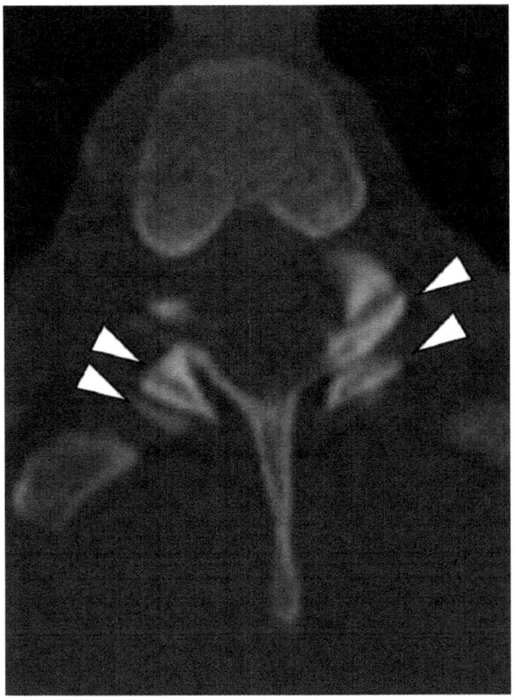

**Fig. 28** Same patient as in Fig. 25. The Reversed Hamburger bun sign represents the blocked bilateral facet joint luxation with a convex appearance of the facets' articular surfaces (arrowheads). NECT, axial reconstruction

## 4.1 Low-Risk Patients

The most significant studies about risk stratification of CSI are the National Emergency X-radiography Utilization Study (NEXUS) (Hoffman et al. 2000) and the Canadian Cervical Spine Prediction Rule Study (CCSPR) (Stiell et al. 2001). Both studies, taken together, comprised more than 43,000 patients. Data revealed comparable high sensitivities for identifying patients at risk for significant spine injury. This means that patients who meet the dedicated low-risk criteria that have been established by these studies (i.e., no midline cervical tenderness; no focal neurologic deficits; no intoxication or indication of brain injury; no painful distracting injuries; normal alertness) do not need imaging (Hoffman et al. 2000; Stiell et al. 2001) (Fig. 34).

Flexion and extension views are considered not cost-effective in imaging the traumatized spine (Anglen et al. 2002). However, flexion and extension imaging of the cervical spine could be useful in evaluating potential ligamentous injury in patients with normal or inconclusive MR imaging findings.

## 4.2 High-Risk Patients

However, adults who do not fulfil these low-risk criteria require comprehensive imaging. In a meta-analysis of seven studies, the pooled sensitivity of radiography for detecting patients with CSI was as low as 52%, while the combined sensitivity of CT was 98% (Holmes and Akkinepalli 2005). Thus, C should be the primary screening study for CSI.

Radiography fails to detect about 30% of potentially lethal cervical spine trauma. In the lower cervical spine, this number raises to 50% in adult patients and to 90% regarding the cranio-cervical junction (Hunter et al. 2014). The second most region of false-negative radiographical results is in the cervicothoracic junction (Inaoka et al. 2012).

CT imaging is necessary to comprehensively evaluate patients with the clinical suspicion of significant cervical injury, regardless whether radiography is positive or negative. Among other findings, even a subtle malalignment of the spinolaminar line on lateral radiographs should prompt CT imaging (Fig. 8). In addition, CT imaging reveals early or subtle haemorrhage of the cervical spinal canal (Fig. 35). The literature does not define a minimum section thickness, maximum voxel dimensions, or other technical factors for CT imaging. Thin section reconstructions of about 1 mm in all three dimensions are usually obtained in the bone as well as in the soft tissue windows.

## 4.3 Infants

To date, there is some data about the reliability of the NEXUS criteria in children. In their study, Oman and co-workers enrolled 1666

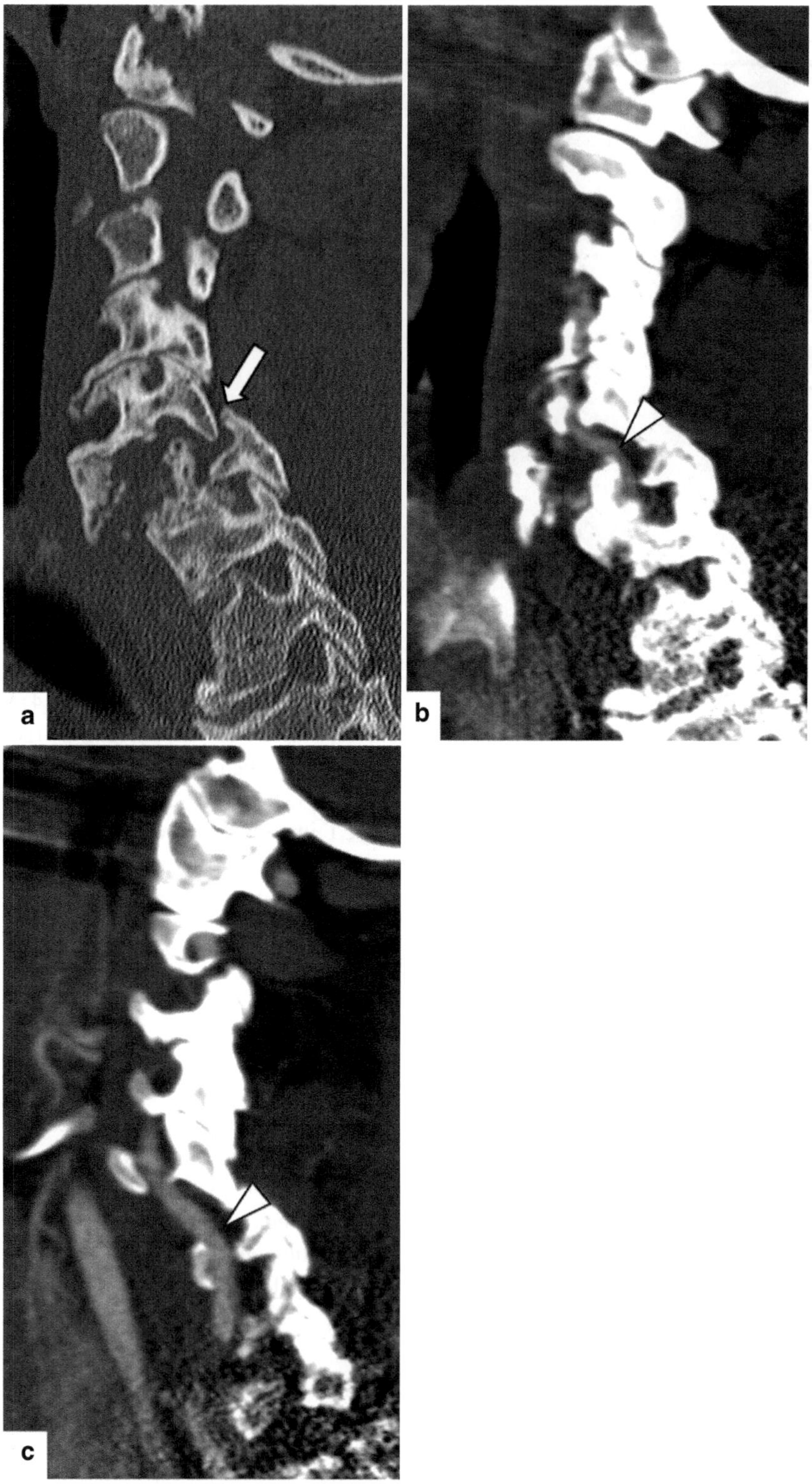


**Fig. 29** Fracture-dislocation of C5/C6 in a 72-year-old pedestrian struck by a car. Bilateral facet joint luxation is noted (arrows; right side is shown). CT angiography demonstrates intact vertebral arteries on both sides (arrowheads). Sagittally reconstructed NECT (**a**) and CT angiography (**b**, **c**)

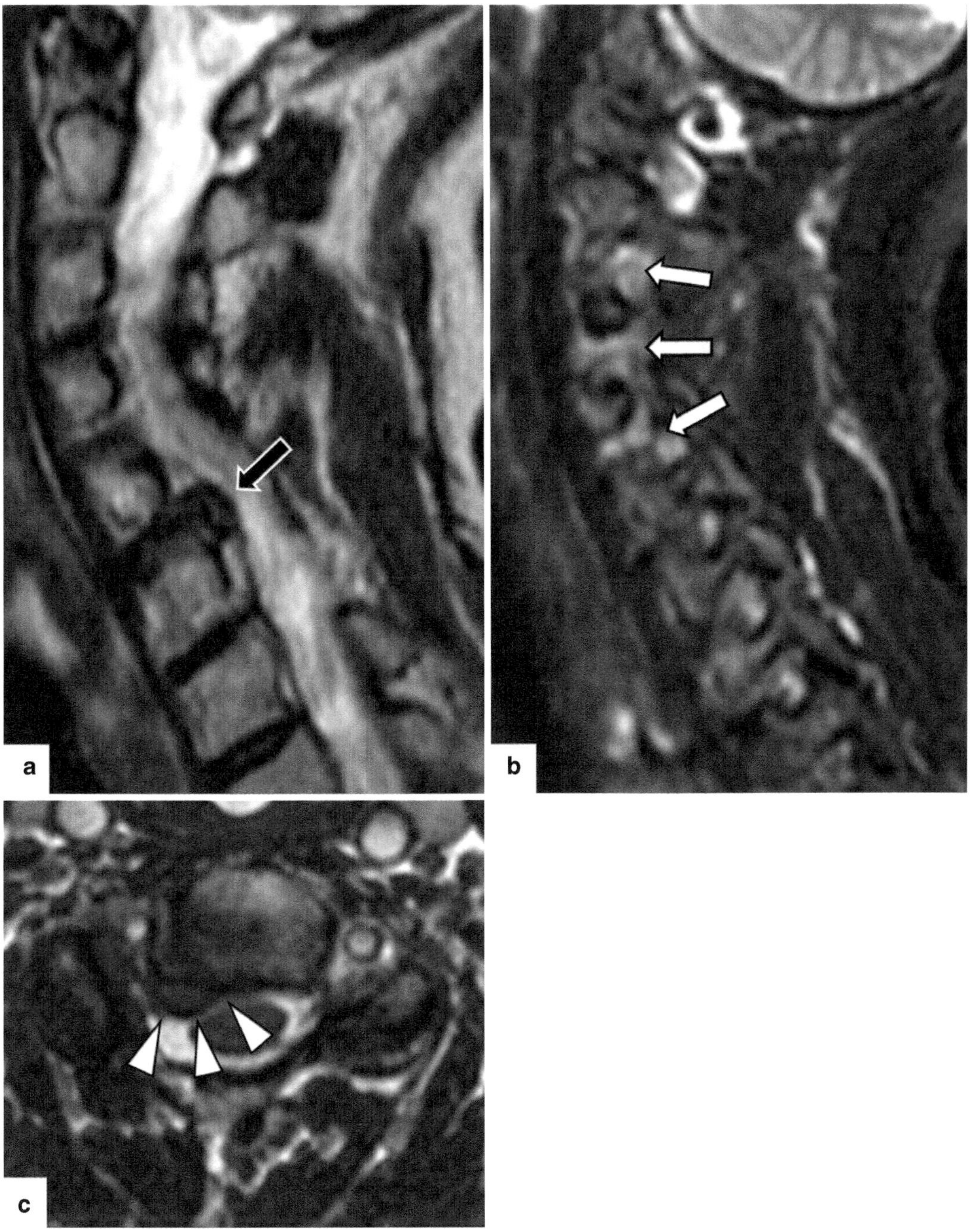


**Fig. 30** Traumatic disc herniation of C5/C6 on the right (black arrow) in a 57-year-old female after a fall. The herniated disc effaces the lateral recess as well as the epidural space on the right (arrowheads). Marked ligamentous strain and intervertebral oedema is from C3 to C5 (arrows). 1.5 Tesla T2-weighted sagittal (**a**), axial (**c**), and sagittal STIR (**b**) MR imaging

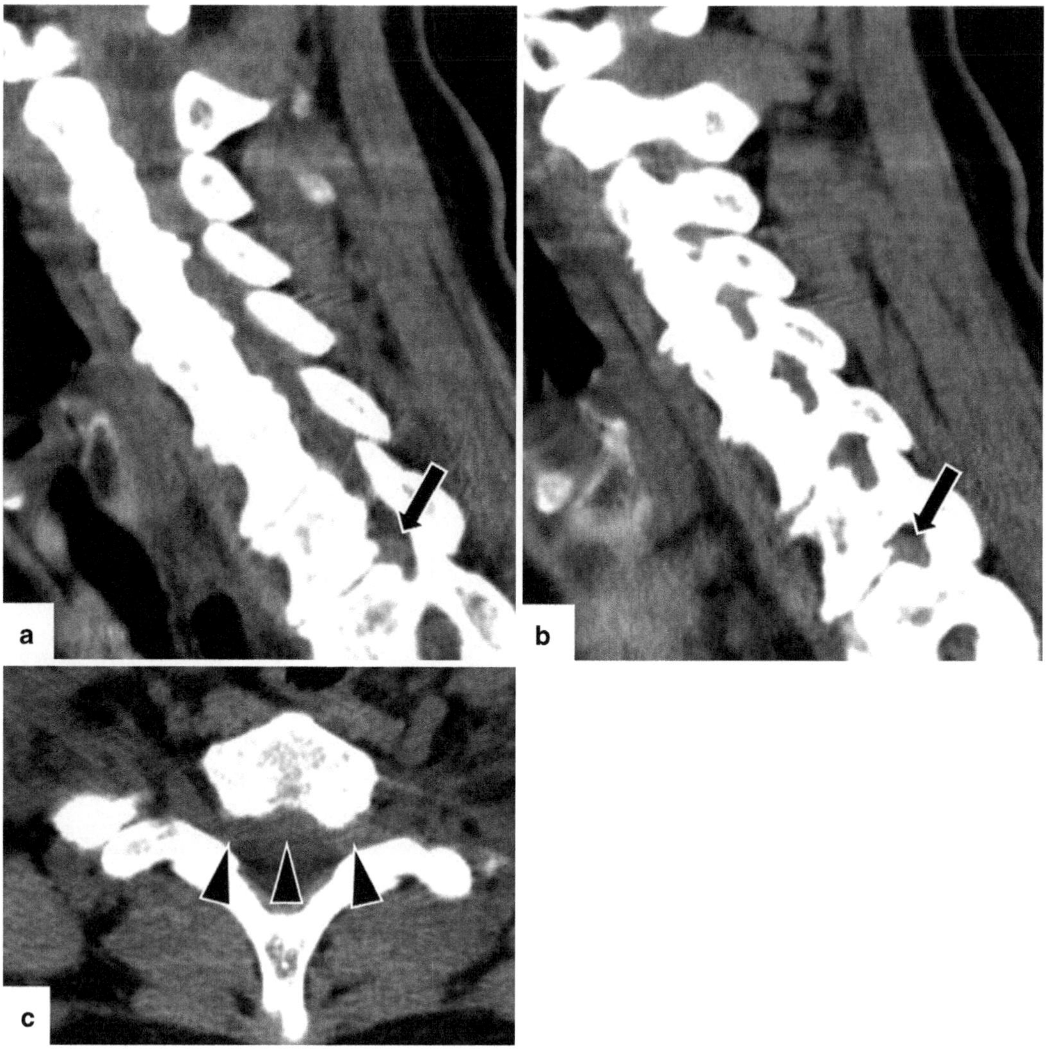


**Fig. 31** Traumatic disc herniation of C6/C7 on the left in a 68-year-old male. NECT reveals a stenosis of the ipsilateral neuroforamen and of the lateral recesses (arrows), more pronounced on the left than on the right (arrowheads). Sagittal (**a**, **b**) and axial (**c**) reconstructions in soft tissue windows

children with suspected spinal injury (Oman et al. 2006). The authors retrospectively applied the NEXUS criteria and found them to be reliable in children. The recommended protocol for cervical spine clearance included radiography as the first-line imaging study, while CT and MR imaging is reserved for patients with inconclusive findings. The prospective study of Viccellio and co-workers included 3065 patients younger than 18 years with blunt cervical spine trauma. The study revealed that the NEXUS decision instrument worked well in children and that its use could reduce cervical spine imaging by nearly 20% (Viccellio et al. 2001).

Radiography is supposed to be of sufficiently high accuracy in imaging the paediatric population. One of the reasons may be that children suffer from CSI different from adults, since the atlanto-occipital as well as the atlanto-dental seg-

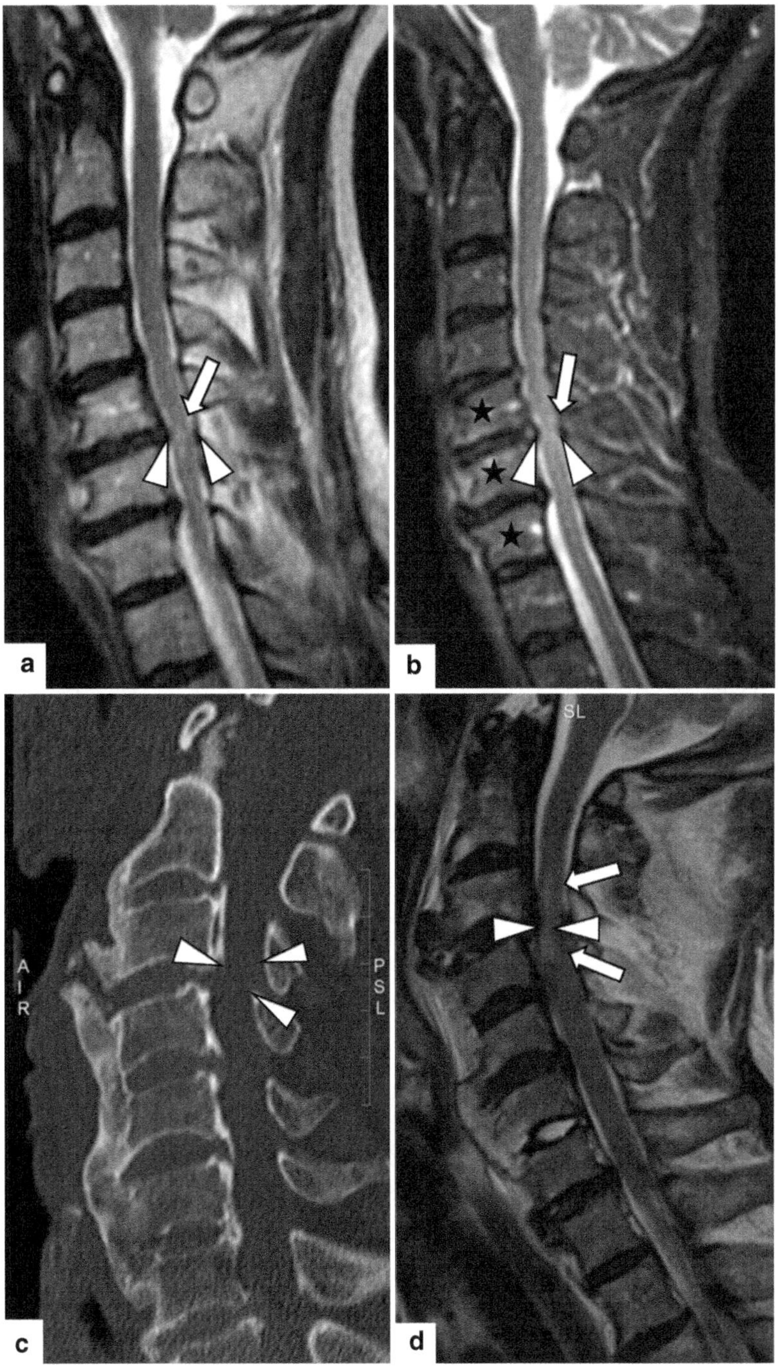


**Fig. 32** Acute spinal cord oedema and underlying chronic degenerative disease of C5/C6 in a 64-year-old female after a fall from 2 m (**a**, **b**), and in an 83-year-old male after an unobserved fall. Cord oedema (arrows) of C5/C6 (**a**, **b**) and of C2/C3 (**d**) is present at the maximum of pre-existing osseous and discogenic spinal canal stenosis (arrowheads). Moderate bone bruise is noted in the vertebral bodies from C5 to C7 (asterices), associated with trauma. 3.0 Tesla sagittal T2-weighted (**a**, **d**) and STIR (**b**) MR imaging. NECT, sagittal reconstruction (**c**)

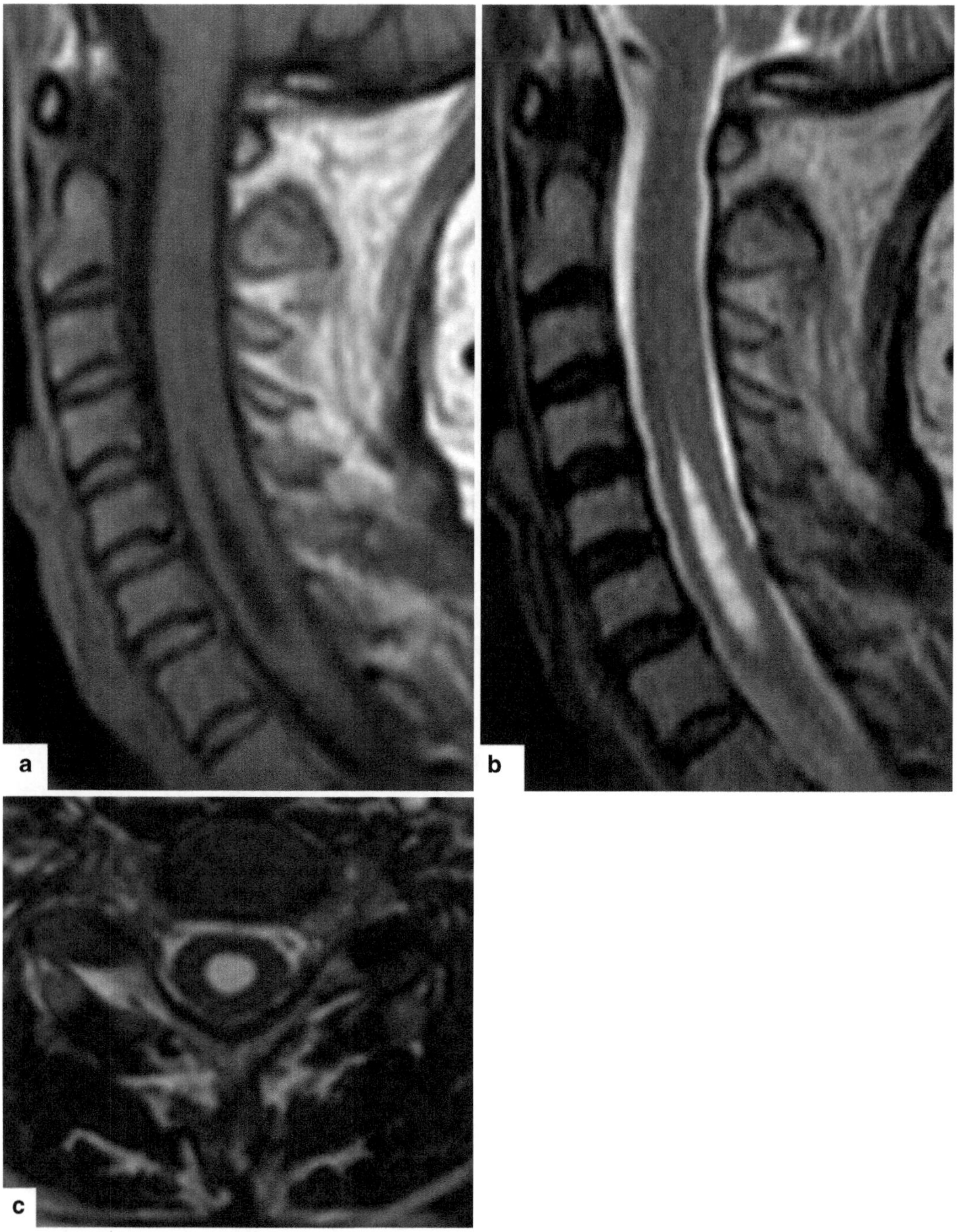

**Fig. 33** Blunt cervical spine trauma in an 18-year-old female with persistent, unspecific paresthesia in both hands. A pre-existing syringomyelia from C4 to C7 is seen. It is 6 mm wide. Findings associated with an acute trauma are absent. 1.5 Tesla sagittal (**a**, **b**) and axial (**c**) T1 weighted (**a**) and T2 weighted (**b**, **c**) MR imaging

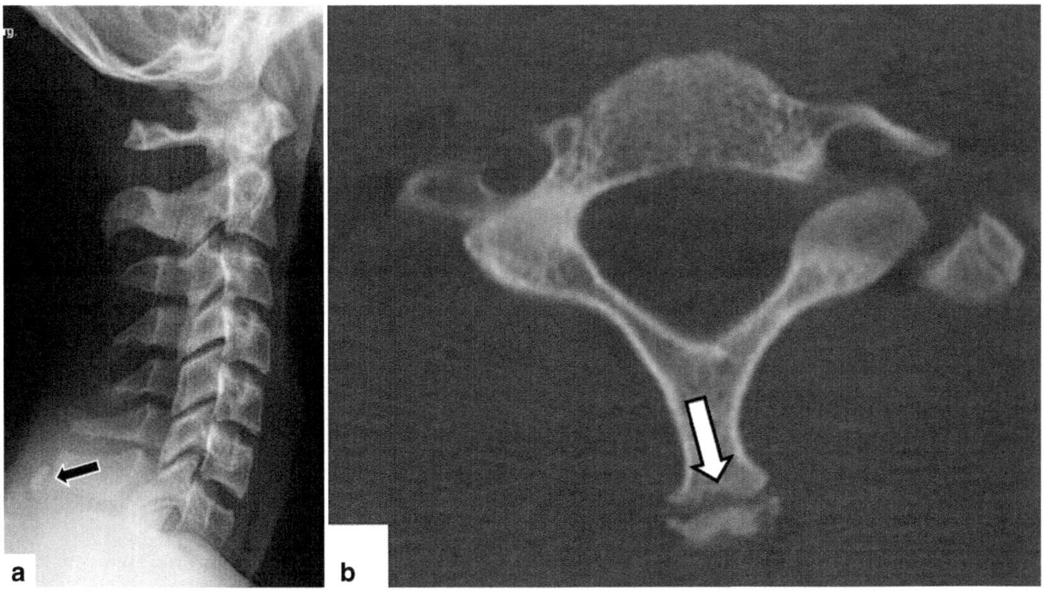


**Fig. 34** No findings related to an acute trauma are observed in a 21-year-old female after a fall from 1 m. NEXUS low-risk criteria (Hoffman et al. 2000; Stiell et al. 2001) are met. However, radiographs (lateral radiograph (**a**); AP view not shown) were obtained and reveal a 10 mm bone calcification next to the spinous process of C7 (arrows). It was mistaken for an acute fracture by the referring clinicians. NECT axial reconstruction confirmed the presence of a non-ossified apophyseal remnant and ruled out an acute fracture (**b**). NECT was unnecessarily performed, as was radiography in this patient

ments are more often involved than the lower cervical spine. In turn, the cranio-cervical junction obviously is well depicted by radiographs in infants.

## 4.4 Neurological Impairment

MR imaging is considered a standard of imaging neurological deficits (Wood et al. 2014). Its role in imaging the traumatic cervical spine is determined by the capabilities of direct visualization of the nerves and the cord. According to the criteria established by the American College of Roentgenology (ACR), it should be performed within 48 h, if the neurological conditions of a patient cannot be fully explained by other examinations, including those with normal CT findings (Fisher et al. 2013; Hogan et al. 2005; Pourtaheri et al. 2014). MR imaging is also indicated when clinical conditions remain deteriorated several weeks after a spinal cord injury (Stiell et al. 2001). There is no clear evidence that MR imaging performed more than 48 h after an injury has a lower sensitivity than acute MR imaging. Instead, the recommendation to perform MR imaging within 48 h rather is due to concerns about keeping patients in collars unnecessarily for a prolonged period of time.

MR imaging is highly accurate in the delineation of traumatic disc herniation, soft tissue injury, and cord injury (see above). MR imaging detects up to about 25% of soft tissue injuries more than CT (Fisher et al. 2013). Unfortunately, it cannot be considered an unequivocal trouble-shooter, since, on the one hand, it potentially misses significant lesions well recognized on CT images and, on the other, clinically insignificant lesions may also be detected.

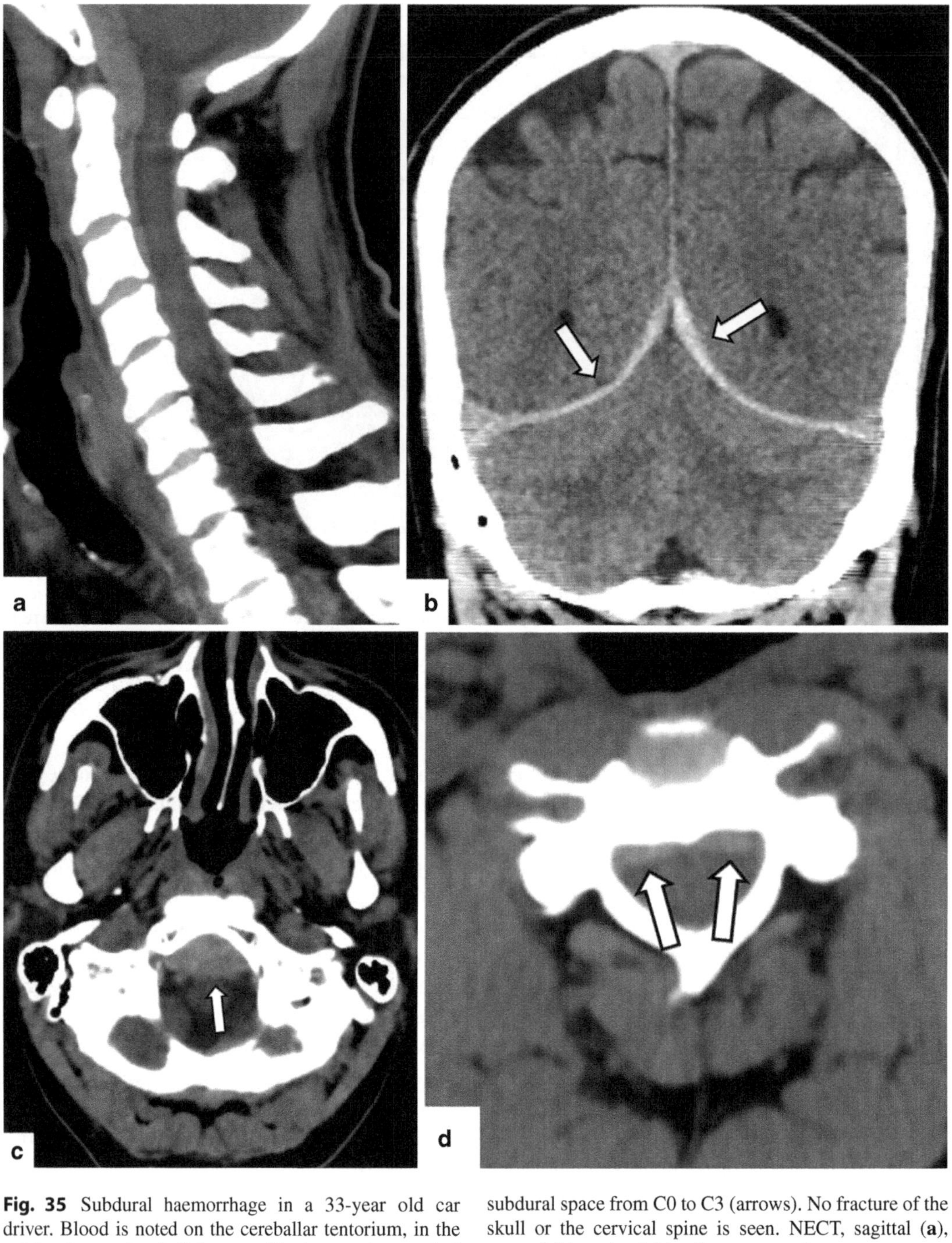


**Fig. 35** Subdural haemorrhage in a 33-year old car driver. Blood is noted on the cereballar tentorium, in the subdural posterior skull base, and in the anterior cervical subdural space from C0 to C3 (arrows). No fracture of the skull or the cervical spine is seen. NECT, sagittal (**a**), coronal (**b**), and axial (**c**, **d**) reconstructions

## 5 Conclusion

In CSI, key variables, such as the delineation of instability as well as the affection of nerve roots and the spinal cord, have implications for the patients' treatment and outcome. An appropriate collaboration of radiologists and clinicians is vitally important. Accordingly, the interpretation of the trauma classifications must be unified among all members of the trauma team in order to provide comprehensive communication in the daily practise. The essential understanding of the subaxial cervical trauma relies on biomechanical considerations of osseous and ligamentous contributors to stability and on the knowledge of stereotypical injury patterns occurring subsequent to specific force vectors sustained to the spine. Despite the fact that radiography is still in use as a first-line modality in a number of institutions, it is cross-sectional imaging which provides an adequate analysis of the traumatized cervical spine. The principles summarized in this chapter may be of good help for the emergency radiologists′ workup of CSI around the clock.

**Conflict of Interest** The authors state that there is no conflict of interest.

## References

Anderson PA, Montesano PX (1988) Morphology and treatment of occipital condyle fractures. Spine 13:731–736

Anglen J, Metzler M, Bunn P, Griffiths H (2002) Flexion and extension views are not cost-effective in a cervical spine clearance protocol for obtunded trauma patients. J Trauma 52:54–59

Bogduk N, Yoganandan N (2001) Biomechanics of the cervical spine part 3: minor injuries. Clin Biomech 16:267–275

Bondurant FJ, Cotler HB, Kulkarni MV, McArdle CB, Harris JH Jr (1990) Acute spinal cord injury. A study using physical examination and magnetic resonance imaging. Spine 15:161–168

Chilvers G, Janjua U, Choudhary S (2017) Blunt cervical spine injury in adult polytrauma: incidence, injury patterns and predictors of significant ligament injury on CT. Clin Radiol 72:907–914

Clayton JL, Harris MB, Weintraub SL, Marr AB, Timmer J, Stuke LE et al (2012) Risk factors for cervical spine injury. Injury 43:431–435

Daffner SD, Daffner RH (2002) Computed tomography diagnosis of facet dislocations: the "hamburger bun" and "reverse hamburger bun" signs. J Emerg Med 23:387–394

Denis F (1983) The three column spine and its significance in the classification of acute thoracolumbar spinal injuries. Spine 8:817–831

Denis F (1984) Spinal instability as defined by the three-column spine concept in acute spinal trauma. Clin Orthop Relat Res 189:65–76

Dvorak MF, Fisher CG, Fehlings MG, Rampersaud YR, Oner FC, Aarabi B, Vaccaro AR (2007) The surgical approach to subaxial cervical spine injuries: an evidence-based algorithm based on the SLIC classification system. Spine 32:2620–2629

Effendi B, Roy D, Cornish B, Dussault RG, Laurin CA (1981) Fractures of the ring of the axis. A classification based on the analysis of 131 cases. J Bone Joint Surg Am 63-B:319–327

Fisher BM, Cowles S, Matulich JR, Evanson BG, Vega D, Dissanaike S (2013) Is magnetic resonance imaging in addition to a computed tomographic scan necessary to identify clinically significant cervical spine injuries in obtunded blunt trauma patients? Am J Surg 206:987–993

Gehweiler JA, Duff DE, Martinez S, Miller MD, Clark WM (1976) Fractures of the atlas vertebra. Skelet Radiol 1:97–102

Groves CJ, Cassar-Pullicino VN, Tins BJ, Tyrrell PN, McCall IW (2005) Chance-type flexion-distraction injuries in the thoracolumbar spine: MR imaging characteristics. Radiology 236:601–608

Han SY, Witten DM, Mussleman JP (1976) Jefferson fracture of the atlas. Report of six cases. J Neurosurg 44:368–371

Hawighorst H, Huisman T, Berger MF, Zach GA, Michel D (2001) MRI in spinal injuries. Radiologe 41:1033–1037

Hendey GW, Wolfson AB, Mower WR, Hoffman JR (2002) Spinal cord injury without radiographic abnormality: results of the National Emergency X-Radiography Utilization Study in blunt cervical trauma. J Trauma 53:1–4

Hills MW, Deane SA (1993) Head injury and facial injury: is there an increased risk of cervical spine injury? J Trauma 34:549–553

Hoffman JR, Mower WR, Wolfson AB, Todd KH, Zucker MI (2000) Validity of a set of clinical criteria to rule out injury to the cervical spine in patients with blunt trauma. National Emergency X-Radiography Utilization Study Group. N Engl J Med 343:94–99

Hogan GJ, Mirvis SE, Shanmuganathan K, Scalea TM (2005) Exclusion of instable cervical spine injury in obtunded patients with blunt trauma: is MR imaging needed when multi-detector row CT findings are normal? Radiology 237:106–113

Holdsworth F (1970) Fractures, dislocations, and fracture-dislocations of the spine. J Bone Joint Surg Am 52:1534–1551

Holmes JF, Akkinepalli R (2005) Computed tomography versus plain radiography to screen for cervical spine injury: a meta-analysis. J Trauma 58:902–905

Hunter BR, Keim SM, Seupaul RA, Hern G (2014) Are plain radiographs sufficient to exclude cervical spine injuries in low-risk adults? J Emerg Med 46:257–263

Inaoka T, Ohashi K, El-Khoury GY, Singh H, Berbaum KS (2012) Clinical role of radiography for thoracic spine fractures in daily practice in the MDCT era: a retrospective review of 255 trauma patients. Jpn J Radiol 30:617–623

Jain NB, Ayers GD, Peterson EN, Harris MB, Morse L, O'Connor KC, Garshick E (2015) Traumatic spinal cord injury in the United States 1993–2012. JAMA 313:2236–2243

Kattail D, Furlan JC, Fehlings MG (2009) Epidemiology and clinical outcomes of acute spine trauma and spinal cord injury: experience from a specialized spine trauma center in Canada in comparison with a large national registry. J Trauma 67:936–943

Langner S, Fleck S, Kirsch M, Petrik M, Hosten N (2008) Whole-body CT trauma imaging with adapted and optimized CT angiography of the craniocervical vessels: do we need an extra screening examination? AJNR Am J Neuroradiol 29:1902–1907

Leucht P, Fischer K, Muhr G, Mueller EJ (2009) Epidemiology of traumatic spine fractures. Injury 40:166–172

Lowery DW, Wald MM, Browne BJ, Tigges S, Hoffman JR, Mower WR (2001) Epidemiology of cervical spine injury victims. Ann Emerg Med 38:12–16

Magerl F, Aebi M, Gertzbein SD, Harms J, Nazarian S (1994) A comprehensive classification of thoracic and lumbar injuries. Eur Spine J 3:184–201

Malhotra AK, Camacho M, Ivatury RR, Davis IC, Komorowski DJ, Leung DA, Grizzard JD, Aboutanos MB, Duane TM, Cockrell C, Wolfe LG, Borchers CT, Martin NR (2007) Computed tomographic angiography for the diagnosis of blunt carotid/vertebral artery injury: a note of caution. Ann Surg 246:632–642

Martinez-Perez R, Jimenez-Roldan L, Lagares A (2014) Ligaments disruption: a new perspective in the prognosis of spinal cord injury. Neural Regen Res 9:456–457

Maynard FM Jr, Bracken MB, Creasey G, Ditunno JF Jr, Donovan WH, Ducker TB, Garber SL, Marino RJ, Stover SL, Tator CH, Waters RL, Wilberger JE, Young W (1997) International standards for neurological and functional classification of spinal cord injury. American Spinal Injury Association. Spinal Cord 35:266–274

Michael DB, Guyot DR, Darmody WR (1989) Coincidence of head and cervical spine injury. J Neurotrauma 6:177–189

Mulligan RP, Friedman JA, Mahabir RC (2010) A nationwide review of the associations among cervical spine injuries, head injuries, and facial fractures. J Trauma 68:587–592

O'Callaghan JP, Ullrich CG, Yuan HA, Kieffer SA (1980) CT of facet distraction in flexion injuries of the thoracolumbar spine: the "naked" facet. AJR Am J Roentgenol 134:563–568

O'Malley KF, Ross SE (1988) The incidence of injury to the cervical spine in patients with craniocerebral injury. J Trauma 28:1476–1478

Oman JA, Cooper RJ, Holmes JF, Viccellio P, Nyce A, Ross SE, Hoffman JR, Mower WR, Investigators NEXUSII (2006) Performance of a decision rule to predict need for computed tomography among children with blunt head trauma. Pediatrics 117:238–246

Palmieri F, Cassar-Pullicino VN, Dell'Atti C, Lalam RK, Tins BJ, Tyrrell PN, McCall IW (2006) Uncovertebral joint injury in cervical facet dislocation: the headphones sign. Eur Radiol 16:1312–1315

Pang D, Wilberger JE Jr (1982) Spinal cord injury without radiographic abnormalities in children. J Neurosurg 57:114–129

Pourtaheri S, Emami A, Sinha K, Faloon M, Hwang K, Shafa E, Holmes L Jr (2014) The role of magnetic resonance imaging in acute cervical spine fractures. Spine J 14(11):2546–2553

Raniga SB, Menon V, Al Muzahmi KS, Butt S (2014) MDCT of acute subaxial cervical spine trauma: a mechanism-based approach. Insights Imaging 5:321–328

Reinhold M, Blauth M, Rosiek R, Knop C (2006) Lower cervical spine trauma: classification and operative treatment. Unfallchirurg 109:471–480

Roberge RJ, Wears RC, Kelly M, Evans TC, Kenny MA, Daffner RD et al (1988) Selective application of cervical spine radiography in alert victims of blunt trauma: a prospective study. J Trauma 28:784–788

Ronnen HR, de Korte PJ, Brink PR, van der Bijl HJ, Tonino AJ, Franke CL (1996) Acute whiplash injury: is there a role for MR imaging? — A prospective study of 100 patients. Radiology 201:93–96

Ryan MD, Henderson JJ (1992) The epidemiology of fractures and fracture-dislocations of the cervical spine. Injury 23:38–40

Sanchez B, Waxman K, Jones T, Conner S, Chung R, Becerra S (2005) Cervical spine clearance in blunt trauma: evaluation of a computed tomography-based protocol. J Trauma 59:179–183

Schueller G (2010) Who is who revisited: spinal trauma. Radiologe 50:1084–1095

Schueller G, Schueller-Weidekamm C (2014) The traumatized vertebral spine reloaded: injury mechanisms and their radiological patterns. Semin Muskuloskelet Radiol 18:240–245

Stiell IG, Wells GA, Vandemheen KL, Clement CM, Lesiuk H, De Maio VJ, Laupacis A, Schull M, McKnight RD, Verbeek R, Brison R, Cass D, Dreyer J, Eisenhauer MA, Greenberg GH, MacPhail I, Morrison L, Reardon M, Worthington J (2001) The Canadian C-spine rule for radiography in alert and stable trauma patients. JAMA 286:1841–1848

Thompson WL, Stiell IG, Clement CM, Brison RJ (2009) Association of injury mechanism with the risk of cervical spine fractures. CJEM 11:14–22

Vaccaro AR, Madigan L, Schweitzer ME, Flanders AE, Hilibrand AS, Albert TJ (2001) Magnetic resonance imaging analysis of soft tissue disruption after flexion-distraction injuries of the subaxial cervical spine. Spine 26:1866–1872

Vaccaro AR, Hulbert RJ, Patel AA, Fisher C, Dvorak M, Lehman RA Jr et al (2007) The subaxial cervical spine injury classification system: a novel approach to recognize the importance of morphology, neurology, and integrity of the disco-ligamentous complex. Spine 32:2365–2374

Viccellio P, Simon H, Pressman BD, Shah MN, Mower WR, Hoffman JR, NEXUS Group (2001) A prospective multicenter study of cervical spine injury in children. Pediatrics 108:E20

White AA 3rd, Johnson RM, Panjabi MM, Southwick WO (1975) Biomechanical analysis of clinical stability in the cervical spine. Clin Orthop Relat Res 109:85–96

Willen J, Anderson J, Toomoka K, Singer K (1990) The natural history of burst fractures at the thoracolumbar junction. J Spinal Disord 3:39–46

Wood KB, Li W, Lebl DS, Ploumis A (2014) Management of thoracolumbar spine fractures. Spine J 14:145–164

Yanar H, Demetriades D, Hadjizacharia P, Nomoto S, Salim A, Inaba K et al (2007) Pedestrians injured by automobiles: risk factors for cervical spine injuries. J Am Coll Surg 205:794–799

# Thoraco-Lumbar Spine

E. A. Dick, M. Naik, and R. Mobasheri

## Contents



**Key Points**

- Imaging is the key to prompt diagnosis and treatment in thoracolumbar (TL) trauma.
- CT is the ideal first investigation, preferably as part of a trauma PanCT. This can be followed by MRI if required.
- Sagittal and coronal bony reconstructions are useful for clinicians who may not have access to multiplanar reconstruction on their viewing platforms.
- Three main classification systems exist for TL injuries: Denis' 3 column model, the TLICS (Thoracolumbar Injury Classification System), and the modified AO (Arbeitsgemeinschaft fur Osteosynthesefragen) classification.
- The radiologist needs to be familiar with all three classification systems but should tailor the classification used in their report to suit the clinical team they work with.
- The radiologist should discuss instability and stability in their report according to local preferences.


E. A. Dick (✉) · M. Naik
Department of Radiology, Imperial College Healthcare NHS Trust, London, UK
e-mail: elizabeth.dick1@nhs.net

R. Mobasheri
Department of Orthopaedic Surgery, Imperial College Healthcare NHS Trust, London, UK




M. Scaglione et al. (eds.), *Emergency Radiology of the Head and Spine*, Medical Radiology Diagnostic Imaging, https://doi.org/10.1007/978-3-030-91047-1_14

## 1 Introduction

Imaging is the key to diagnosis of spinal injury and therefore the radiologist has a crucial early role in the management of a potential spinal patient (Anderson 2010). An important consideration for the radiologist reporting patients with thoracolumbar (TL) spinal trauma is to ensure they are speaking the same language as the spinal surgeons and trauma team. This chapter will set out how to image the TL trauma patient and how to report the findings, answering the questions the spinal surgeon may have regarding stability, morphology, mechanism and associated injuries.

## 2 Stability

A fundamental question is whether the spine is stable or unstable. Stability is defined as the ability to withstand physiological loads without producing mechanical deformity or progressive neurology or pain (Bernstein 2010). An unstable injury is one where there is risk of progression of a skeletal deformity or neurological deficit under normal physiological conditions (Daffner et al. 1990). For example a compression fracture may progress resulting in further loss of height without neurological deficit, whereas in a burst fracture the middle column fracture may cause progressive neurological deficit due to continuous compression of the cord or cauda equina during axial loading (Daffner et al. 1990; Denis 1983). As stability is dependent on bony and soft tissue/ligamentous structures and both of these are visualised on imaging, the radiologist should be able to give an opinion on the likelihood of the injury being stable or unstable. However, individual surgeons have individual preferences as to whether they want the radiologist to state if the TL spine is stable, unstable, or even suggest that it is 'likely' to be stable or unstable. The surgeon will certainly be considering stability, not just in the short term but also in the long term as it is imperative to avoid long-term pain, neurological deficit and deformity.

## 3 Who, Where and How to Image

TL spine fractures commonly arise from high energy mechanisms such as motor vehicle accidents or in the elderly, low energy mechanisms (Anderson 2010). The threshold for imaging should generally be lower for the elderly (Atinga et al. n.d.). In high energy mechanisms, if there is a TL spine fracture, it is relatively likely to result in spinal cord injury (Diaz Jr. et al. 2007). There is a general consensus across the literature over which patients need to be imaged. The features listed in Table 1 will ensure almost all patients with TL spine injury are identified (Anderson 2010; Van Goethem et al. 2005). It is crucial to avoid a delay in imaging as this results in higher incidence of neurological deficit (Anderson 2010; Bernstein 2010; Van Goethem et al. 2005).

The role of the plain radiograph in trauma imaging is questionable (unless there is no access to CT). CT has a sensitivity of 94–100% compared to radiographs with a sensitivity of 33–73% for TL fractures. Even if a radiograph demonstrates a fracture, it is likely to underestimate its severity. For example, 20% of burst fractures are misdiagnosed as simple anterior compression fractures on radiographs alone (Ballock et al. 1992). It follows that if a fracture is detected with a radiograph, CT is indicated anyway; therefore if CT is available, it should be the first-line screening tool for blunt trauma patients (Anderson 2010; Hauser et al. 2003). CT has the further advantage of identifying non-contiguous fractures and soft tissue injury (as part of the trauma PanCT) ((Keenen et al.

**Table 1** Who should be imaged? (Anderson 2010)

| Who should be imaged? |
|---|
| • Who needs imaging?<br>– High energy mechanism (fall>10 ft., ejected from car, pedestrian v car).<br>– Altered level of consciousness.<br>– Major distracting injury.<br>– A known fracture anywhere in the spine.<br>– Focal pain/tenderness to palpation of spine.<br>– Neurological deficit. |
| • Avoid delay in imaging as it results in higher incidence of neurological injury. |

1990). If performed promptly, CT will avoid further radiation that can occur with piecemeal imaging. Dedicated bony reconstructions are required with the provision of sagittal and coronal reconstructions advisable in our opinion, in case a clinician using a remote viewing platform does not have multiplanar reconstruction capability.

# 4 Imaging Evaluation on CT & MRI (Anderson 2010)

Tables 2 and 3 provide a framework for reviewing trauma CT and MRI studies in the context of trauma.

MRI is indicated in patients with a neurological deficit or suspicion of a ligamentous injury (due to clinical findings). The value of MRI lies in its direct demonstration of soft tissue including ligaments (both anterior and posterior), disc material, epidural space, cord and nerve roots (Diaz Jr. et al. 2007).

**Table 2** Suggested CT imaging checklist

| |
|---|
| Vertebral and facet alignment |
| Vertebral body morphology including posterior cortical margins |
| • Compression, burst, translation, distraction |
| Vertebral height loss |
| Retropulsion |
| Canal narrowing |
| Kyphosis |
| Intervertebral disc space widening |
| Posterior ligamentous complex injury predictors |
| • Facet joint widening |
| • Interspinous distance widening |
| • Spinous process avulsion |
| • Vertebral body subluxation |
| Paravertebral soft tissues including epidural fat (on soft tissue windows) for indirect detection of epidural haematoma and disc protrusion |

**Table 3** Suggested MRI imaging checklist

| |
|---|
| Bony Injury—as for CT |
| Soft tissue: |
| ALL: anterior longitudinal ligament |
| PLL: posterior longitudinal ligament |
| Discs |
| Spinal cord and nerve roots |
| Epidural haematoma |
| PLC: Posterior ligamentous complex (intact, indeterminate, disrupted) |
| • Supraspinous ligaments |
| • Ligamentum flavum |
| • Interspinous ligaments |
| • Facet capsule |

# 5 General Considerations

At T1 to T10 the protection of the ribs and sternum means that high energy is required to disrupt the vertebral bodies and therefore injuries are relatively uncommon but, if they occur, a fracture or dislocation is relatively likely. The T11 to L2 levels are the most common sites of injury as there is a transition between the thoracic kyphosis and the lumbar lordosis without the chest wall stability of the upper thoracic vertebrae. Compression fractures are most common at this level. In the lower lumbar spine (L3-L5), compression injury causes burst fractures (Bernstein 2010).

# 6 Classification Systems

## 6.1 Three Column Spine

In 1983, Francis Denis published his landmark single-author paper introducing the concept of a three column spine and proposing the middle column as the key to understanding stability (Denis 1983). Denis suggested that the spinal column be divided into three with the middle column formed by the posterior wall of the vertebral body, the posterior longitudinal ligament (PLL) and the posterior annulus fibrosis. Denis postulated that the middle column is crucial as its failure predicts associated mechanical or neurological instability. The three columns are demonstrated in Fig. 1.

He proposed that severe compression fractures and seat belt–type injuries have ‘instability of the first degree’ (mechanical instability), due to buckling around the middle or anterior column respectively. ‘Instability of the second degree’ relates to neurological instability. He argued that in the burst fracture, by definition the middle column has ruptured, and with early ambulation the patient would be at increased risk of developing a neurological deficit due to the retropulsed burst

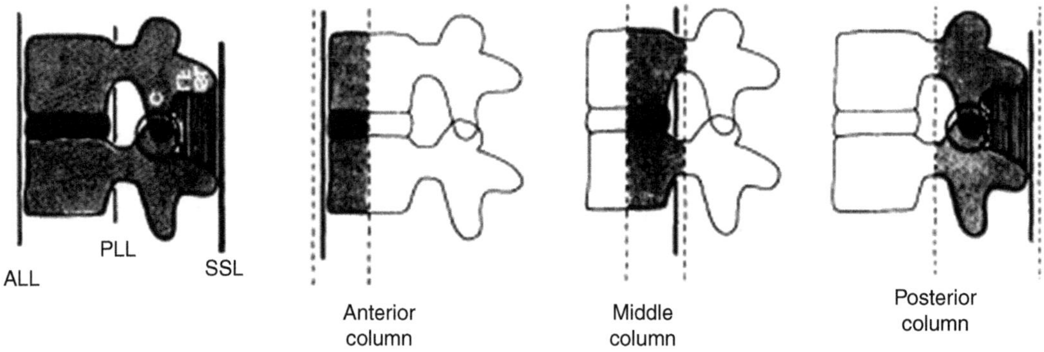


**Fig. 1** The anterior, middle and posterior column are illustrated (Adapted from Denis 1983). Anterior column: ALL (Anterior longitudinal ligament), anterior 2/3rds of the vertebral body and adjacent disc. Middle column: posterior 1/third of the vertebral body and adjacent discs along with the PLL (posterior longitudinal ligament) and posterior annulus fibrosis. Posterior column: osseous and ligamentous structures posterior to the PLL and annulus fibrosis

**Table 4** Basic modes of failure of the three columns in the four major types of spinal injury (Denis 1983)

| Type of fracture | Anterior column | Middle column | Posterior column |
|---|---|---|---|
| Compression | Compression | None | None or distraction (severe) |
| Burst | Compression | Compression | None |
| Seat-belt type | None or compression | Distraction | Distraction |
| Fracture dislocation | Compression rotation shear | Distraction rotation shear | Distraction rotation shear |

fracture fragment. 'Instability of the third degree' (neurological AND mechanical instability) is related to a fracture dislocation or severe burst fracture which is usually treated with surgical decompression and stabilisation (Denis 1983).

While there has been debate over these concepts, including the stability/instability of a burst fracture and the importance of the posterior versus the middle column (which will be discussed later), the morphology Denis described is almost universally recognised by spinal surgeons and generalists alike. The language therefore provides a very useful starting point.

Denis devised his classification based on a retrospective review of patients with 412 spinal injuries. He classified the fractures into major and minor. Minor fractures included isolated fractures of the transverse process, fractures of the pars and articular process and fractures of the spinous process. If these injuries occurred in isolation (affecting only one column), they were considered minor. If they were associated with major fractures of >1 column, they were considered to be part of the major injury complex. Denis divided the four major fracture types on the basis of biomechanics and columnar injury (Table 4).

### 6.1.1 Compression Fractures

These are considered to be due to a failure of the anterior column under compression with the middle column remaining intact and acting as a hinge. The neural canal is not transgressed by this injury. The key radiographic feature is loss of anterior vertebral body height, although the fracture line may extend to the posterior cortex (Fig. 2a).

On MRI, the fracture line will be visible as horizontal low signal on T1 and high signal on T2, with associated bone marrow oedema if it is acute (Fig. 2b).

### 6.1.2 Burst Fractures

Burst fractures are due to failure of the vertebral body under axial compressive load, affecting both the anterior and middle columns. On CT, the break in the posterior vertebral body wall is accompanied by retropulsion causing variable canal narrowing and variable cord or cauda equina damage

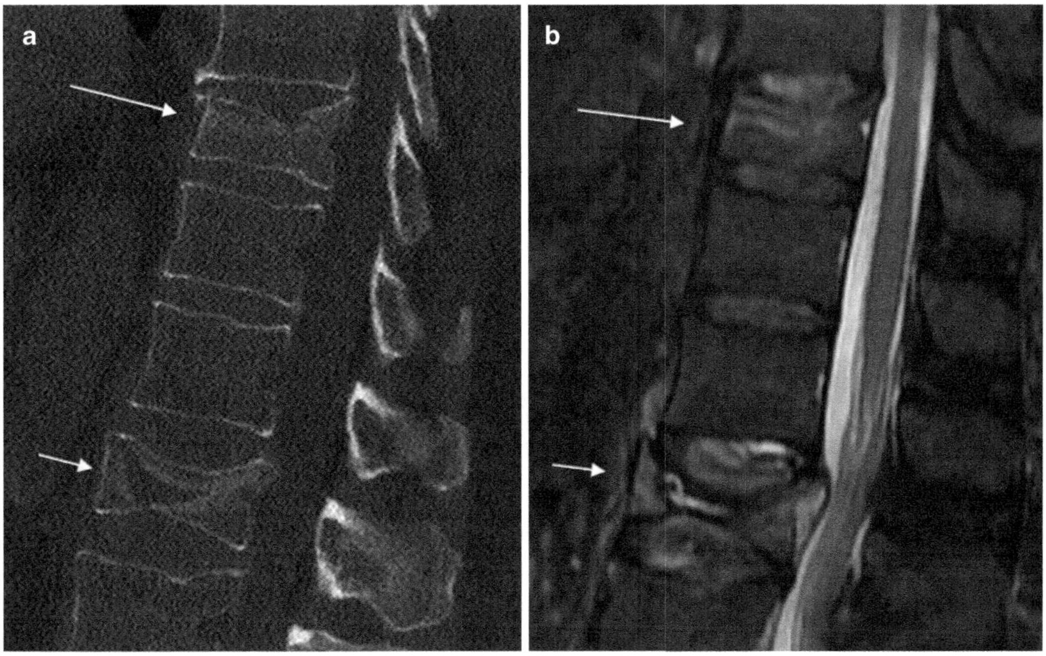


**Fig. 2** Sagittal CT (**a**) and T2 fat-saturated MRI (**b**) images of T10 and L1 compression fractures (white arrows). Axial loading on the flexed spine causes anterior column failure and anterior vertebral body height loss. The posterior cortex and posterior elements are intact (although the posterior cortex may be buckled). MRI demonstrates linear bone marrow oedema

(Fig. 3). Denis had a high index of suspicion for instability. Just fewer than 50% of his series of burst fracture patients had a neurological deficit, mostly due to the initial traumatic impaction on the cord and nerve roots, and later from continued compression by the middle column fragment on the neural elements. Denis argued that even when patients present without neurological deficit, there is a risk of developing neurological compromise due to axial loading during ambulation in a cast. In his series 20% of these patients initially treated non-operatively developed a focal neurological deficit requiring surgery. Subsequent modification of the Denis classification has recognised that burst fractures can be stable (Khurana et al. 2013).

Denis described how it is key to recognise if the burst fracture extends to both the superior and inferior endplate as decompression is required at both the involved vertebra and the adjacent levels (Fig. 4). He also highlighted the importance of which level the burst fracture occurs at. If at the upper lumbar or lower thoracic level, the burst fracture tends to have a kyphotic component, but if at the L3 to L5 level, there is mainly loss of height and little kyphosis.

A further consideration relevant to surgeons is the configuration of the posterior fragment. If there is rotational malalignment, meaning that the posterior fragment is rotated, the fracture will not be reduced by posterior distraction and fixation (Fig. 5).

### 6.1.3 Seat Belt–Type Fracture

The third type of morphology which Denis described is the seat belt–type injury (which included the 'chance' fracture). This is often referred to by others as a flexion-distraction injury, but Denis did not like this description as it is mechanistic. This occurs with flexion and compression of the anterior and middle column ± superadded dislocation of the posterior column. In this injury, there is increased interspinous distance and there can be horizontal split of the transverse process, pedicles or pars interarticularis. The fracture line can be one or more than one level and can traverse bone or ligaments (see

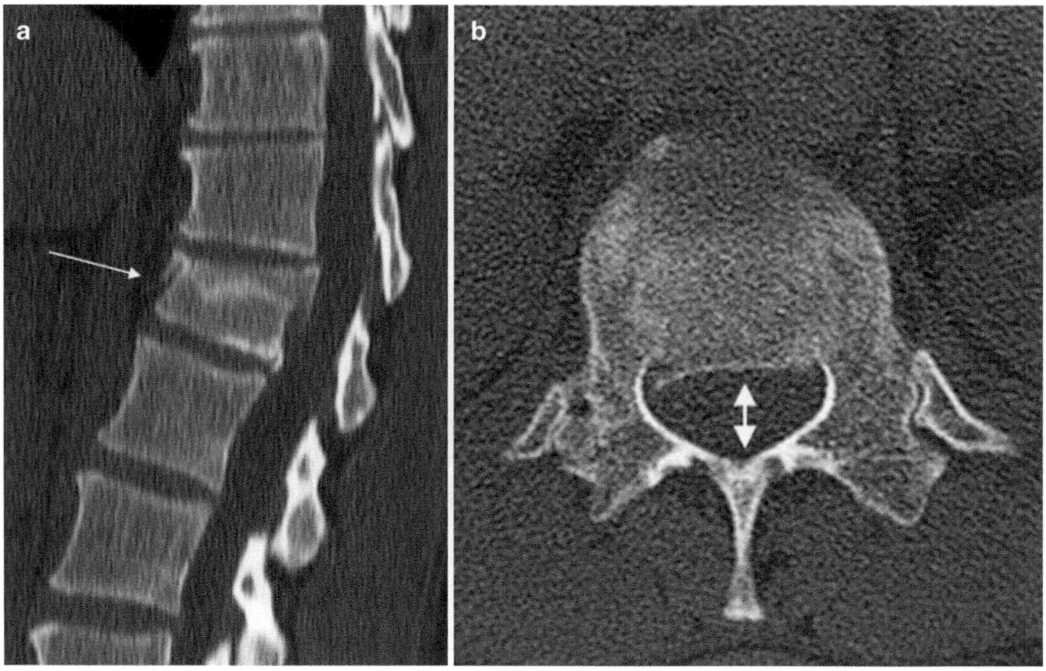


**Fig. 3** Sagittal (**a**) and axial (**b**) CT images of a T12 burst fracture in a patient who fell three metres. There is loss of vertebral body height (<50%), minimal retropulsion (<50%) and spinal canal narrowing (double arrow). However Progressive kyphosis developed over serial radiographs (not shown) hence, patient managed with posterior decompression and fixation

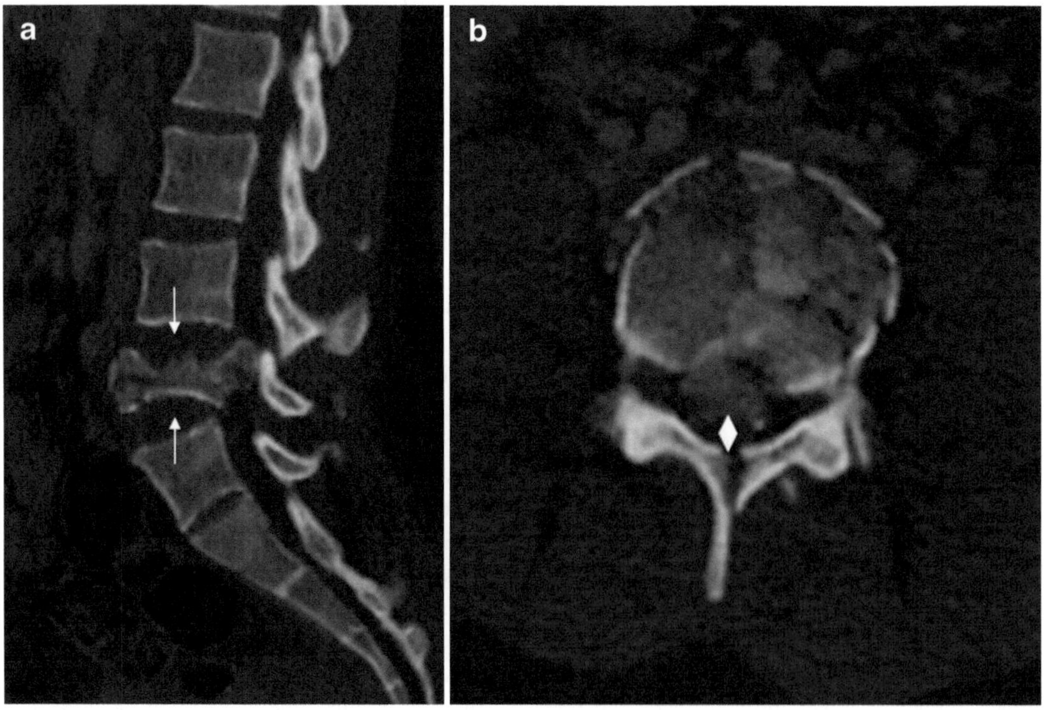


**Fig. 4** Sagittal (**a**) and axial (**b**) CT images of a L4 burst fracture involving the superior and inferior endplates (white arrow). In this instance there is >50% loss of vertebral body height and >50% spinal canal narrowing (short double arrow). This was treated with posterior decompression and distraction

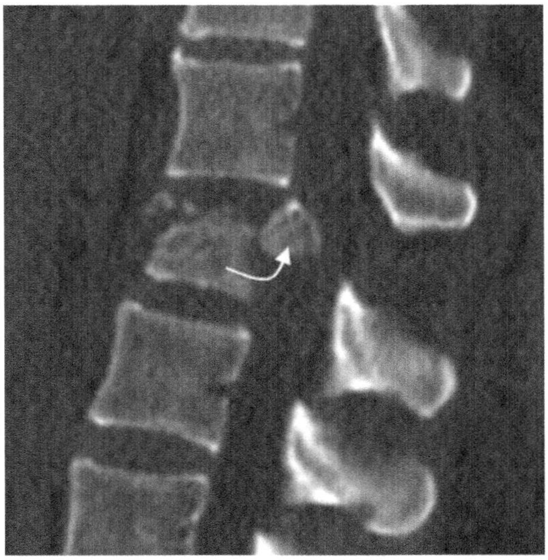

**Fig. 5** Sagittal CT image of an L1 burst fracture with rotational malalignment (curved arrow) of the posterior fragment, an indication for surgery. Posterior distraction of the L1 vertebral body will not be sufficient to realign, and the posterior longitudinal ligament is likely interrupted

Fig. 6). As the fulcrum of flexion lies anterior to the vertebral body, there is an incidence of associated intraabdominal injuries (up to 40%). Figure 7 demonstrates a two-level seat belt–type fracture on CT.

#### 6.1.4 Fracture Dislocation

The fourth and most severe type of fracture is the fracture dislocation, in which all columns fail under compression, tension, rotation or shear (Fig. 8a). This is often associated with other fractures.

Finally Denis argued strongly that an isolated posterior column/posterior ligamentous complex injury did not mean instability, unless there is associated disruption of at least the PLL and posterior annulus fibrosis. His thesis was: 'The posterior ligamentous complex has only a modest role in spine stability when compared to the middle column complex' (Denis 1983).

### 6.2 TLICS (Thoracolumbar Injury Classification and Severity Score)

Denis' classification was widely adopted, with the language he used a basis for subsequent classifications. However subsequent classifications including the Thoracolumbar Injury Classification and Severity Score (TLICS) system evolved for a number of reasons, including that interpretation of Denis' system, became oversimplified to state that instability exists if two out of three columns are disrupted (Lee et al. 2005). While it is likely that injury of two out of three columns will require operative stabilisation, it is not always the case (Khurana et al. 2013; Agus et al. 2005; Wood et al. 2003). A further limitation in Denis' classification was that, as it was published in 1983, it necessarily did not include MRI findings and therefore had no direct imaging of ligamentous injury. Finally, although Denis commented on the likelihood of neurological deficit, the classification did not provide prognostic information or consider the neurological status of the patients and therefore could not act as a guide to surgical intervention (Khurana et al. 2013; Joaquim et al. 2011; Oner et al. 2002). For all of these reasons, the TLICS system was introduced to take into account current understanding of the biomechanics of injury, both MRI and CT imaging features, and to help to guide treatment planning.

The TLICS classification is based on: (i) morphology; (ii) integrity of the posterior ligamentous complex; and (iii) neurological status of the patient, as shown in Table 5 (Lee et al. 2005; Vaccaro et al. 2005). Specific points are allocated for each category and based on the total TLICS score; the patient is more or less likely to need surgery (Table 6).

The morphology is classified into three main subgroups: 1. compression fractures, 2. translation/rotation injuries and 3. distraction injuries. If injuries are multilevel, the most severe level is selected for the assessment (i.e. the injuries are not additive).

#### 6.2.1 Morphology

##### 6.2.1.1 Compression Injuries

This category includes both compression fractures (where the anterior vertebral body deforms into a wedge with the posterior vertebral body remaining intact) and the burst fracture, where both anterior and posterior vertebral body cortex are disrupted with retropulsion of the bone into the spinal canal.

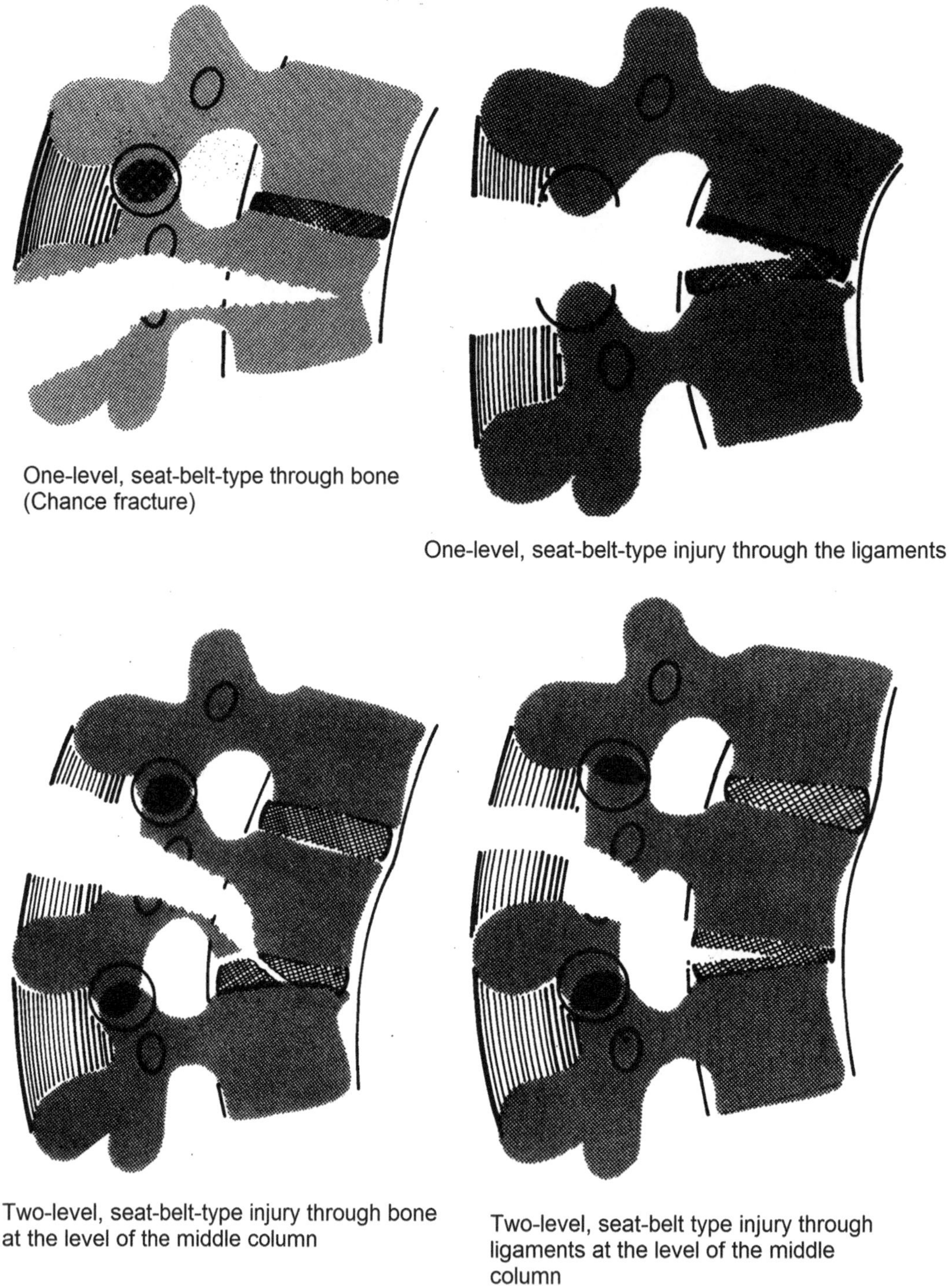


**Fig. 6** Subtypes of seat belt–type injuries (Denis 1983). Injuries can be across one or two levels, and can involve the bone or ligament

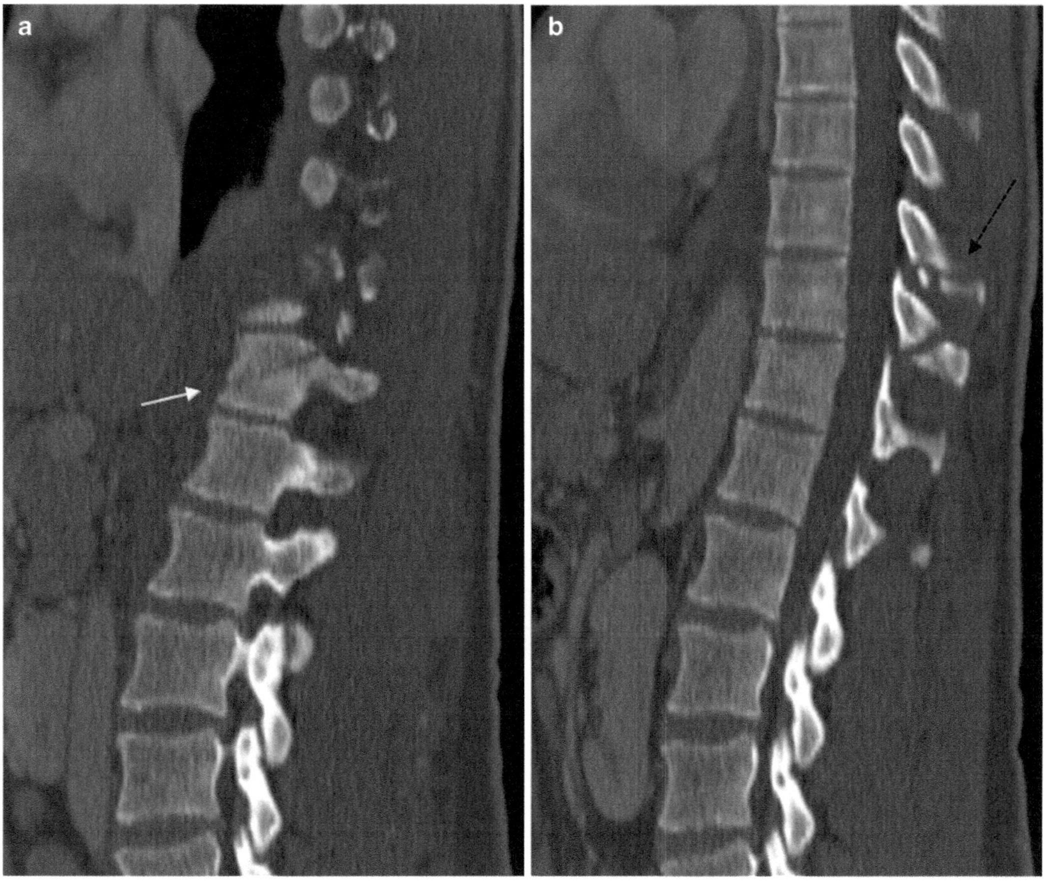


**Fig. 7** Sagittal CT images of a T11 chance fracture (**a**, white arrow) with extension into the T9 and T10 spinous processes (**b**, black arrow)

#### 6.2.1.2 Translation/Rotation Injuries

These usually cause an unstable spine and therefore have a higher score.

#### 6.2.1.3 Distraction Injuries

This includes 'chance' or flexion-distraction or 'seat-belt' injuries and result in circumferential instability which scores four points. However, there needs to be clear posterior ligamentous complex (PLC) disruption for the injury to be assigned the distraction morphology.

#### 6.2.1.4 Neurological Status

The neurological status is assessed clinically but cord or nerve root injury can also be commented on from the MRI (Khurana et al. 2013). Clinical neurological status will also be affected by the presence and extent of cord oedema and presence of haemorrhage in the cord. There is no direct correlation between neurological signs and the degree of canal encroachment at the time of imaging, likely because the maximal neural encroachment occurs at the time of injury and the final position of bony fragments cannot be used to infer the degree of neural encroachment at the time of injury (Anderson 2010). However the following should be observed (Bernstein 2010; Khurana et al. 2013; Sansur 2010): (Table 7).

#### 6.2.1.5 Integrity of the Posterior Ligamentous Complex

The PLC is assessed via indirect signs on XR or CT or direct signs on MRI. The signs on XR/CT include interspinous widening, spinous process avulsion fractures, widened, perched or dislocated facet joints and vertebral body translation or

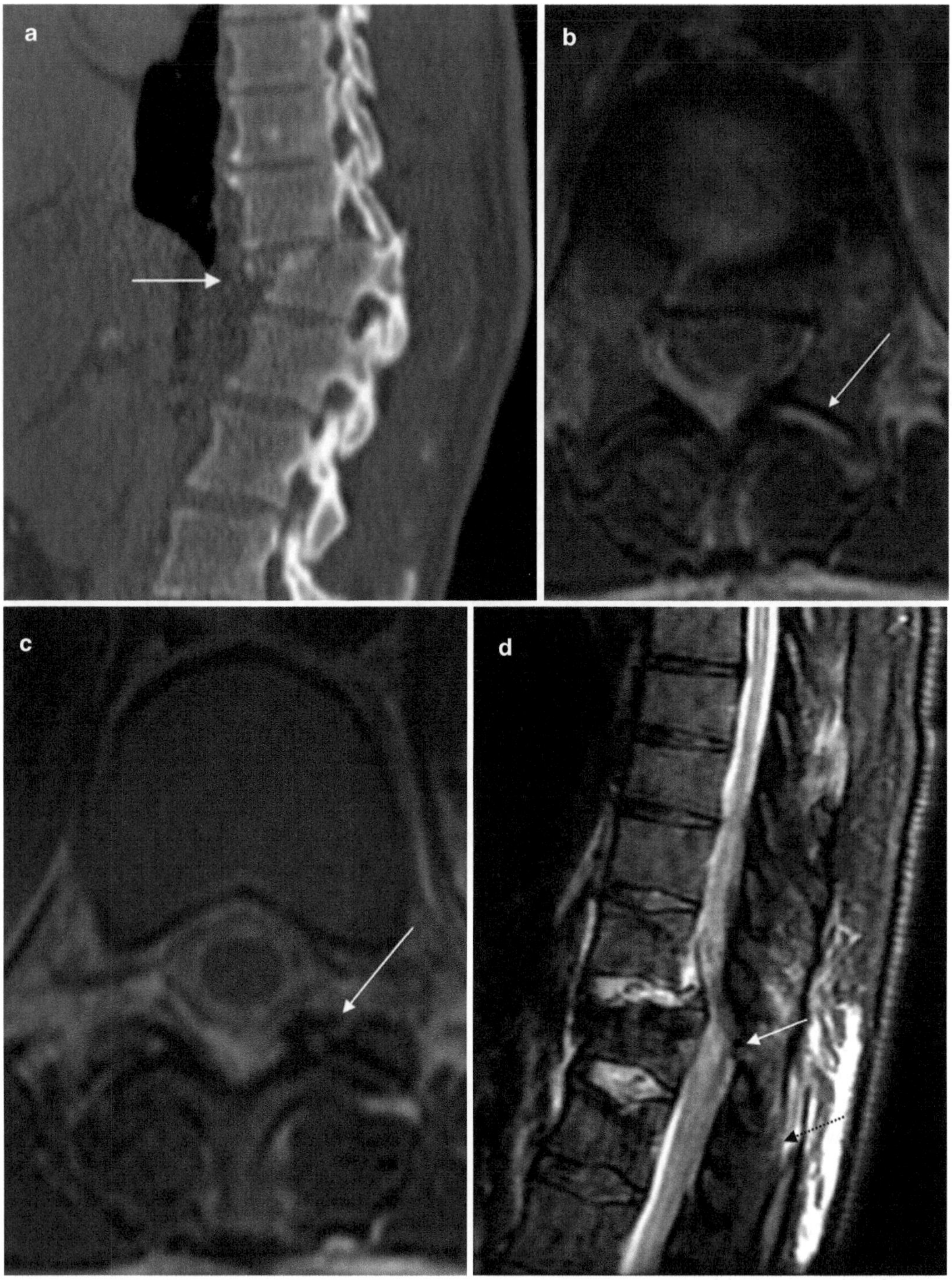


**Fig. 8** (**a**) Sagittal CT image of a patient who fell from a height, demonstrating a T12 fracture with a three-column dislocation at T11-T12 (white arrow). Axial T2 fat-saturated MRI images at T11-T12 showing (**b**) fluid in the left facet joint and (**c**) avulsion of the facet joint capsule (white arrows). Sagittal T2 fat-saturated MRI image (**d**) demonstrating a T11-T12 fracture-dislocation with interruption of the ligamentum flavum (white arrow) and supraspinous ligaments (black arrow) indicating PLC injury

**Table 5** TLICS classification scoring (Lee 2005)

| Parameter | Points |
|---|---|
| *Morphology* | |
| Compression fracture | 1 |
| Burst fracture | 2 |
| Translational/rotational | 3 |
| Distraction | 4 |
| *Neurologic involvement* | |
| Intact | 0 |
| Nerve root | 2 |
| Cord, conus medullaris | |
| Incomplete | 3 |
| Complete | 2 |
| Cauda equina | 3 |
| *Posterior ligamentous complex* | |
| Intact | 0 |
| Injury suspected/indeterminate | 2 |
| Injured | 3 |

**Table 6** Management as per TLICS score (Lee 2005)

| Management | Points |
|---|---|
| Non-operative | 0–3 |
| Non-operative or operative | 4 |
| Operative | ≥5 |

**Table 7** Features that suggest surgical management may be required (brackets denote percentage or findings which make surgery more likely)

1. Anterior vertebral body compression (>50% significant).
2. Kyphosis (>25% or progressive kyphosis).
3. Sagittal canal narrowing (>50% significant).
4. Retropulsion (distance of a line drawn between posterior margins of adjacent vertebral bodies and the most posterior margin of the bone fragment).
5. Rotational malalignment (if present, likely to require surgery).

rotation (Khurana et al. 2013). MRI is the imaging gold standard of reference for identifying PLC injury with higher sensitivity, specificity and accuracy than CT (Khurana et al. 2013; Vaccaro et al. 2013). Each component of the PLC should be individually analysed. The ligamentum flavum and supraspinous ligaments are best seen on sagittal T1 and T2 as continuous low signal intensity stripes. The interspinous ligaments are best seen on sagittal fluid sensitive MRI (e.g. T2 fat saturated sequence or STIR). Axial fat saturated T2 imaging demonstrates facet capsule oedema or fluid (Fig. 8b). MRI is most reliable at identifying the interruption of the supraspinous ligament and ligamentum flavum and slightly less reliable for interspinous ligament or facet capsule disruption which tend to be overestimated on MRI compared with surgical findings. As always, clear dialogue with the surgeons is the key (Khurana et al. 2013; Pizones et al. 2011).

On MRI signs include PLC hyperintensity on T2 fat saturated sequence and interruption of the supraspinous ligament and ligamentum flavum on T1 or T2 sequences (Khurana et al. 2013; Lee et al. 2005), as shown in Fig. 8c and d.

#### 6.2.1.6 Understanding the PLC

The vertebral bodies and discs act to resist compressive loading and circumferential tensile stress (Khurana et al. 2013; Nordin 2001). The PLC guides movement and acts as a posterior tension band balancing a compressive force through the vertebral bodies. Disruption of the PLC interrupts this balance and, if disrupted, the PLC usually requires surgical intervention because of its poor healing potential. The intact PLC protects the spine from excess flexion, rotation, translation and distraction so that without surgery progressive kyphosis and vertebral collapse can occur (Rihn et al. 2008). The TLICS score therefore addresses: (1) immediate mechanical stability (related to injury morphology); (2) long-term stability (related to PLC status); and (3) neurological stability (depend on neurological deficit) (Khurana et al. 2013).

The total TLICS score indicates likelihood to require operative stabilisation with patients with a score of 4 being in the indeterminate category; those above 4 should have operative management (Lee et al. 2005). The posited advantage of the TLICS system is high interobserver and intraobserver reliability (Lee et al. 2005).

TLICS certainly has the advantage of simplicity and being comprehensive; however, interobserver reliability is variable: between 0.4 and 0.7 for MRI interpretation of the PLC injury depending on the study and who is doing the evaluation (spinal surgeon or radiologist) (Rihn et al. 2010; Whang et al. 2007). Contributing to this, optimal

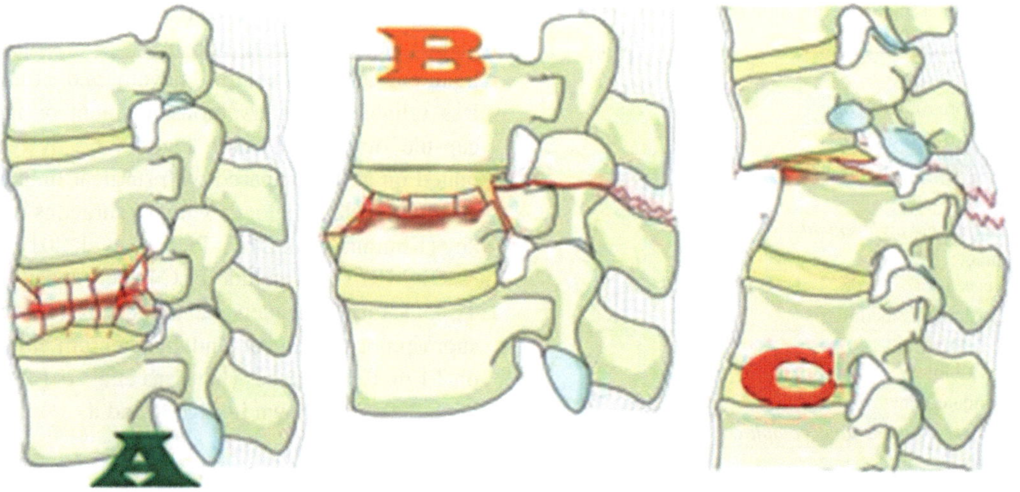


**Fig. 9** The three basic AO categories. Type A: compression injuries. Failure of anterior structures under compression with intact tension band. Type B: failure of the posterior or anterior tension band. Type C: failure of all elements leading to dislocation or displacement (Vaccaro et al. 2013). © AOSpine International, Switzerland

surgical management of PLC injury is still an area of debate among the international spine surgery community (Vaccaro et al. 2013).

## 6.3 Arbeitsgemeeinschaft fur Osteosynthesefragen/AO Classification

The third classification system that clinicians may use is termed the AO system and was originally outlined in 1994. The AO system divides injuries into three categories as shown in Fig. 9: Group A: compression; Group B: tension band injuries; and Group C: translational, originally with up to nine subtypes in each group. The detailed subclassification led to poorer interobserver reliability and the original classification also did not include neurological status, although it did recognise the importance of soft tissue injuries (from the ALL to the PLC) (Sethi et al. 2009). However a revised and simplified AO version (Vaccaro et al. 2013; Reinhold et al. 2013) had greater interobserver reliability when evaluated by spinal surgeons (between 0.69 and 0.90 kappa correlation co-efficient (Reinhold et al. 2013)), which is shown in Table 8. Yacoub et al. compared external validity between AOSpine and

**Table 8** AOSpine fracture classifications, modifiable factors and thoracolumbar AOSpine injury score (Astolfi et al. 2018)

| Fracture classifications | | | |
|---|---|---|---|
| Type/subtype | | Description | TL AOSIS |
| Type A: compression fractures | A0 | Fracture that does not have a possibility of impacting structural integrity of the spine, or no fracture | 0 |
| | A1 | Fracture through 1 endplate without extension into the posterior wall | 1 |
| | A2 | Fracture through both endplates without extension into the posterior wall | 2 |
| | A3 | Incomplete burst (fracture through the single endplate with extension through the posterior wall) | 3 |
| | A4 | Burst (fracture through both endplates with extension through the posterior wall) | 4 |

(continued)

**Table 8** (continued)

| Fracture classifications | | | |
|---|---|---|---|
| Type/subtype | | Description | TL AOSIS |
| Type B: tension band injuries | B1 | A full osseous posterior tension band injury | 5 |
| | B2 | Injury involving the disruption of ligamentous posterior tension components, with or without bony involvement | 6 |
| | B3 | Fracture with the disruption of the anterior tension components, intact posterior tension band | 7 |
| Type C: translational injuries | C | Displacement of the spinal column in any plane | 8 |
| *Modifiable factors* | | | |
| Neurologic status | N0 | Neurologically intact | 0 |
| | N1 | Temporary neurologic injury, resolved | 1 |
| | N2 | Nerve root damage | 2 |
| | N3 | Cauda equina syndrome of incomplete spinal cord injury | 4 |
| | N4 | Complete spinal cord injury | 4 |
| | Nx | Reliable examination cannot be completed | 3 |
| Patient-specific modifiers | M1 | Ambiguity of integrity of the PLC | 1 |
| | M2 | Patient-specific factors impacting the treatment algorithm (e.g. severe burns and ankylosing spondylitis) | 0 |

TLICS with comparable results for morphology groups (Yacoub et al. 2017; Astolfi et al. 2018) however lower reliability for determining AO subgroups.

The entire range of AO classification is illustrated in an overview published by aospine.org (Fig. 10).

### 6.3.1 Type A

This involves the anterior elements and can include clinically insignificant injuries such as transverse or spinous process fractures (subtype A0, as shown in Fig. 11). Subtype A1 is a wedge compression or impaction fracture of a single endplate without the involvement of the posterior wall of the vertebral body (Fig. 12). Subtle A2 is a 'pincer' type fracture which does not extend to the posterior vertebral body wall (Fig. 13). For example, a T12 pincer fracture would be coded: T12-A2. Subtype A3 (also called an incomplete burst fracture) affects a single endplate plus vertebral body wall AND the spinal canal (Fig. 14), such as a non-displaced laminar fracture. However, the posterior tension band remains intact. Subtype A4, also called a complete burst fracture, is similar to A3 but involve *both* superior and inferior endplates, as shown in Fig. 15 (Vaccaro et al. 2013; Reinhold et al. 2013).

### 6.3.2 Type B

Type B injuries involve the anterior or posterior tension band and may be seen in combination with Type A injuries. Subtype B1 is a transosseous failure of the posterior tension band at one vertebral body level (so called 'chance fracture', Fig. 16). Subtype B2 disrupts the ligamentous posterior tension band with or without osseous involvement, demonstrated in Fig. 17. If there is an associated vertebral body compression fracture, this should be specified separately. For example an L2 burst fracture with the disruption of the PLC would be classified as A3 (incomplete burst) or A4 (complete burst) WITH B2 injury i.e. L2-A3 (L2-B2).

Subtype B3 (Fig. 18) disrupts the anterior tension band of the spine with or without bony involvement. The injury involves the anterior longitudinal ligament and can pass through disc or vertebral body and disc (for example in the ankylosed spine) but the posterior elements are intact. If the posterior elements are interrupted, this is a type C injury.

### 6.3.3 Type C

Type C injuries have no subtypes, and are translation injuries in any plane (Fig. 19). There is dis-

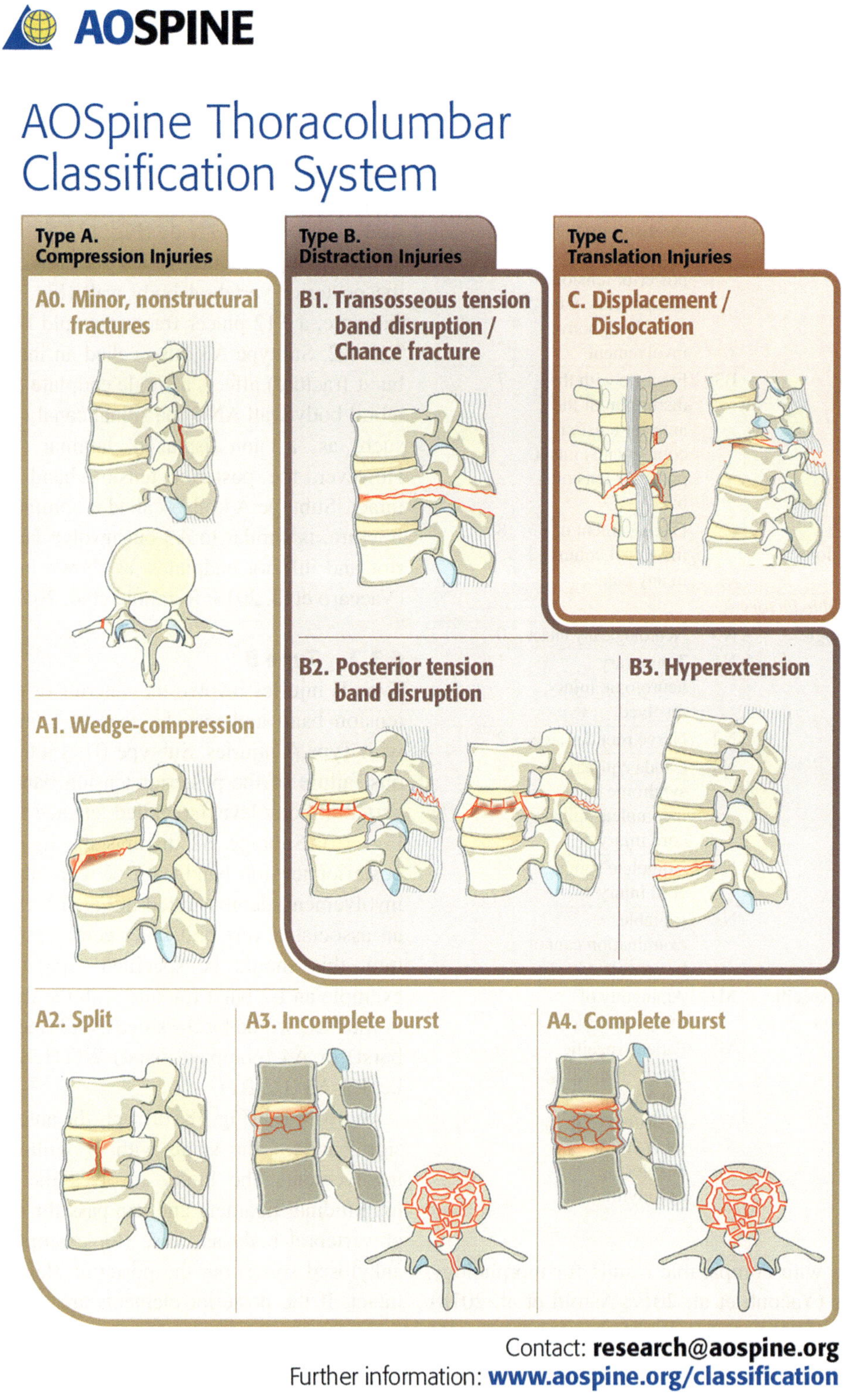


**Fig. 10** Overview of AOSpine thoracolumbar classification system (www.aospine.org/classification). © AOSpine International, Switzerland

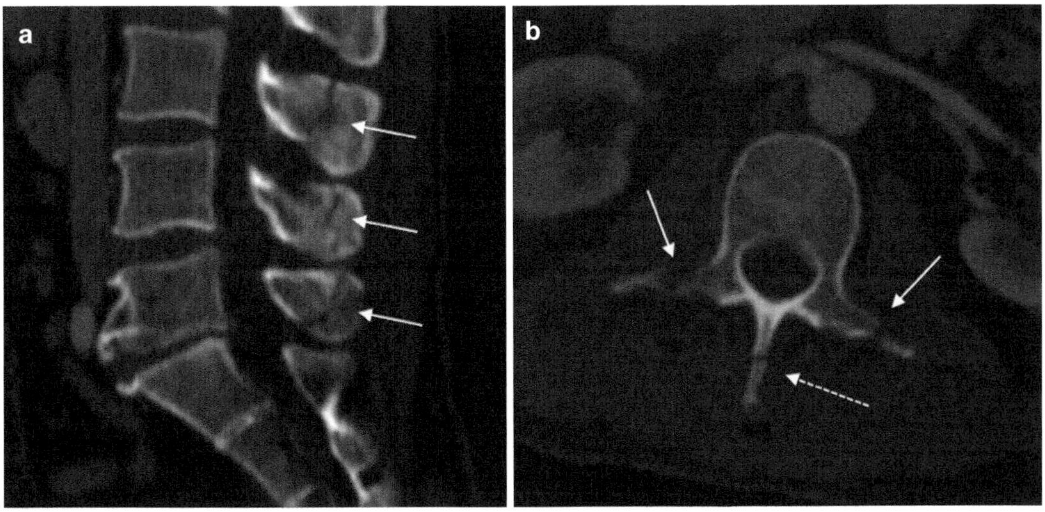


**Fig. 11** (**a**) Sagittal CT images of multiple spinous process fractures between L3 and L5 (white arrows); (**b**) axial CT images of the same patient showing bilateral transverse process fractures (white arrows) in addition to the spinous process fracture (white dotted arrow) at L3 (AO subtype A0)

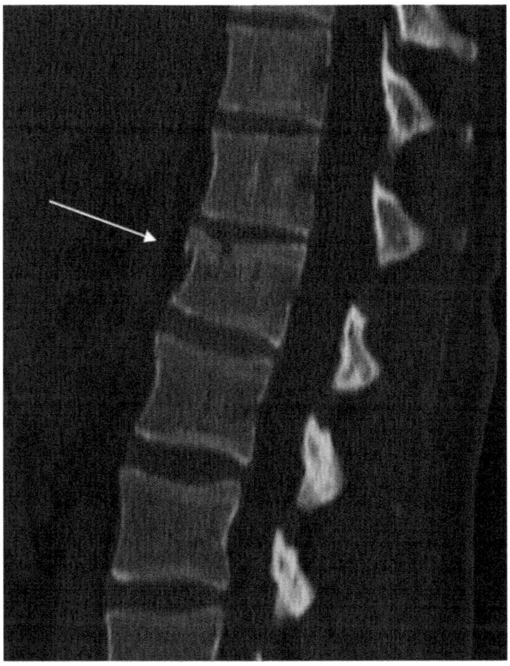

**Fig. 12** Sagittal CT image of a T12 compression fracture (white arrow), with no involvement of the posterior cortex (AO subtype A1)

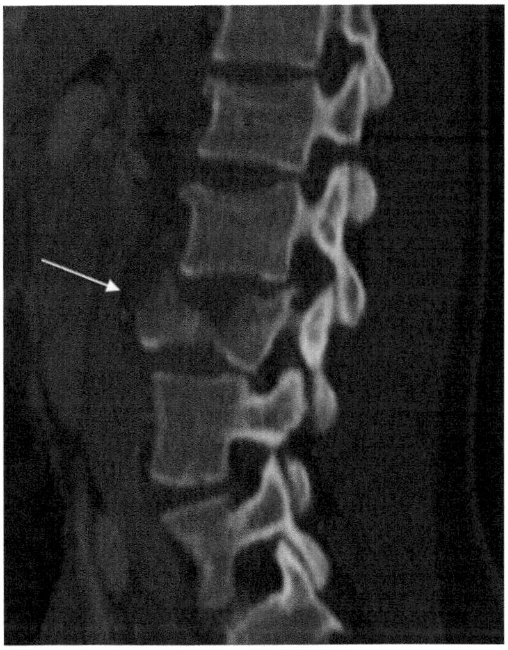

**Fig. 13** Sagittal CT image demonstrating the configuration of a coronal split, or pincer fracture of the L3 vertebral body (AO subtype A2)

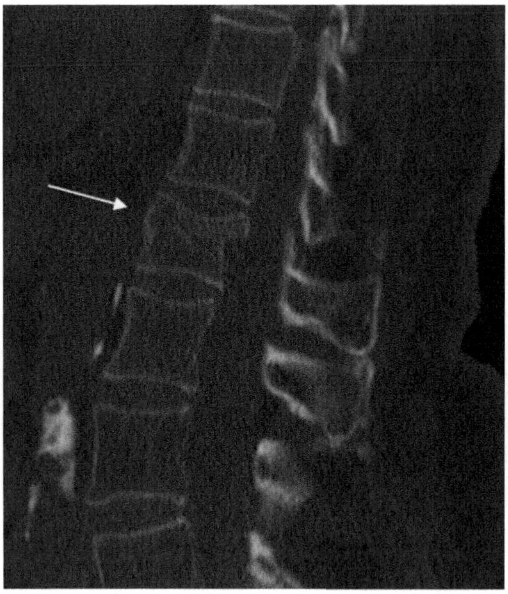

**Fig. 14** Sagittal CT image of an incomplete burst fracture at T12, with the involvement of the superior end plate but not the inferior (AO subtype A3)

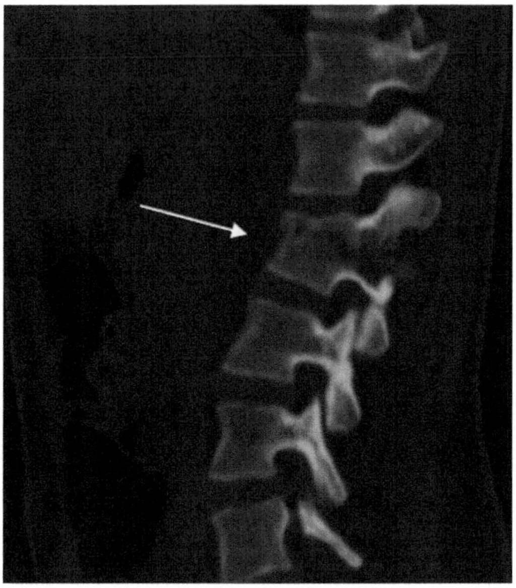

**Fig. 16** Sagittal CT image showing a fracture extending through the L2 vertebral body and the right pedicle into the lamina and spinous process (AO subtype B1)

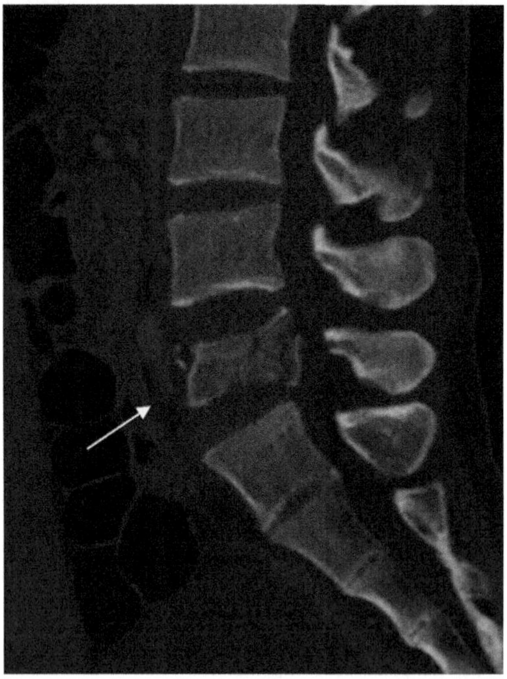

**Fig. 15** Sagittal CT image of a complete burst fracture at L5 (white arrow), with the involvement of both superior and inferior endplates and preservation of the posterior elements (AO subtype A4)

placement of the fracture beyond the physiological range of the spinal column in any plane. Type C also includes distraction of anterior and posterior structures. Type C injuries have to be described in conjunction with an associated vertebral body fracture (e.g. A0 or A4) and associated tension band injury (e.g. B1). For example a patient with the disruption of the posterior tension band at T12/L1 and an incomplete burst fracture affecting one endplate only will be described as T12/L1-B2 (L1-A3) (Vaccaro et al. 2013). A 'chance' fracture through the L1/L2 intervertebral disc level with ALL disruption and displacement would be described as L1/L2 B3 (L1/L2 C).

### 6.3.4 Modifiable Factors

Two additional modifiers may be relevant in some patients. Neurological deficit is graded N0 (intact) to N4 (complete spinal injury) with N1 representing transient neurological deficit, N2 radiculopathy, N3 incomplete spinal cord injury or cauda equina injury. NX indicates that neurological status cannot be designated.

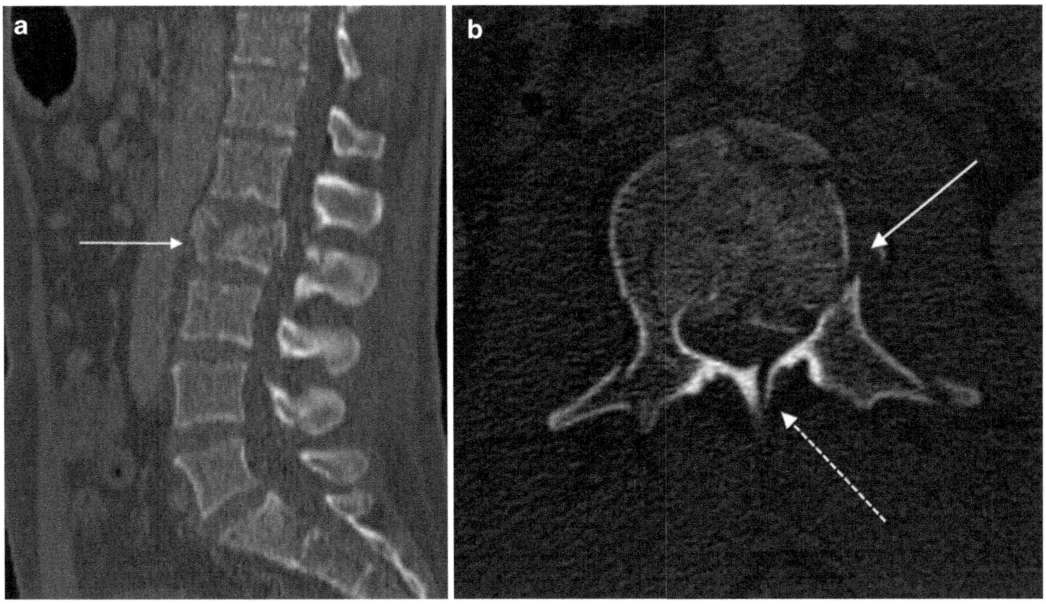


**Fig. 17** Sagittal CT image (**a**) shows a burst fracture through the L2 vertebral body with the involvement of the posterior cortex. Axial CT image at L2 of the same patient (**b**) shows extension of the fracture to the left pedicle (white arrow) and a left lamina fracture (white dotted arrow) suggesting the involvement of the posterior tension band/PLC making this an AO subtype B2 injury

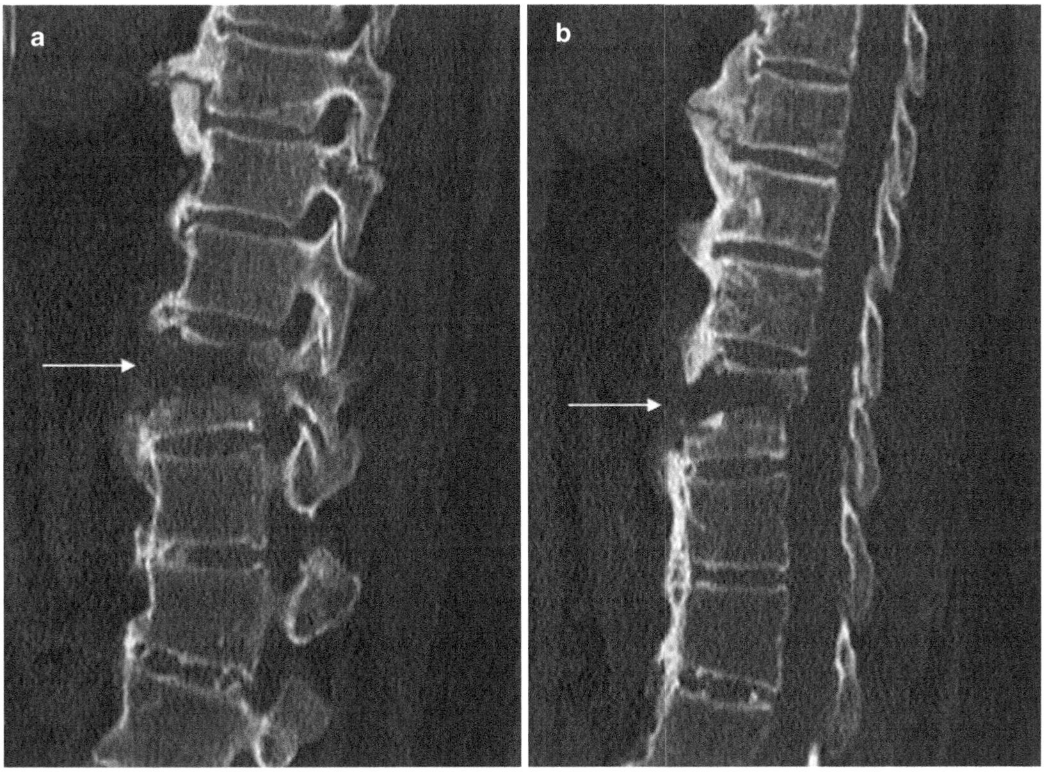


**Fig. 18** Two sagittal CT images (**a**) and (**b**) demonstrating a hyperextension injury at T11 (white arrows), with failure of the anterior tension band in a patient with diffuse idiopathic skeletal hyperostosis (AO subtype B3)

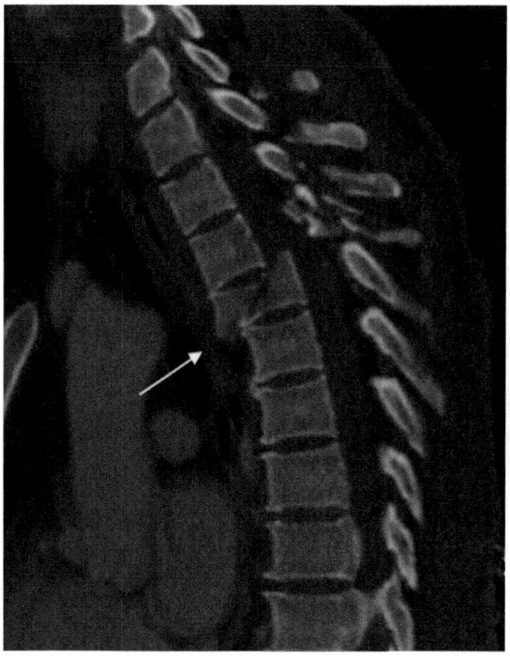

**Fig. 19** Sagittal CT image following a high-energy traumatic injury resulting in a complete translation of the spine at T4 (white arrow) with the distraction of both anterior and posterior structures (AO subtype C)

Finally M1 indicates an indeterminate injury to the tension band, which requires clinical evaluation on a case-by-case basis (Vaccaro et al. 2013; Reinhold et al. 2013).

## 7 Conclusion

All the classification systems described strike a balance between simplicity and complexity with TLICS and AO necessarily relying more on advanced imaging findings and Denis relying more on radiographic or CT findings. The radiologist needs to be familiar with all three classifications so they can converse accurately and precisely with clinicians and ultimately adjust their reporting style to suit the clinical team who they are working with.

**Acknowledgements and Notes** AOSpine is a clinical division of the AO Foundation—an independent medically guided nonprofit organization.

The AOSpine Knowledge Forums are pathology focused working groups acting on behalf of AOSpine in their domain of scientific expertise. Each forum consists of a steering committee of up to 10 international spine experts who meet on a regular basis to discuss research, assess the best evidence for current practices and formulate clinical trials to advance spine care worldwide. Study support is provided directly through AOSpine's Research Department and AO's Clinical Investigation and Documentation unit.

We thank Dr. Francis Denis for permission to adapt and reproduce Figs. 1 and 6.

## References

Agus H, Kayali C, Arslantas M (2005) Nonoperative treatment of burst-type thoracolumbar vertebra fractures: clinical and radiological results of 29 patients. Eur Spine J 14(6):536–540

Anderson M (2010) Imaging of Thoracic and Lumbar Spine. Semin Spine Surg 22:8–19

Astolfi MMMP, Murphy H, Schroeder G, Vaccaro AR (2018) Thoracolumbar Fracture Classifications: Pros and Cons of the TLICS and AOSpine classification systems. Contemp Spine Surg 19(1):1–8

Atinga A, Shekkeris A, Fertleman M, Batrick N, Kashef E, Dick E (n.d.) Trauma in the elderly patient. Br J Radiol 91(1087):20170739

Ballock RT, Mackersie R, Abitbol JJ, Cervilla V, Resnick D, Garfin SR (1992) Can burst fractures be predicted from plain radiographs? J Bone Joint Surg Br 74(1):147–150

Bernstein M (2010) Easily missed thoracolumbar spine fractures. Eur J Radiol 74(1):6–15

Daffner RH, Deeb ZL, Goldberg AL, Kandabarow A, Rothfus WE (1990) The radiologic assessment of post-traumatic vertebral stability. Skelet Radiol 19(2):103–108

Denis F (1983) The three column spine and its significance in the classification of acute thoracolumbar spinal injuries. Spine (Phila Pa 1976) 8(8):817–831

Diaz JJ Jr, Cullinane DC, Altman DT, Bokhari F, Cheng JS, Como J et al (2007) Practice management guidelines for the screening of thoracolumbar spine fracture. J Trauma 63(3):709–718

Hauser CJ, Visvikis G, Hinrichs C, Eber CD, Cho K, Lavery RF et al (2003) Prospective validation of computed tomographic screening of the thoracolumbar spine in trauma. J Trauma 55(2):228–234. discussion 234-5

Joaquim AF, Fernandes YB, Cavalcante RA, Fragoso RM, Honorato DC, Patel AA (2011) Evaluation of the thoracolumbar injury classification system in thoracic and lumbar spinal trauma. Spine (Phila Pa 1976) 36(1):33–36

Keenen TL, Antony J, Benson DR (1990) Non-contiguous spinal fractures. J Trauma 30(4):489–491

Khurana B, Sheehan SE, Sodickson A, Bono CM, Harris MB (2013) Traumatic thoracolumbar spine injuries: what the spine surgeon wants to know. Radiographics 33(7):2031–2046

Lee JY, Vaccaro AR, Lim MR, Oner FC, Hulbert RJ, Hedlund R et al (2005) Thoracolumbar injury classification and severity score: a new paradigm for the treatment of thoracolumbar spine trauma. J Orthop Sci 10(6):671–675

Nordin MWS (2001) Biomechanics of the lumbar spine. In: Nordin MFV (ed) Basic bio-mechanics of the musculoskeletal system. Lippincott Williams & Wilkins, Philadelphia, pp 256–285

Oner FC, Ramos LM, Simmermacher RK, Kingma PT, Diekerhof CH, Dhert WJ et al (2002) Classification of thoracic and lumbar spine fractures: problems of reproducibility. A study of 53 patients using CT and MRI. Eur Spine J 11(3):235–245

Pizones J, Izquierdo E, Alvarez P, Sanchez-Mariscal F, Zuniga L, Chimeno P et al (2011) Impact of magnetic resonance imaging on decision making for thoracolumbar traumatic fracture diagnosis and treatment. Eur Spine J 20 Suppl 3:390–396

Reinhold M, Audige L, Schnake KJ, Bellabarba C, Dai LY, Oner FC (2013) AO spine injury classification system: a revision proposal for the thoracic and lumbar spine. Eur Spine J 22(10):2184–2201

Rihn JA, Anderson DT, Harris E, Lawrence J, Jonsson H, Wilsey J et al (2008) A review of the TLICS system: a novel, user-friendly thoracolumbar trauma classification system. Acta Orthop 79(4):461–466

Rihn JA, Yang N, Fisher C, Saravanja D, Smith H, Morrison WB et al (2010) Using magnetic resonance imaging to accurately assess injury to the posterior ligamentous complex of the spine: a prospective comparison of the surgeon and radiologist. J Neurosurg Spine 12(4):391–396

Sansur CSC (2010) Diagnosis and Management of Low Lumbar Burst Fractures. Semin Spine Surg 22:33–37

Sethi MK, Schoenfeld AJ, Bono CM, Harris MB (2009) The evolution of thoracolumbar injury classification systems. Spine J 9(9):780–788

Vaccaro AR, Zeiller SC, Hulbert RJ, Anderson PA, Harris M, Hedlund R et al (2005) The thoracolumbar injury severity score: a proposed treatment algorithm. J Spinal Disord Tech 18(3):209–215

Vaccaro AR, Oner C, Kepler CK, Dvorak M, Schnake K, Bellabarba C et al (2013) AOSpine thoracolumbar spine injury classification system: fracture description, neurological status, and key modifiers. Spine (Phila Pa 1976) 38(23):2028–2037

Van Goethem JW, Maes M, Ozsarlak O, van den Hauwe L, Parizel PM (2005) Imaging in spinal trauma. Eur Radiol 15(3):582–590

Whang PG, Vaccaro AR, Poelstra KA, Patel AA, Anderson DG, Albert TJ et al (2007) The influence of fracture mechanism and morphology on the reliability and validity of two novel thoracolumbar injury classification systems. Spine (Phila Pa 1976) 32(7):791–795

Wood K, Buttermann G, Mehbod A, Garvey T, Jhanjee R, Sechriest V (2003) Operative compared with nonoperative treatment of a thoracolumbar burst fracture without neurological deficit. A prospective, randomized study. J Bone Joint Surg Am 85-A(5):773–781

Yacoub AR, Joaquim AF, Ghizoni E, Tedeschi H, Patel AA (2017) Evaluation of the safety and reliability of the newly-proposed AO spine injury classification system. J Spinal Cord Med 40(1):70–75

# Part IV

# Spine: Non-traumatic Emergent Injuries (J. Van Goethem, L. Van der Hauwe, Belgium – M. Thurnher, Austria)

# Spine: Non-traumatic Emergent Injuries. Introduction

Alfredo Bucciero

## Contents



Non-traumatic spinal emergent injuries (NTSEI) are all those conditions which present with acute signs and symptoms of spinal cord involvement not because of trauma, can potentially lead to death or prolonged or permanent disability, and therefore need immediate management. Reported prevalence ranges from 367 to 1227 per million population (WHO, 2013). Two types of NTSEI are recognized (Sanchez et al. 2011):

- NTSEI from intrinsic cord damage.
- NTSEI from extrinsic cord compression.

NTSEI due to ***intrinsic cord damage*** (non-compressive myelopathy) can be divided into acute inflammatory myelopathies and acute non-inflammatory myelopathies (Cree 2014; Mark 1996; Jacob and Weinshenker 2008). *Acute inflammatory myelopathies* or *acute myelites* can be classified with regard to their aetiology, location, and histopathology (Loeb and Dagnino 1984). Regarding their aetiology, acute inflammatory myelopathies can be distinguished into infective and non-infective. Infective acute inflammatory myelopathies can be due to viral, bacterial, fungal, or parasitic infections whereas non-infective acute inflammatory myelopathies can be due to primary diseases of the central nervous system, paraneoplastic disease or systemic inflammatory disease (Cree 2014). Regarding their location, acute inflammatory myelopathies can be distinguished into grey matter myelitis or poliomyelitis, white matter myelitis or leukomyelitis, grey and white matter myelitis, focal myelitis, disseminated myelitis, and transverse myelitis (Table 1). Regarding their histopathology, acute inflammatory myelopathies can be distinguished into necrotizing myelitis, demyelinating myelitis, haemorrhagic myelitis, granulomatous myelitis, suppurative myelitis, and non-specific myelitis (Table 2).

*Acute non-inflammatory myelopathies* (Table 3) can be due to (Hunderfund and Wijdicks 2009; Kadir et al. 2012; Riva et al. 2007; Sanchez et al. 2011; Sharma et al. 2018; Tariq et al. 2018; Vargas et al. 2015):

A. Bucciero (✉)
Department of Neurosurgery, Pinetagrande, Castel Volturno, Italy



M. Scaglione et al. (eds.), *Emergency Radiology of the Head and Spine*, Medical Radiology Diagnostic Imaging, https://doi.org/10.1007/978-3-030-91047-1_15

**Table 1** Location of acute inflammatory myelopathies

| Types | Causes |
|---|---|
| Gray matter myelitis (poliomyelitis) | Poliovirus |
| White matter myelitis (leukomyelitis) | Multiple sclerosis |
| Gray and white matter myelitis | *Staphylococcus aureus*, idiopathic transverse myelitis, paraneoplastic disease |
| Focal myelitis | *Mycobacterium tuberculosis*, fungal infections |
| Disseminated myelitis | Acute disseminated encephalomyelitis, multiple sclerosis |
| Transverse myelitis | *Staphylococcus aureus*, idiopathic transverse myelitis |

**Table 2** Histopathology of acute inflammatory myelopathies

| Types | Features | Causes |
|---|---|---|
| Necrotizing myelitis | • Coagulative necrosis<br>• Thickening and hyalinization of the vascular walls | Herpes simplex virus, systemic lupus erythematosus, paraneoplastic disease |
| Demyelinating myelitis | • Fragmentation of myelin with axonal preservation<br>• Microglial proliferation | Multiple sclerosis, acute disseminated encephalomyelitis |
| Haemorrhagic myelitis | • Perivascular haemorrhages<br>• Fibrinoid necrosis<br>• Confluent oedema<br>• Foci of demyelination<br>• Leukocyte infiltration | Varicella-zoster virus |
| Granulomatous myelitis | • One or more collections of macrophages, epithelioid cells and multinucleated giant cells<br>• Perifocal reactive gliosis<br>• Necrotizing, non-necrotizing or suppurative evolution | *Mycobacterium tuberculosis*, *Brucella melitensis*, *Coccidiodes immitis*, *Blastomyces dermatides*, *Toxoplasma gondii*, Sarcoidosis |
| Suppurative myelitis | • One or more fibrino-purulent, purulent, or purulent-necrotic collections<br>• Leukocyte infiltration | *Staphylococcus aureus* |
| Non-specific myelitis | • Perivascular leukocyte infiltration<br>• Microglial proliferation<br>• Neuronal degeneration | Poliovirus |

- Intramedullary infarction from disruption of blood flow in the spinal cord (atherosclerosis, aortic dissection, Takayasu's arteritis, atheromatous emboli, thromboemboli, fibrocartilaginous emboli, decompression sickness, hypotensive-hypoperfusion, fat embolism, cardiac surgery, spinal procedures, vascular malformations, epidural infection leading to epidural venous thrombosis).
- Intramedullary haematoma (haematomyelia) from bleeding in the substance of the spinal cord (rupture of spinal vascular malformations, anticoagulation or thrombolysis, hereditary or acquired bleeding disorders).
- Infarction or haemorrhage in the core of primary or metastatic intramedullary tumours.
- Intrasyrinx bleeding (haemorrhagic syringomyelia).
- Ionizing radiation (radiation myelopathy) or electrical current.
- Drugs or chemical agents, such as methotrexate, heroin, or konzo (toxic myelopathy).

NTSEI due to ***extrinsic cord compression*** (compressive myelopathy) can be caused by extra-axial (extradural or subdural) space occupying lesions, including:

- Degenerative or reactive osteo-articular processes (herniated nucleus pulposus, osteophytes, calcification and ossification of the posterior longitudinal ligament, calcifying pseudoneoplasm of the neuroaxis).
- Primary or metastatic tumours.
- Abscesses (*Staphylococcus aureus*, *Escherichia coli*, *Pseudomonas aeruginosa*).

**Table 3** Non-inflammatory acute myelopathies

| Patterns | Pathological features |
|---|---|
| Intramedullary infarction | • Coagulative necrosis<br>• Erytrhrodiapedesis<br>• Perifocal oedema |
| Intramedullary haemorrhage | • Haematoma dissecting longitudinally above and below the area of initial haemorrhage, and disrupting gray matter more than white matter<br>• Perifocal oedema |
| Infarction or haemorrhage in the core of intramedullary tumors | • Primary or metastatic tumor harbouring coagulative necrosis or haematoma<br>• Perifocal oedema |
| Haemorrhagic syringomyelia | • Haematoma in a syringomyelic cavity<br>• Possible coexistence of Chiari marformation or hydrocephalus |
| Radiation myelopathy | • Myelin degeneration<br>• Erytrhrodiapedesis<br>• Focal astrocytosis<br>• Perifocal oedema |
| Myelopathy from electrical current | • Neuronal necrosis<br>• Necrosis of the vascula wall<br>• Thrombosis and vasospasm<br>• Perifocal oedema |
| Toxic myelopathy | • Myelin degeneration<br>• Neuronal necrosis<br>• Thrombosis<br>• Endothelial proliferation<br>• Vacuolization |

- Haematomas (rupture of spinal vascular malformations, anticoagulation or thrombolysis, hereditary or acquired bleeding disorders, spinal procedures.
- Vascular malformations.
- Granulomas (*Mycobacterium tuberculosis*, *Brucella melitensis*).
- Non-neoplastic cysts (synovial cyst, arachnoid cyst) (Mark 1996; Ropper and Ropper 2017).

It may or may not coexist with spinal stenosis. When it is present spinal stenosis increases extrinsic cord compression because it reduces up to make null the perimedullary reserve space (cerebrospinal fluid, meninges, epidural soft tissue), which normally provides mechanical protection for the spinal cord (Freedman et al. 2015). The compression site can be anterior, anterolateral, lateral, posterior, or circumferential (Sanchez et al. 2011). Cord compression may or may not cause intramedullary oedema, transient ischemia, and ultimately myelomalacia: both severity and duration of compression are determining factors for the occurrence and gravity of cord damage (Alshareef et al. 2014; Dolan et al. 2016).

NTSEI are thus associated with numerous and different aetiologies. Each pathogen noxa primary acts on one or both subsystems of the spinal cord (i.e. neural/glial cells subsystem and vascular subsystem) through mechanical injury (compression, irritation, displacement, strangulation, obstruction, occlusion) and/or non-mechanical injury (biochemical, metabolic, immunologic) (Dolan et al. 2016). Any change in one subsystem can subsequently affect the other subsystem.

Clinical signs and symptoms of NTSCI can manifest abruptly or can develop rapidly over minutes or hours. They include impairment of motor, sensory, or autonomic functions below the level of cord injury and can correspond to a new acute onset disease or an acute exacerbation of a pre-existing unsuspected or unknown non-compressive or compressive myelopathy (Chakravarty 2010). Functional impairment of spinal cord can be complete and incomplete. Complete impairment corresponds to grade A of ASIA Impairment Scale (Kirshblum et al. 2011) and configures a complete transverse cord syndrome. Incomplete impairment corresponds to grades B, C, or D of ASIA Impairment Scale (Kirshblum et al. 2011), and configures different spinal cord syndromes (Jacob and Weinshenker 2008; Pastorino 1984; Ropper and Ropper 2017):

- Anterior horn cell syndrome (mono- or bilateral anterior horn).
- Posterior horn cell syndrome (mono- or bilateral posterior horn).
- Brown-Sequard hemicord syndrome (ipsilateral cortico-spinal, posterior columns, contralateral spino-thalamic).
- Anterior cord syndrome (bilateral anterior horn cells, contralateral spino-thalamic).
- Posterior cord syndrome (bilateral posterior columns).
- Central cord syndrome (crossing spino-thalamic, cortico-spinal, and autonomic fibres).
- Tractopathies (selective tract involvement).

Both complete and incomplete spinal cord impairments depend on the level of medullary involvement: upper cervical (C1-C4), lower cervical (C5-Th1), thoracic (Th2-Th12), lumbosacral (L1-S2), conus medullaris (S3-S5), and cauda equina (L2-S5 nerve roots) (Pastorino 1984; Ropper and Ropper 2017).

The differential diagnosis of NTSCI is therefore broad and can be challenging. Nevertheless, it must be appropriate and timely in order to allow an adequate and effective treatment. As a matter of fact, therapeutic strategy differs depending on the kind and topography of pathology. Radical or partial resection, biopsy, decompressive laminectomy (with or without durotomy and duroplasty) are reasonable options.

## References


Alshareef M, Krishna V, Ferdous J et al (2014) Effect of spinal cord compression on local vascular blood flow and perfusion capacity. PLoS One 9:e108820

Chakravarty A (2010) The challenge of acute non-compressive transverse myelopathies. Front Neurol 1:6. https://doi.org/10.3389/fneur.2010.00006

Cree BAC (2014) Acute inflammatory myelopathies. In: Goodin DS (ed) Handbook of clinical neurology, vol 122. Elsevier BV, Amsterdam. (3rd series)

Dolan RT, Butler JS, O'Byrne JM et al (2016) Mechanical and cellular processes driving cervical myelopathy. World J Orthop 7:20–29

Freedman BA, Hoffler CE, Cameron BM et al (2015) A comparison of computed tomography measures for diagnosing cervical spinal stenosis associated with myelopathy: a case-control study. Asian Spine J 9:22–29

Hunderfund ANL, Wijdicks EFM (2009) Intramedullary spinal cord hemorrhage (hematomyelia). Rev Neurol Dis 6:E54–E60

Jacob A, Weinshenker B (2008) An approach to the diagnosis of acute transverse myelitis. Semin Liver Dis 28:105–120

Kadir T, Sarica FB, Ozgur K et al (2012) Delayed radiation myelopathy: differential diagnosis with positron emission tomography/computed tomography examination. Asian J Neurosurg 7:206–209

Kirshblum SC, Burns SP, Biering-Sorensen F et al (2011) International standards for neurological classification of spinal cord injury (Revised 2011). J Spinal Cord Med 34:535–546

Loeb C, Dagnino N (1984) Mieliti e mielopatie. In: Fazio C, Loeb C (eds) Neurologia. Società Editrice Universo, Roma

Mark AS (1996) Infectious and inflammatory disease of the spine. In: Atlas SW (ed) Magnetic resonance imaging of the brain and spine. Lippincott-Raven, Philadelphia, PA

Pastorino P (1984) Sindromi midollari. In: Fazio C, Loeb C (eds) Neurologia. Società Editrice Universo, Roma

Riva N, Morana P, Cerri F et al (2007) Acute myelopathy selectively involving lumbar anterior horns following intranasal insufflation of ecstasy and heroin. J Neurol Neurosurg Psychiatry 79:908–909

Ropper AE, Ropper AH (2017) Acute spinal cord compression. N Engl J Med 376:1358–1369

Sanchez AMG, Posada LMG, Toscano CAO et al (2011) Diagnostic approach to myelopathies. Rev Colomb Radiol 22:1–21

Sharma SR, Hussain M, Hibong H (2018) Cervical myelopathy after high-voltage electrical burn of the head: report of an unusual case. Ann Indian Acad Neurol 21:76–79

Tariq H, Gilbert A, Sharkey FE (2018) Intrathecal methotrexate-induced necrotizing myelopathy: a case report and review of histologic features. Clin Med Insights Pathol 11:1–5

Vargas MI, Gariani J, Sztajzel R et al (2015) Spinal cord ischemia: pratical imaging tips, pearls, and pitfalls. AJNR Am J Neuroradiol 36:825–830

World Health Organization. International perspectives on spinal cord injury. WHO Library Cataloguing, 2013

# Emergent Degenerative and Disc Diseases

Nuria Santamaria, Maria del Carmen Polidura, George Bunea, and Jonathan Spratt

## Contents



N. Santamaria (✉)
Radiology Department, South Tyneside and Sunderland Foundation Trust, Sunderland, UK

Division Radiology Department, University Clatterbridge Cancer Center, Liverpool, UK

M. d. C. Polidura
Radiology Department, Hospital Clinico San Carlos, Madrid, Spain

G. Bunea · J. Spratt
Radiology Department, South Tyneside and Sunderland Foundation Trust, Sunderland, UK


M. Scaglione et al. (eds.), *Emergency Radiology of the Head and Spine*,
Medical Radiology Diagnostic Imaging, https://doi.org/10.1007/978-3-030-91047-1_16

**Abstract**

Aged-related changes in the spine are initiated in the discovertebral complex and will extend to the adjacent vertebral bone marrow, cervical uncovertebral and facet joints and spinal ligaments. These occur in response to a wide range of insults, repetitive low-level mechanical trauma being the most important. Degenerative spinal stenosis represents a significant cause of pain and disability in the elderly population. Age-related changes and disc herniation may narrow the central canal and neuroforamina, causing cord compression and myelopathy, cauda equina compromise or individual radiculopathy.

Accurate and comprehensive interpretation of age-related spinal imaging findings can be challenging because often there is poor correlation with symptoms. Imaging may confirm the diagnosis of spinal canal stenosis and identify exactly the affected levels and anatomic structures involved, therefore enabling clinical correlation and treatment planning.

Plain film imaging remains the first line technique in the evaluation of spinal degenerative changes, being useful in assessing the morphology and alignment of the vertebrae, including the assessment of instability where needed using flexion and extension lateral radiographs and the degree of disc/facet joint degeneration and reactive osteophytosis. Computer tomography (CT) imaging provides more detailed information on the bony components of the spinal degenerative process but suboptimally assesses protrusive disc disease. CT myelography is an invasive procedure mainly restricted to cases in which MR is contraindicated. Magnetic resonance imaging (MRI) is the preferred imaging technique for spinal pathologies as it can clearly delineate the soft tissue contents of the spinal canal and neuroforamina to define both annuloprotrusive and neural pathology.

## Abbreviation

| | |
|---|---|
| CSF | Cerebrospinal fluid |
| CT | Computed tomography |
| DCM | Degenerative cervical myelopathy |
| DISH | Diffuse idiopathic skeletal hyperostosis |
| DTI | Diffusion tensor imaging |
| FSU | Functional spinal unit |
| LF | Ligamentum flavum |
| MR | Magnetic resonance |
| PLL | Posterior longitudinal ligament |

## 1 Introduction

The main functions of the osseoligamentous and discogenic complexes of the spinal column are to give structural support, allow trunk mobility, shock absorb compressive axial forces and protect the neuraxis (Oxland 2016). The cervical spine is designed to allow a great range of movement for the cranium, the thoracic spine to aid respiration via its costovertebral articulations, whereas the lumbar spine is primarily designed for weight bearing (Bland and Boushey 1990).

The basic biomechanical element of the spine is the functional spinal unit (FSU) composed by two contiguous vertebrae, the intervertebral disc, the facet joints and the spinal ligaments.

### 1.1 Discovertebral Complex

The discovertebral complex is an amphiarthrosis composed by the adjacent vertebral body endplates and the intervertebral disc. Its function is to transmit mechanical loads to the underlying vertebra and facilitate the motion of the spine.

The intervertebral disc is formed by the central nucleus pulposus constrained by the peripheral anulus fibrosus. The nucleus pulposus, a remnant of the notochord, is a gelatinous structure rich in proteoglycans and water. Aggrecan is the most abundant proteoglycan delivering osmotic properties essential to resist compression. The anulus fibrosus surrounds the nucleus pulposus and is composed by collagen fibres arranged in concentric rings called lamellae, with an inner fibrocartilage portion which blends with the nucleus pulposus. The external lamellae are connected to the longitudinal ligaments and vertebral bodies (Sharpey fibres). The lamellae of the anulus fibrosus are thinner posteriorly than anteriorly, and this anatomic disposition may explain the propensity for posterior disc herniation. It provides reinforcement during axial loading, bending and torsion, as well as maintaining the nucleus pulposus osmotic pressure.

The vertebral endplates are composed of a central bony disc covered by hyaline cartilage and an elevated bony rim called the ring apophysis. The cartilaginous endplate is strongly fixed to the intervertebral disc, more loosely bound to the underlying subchondral vertebral bone (Hukins 1988).

The intervertebral discs are the largest nonvascularised structures in the body, and their nutrition is based largely on diffusion across the vertebral endplates (Holm et al. 1981).

Only the outer third of the anulus fibrosus is innervated (Ashton et al. 1994), more abundantly in the posterior and posterolateral margins of the intervertebral disc.

Spinal degeneration occurs in response to a wide range of insults, mechanical trauma being the most important aetiologic factor, including chronic overuse and sequelae of vertebral fracture or surgery (Gallucci et al. 2005; Bogduk 2012). Other causes include metabolic disease, e.g. diabetes mellitus and ochronosis (Aufdermaur et al. 1980; Robinson et al. 1998; Millucci et al. 2017), nutritional and genetic factors.

## 2 Aging of the Intervertebral Disc

Increasing age is associated with disc degeneration in the cervical and lumbar spine (Boden et al. 1990a, b; Cheung et al. 2009). The process of intervertebral disc aging is called intervertebral chondrosis, and when affects the adjacent vertebral body, osteochondrosis.

Notochordal cells disappear before maturity and are substituted by chondrocyte-like cells that synthetize a collagen-rich and less hydrated matrix (Trout et al. 1982; Hunter et al. 2003). The aging cartilaginous endplate sustains calcification followed by resorption and bony replacement (Bernick and Caillet 1982), disrupting nutrient exchange (Roberts et al. 1997).

A majority of the studies of the aging intervertebral disc relate to the lumbar spine, but the morphology and functions of the intervertebral discs differ by spinal level (Mercer and Bogduk 1994) and so does their response to aging.

The cervical intervertebral discs show progressive disappearance of the nucleus pulposus, being replaced by fibrocartilage and dense fibrous tissue, known as "dry" disc (Bland and Boushey 1990). During early adulthood, the cervical discs develop cracks and fissures that are believed to be physiological (Bland and Boushey 1990) and thought to allow rotational movement (Bogduk and Mercer 2000).

The aging lumbar intervertebral discs undergo biochemical changes with loss of water and proteoglycans in the nucleus pulposus (Gower and Pedrini 1969) accompanied by an increase in collagen within the disc (Olczyk 1992). On MRI, these biochemical changes translate into loss of intranuclear hyperintensity on T2 WI and subsequent loss of disc height. A number of morphological grading systems to evaluate degeneration of cervical (Matsumoto et al. 1998; Miyazaki et al. 2008; Nakashima et al. 2015) and lumbar (Pfirrmann et al. 2001; Griffith et al. 2007) intervertebral discs have been proposed.

These changes lead to altered biomechanics of the disc resulting in mechanical load transfer into the anulus fibrosus (Adams et al. 1996) and facet joints. Hence age-related changes comprise disc desiccation and fibrosis, disc space loss, diffuse annular bulging and fissuring, intradiscal fluid and vacuum phenomena (see below), ligamentous hypertrophic changes, bone marrow changes, disc herniation, marginal vertebral osteophyte formation, malalignment and stenosis (Modic and Ross 2007).

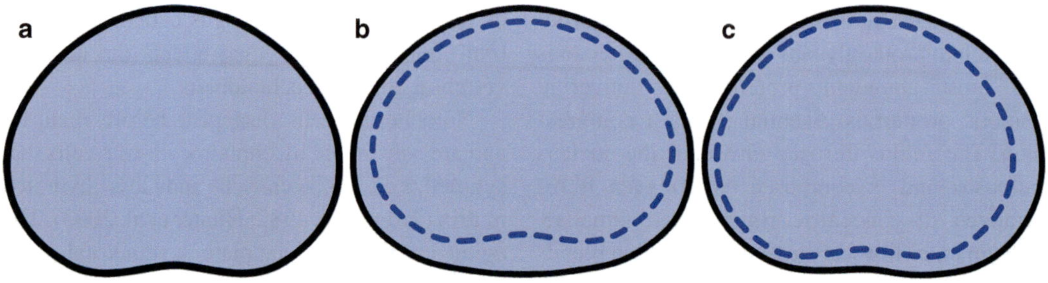


**Fig. 1** Schematic drawings of normal-appearing intervertebral disc in axial plane (**a**), and diffuse (**b**) and asymmetric (**c**) disc bulging. Black line represents the margin of the intervertebral disc whereas blue dashed line depicts the vertebral ring apophysis

## 3 Anular Fissures

Anular fissures are separations between the anular fibres or separations of anular fibres from their insertions to the vertebrae. According to their orientation, they are classified into concentric, radial and transverse fissures. These lesions are present in the majority of degenerated discs (Yu et al. 1988). T2 WI demonstrates localised high signal intensity zones (HIZ) within the anulus (Modic et al. 1988a, b; Carragee et al. 2000; Schellhas et al. 1996) representing fluid and granulation tissue and may show enhancement on post-gadolinium T1 WI. Its appearances may remain stable over years (Munter et al. 2002) and therefore they do not denote acute injury.

As disc degeneration evolves, vacuum phenomenon, intradiscal fluid accumulation and intradiscal calcification may happen. Vacuum phenomenon refers to gas collection, mainly nitrogen within clefts in aged discs with intradiscal negative pressure.

## 4 Disc Displacement

### 4.1 Disc Bulging

Disc bulging describes the contour of the outer anulus extending beyond the edges of the ring apophyses symmetrically throughout the disc circumference, usually by less than 3 mm as seen on axial imaging—it is not considered a form of herniation. There are two types of disc bulging—diffuse and asymmetric. Asymmetric disc bulging describes the contour of the outer anulus extending beyond the edges of the ring apophyses greater than 25% of the disc circumference (Fardon et al. 2014) (Fig. 1). It is believed that disc bulging is an asymptomatic lesion (Jensen et al. 1994).

### 4.2 Disc Herniation

Disc herniation is defined as a localized or focal displacement of disc material beyond the limits of the intervertebral disc space (Fardon et al. 2014). Acute disc herniation may happen within age-related discogenic changes in trauma or heavy lifting settings due to acute increase in intradiscal pressure (Kushchayev et al. 2018). In subacute disc herniations, there is fluctuating displacement of disc material according to intradiscal pressure variations with patient position. In chronic disc herniations, there is a static displacement of the disc material (Kushchayev et al. 2018). There are no specific imaging criteria to differentiate between acute, subacute or chronic herniations (Fardon et al. 2014).

Based on the shape of the herniated disc material, it can be categorised into protrusion, extrusion or extrusion with sequestration. Protrusion is a focal displacement of disc material involving less than 25% of the disc circumference; the greatest diameter of the herniated disc is less than its base at the site of herniation (Fardon et al. 2014). Extrusion is present when at least in one plane the maximum diameter of the herniated disc is greater than its base. Extrusion with

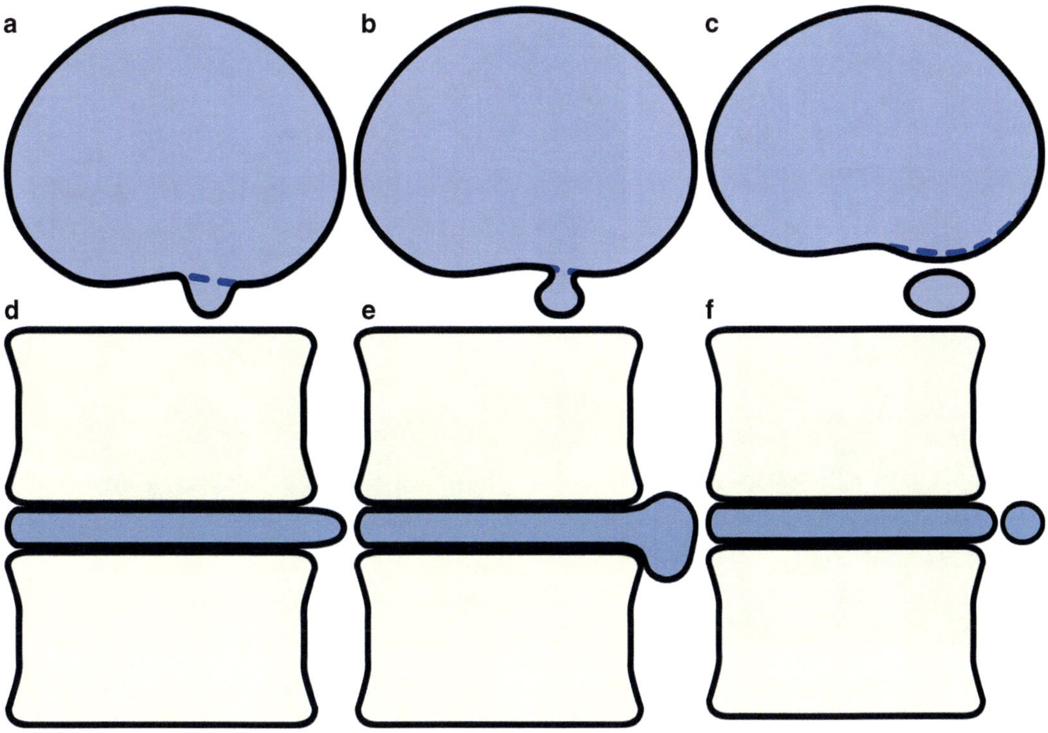


**Fig. 2** Schematic drawings of disc herniation classifications. Disc protrusion is demonstrated in axial (**a**) and sagittal (**d**) planes. Disc extrusion in axial (**b**) and sagittal (**e**) planes. Disc sequestration in axial (**c**) and sagittal (**f**) planes

sequestration is present if there is no connection of the herniated disc material to the parent disc (Fig. 2). The term 'migration' implies displacement of disc material away from the site of extrusion craniocaudally or mediolaterally. Disc herniations may be further categorised by containment as well as referenced by size, location and neural relationships. Those covered by outer anulus fibres and/or the posterior longitudinal ligament are named contained or subligamentous disc herniations. If this covering is absent, they are called uncontained or transligamentous.

The location of the herniated disc may be expressed using anatomic landmarks in the axial (zones) and sagittal (levels) planes (Wiltse et al. 1997). Within the transverse plane, the disc is divided into five zones—posterocentral, paracentral (subarticular), foraminal (lateral), extraforaminal (far lateral) and anterior (Fig. 3). The location of the disc herniation foresees

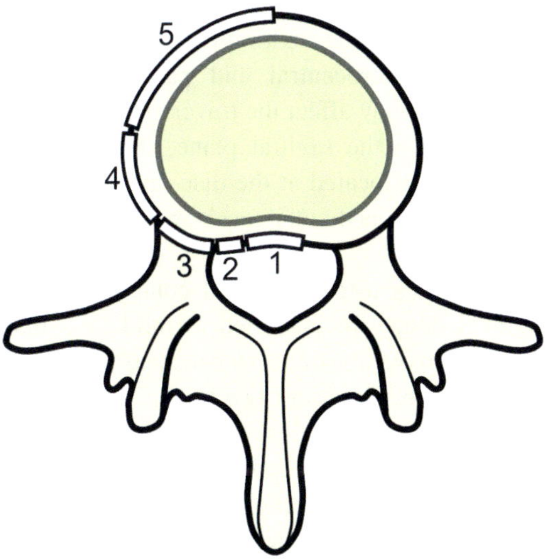


**Fig. 3** Schematic drawing of a lumbar vertebra showing the five anatomic zones of disc herniations—posterocentral (**1**), subarticular (**2**), foraminal (**3**), extraforaminal (**4**) and anterior (**5**)

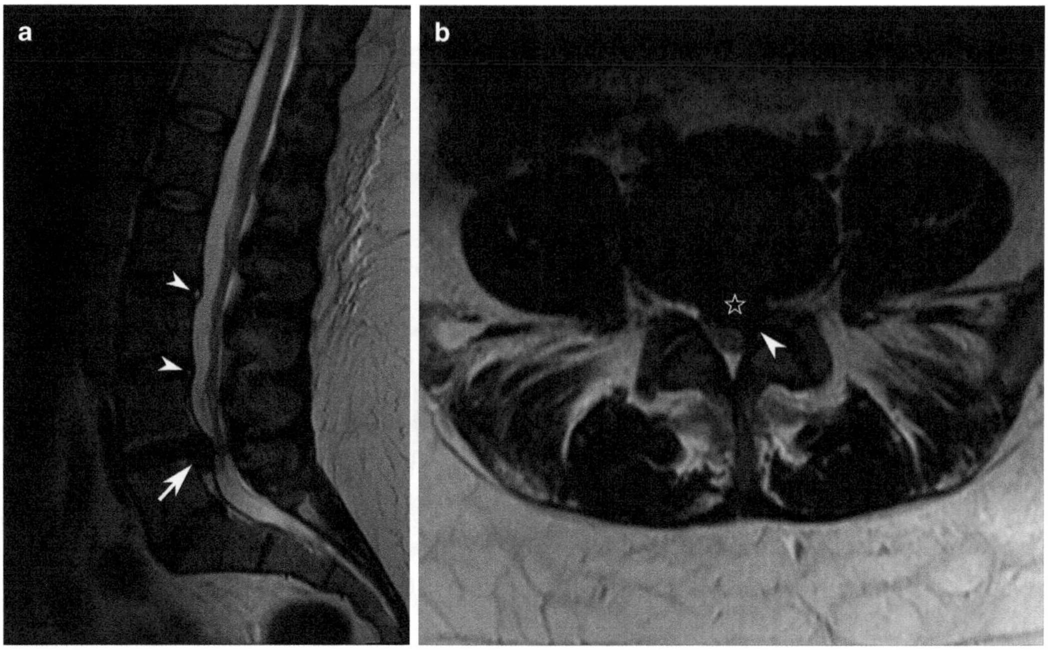


**Fig. 4** A 34-year-old woman with lower back pain and new urinary incontinence. Sagittal midline (**a**) and axial (**b**) T2 WI demonstrates a L4–5 posterocentral disc extrusion (**a**, white arrow) (**b**, star), causing left L5 nerve root compression (**b**, white arrowhead). Anular fissures and disc bulging at L2–3 and L3–4 are also seen (**a**, small white arrowheads). The patient underwent lumbar L4–5 discectomy

which nerve is most likely to be affected; e.g. foraminal and extraforaminal disc herniations may impinge the exiting/exited nerve root whereas posterocentral and paracentral disc herniations may affect the traversing nerve root (Fig. 4). On the sagittal plane, the herniated disc may be located at the disc level, suprapedicular level, pedicular level or infrapedicular level (Fig. 5).

According to central canal compromise, the herniation may be classified as mild (less than one-third reduction of the spinal canal), moderate (between one-third and two-thirds reduction of the spinal canal) and severe (more than two-thirds reduction of the spinal canal).

To describe the effect of the disc herniation on the lumbar nerves, a grading system of four categories can be used, ranging from grades 0 to 3 (Pfirrmann et al. 2004). Grade 0 where there is no herniated disc neural contact; grade 1 where there is contact between the undisplaced nerve root and the herniated disc; grade 2 where there is dorsal displacement of the nerve root by the herniated disc; grade 3 where the nerve root is compressed between the herniated disc and other elements of the spinal canal.

To describe the compromise of the exiting nerve roots within their neuroforamina, a dichotomous system of no root compression and root compression (obliteration of the periradicular fat) can be used (van Rijn et al. 2005).

Disc herniations may cause neurological, vascular or focal complications. Disc herniation is the most common cause of radicular pain (Izzo et al. 2015). Neurological complications are secondary to spinal cord, cauda equina or more peripheral nerve root impingement potentially warranting surgical intervention. Vascular complications occur after the compression of the spinal arteries and veins. Focal complications refer to epidural scarring developed in subacute or chronic disc herniations due to ongoing inflammation.

Disc herniations can regress spontaneously over time (Bozzao et al. 1992; Borota et al. 2008; Bush et al. 1992) with sequestered disc hernia-

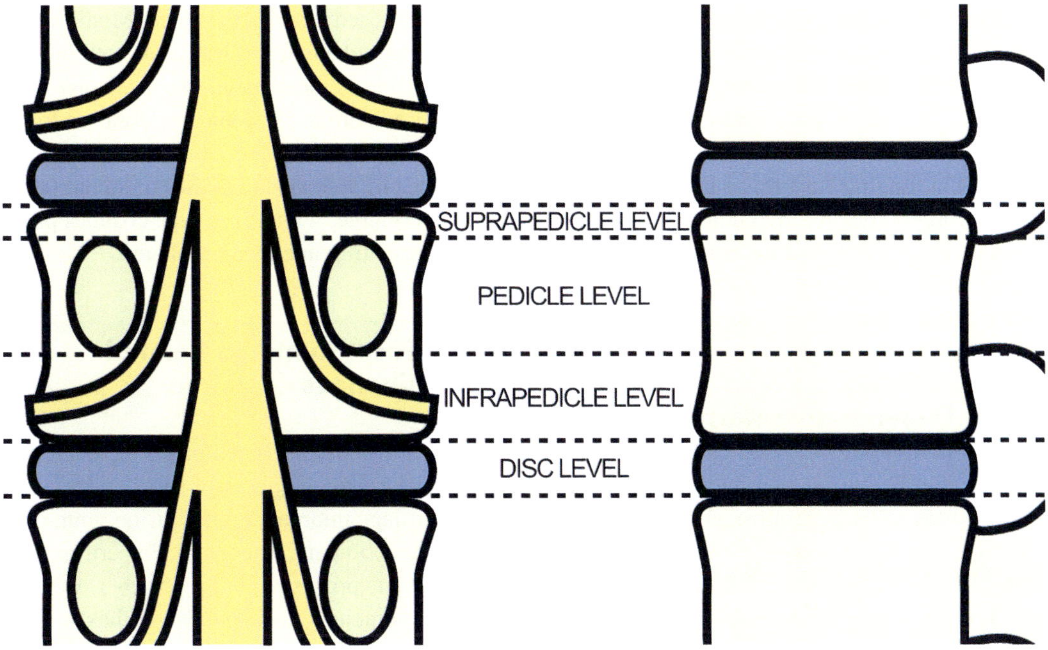


**Fig. 5** Schematic drawings of two lumbar vertebrae in coronal and sagittal planes illustrating suprapedicular, pedicle, infrapedicle and disc levels

tions usually demonstrating greater morphologic decrease in size (Ahn et al. 2000). It is hypothesized that there is an absorption process with neovascularisation, inflammatory cell infiltration and phagocytosis of the disc herniated material (Ikeda et al. 1996).

## 5 Osteophyte Formation

Spinal osteophyte formation (spondylosis deformans) is believed to represent an attempt to increase joint surface and reduce the pressure within an aging spinal joint (Bogduk 2012). Osteophytes arising from the anterior aspect of the lumbar vertebral bodies are classified into traction and claw osteophytes. Traction osteophytes are more common than claw osteophytes, but both may be part of the same process. Traction osteophytes are a marker of spinal instability (Pate et al. 1988).

Osteophytes arising from the posterior endplates of the vertebrae contribute to central canal stenosis. Uncovertebral spurs may impinge upon the V2 segment of the vertebral artery, radicular artery and spinal nerve roots. Osteophytes arising from the facet joints are more prominent in the lumbar spine, and they may cause compression of the lateral recess and neuroforamen.

In addition to impingement of the spinal canal and neuroforamina, osteophytes may be compress neighbouring structures along the spine, causing dysphagia, compression of main bronchus and neural or vascular complications (Klaassen et al. 2011; Ullman et al. 2016). Endplate osteophytes and herniated discs have been associated with ventral dural sac tears resulting in spontaneous intracranial hypotension (Thielen et al. 2015; Hoxworth et al. 2012; Eross et al. 2002).

## 6 Vertebral Endplate Changes

MRI classification of degenerative changes of the vertebral endplates uses a six-stage system from normal appearances to extensive changes (Rajasekaran et al. 2008). The initial aging changes include endplate thinning and focal defect without subchondral bone marrow changes. Associated with Modic endplate changes, more extensive endplate damage can be seen with less than 25%, up to 50% or complete destruction of the endplate surface. Intravertebral herniation (Schmorl's node) occurs when the disc herniates through a fracture in the endplate into the vertebral body with MRI demonstrating bone marrow oedema in the acute setting—such acute intravertebral herniation may be an underestimated cause of back pain (Takahashi et al. 1995).

## 7 Degenerative Marrow Changes

Three forms of degenerative change involving the bone marrow adjacent to the vertebral endplates have been described (Modic et al. 1988a, b). Type 1 consists of fibrovascular tissue, type 2 fatty bone marrow and type 3 bone sclerosis. Mixed types 1/2 and 2/3 may also be seen.

Modic type 1 changes are strongly associated with non-specific low back pain (Modic et al. 1988a, b) with characteristic low signal on T1 WI and high signal on T2 WI with enhancement on postcontrast imaging. These appearances may mimic infective spondylodiscitis or rarely malignancy—characteristic morphological changes of the disc, endplates and adjacent soft tissues may help in differentiating between these conditions.

In Modic type 1 change, the disc is often normal or exhibits low signal on T2 W2 whereas in infectious spondylodiscitis it returns high signal (James and Davies 2006; Diehn 2012). Prominent destruction of the endplates is often characteristic of infective spondylodiscitis (James and Davies 2006, Diehn 2012). Modic type 1 changes often reveal the claw sign on DWI, well-defined usually symmetrical high signal areas around the affected disc, whereas this sign is absent in infectious spondylodiscitis (Patel et al. 2014). The presence of perivertebral/epidural soft tissue thickening or collection should suggest infective spondylodiscitis (James and Davies 2006, Diehn 2012). Modic type 2 endplate change correlates with high signal on T1 WI and isointense to high signal on T2 WI, without enhancement after contrast administration. Modic type 3 endplate change demonstrates low signal on both T1 and T2 WI.

The proposed theories to explain Modic vertebral endplate changes are based on both biomechanical and biochemical mechanisms. The temporal evolution of Modic vertebral endplate changes is uncertain, and conversion of type 1 into type 2 or vice versa in cases of spinal instability is possible, with mixed type changes probably representing intermediate stages.

## 8 Facet Joint Age-Related Changes

Facet joint osteoarthritis comprises a complex of joint space narrowing, erosive subchondral sclerosis, cartilage thinning, joint effusion, joint capsule calcification and osteophytic hypertrophy of the articular processes with possible vacuum joint phenomenon and spondylolisthesis. It is associated with ligamentum flavum thickening.

There is a high prevalence of facet joint osteoarthritis in the population (Kalichman et al. 2008), and as L4–5 is the level of maximum mobility, it is the most affected level (Eubanks et al. 2007). This may cause stenosis of the central spinal canal, lateral recesses and neuroforamina (Modic and Ross 2007).

### 8.1 Facet Joint Syndrome

Facet joint syndrome is defined as unilateral or bilateral back pain radiating to one or both buttocks, groin and thighs stopping above the knee (Manchikanti et al. 2001). The prevalence of facet joint pain is unknown, but it has been estimated from 27 to 40% in patients with chronic lumbar back pain (Datta et al. 2009). The diagnosis of facet joint syndrome based on history and clinical examination is difficult (Jackson 1992). The most common cause of facet joint pain is osteoarthritis (Kalichman et al. 2008); other causes include septic and inflammatory arthropathies. Pain is thought to be caused by inflammation from degeneration of the facet joints and adjacent tissues. In the differential diagnosis, sciatica and hip or sacroiliac pathology need to be considered (Perolat et al. 2018). The initial radiographic assessment should include AP, lateral and oblique views of the lumbar

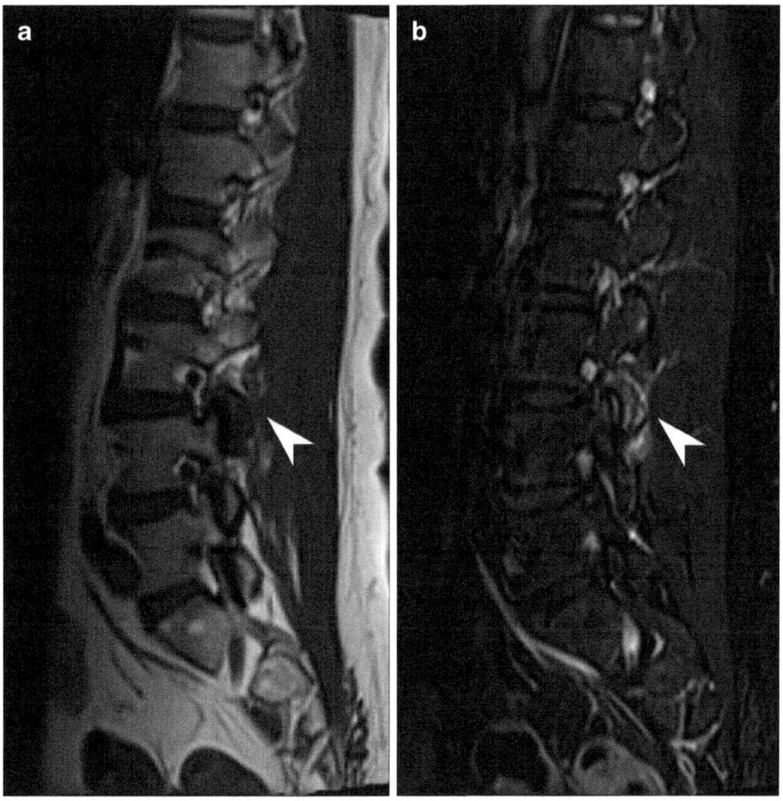

**Fig. 6** Facet joint syndrome. Parasagittal T1-weighted (**a**) and STIR (**b**) images showing oedema within the left facet joint and surrounding tissues (white arrowheads), better depicted on STIR images

spine (Varlotta et al. 2011) and may be useful to detect facet joint osteoarthritis, spondylolisthesis and defects of the pars interarticularis. CT and MRI are more efficient in demonstrating facet osteoarthritis (Weishaupt et al. 1999). CT better depicts bony anatomy (Varlotta et al. 2011) but MRI is able to show synovitis and oedema of the articular processes of the facet joints (D'Aprile et al. 2006) (Fig. 6). Facet joint synovitis is demonstrated after the enhancement of the capsule on postcontrast imaging.

Bone scans, particularly SPECT-CT, shows good agreement in detecting symptomatic facet or disc disease prior to surgery or facet injection (Malham et al. 2015).

### 8.2 Synovial Cysts of the Facet Joints

Synovial cysts are herniations of the synovium through the capsule of a degenerated facet joint, and they represent the most common cause of juxta-articular cysts. Their development is associated with degenerative changes of the facet joints (Banning et al. 2001; Hsu et al. 1995; Pirotte et al. 2003), spinal instability and spondylolisthesis (Reust et al. 1988; Parlier-Cuau et al. 1999).

A majority of the synovial cysts are incidental findings (Hemminghytt et al. 1982). They have been reported anywhere in the spine, but there is a marked lumbar predominance; the most common location is L4–5 level, followed by L5-S1 level. They may be lateral or medial to the facet joint, and if there is intracanalicular growth of synovial cyst, it may cause compression of neural structures leading to back or radicular pain (Howington et al. 1999) and neurological deficits.

On imaging, synovial cysts appear as a well-defined mass adjacent to a degenerated facet joint. MRI is the preferred imaging technique and typically will demonstrate low signal on T1WI and high signal intensity on T2WI. However, cysts with high proteinaceous content fluid as a

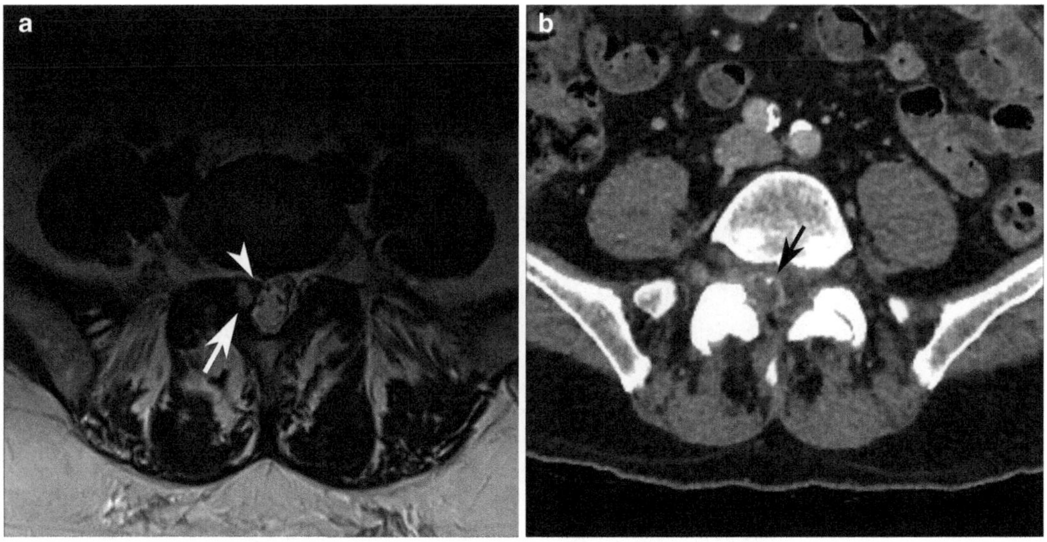


**Fig. 7** Juxta-articular cysts. Axial T2 WI (**a**) demonstrates an epidural cystic lesion (**a**, white arrow) adjacent to an osteoarthritic facet joint. The traversing right nerve root (**a**, white arrowhead) is mildly displaced. CT image (**b**, different patient) demonstrates facet joints osteoarthritis and a synovial cyst arising from the right facet joint with a hyperdense rim and a punctate calcification (**b**, black arrow) causing stenosis of the spinal canal

result of internal debris or haemorrhage may exhibit heterogeneously high T1 and low T2 signal (Khan and Girardi 2006). Rarely they may present with acute haemorrhage (Cicuendez et al. 2010). Peripheral rim enhancement may be seen on postcontrast imaging. CT may reveal dense rim or calcification of the wall or gas within the cyst (Wang et al. 1987) (Fig. 7).

## 9 Posterior Longitudinal Ligament and Ligament Flavum Changes

The spinal canal ligaments, posterior longitudinal ligament (PLL) and ligamentum flavum (LF) fill a small space in the healthy spine. However, abnormally thickened spinal ligaments may contribute to decreasing the spinal canal size.

### 9.1 Posterior Longitudinal Ligament Changes

PLL ossification may narrow the spinal canal anteriorly, particularly in the cervical spine leading to radiculopathy and myelopathy, more commonly affecting men in their 50s and 60s, especially of Japanese descent. There are four types of PLL ossification—continuous, segmental, mixed or localised. Multilevel effacement of the anterior CSF space and spinal cord compression may be observed with a low signal intensity band between the posterior surface of the vertebral bodies and the thecal sac on both T1 and T2 WI (Luetkehans et al. 1987). Sometimes T1 WI demonstrates high or intermediate signal within the ossified lesions secondary to its fatty marrow content (Yamashita et al. 1990). Thin ossification of the PLL is difficult to identify on MRI, and plain X-rays and CT are more sensitive (Wong et al. 2011). It has been associated with diffuse idiopathic skeletal hyperostosis (DISH) and ligamentum flavum (LF) calcification (referred to as tandem ossification, Guo et al. 2009) and ankylosing spondylitis.

DISH (also known as Forestier's disease) is a systemic noninflammatory entity causing ossification and calcifications of entheses and ligaments. It characteristically mainly involves the thoracic spine and consists of flowing ossification along the anterior or right anterolateral

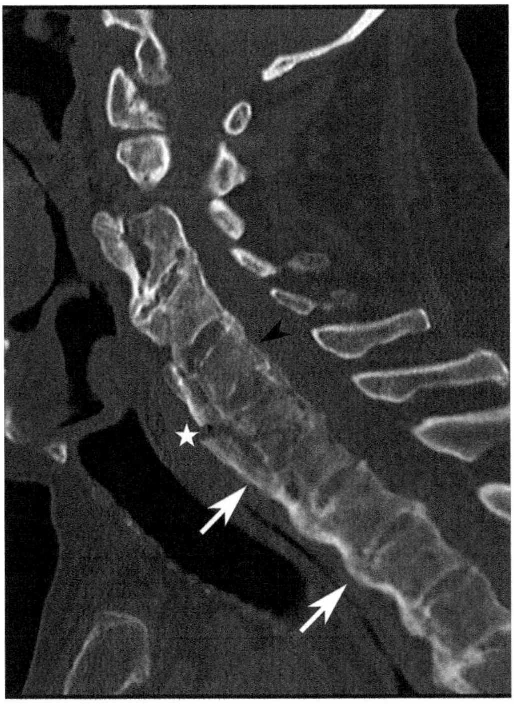

**Fig. 8** Sagittal midline reformatted CT of an 80-year-old man complaining of cervical spine tenderness and confusion after collapse shows DISH (white arrow) and C6 fracture (white star). PLL ossification is also noted (black arrowhead)

aspect of at least four contiguous vertebrae in the absence of intervertebral disc age–related changes and sacroiliitis (Resnick and Niwayama 1976). The estimated prevalence is roughly 10% of those aged 50 years and over with male predominance and is largely asymptomatic. Spinal involvement in DISH may lead to dysphagia, dyspnoea, stridor, myelopathy, atlantoaxial pseudoarthrosis or subluxation and low-energy vertebral fractures (Mader 2002; Westerveld et al. 2009; Caron et al. 2010) (Fig. 8).

### 9.2 Ligamentum Flavum Hypertrophy and Cysts

Disc degeneration and facet joint arthrosis cause mechanical stress and spinal instability that correlate with LF infolding, hypertrophy and fibrosis (Fukuyama et al. 1995; Okuda et al. 2004). LF thickness increases with aging (Okuda et al. 2004; Altinkaya et al. 2011; Twomey and Taylor 1988) and it plays a key role in the development of lumbar spinal canal stenosis. The normal LF is 2–4 mm thick. In the lower lumbar spine, the LF is said to be hypertrophic if it is thicker than 5 mm (Grenier et al. 1987). As the LF is thinnest at midline, the reduction of canal size is most prominent on parasagittal images. The LF may suffer from ossification and calcification, and it may rarely lead to myelopathy (Miyasaka et al. 1983) (Fig. 9).

LF cysts are an uncommon cause of juxta-articular ganglion cysts (Chimento et al. 1995) arising from an aged LF, mostly within the lumbar spine, particularly at L4–5 level. Rarely symptomatic, they may represent an unusual cause of age-related spinal stenosis. It may be difficult to differentiate from synovial facet joint cysts on imaging, but there is no communication with the facet joint.

## 10 Baastrup's Disease

Baastrup's disease ('kissing spine') is characterized by excessive abnormal contact between adjacent spinous processes resulting in their enlargement, flattening and sclerosis often with interspinous bursitis. Clinically there is focal pain alleviated during flexion and worsening during extension (Hazlett 1964). Large interspinous collections may project into the posterior epidural space (Chen et al. 2004).

## 11 Degenerative Intervertebral Instability

Degenerative intervertebral instability is due to the combined failure of the intervertebral complex, facet joints and ligaments in maintaining the alignment of the involved functional spinal unit; and it will extend to adjacent levels, evolving from a segmental into a regional pathology. Patients with degenerative instability present with back pain exacerbated by movement, affecting the cervical and lumbar spine (the thoracic spine is almost always spared).

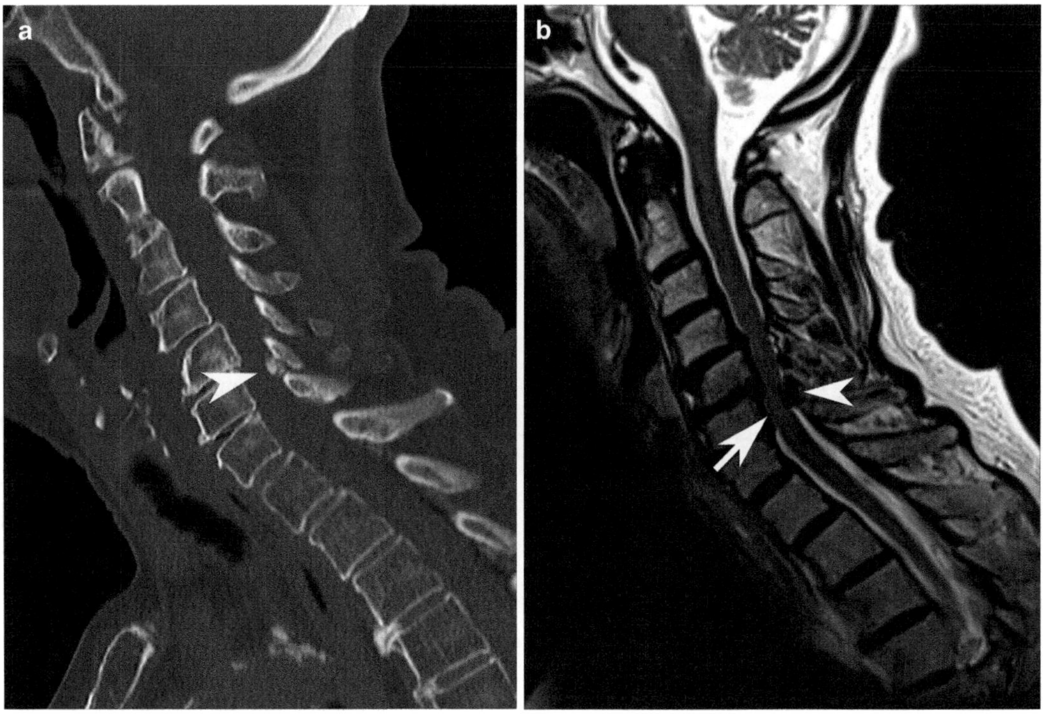


**Fig. 9** Reformatted sagittal CT (**a**) and T2-weighted (**b**) images showing spinal age-related changes of an elderly lady resulting in stenosis of the cervical canal at C5–6 due to degenerative listhesis and calcification of the ligamentum flavum (**a**, white arrowhead). There is subtle degenerative cervical myelopathy at C6 level (**b**, white arrow)

The cascade of degenerative instability is classified into dysfunction, instability and restabilisation (Kirkaldy-Willis and Farfan 1982). During the initial dysfunction phase, age-related changes of the intervertebral disc and facet joints occur. This is followed by the instability phase, characterised by abnormal motion leading to anterolisthesis or retrolisthesis. On imaging Modic type 1 endplate changes, pedicle and isthmus bone marrow oedema, traction osteophytes, discal vacuum phenomenon, facet joint effusion or intraarticular vacuum phenomenon (Chaput et al. 2007), synovial cysts, anular fissure, and listhesis can be found (Kirkaldy-Willis and Farfan 1982). During the final restabilisation phase, there is decreasing mobility with rigidity development. On imaging marked loss of height of the disc, Modic type 3 end plate changes, 'claw' osteophytes of the vertebral bodies, 'wrap around bumper' osteophytes of the facet joints, and Baastrup's disease.

## 11.1 Degenerative Spondylolisthesis

Degenerative spondylolisthesis is the displacement of one vertebra to another in the sagittal plane, as a result of subluxation of osteoarthritic facet joints (Cavanaugh et al. 1996). It is classified into two categories, dynamic and static, according to radiological evidence of instability on flexion/extension radiographs (Even et al. 2014), the diagnostic technique of choice. Ancillary findings of instability are facet joint effusion or osteoarthritis, facet synovial cysts and intradiscal vacuum phenomenon. Aged-related changes of the intervertebral disc can result in vertebral displacement in the coronal plane—lateral listhesis—which together with lateral wedging of the vertebral body and asymmetric facet joint osteoarthrosis may cause degenerative scoliosis.

Cervical degenerative spondylolisthesis most commonly occurs at C3–4 and C4–5 levels and may be more frequent than previously recognised (Jiang et al. 2011). Different classifications have been proposed to describe cervical degenerative spondylolisthesis. One of these systems is based on the degree of disc degeneration and spondylosis at adjacent levels, type I or adjacent spondylolisthesis at the transition between a more mobile segment to a more rigid one and type II or spondylotic spondylolisthesis related to advanced disc degeneration (Dean et al. 2009). Another system employs maximum slippage on flexion/extension radiographs (Kawasaki et al. 2007) classified as mild (less than 2.0 mm), moderate (2.0–3.4 mm) and severe (3.5 mm or more). Degenerative retrolisthesis is more commonly seen in the cervical and upper lumbar levels (Gallucci et al. 2007).

Degenerative lumbar spondylolisthesis most often occurs at the L4–5 level (Kalichman et al. 2008), and it is significantly more frequent in women (Kauppila et al. 1998). Lumbar spondylolisthesis is described employing the Meyerding classification (Meyerding 1932) based on the position of the posterior margin of the displaced superior vertebral body to the superior endplate of the vertebra below which is divided into four quarters—grade I, displacement less than 25%; grade II, 25–50%; grade III, 50–75%; grade IV, 75–100%; grade V or spondyloptosis. Degenerative spondylolisthesis is usually a grade 1. Sagittal planes are useful to assess the resultant degree of central canal and neuroforaminal stenosis.

## 12 Degenerative Stenosis of the Spine

Spinal stenosis is the consequence of congenital or acquired narrowing of the spinal canal. The former type includes achondroplastic syndromes and developmentally narrowed spinal canal. Acquired narrowing of the spine comprises degenerative changes, iatrogeny, systemic processes and trauma. Mixed stenosis refers to degenerative stenosis in patients with developmentally narrowed spinal canal (Gallucci et al. 2005), and in these cases, the contribution of age-related changes on a pre-existing developmentally narrowed canal may cause stenosis at an earlier age. The aging spine may be narrowed anteriorly by disc bulge or herniation, osteophytes or PLL ossification; posterolaterally by facet joint osteoarthritis and ligamentum flavum hypertrophy; anterolaterally in the cervical spine by uncovertebral joint hypertrophy which may compromise the cervical neuroforamina. In addition to the combination of these factors, degenerative spondylolisthesis may further reduce the spinal canal and neuroforaminal dimensions.

Stenosis of the spinal canal is a frequent observation in asymptomatic population with prevalence increasing with age (Boden et al. 1990a, b), and a distinction between morphological stenosis and clinically stenosis must be drawn. The role of imaging techniques is to assist the clinician in confirming the diagnosis of spinal canal stenosis, identifying the affected levels and anatomic structures involved, and to aid in treatment planning.

The symptoms are related to the location of stenosis—vague manifestations and ill-defined pain are present in central spinal stenosis whereas well-defined pain pattern is common in neuroforaminal stenosis. Cervicothoracic spinal stenosis can lead to spinal cord and radicular compression, resulting in pain, myelopathy, radiculopathy or myeloradiculopathy. Lumbar spinal stenosis causes nerve compression, resulting in neurogenic claudication or radicular leg pain. Neurogenic claudication refers to pain and weakness in the legs and calves when walking and may lessen when sitting, bending forward or lying down. Cauda equina syndrome is caused by the dysfunction of multiple sacral and lumbar nerve roots in the lumbar spinal canal with impairment of bladder, bowel, or sexual function, and perianal or "saddle" numbness. The most common aetiology of cauda equina syndrome is spinal canal stenosis secondary to large central disc herniation at the L4/5 and L5/S1 level (Ahn et al. 2000) (Fig. 10).

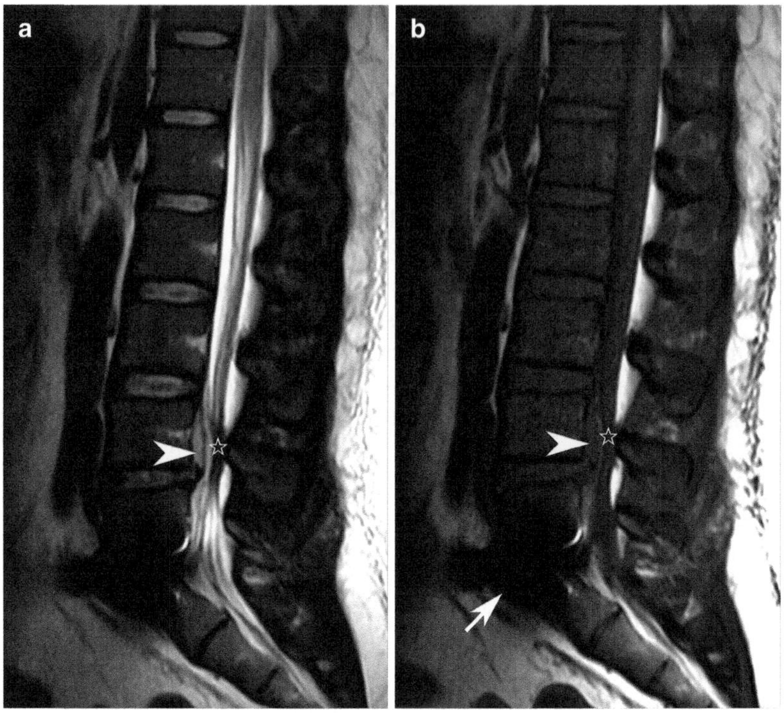


**Fig. 10** Sagittal midline T2- (**a**) and T1 (**b**)-weighted images of a young man with cauda equina syndrome on presentation after lifting weights. A L4–5 disc extrusion (white arrowhead) causing severe stenosis of the thecal sac (star) is demonstrated. Magnetic susceptibility artefact due to prior L5-S1 discectomy noted (**b**, white arrow)

## 12.1 Degenerative Cervical Spinal Canal Stenosis

Degenerative stenosis of the cervical canal is secondary to disc degeneration, uncovertebral and facet joint osteoarthritis, thickening of the ligamentum flavum, and ossification of the posterior longitudinal ligament.

The normal developmental segmental sagittal diameter is the distance from the posterior vertebral body to the nearest point of the corresponding spinolaminar line. Individuals with developmentally narrowed mid-cervical sagittal diameters smaller than 10 mm frequently have degenerative cervical myelopathy (DCM) and individuals with central canals from 13 to 17 mm often have symptomatic degenerative change often without myelopathy (Edwards and LaRocca 1983). In patients with developmentally narrowed cervical canal in addition to the restricted available space, there is more segmental mobility from C4–5 to C6–7 compared to individuals with normal cervical diameters, with more marked age-related changes at these levels (Morishita et al. 2009).

The pathophysiology of DCM encompasses static factors leading to stenosis of the cervical canal and dynamic factors causing repetitive cord damage due to spinal instability. Mechanical cord compression causes direct damage to the cord; and in addition to this ischemia, inflammation, and apoptosis are secondary causes of DCM (Baptiste and Fehlings 2006).

Clinically degenerative changes in the cervical spine may result in neck pain, myelopathy and radiculopathy. DCM is a clinical syndrome characterised by gait imbalance, loss of hand dexterity and sphincter dysfunction (Tetreault et al. 2015) with a progressive course. It represents the most common cause of spinal cord dysfunction in adults (Kalsi-Ryan et al. 2013; Fehlings et al. 2013).

Imaging in cervical degenerative stenosis is indicated to demonstrate the cause and level of stenosis and presence or absence of myelopathy. Previously lateral X-ray of the cervical spine has been employed to measure the developmental segmental sagittal diameter (distance from the posterior vertebral body to the nearest point of the corresponding spinolaminar line) and the ver-

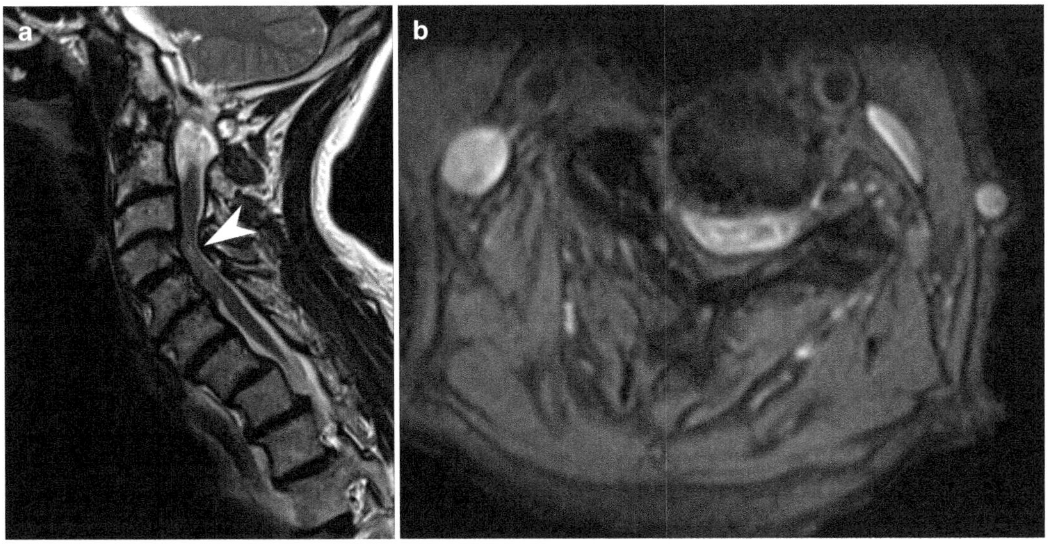


**Fig. 11** An 86-year-old woman with acute deterioration, subacute urinary retention and high clinical suspicion of cervical myelopathy. Age-related changes causing spinal canal stenosis and focal high signal of the spinal cord on T2 WI (**a**, arrowhead). Axial GRE T2 images at C4–5 level (**b**) shows posterior disc osteophyte complex, myelopathy and bilateral neural foraminal stenosis

tebral body ratio method or Pavlov ratio (the sagittal diameter of the spinal canal is divided by the sagittal diameter of the corresponding vertebral body, stenotic canal if $\leq$0.82) (Pavlov et al. 1987). Flexion-extension lateral X-rays are useful in demonstrating spinal instability.

MRI is the gold standard imaging method to assess spinal canal stenosis (Al-Mefty et al. 1988) and along with CT is the preferred imaging method to assess the dimensions of the cervical canal. Grading systems to describe central spinal canal have been proposed (Kang et al. 2011). Sagittal T1 WI and FSE T2 WI, and axial T2 gradient recalled echo (GRE) sequences are routinely used. Axial T2 GRE sequences can differentiate between disc-osteophyte complex and disc herniation and are useful in assessing the morphology of the neuroforamina. However, T2 GRE sequences may overestimate the degree of neuroforaminal narrowing because of magnetic susceptibility artefacts (Czervionke et al. 1988).

Intramedullary signal changes may reflect a wide spectrum of pathological changes from reversible oedema to established structural changes (Mizuno et al. 2003; Al-Mefty et al. 1988; Ohshio et al. 1993) (Fig. 11). Faint and ill-defined intramedullary T2 high signal more likely reflects reversible oedema. Strong and well-demarcated intramedullary T2 high signal is suggestive irreversible gliosis or cystic necrotic change correlating with hypointensity on T1 WI. Usually no postcontrast imaging in patients with suspected DCM is obtained; however, in a minority of patients (7.3%), intramedullary enhancement can be seen, and it has been associated with worse prognosis after decompressive surgery. Spinal cord enhancement is located between the intervertebral disc at the level of the maximal stenosis and the superior half of the lower vertebral body. Peripheral or scattered enhancing areas are the most prevalent pattern of enhancement seen on axial images. After surgery, the enhancement of the spinal cord may disappear or decrease (Ozawa et al. 2010). Some cases of DCM may be misdiagnosed as inflammatory or neoplastic diseases, as MRI demonstrates a long fusiform T2-signal abnormality and enlargement of the spinal cord, with enhancement just caudal to the point of maximal narrowing of the thecal sac (Flanagan et al. 2014). There is increasing interest in the evaluation of DCM with advanced MRI techniques—diffusion tensor imaging (DTI), MR spectroscopy and magnetization transfer—and the strongest correlation with symptoms has been found with DTI metric fractional anisotropy (Martin et al. 2015).

CT scanning better depicts bone anatomy, osteophytes and ossification of the posterior longitudinal ligament and flavum ligament. Myelogram and CT myelogram are used in selected cases when MR is contraindicated and the cause or the site of neural impingement is not depicted on conventional CT. As well it has an important role in showing the site of osteophyte-related CSF leaks (Yoshida et al. 2014).

## 12.2 Foraminal Stenosis in the Cervical Spine

Osteophytes at the uncovertebral joints (joints of Lushka) or posterior vertebral body, osteoarthritis of the facet joints or lateral disc herniations may lead to neuroforaminal stenosis (Wainner and Gill 2000; Yousem et al. 1991; Abbed and Coumans 2007). Uncovertebral joint hypertrophic spurs are the most common cause of neuroforaminal stenosis usually narrowing the superior aspect of the foramen—the nerve root sits in the lower aspect of the neuroforamen. Many papers have evaluated neuroforaminal stenosis (Park et al. 2013; Kim et al. 2015) but there is no universally accepted classification.

## 12.3 Degenerative Thoracic Spinal Canal Stenosis

Degenerative stenosis of the thoracic spine is less common than cervical or lumbar stenosis, as the thoracic spine is attached to the rib cage, thus limiting its motion range (Girard et al. 2004). It can occur associated with lumbar canal stenosis (Palumbo et al. 2001). Degenerative stenosis and disc herniations may impinge upon the spinal cord, causing localised back pain, myelopathy and sensory level. Symptomatic disc herniations are less frequently encountered in the thoracic spine than in other spinal levels (Arce and Dohrmann 1985). The majority of the thoracic herniations requiring surgery are located in the lower half of the thoracic spine (Oppenheim et al. 1993; Stillerman et al. 1998; Gille et al. 2006; Cornips et al. 2011) and are typically large and exhibit calcification (Stillerman et al. 1998; Cornips et al. 2011; Gille et al. 2006) (Fig. 12).

## 12.4 Lumbar Spinal Canal Stenosis

Degenerative stenosis of the lumbar spinal canal is secondary to bulging or herniated disc, osteophytes, hypertrophy of the facet joints and flavum ligament. In patients with vertebral instability and listhesis, the severity of stenosis may increase in upright position.

As a general rule, sagittal diameter of the central canal less than 12 mm in the lumbar spine is considered stenotic (Mamisch et al. 2012), and less than 10 mm is considered absolute stenosis.

Lateral recess stenosis is usually secondary to hypertrophy of the superior articular facet, although any other degenerative changes may coexist. The lateral recess height is the distance between the anterior superior articular facet and the posterior vertebral body. The cut-off value for stenosis of the lateral recess height is 3 mm (Mamisch et al. 2012).

Foraminal stenosis is secondary to osteophytes, disc bulging or herniation or spondylolisthesis. The cut-off value for stenosis of the lumbar neural foramen is 3 mm (Mamisch et al. 2012).

The role of imaging in patients with acute back pain is to exclude 'red flag indications'—suspicion of aortic pathology, neoplasm, infection, cauda equina syndrome, fracture or motor weakness (Lateef and Patel 2009). Imaging studies are to be considered in those patients who had no improvement of acute low back pain or radiculopathy after 4–6 weeks after conservative management.

## 12.5 Redundant Nerve Roots of the Cauda Equina

Redundant nerve roots of the cauda equina is a frequent finding in patients with lumbar spinal canal stenosis. Elongated, enlarged and serpigi-

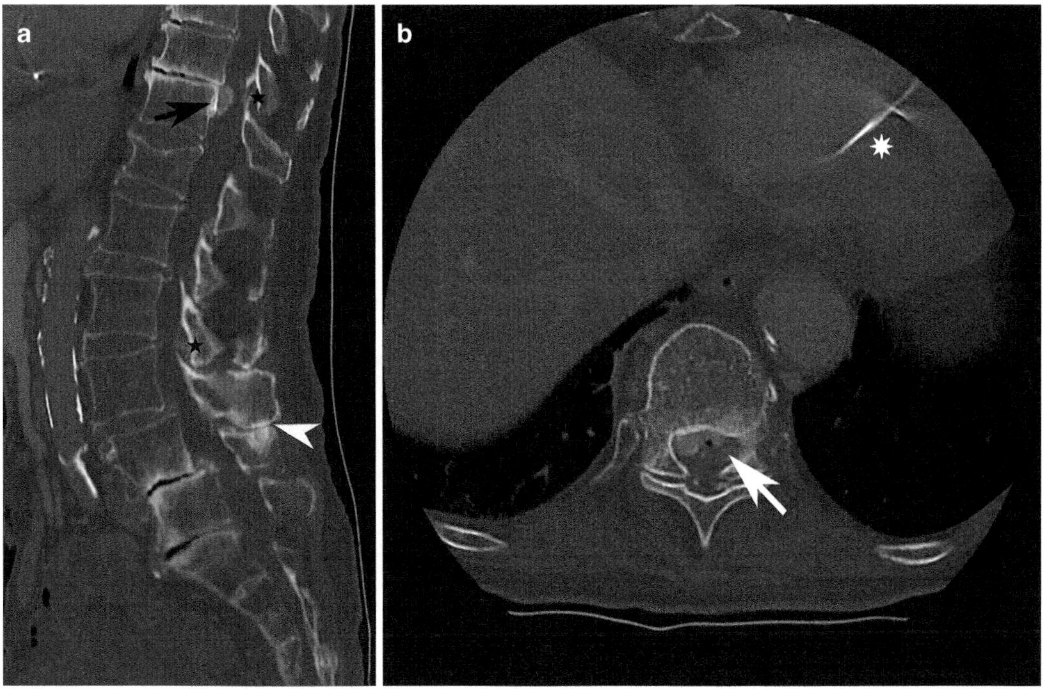

**Fig. 12** An 80-year-old woman with a pacemaker and clinical suspicion of thoracic myelopathy. Sagittal midline reformatted (**a**) and axial (**b**) CT images of the spine showing a calcified lesion posterior to T11 vertebral body (**a**, black arrow) and ossification of the ligamentum flavum (**a**, black star). There is gas within the calcified material (**b**, white arrow) consistent with calcified thoracic disc herniation. Multilevel intervertebral vacuum gas phenomena noted, including T10–11 disc. Lumbar degenerative listhesis, central canal stenosis and Baastrup's disease (**a**, white arrowhead) are also seen

nous nerve roots within the thecal sac are seen on sagittal T2 WI (Fig. 13). Its main differential diagnosis on MRI must done with spinal dural arteriovenous fistula or spinal extradural arteriovenous fistulas, in which spinal cord oedema or serpentine flow voids on the dorsal surface of the spinal cord are seen (Jeng et al. 2015). Patients with redundant nerve roots on imaging have more severe clinical symptoms than patients without this imaging feature (Ono et al. 2007). After decompressive surgery, the outcome of this group of patients may also be worse in comparison with no redundant nerve roots (Min et al. 2008).

## 13 Epidural Lipomatosis

Epidural lipomatosis is characterized by excessive presence of fat in the spinal epidural space reducing the size of the thecal sac. The symptomatology depends on the spinal levels affected, with spinal cord, conus medullaris or radicular compression. Epidural lipomatosis may aggravate spinal canal narrowing in patients with degenerative spinal canal stenosis. It is most commonly found in patients on long-term steroid treatment but can be found in obese patients, patients with endocrinopathies and some idiopathic cases (Fogel et al. 2005). Thoracic epidural lipomatosis is slightly more common than lumbar involvement (Fessler et al. 1992; Stern et al. 1994). In patients with thoracic epidural lipomatosis, the posterior epidural fatty tissue impinges upon the thecal sac, with effacement of the peri medullary CSF and flattening of the spinal cord. At the lumbar spine, the excessive fat tissue causes geometric thecal sac deformation, with polygonal, stellate or 'Y' sign (Kuhn et al. 1994) on axial MR or CT images. The cause for this anatomical configuration can be explained due to mass effect of the hypertrophic epidural fat on the thecal sac and meningovertebral ligaments (Geers et al. 2003).

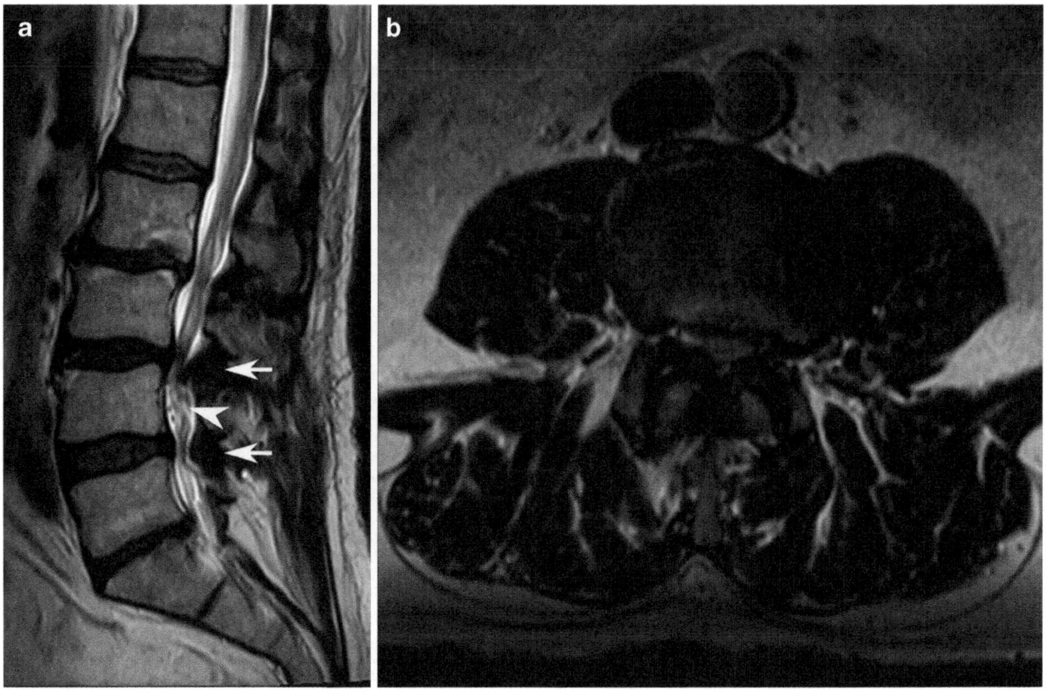


**Fig. 13** Sagittal T2 WI (**a**) shows age-related changes in the lumbar spine with multilevel stenosis of the central spinal canal, listhesis, hypertrophy of the ligamentum flavum (**a**, white arrows) and redundant nerve roots of the cauda equina (**a**, white arrowhead). Axial T2 WI (**b**) at L3–4 level shows severe stenosis of the central spinal canal and lateral recesses with facet joint osteoarthritis and hypertrophy of the ligamentum flavum

## 14 Conclusion

Spinal degeneration occurs naturally with age and is exacerbated in response to different aetiologies, mainly mechanical insults. They are routinely encountered in radiological examinations and are a common cause of pain and disability. Back pain is the second most common reason for a doctor's visit, second only to common cold. The degenerative process will be initiated in the discovertebral complex and will spread to the adjacent vertebral bone marrow, cervical uncovertebral and facet joints and spinal ligaments. Age-related changes and disc herniation may cause stenosis of the spinal canal and neural foramina with subsequent cord compression and myelopathy, cauda equina syndrome or radiculopathy. Other spinal conditions, some age-related such as facet joint syndrome, Baastrup's disease and others such as DISH and epidural lipomatosis have also been described. Imaging examinations are to be interpreted cautiously in relation with the clinical picture, as often there is poor correlation between symptoms and radiological findings. Plain films, CT and MR exams are routinely employed in the assessment of these patients while more specialised exams like myelogram or bone scans are used in selected patients. MRI is the preferred imaging technique due to its superior soft tissue resolution; it is particularly useful in confirming suspected disc herniations, nerve root entrapment, cord compression and spinal canal stenosis.

## References

Abbed KM, Coumans JV (2007) Cervical radiculopathy: pathophysiology, presentation, and clinical evaluation. Neurosurgery 60(1 Suppl 1):S28–S34

Adams MA, McNally DS, Dolan P (1996) 'Stress' distributions inside inter-vertebral discs. The effects of age and degeneration. J Bone Joint Surg Br 78:965–972

Ahn UM, Ahn NU, Buchowski JM et al (2000) Cauda equina syndrome secondary to lumbar disc herniation: a meta-analysis of surgical outcomes. Spine 25:1515–1522

Al-Mefty O, Harkey LH, Middleton TH et al (1988) Myelopathic cervical spondylotic lesions demonstrated by magnetic resonance imaging. J Neurosurg 68:217–222

Altinkaya N, Yildirim T, Demir S et al (2011) Factors associated with the thickness of the ligamentum flavum: is ligamentum flavum thickening due to hypertrophy or buckling? Spine (Phila Pa 1976) 36(16):E1093–E1097

Arce CA, Dohrmann GJ (1985) Herniated thoracic disks. Neurol Clin 3(2):383–392

Ashton IK, Roberts S, Jaffray DC et al (1994) Neuropeptides in the human intervertebral disc. J Orthop Res 12(2):186–192

Aufdermaur M, Fehr K, Lesker P et al (1980) Quantitative histochemical changes in intervertebral discs in diabetes. Exp Cell Biol 48:89–94

Banning CS, Thorell WE, Leibrock LG (2001) Patient outcome after resection of lumbar juxtafacet cysts. Spine 26(8):969–972

Baptiste DC, Fehlings MG (2006) Pathophysiology of cervical myelopathy. Spine J 6(6 Suppl):190S–197S

Bernick S, Caillet R (1982) Vertebral end-plate changes with aging of human vertebrae. Spine 7:97–102

Bland JH, Boushey DR (1990) Anatomy and physiology of the cervical spine. Semin Arthritis Rheum 20:1–20

Boden SD, Davis DO, Dina TS et al (1990a) Abnormal magnetic-resonance scans of the lumbar spine in asymptomatic subjects. A prospective investigation. J Bone Joint Surg Am 72(3):403–408

Boden SD, McCowin PR, Davis DO et al (1990b) Abnormal magnetic-resonance scans of the cervical spine in asymptomatic subjects. A prospective investigation. J Bone Joint Surg Am 72(8):1178–1184

Bogduk N (2012) Degenerative joint disease of the spine. Radiol Clin N Am 50(4):613–628

Bogduk N, Mercer SR (2000) Biomechanics of the cervical spine. I: Normal kinematics. Clin Biomech 15:633–648

Borota L, Jonasson P, Agolli A (2008) Spontaneous resorption of intradural lumbar disc fragments. Spine J 8(2):397–403

Bozzao A, Gallucci M, Masciocchi C et al (1992) Lumbar disk herniation: MR imaging assessment of natural history in patients treated without surgery. Radiology 185(1):135–141

Bush K, Cowan N, Katz DE et al (1992) The natural history of sciatica associated with disc pathology. A prospective study with clinical and independent radiologic follow-up. Spine 17(10):1205–1212

Caron T, Bransford R, Nguyen Q et al (2010) Spine fractures in patients with ankylosing spinal disorders. Spine 35:E458–E464

Carragee EJ, Paragioudakis SJ, Khurana S (2000) Lumbar high-intensity zone and discography in subject without low back problems. Spine 25:2987–2992

Cavanaugh JM, Ozaktay AC, Yamashita HT et al (1996) Lumbar facet pain: biomechanics, neuroanatomy and neurophysiology. J Biomech 29(9):1117–1129

Chaput C, Padon D, Rush J et al (2007) The significance of increased fluid signal on magnetic resonance imaging in lumbar facets in relationship to degenerative spondylolisthesis. Spine 32(17):1883–1887

Chen CK, Yeh L, Resnick D et al (2004) Intraspinal posterior epidural cysts associated with Baastrup's disease: report of 10 patients. AJR 182:191–194

Cheung KM, Karppinen J, Chan D et al (2009) Prevalence and pattern of lumbar magnetic resonance imaging changes in a population study of one thou-sand forty-three individuals. Spine (Phila Pa 1976) 34(9):934–940

Chimento GF, Ricciardi JE, Whitecloud TS 3rd (1995) Intraspinal extradural ganglion cyst. J Spinal Disord 8:82–85

Cicuendez M, Alen JF, Ramos A et al (2010) Spontaneous hemorrhage into a lumbar synovial cyst. Eur Spine J 19(Suppl 2):190–192

Cornips EM, Janssen ML, Beuls EA (2011) Thoracic disc herniation and acute myelopathy: clinical presentation, neuroimaging findings, surgical considerations, and outcome. J Neurosurg Spine 14(4):520–528

Czervionke L, Daniels D, Wehrli F et al (1988) Magnetic susceptibility artefacts in gradient-recalled echo MR imaging. AJNR Am J Neuroradiol 9:1149–1155

D'Aprile P, Tarantino A, Lorusso V et al (2006) Fat saturation technique and gadolinium in MRI of lumbar spinal degenerative disease. Neuroradiol J 19(5):654–671

Datta S, Lee M, Falco FJ et al (2009) Systematic assessment of diagnostic accuracy and therapeutic utility of lumbar facet joint interventions. Pain Physician 12(2):437–460

Dean CL, Gabriel JP, Cassinelli EH et al (2009) Degenerative spondylolisthesis of the cervical spine: analysis of 58 patients treated with anterior cervical de-compression and fusion. Spine J 9:439–446

Diehn FE (2012) Imaging of spinal infection. Radiol Clin N Am 50(4):777–798

Edwards WC, LaRocca H (1983) The developmental segmental sagittal diameter of the cervical spinal canal in patients with cervical spondylosis. Spine 8(1):20–27

Eross EJ, Dodick DW, Nelson KD et al (2002) Orthostatic headache syndrome with CSF leak secondary to bony pathology of the cervical spine. Cephalalgia 22:439–443

Eubanks JD, Lee MJ, Cassinelli E et al (2007) Prevalence of lumbar facet arthrosis and its relationship to age, sex, and race: an anatomic study of cadaveric specimens. Spine (Phila Pa 1976) 32(19):2058–2062

Even JL, Chen AF, Lee JY (2014) Imaging characteristics of "dynamic" versus "static" spondylolisthesis: analysis using magnetic resonance imaging and flex-ion/extension films. Spine J 14(9):1965–1969

Fardon DF, Williams AL, Dohring EJ et al (2014) Lumbar disc nomenclature: Version 2.0 Recommendations of the combined task forces of the North American Spine Society, the American Society of Spine Radiology and the American Society of Neuroradiology. Spine J 14(11):2525–2545

Fehlings MG, Tetreault LA, Wilson JR et al (2013) Cervical spondylotic myelopathy: current state of the

art and future directions. Spine (Phila Pa 1976) 38(22 suppl 1):S1–S8
Fessler RG, Johnson DL, Brown FD et al (1992) Epidural lipomatosis in steroid-treated patients. Spine 17:183–188
Flanagan EP, Krecke KN, Marsh RW et al (2014) Specific pattern of gadolinium enhancement in spondylotic myelopathy. Ann Neurol 76:54–65
Fogel GR, Cunningham PY 3rd, Esses SI (2005) Spinal epidural lipomatosis: case reports, literature review and meta-analysis. Spine J 5(2):202–211
Fukuyama S, Nakamura T, Ikeda T et al (1995) The effect of mechanical stress on hypertrophy of the lumbar ligamentum flavum. J Spinal Disord 8(2):126–130
Gallucci M, Puglielli E, Splendiani A et al (2005) Degenerative disorders of the spine. Eur Radiol 15:591–598
Gallucci M, Limbucci N, Paonessa A et al (2007) Degenerative disease of the spine. Neuroimaging Clin N Am Feb 17(1):87–103
Geers C, Lecouvet FE, Begets C et al (2003) Polygonal deformation of the dural sac in lumbar epidural lipomatosis: anatomic explanation by the presence of meningovertebral ligaments. AJNR Am J Neuroradiol 24(7):1276–1282
Gille O, Soderlund C, Razafimahandri HJC et al (2006) Analysis of hard thoracic herniated discs: review of 18 cases operated by thoracoscopy. Eur Spine J 15(5):537–542
Girard CJ, Schweitzer ME, Morrison WB et al (2004) Thoracic spine disc-related abnormalities: longitudinal MR imaging assessment. Skeletal Radiol 33(4):216–222
Gower WE, Pedrini V (1969) Age-related variations in protein polysaccharides from human nucleus pulposus, annulus fibrosus, and costal cartilage. J Bone Joint Surg Am 51(6):1154–1162
Grenier N, Kressel HY, Schiebler ML et al (1987) Normal and degenerative posterior spinal structures: MR imaging. Radiology 165(2):517–525
Griffith JF, Wang YX, Antonio GE et al (2007) Modified Pfirrmann grading system for lumbar intervertebral disc degeneration. Spine 32(24):E708–E712
Guo JJ, Yang HL, Cheung KM et al (2009) Classification and management of the tandem ossification of the posterior longitudinal ligament and flaval ligament. Chin Med J (Engl) 122(2):219–224
Hazlett J (1964) Kissing spines. J Bone Joint Surg Br 46:1368–1369
Hemminghytt S, Daniels DL, Williams AL et al (1982) Intraspinal synovial cysts: natural history and diagnosis by CT. Radiology 145:375–376
Holm S, Maroudas A, Urban JPG et al (1981) Nutrition of the intervertebral disc. Solute transport and metabolism. Connect Tissue Res 8:101–119
Howington JU, Connolly ES, Voorhies RM (1999) Intraspinal synovial cysts: 10-year experience at the Ochsner Clinic. J Neurosurg 91.2(Suppl):193–199
Hoxworth JM, Trentman TL, Kotsenas AL et al (2012) The role of digital subtraction myelography in the diagnosis and localization of spontaneous spinal CSF leaks. AJR 99:649–653
Hsu KY, Zucherman JF, Shea WJ et al (1995) Lumbar intraspinal synovial and ganglion cysts (facet cysts). Ten-year experience in evaluation and treatment. Spine (Phila Pa 1976) 20(1):80–89
Hukins DWL (1988) Disc structure and function. In: Ghosh P (ed) The biology of the intervertebral disc, vol 1. CRC Press Inc, Boca Raton, FL, pp l–37
Hunter CJ, Matyas JR, Duncan NA (2003) The notochordal cell in the nucleus pulposus: a review in the context of tissue engineering. Tissue Eng 9:667–677
Ikeda T, Nakamura T, Kikuchi TJ et al (1996) Pathomechanism of spontaneous regression of the herniated lumbar disc: histologic and immunohistochemical study. Spinal Disord 9(2):136–140
Izzo R, Popolizio T, D'Aprile P et al (2015) Spinal pain. Eur J Radiol 84(5):746–756
Jackson RP (1992) The facet syndrome. Myth or reality? Clin Orthop Relat Res 279:110–121
James SL, Davies AM (2006) Imaging of infectious spinal disorders in children and adults. Eur J Radiol 58:27–40
Jeng Y, Chen DY, Hsu HL et al (2015) Spinal dural arteriovenous fistula: imaging features and its mimics. Korean J Radiol 16(5):1119–1131
Jensen MC, Brant-Zawadski MN, Obuchowski N et al (1994) Magnetic resonance imaging of the lumbar spine in people without back pain. N Engl J Med 331:69–73
Jiang SD, Jiang LS, Dai LY (2011) Degenerative cervical spondylolisthesis: a systematic review. Int Orthop 35(6):869–875
Kalichman L, Li L, Kim DH et al (2008) Facet joint osteoarthritis and low back pain in the community-based population. Spine (Phila Pa 1976) 33(23):2560–2565
Kalsi-Ryan S, Karadimas SK, Fehlings MG (2013) Cervical spondylotic myelopathy: the clinical phenomenon and the current pathobiology of an increasingly prevalent and devastating disorder. Neuroscientist 19:409–421
Kang Y, Lee JW, Koh YH et al (2011) New MRI grading system for the cervical canal stenosis. Am J Roentgenol 197(1):W134–W140
Kauppila LI, Eustace S, Kiel D et al (1998) Degenerative displacement of lumbar vertebrae: a 25-year follow up study in Framingham. Spine 23:1868–1873
Kawasaki M, Tani T, Ushida T et al (2007) Anterolisthesis and retrolisthesis of the cervical spine in cervical spondylotic myelopathy in the elderly. J Orthop Sci 12:207–213
Khan AM, Girardi F (2006) Spinal lumbar synovial cysts. Diagnosis and management challenge. Eur Spine J 15(8):1176–1182
Kim S, Lee JW, Chai JW et al (2015) A new MRI grading system for cervical foraminal stenosis based on axial T2-weighted images. Korean J Radiol 16(6):1294–1302
Kirkaldy-Willis WH, Farfan HF (1982) Instability of the lumbar spine. Clin Orthop Relat Res 165:110–123

Klaassen Z, Tubbs RS, Apaydin N et al (2011) Vertebral spinal osteophytes. Anat Sci Int 86(1):1–9

Kuhn MJ, Youssef HT, Swan TL et al (1994) Lumbar epidural lipomatosis: the "Y" sign of thecal sac compression. Comput Med Imaging Graph 18(5):367–372

Kushchayev SV, Glushko T, Jarraya M et al (2018) ABCs of the degenerative spine. Insights Imaging 9(2):253–274

Lateef H, Patel D (2009) What is the role of imaging in acute low back pain? Curr Rev Musculoskelet Med 2(2):69–73jeng

Luetkehans TJ, Coughlin BF, Weinstein MA (1987) Ossification of the posterior longitudinal ligament diagnosed by MR. AJNR Am J Neuroradiol 8:924–925

Mader R (2002) Clinical manifestations of diffuse idiopathic skeletal hyperostosis of the cervical spine. Semin Arthritis Rheum 32:130–135

Malham GM, Parker RM, Ballock ZE et al (2015) Bone scans are reliable for the identification of lumbar disk and facet pathology. Global Spine J 5(1):23–30

Mamisch N, Brumann M, Hodler J et al (2012) Radiologic criteria for the diagnosis of spinal stenosis: results of a Delphi survey. Radiology 264(1):174–179

Manchikanti L, Singh V, Pampati V et al (2001) Evaluation of the relative contributions of various structures in chronic low back pain. Pain Physician 4(4):308–316

Martin AR, Aleksanderek I, Cohen-Adad J et al (2015) Translating state-of-the-art spinal cord MRI techniques to clinical use: a systematic review of clinical studies utilizing DTI, MT, MWF, MRS, and fMRI. Neuroimage Clin 10:192–238

Matsumoto M, Fujimura Y, Suzuki N et al (1998) MRI of cervical intervertebral discs in asymptomatic subjects. J Bone Joint Surg Br 80:19–24

Mercer S, Bogduk N (1994) The ligaments and anulus fibrosus of human adult cervical intervertebral discs. Spine 24:619–626

Meyerding HW (1932) Spondylolisthesis. Surg Gynecol Obstet 54:371–377

Millucci L, Bernardini G, Spreafico A et al (2017) Histological and ultra-structural characterization of alkaptonuric tissues. Calcif Tissue Int 101:50–64

Min JH, Jang JS, Lee SH (2008) Clinical significance of redundant nerve roots of the cauda equina in lumbar spinal stenosis. Clin Neurol Neurosurg 110:14–18

Miyasaka K, Kaneda K, Sato S et al (1983) Myelopathy due to ossification or calcification of the ligamentum flavum: radiologic and histologic evaluations. Am J Neuroradiol 4:629–632

Miyazaki M, Hong SW, Yoon SH et al (2008) Reliability of a magnetic resonance imaging-based grading system for cervical intervertebral disc degeneration. J Spinal Disord Tech 21:288–292

Mizuno J, Nakagawa H, Inoue T et al (2003) Clinicopathological study of "snake-eye appearance" in compressive myelopathy of the cervical spinal cord. J Neurosurg Spine 99(2):162–168

Modic MT, Ross JS (2007) Lumbar degenerative disc disease. Radiology 245(1):43–61

Modic MT, Masaryk TJ, Ross JS et al (1988a) Imaging of degenerative disc disease. Radiology 168:177–186

Modic MT, Steinberg PM, Ross JS et al (1988b) Degenerative disk disease: assessment of changes in vertebral body marrow with MR imaging. Radiology 166:193–199

Morishita Y, Naito M, Hymanson H et al (2009) The relationship between the cervical spinal canal diameter and the pathological changes in the cervical spine. Eur Spine J 18(6):877–883

Munter FM, Wasserman BA, Wu HM et al (2002) Serial MR imaging of annular tears in lumbar intervertebral disks. AJNR Am J Neuroradiol 23(7):1105–1109

Nakashima H, Yukawa Y, Suda K et al (2015) Cervical disc protrusion correlates with the severity of cervical disc degeneration: a cross-sectional study of 1,211 relatively healthy volunteers. Spine (Phila Pa 1976) 40:E774–E779

Ohshio I, Hatayama A, Kaneda K et al (1993) Correlation between histopathologic features and magnetic resonance images of spinal cord lesions. Spine (Phila Pa 1976) 18(9):1140–1149

Okuda T, Baba I, Fujimoto Y et al (2004) The pathology of ligamentum flavum in degenerative lumbar disease. Spine 29(15):1689–1697

Olczyk K (1992) Age related changes in collagen of human intervertebral discs. Gerontology 38:196–204

Ono A, Suetsuna F, Irie T et al (2007) Clinical significance of the redundant nerve roots of the cauda equina documented on magnetic resonance imaging. J Neurosurg Spine 7(1):27–32

Oppenheim JS, Rothman AS, Sachdev VP (1993) Thoracic herniated discs: review of the literature and 12 cases. Mt Sinai J Med 60(4):321–326

Oxland TR (2016) Fundamental biomechanics of the spine – what we have learned in the past 25 years and future directions. J Biomech 49(6):817–832

Ozawa H, Sato T, Hyodo H et al (2010) Clinical significance of intramedullary Gd-DTPA enhancement in cervical myelopathy. Spinal Cord 48(5):415–422

Palumbo MA, Hilibrand AS, Hart RA et al (2001) Surgical treatment of thoracic spinal stenosis: a 2- to 9-year follow-up. Spine 26(5):558–566

Park H-J, Kim SS, Lee S-Y et al (2013) A practical MRI grading system for cervical foraminal stenosis based on oblique sagittal images. Br J Radiol 86(1025):20120515

Parlier-Cuau C, Wybier M, Nizard R et al (1999) Symptomatic lumbar facet joint synovial cysts: clinical assessment of facet joint steroid injection after 1 and 6 months and long-term follow-up in 30 patients. Radiology 210(2):509–513

Pate D, Goobar J, Resnick D et al (1988) Traction osteophytes of the lumbar spine: Radiographic-pathologic correlation. Radiology 166(3):843–846

Patel KB, Poplawski MM, Pawha PS et al (2014) Diffusion-weighted MRI "claw sign" improves differentiation of infectious from degenerative Modic type 1 signal changes of the spine. AJNR Am J Neuroradiol 35(8):1647–1652

Pavlov H, Torg JS, Robie B et al (1987) Cervical spinal stenosis: determination with vertebral body ratio method. Radiology 164(3):771–775

Perolat R, Kastler A, Nicot B et al (2018) Facet joint syndrome: from diagnosis to interventional management. Insights Imaging 9(5):773–789

Pfirrmann CW, Metzdorf A, Zanetti M et al (2001) Magnetic resonance classification of lumbar intervertebral disc degeneration. Spine (Phila Pa 1976) 26:1873–1878

Pfirrmann C, Dora C, Schmid M et al (2004) MR image based grading of lumbar nerve root compromise due to disk herniation: reliability study with surgical correlation. Radiology 230(2):583–588

Pirotte B, Gabrovsky N, Massager N et al (2003) Synovial cysts of the lumbar spine: surgery-related results and outcome. J Neurosurg 99(1 Suppl):14–19

Rajasekaran S, Venkatadass K, Naresh Babu J et al (2008) Pharmacological enhancement of disc diffusion and differentiating of healthy, ageing and degenerated discs: results from in-vivo serial post-contrast MRI studies in 365 human lumbar discs. Eur Spine J 17(5):626–643

Resnick D, Niwayama G (1976) Radiographic and pathologic features of spinal involvement in diffuse idiopathic skeletal hyperostosis (DISH). Radiology 119:559–568

Reust P, Wendling D, Lagier R, Pageaut G et al (1988) Degenerative spondylolisthesis, synovial cyst of the zygapophyseal joints, and sciatic syndrome: re-port of two cases and review of the literature. Arthritis Rheum 31(2):288–294

Roberts S, McCall IW, Menage J et al (1997) Does the thickness of the vertebral subchondral bone reflect the composition of the intervertebral disc? Eur Spine J 6:385–389

Robinson D, Mirovsky Y, Halperin N et al (1998) Changes in proteoglycans of intervertebral disc in diabetic patients: a possible cause of increased back pain. Spine 23:849–856

Schellhas KP, Pollei SR, Gundry CR et al (1996) Lumbar disc high intensity zone. Correlation of magnetic resonance imaging and discography. Spine 21:79–86

Stern JD, Quint DJ, Sweasey TA et al (1994) Spinal epidural lipomatosis: two new idiopathic cases and a review of the literature. J Spinal Disord 7:343–349

Stillerman CB, Chen TC, Couldwell WT et al (1998) Experience in the surgical management of 82 symptomatic herniated thoracic discs and review of the literature. J Neurosurg 88(4):623–633

Takahashi K, Miyazaki T, Ohnari H et al (1995) Schmorl's nodes and low-back pain. Analysis of magnetic resonance imaging findings in symptomatic and asymptomatic individuals. Eur Spine J 4:56–59

Tetreault L, Goldstein CL, Arnold P et al (2015) Degenerative cervical myelopathy: a spectrum of related disorders affecting the aging spine. Neurosurgery 77(suppl 4):S51–S67

Thielen KR, Sillery JC, Morris JM et al (2015) Ultrafast dynamic computed tomography myelography for the precise identification of high-flow cerebrospinal fluid leaks caused by spiculated spinal osteophytes. J Neurosurg Spine 22:324–331

Trout JJ, Buckwalter JA, Moore KC et al (1982) Ultrastructure of the human intervertebral disc. I. Changes in notochordal cells with age. Tissue Cell 14:359–369

Twomey L, Taylor J (1988) Age changes in the lumbar spinal and intervertebral canals. Paraplegia 26(4):238–249

Ullman N, Gregg L, Becker D et al (2016) Anterior disco-osteo-arterial conflict as a cause of intersegmental arterial flow impairment and spinal cord ischemia. Neuroradiology 58:1109–1115

van Rijn JC, Klemetso N, Reitsma JB et al (2005) Observer variation in MRI evaluation of patients suspected of lumbar disk herniation. AJR Am J Roentgenol 184:299–303

Varlotta GP, Lefkowitz TR, Schweitzer M et al (2011) The lumbar facet joint: a review of current knowledge: part 1: anatomy, biomechanics and grading. Skelet Radiol 40(1):13–23

Wainner RS, Gill H (2000) Diagnosis and nonoperative management of cervical radiculopathy. J Orthop Sports Phys Ther 30:728–744

Wang AM, Haykal HA et al (1987) Synovial cysts of the lumbar spine: CT evaluation. Comput Radiol 11(5–6):253–257

Weishaupt D, Zanetti M, Boos N et al (1999) MR imaging and CT in osteoarthritis of the lumbar facet joints. Skelet Radiol 28(4):215–219

Westerveld LA, Verlaan JJ, Oner FC (2009) Spinal fractures in patients with ankylosing spinal disorders: a systematic review of the literature on treatment, neurological status and complications. Eur Spine J 18:145–156

Wiltse LL, Berger PE, McCulloch JA (1997) A system for reporting the size and location of lesions in the spine. Spine 22:1534–1537

Wong JJ, Leung OC, Yuen MK (2011) Questionable adequacy of magnetic resonance for the detection of ossification of the posterior longitudinal ligament of the cervical spine. Hong Kong J Radiol 14:78–83

Yamashita Y, Takahashi M, Matsuno Y et al (1990) Spinal cord compression due to ossification of ligaments: MR imaging. Radiology 175(3):843–848

Yoshida H, Takai K, Taniguchi M (2014) Leakage detection on CT myelography for targeted epidural blood patch in spontaneous cerebrospinal fluid leaks: calcified or ossified spinal lesions ventral to the thecal sac. J Neurosurg Spine 21(3):432–441

Yousem DM, Atlas SW, Goldberg HI et al (1991) Degenerative narrowing of the cervical spine neural foramina: evaluation with high-resolution 3DFT gradient-echo MR imaging. AJNR Am J Neuroradiol 12:229–236

Yu S, Haughton VM, Sether LA et al (1988) Anulus fibrosus in bulging inter-vertebral disks. Radiology 169:761–763

# Vascular Injury of the Spinal Cord

Jasmina Boban and Majda M. Thurnher

## Contents



J. Boban (✉)
Department of Radiology, Faculty of Medicine Novi Sad, University of Novi Sad, Novi Sad, Serbia

M. M. Thurnher
Department for Biomedical Imaging and Image-guided Therapy, Medical University of Vienna, Vienna, Austria

**Abstract**

Vascular disorders of the spinal cord are rare entities that are often underdiagnosed. It is important for a radiologist in emergency set-



M. Scaglione et al. (eds.), *Emergency Radiology of the Head and Spine*,
Medical Radiology Diagnostic Imaging, https://doi.org/10.1007/978-3-030-91047-1_17

ting to be familiar with complex vascular supply of the spinal cord. In this chapter, clinical and radiological findings of spinal cord infarction and ischemia, spinal arteriovenous shunts, spinal hemorrhage, and fibrocartilaginous embolism will be discussed in detail. Clinical presentation, as well as prognosis of these entities, is variable, dependent on the affected vessel(s) and the extent of the disorder in the spinal cord. It varies from acute pain and neurological deficit (both motor and sensory disorders) to progressive myelopathy. Since successful treatment is highly influenced by timely and correct diagnosis, based both on clinical and imaging findings, it is essential to recognize these entities in an emergency setting.

# 1 Spinal Cord Infarction/Spinal Cord Ischemia

## 1.1 Definition of Entity and Clinical Highlights

Spinal cord infarction (SCI) respresents a relatively uncommon condition, often clinically and radiologically challeging. This condition is related to a high morbidity due to acute myelopathy. Patients present with severe neurological deficits, but often show satisfactory functional improvement. However, up to 20% of patients present with biphasic strokes, presenting with acute or transitory sensory deficits preceded by radiant pain in the region between the shoulders (Vuong et al. 2016).

Clinical presentation is highly dependent on the affected vessel and the extent of infarction. It usually presents with acute pain, weakness, and sensation loss. The development of symptoms is quick, accounting for a few minutes up to 12 h. In 59% of patients, acute radicular pain along the distribution of radiculomedullary artery occurs (Romi and Naess 2016). Clinical syndromes as commonly observed are the following:

1. Anterior spinal artery syndrome, consisting of flaccid tetra/paraplegia with a loss of pain and temperature (bilaterally), and preserved proprioception and vibration sensations.
2. Incomplete syndrome, the spinal artery syndrome (involving only anterior horns), presenting with acute paraplegia (pseudopoliomyelitic form), painful brachial diplegia ("man-in-the-barrel" syndrome), and progressive distal amyotrophy (chronic phase).
3. Posterior spinal artery syndrome presents with a loss of proprioception and vibration sensations below the level of injury, more commonly unilateral.
4. Brown-Sequard syndrome (central artery syndrome) is ipsilateral spastic paraparesis with loss of pain and temperature sensation on the contralateral side.
5. Transverse infarct presents with bilateral motor deficits and complete sensory loss.

A separate entity is spinal transient ischemic attack lasting for several minutes to a few hours, described in a variety of clinical settings, extremely unusual.

Zalewski and his group recently proposed diagnostic criteria for spinal cord infarctions and divided them into five groups: definite spontaneous, probable spontaneous, and possible spontaneous, as well as definite periprocedural and probable periprocedural (Zalewski et al. 2019). Spontaneous SCI encompasses those not directly associated to trauma or certain procedure; they are considered rare, although often underdiagnosed (recent studies reported that 14–16% of reported transverse myelitis were ultimately diagnosed as SCI) (Barreras et al. 2018; Zalewski et al. 2018). Recently proposed diagnostic criteria include three major components as follows:

1. clinical features,
2. MRI of the spinal cord.
3. cerebrospinal fluid analysis.

Typical clinical features include rapid development of severe neurological deficit (within

12 h). More prolonged onset of neurological deficit associated with spinal cord favors alternative diagnoses. However, the evolution of deficit is commonly slower than that in cerebral infarction due to more powerful arterial collateralization. Nevertheless, small cross-sectional area of the spinal cord makes the surrounding tissue more susceptible to edema and compression that contributes to clinical worsening.

## 1.2 Epidemiology/Demographics

Spinal cord infarction occurs rarely in comparison with cerebral strokes, accounting for 0.3–1% of all insults, 1–2% of all vascular neurologic pathologies, and for approximately 6% of all acute myelopathies (Vargas et al. 2015). Spontaneous ischemic strokes are the most common variant of spinal cord ischemia, presenting in around 86%, while hemorrhagic strokes account for around 9% of cases (Romi and Naess 2011). Patients with spinal cord stroke are younger and more commonly females, compared to cerebral strokes. Mean age at presentation is 56 years (Sullivan and Sundt 2006). Interestingly, less commonly, these strokes are associated with hypertension and concurrent cardiac disease (Jorgensen et al. 1994). However, risk factors associated with accelerated atherosclerosis (diabetes mellitus, smoking, peripheral artery disease, and elevated cholesterol levels) are commonly observed as risk factors (Ghandehari et al. 2010; Naess and Romi 2011). Younger and male patients usually present with more severe clinical findings in the initial phase. However, these patients show much better long-term functional recovery compared to females and older patients, in whom complications during hospital stay (pneumonia, thromboemolic events) are more often encountered (Naess and Romi 2011). There are not many studies on long-term mortality among these patients. Those available report incidence of about 23% in 7 years follow-up period and 9% in 4.5 years follow-up, which is lower than in cerebral stroke patients (Nedeltchev et al. 2004; Hanson et al. 2015). High long-term mortality is associated with higher age at presentation, severity of acute neurological deficits, and the extent of peripheral artery disease (Robertson et al. 2012; Hanson et al. 2015). Up to 80% of patients with spinal cord infarction report chronic pain on long-term follow-up, while symptoms commonly reported in cerebral stroke patients, such as fatigue, depression, and cognitive deficits, occur more seldom (comparable with incidence in healthy individuals) (Naess et al. 2005).

## 1.3 Pathophysiology

Spinal cord infarct is caused by acute restriction of spinal cord arterial blood supply (due to embolus or plaque), leading to depletion in oxygen and glucose delivery to grey and/or white matter, which results in ischemia and infarction. This further causes acute spinal cord-related neurological deficits that are almost always clearly associated with the vascular territory of the affected artery. Perfusion restriction can occur as a result of either global flow insufficiency or occlusion of selective radiculomedullary artery. Venous origin of the infarct is present in the cases of arteriovenous fistula, leading to increased venous pressure and vasogenic edema. If prolonged, it leads to the deprivation of arterial perfusion and cytotoxic edema. Additionally, it can be found in coagulopathies, epidural infections (epidural venous thrombosis), and myelopathy caused by cervical spinal stenosis ("snake-eye" sign).

The mechanism and exact pathogenesis of this disorder remain undetermined due to lack of large populational studies that would include associated vascular diseases and comorbidities that involve vertebral bodies (Kumral et al.). Etiological factors are various and several risk factors have been identified over time: hypertension, smoking, hyperlipidemia, diabetes mellitus, as well as coronary artery disease, peripheral vascular disease, and atrial fibrillation. Mechanisms of infarction reported in the literature also vary, with majority of patients presenting with idiopathic SCI due to atherosclerotic risk factors, followed by fibrocartilaganeous embolism, aortic dissection, hypercoaguability, vertebral artery dissection, systemic hypotension (in shock), cardioembolism, and vasculitis. Iatrogenic factors have to be taken into account, including vascular surgery (aortic cross-clamping, aortic stent-grafting, lumbar sympathectomy, splenectomy, nephrectomy, and others) and anesthetic procedures (epidural anesthesia, intercostal, and coeliac plexus block).

For the interpretation of spinal cord infarctions, it is necessary to be aware of complex vascular supply of the spinal cord. The first region of the spinal cord vascularization is located between craniocervical junction and T3 level. Cervical part of the spinal cord is supplied from one or two segmental radiculomedullary arteries, typically at the level of C3, and accessory artery at C6 and/or C8. These arteries most commonly branch off vertebral arteries, but there are some alternative pathways (the occipital artery, the ascending pharyngeal artery, the deep cervical artery, or the ascending cervical artery). The second region of vascularization extends from T3 to T7 and is supplied from the intercostal arteries. In about 70% of patients, in the upper thoracic region, an additional dominant radiculomedullary artery, called artery of von Haller, can be present. The third region extends from T8 up to the conus medullaris and is supplied by the Adamkiewicz artery (branch of intercostal artery, at the level between T9–12).

Intrinsic arterial circulation of the spinal cord is divided into the central and peripheral system. The central system supplies the gray matter and central parts of the spinal cord and is provided by the penetrating branches of central arteries (branches of the anterior spinal artery). The peripheral system vascularizes primarily white matter via radicular arteries (that are up to 5 times smaller in diameter compared to the central arteries), branches of the posterior spinal arteries. The contribution of anterior spinal arteries is much larger, and comprises about two thirds to four fifths of the transverse cross-sectional area of the spinal cord. What is also interesting is that neither transverse nor rostrocaudal anastomoses between central and peripheral systems are hemodynamically significant, except in the superficial part of conus medullaris (cruciate anastomosis or conus arcade).

Venous system of the spinal cord drains the instrinsic parts in a symmetrical centrifugal manner. Deep central regions are drained symmetrically through anterior median spinal vein and the posterior median spinal vein, while superficial regions (white matter mostly) are drained by radial veins into coronal venous plexus on the pial surface. There are rich anastomoses between these two systems. Deep veins (the anterior and posterior median spinal veins) drain through ventral and dorsal radiculomedullary veins into segmental spinal veins. Radiculomedullary veins are present on several segments only (5–10 both dorsally and ventrally). The extradural intervertebral veins communicate directly with the spinal epidural venous plexus, Batson's plexus. The intervertebral veins drain into the ascending lumbar or azygos venous systems.

At each level of the spinal cord, there is one anterior and two posterior spinal arteries. Additionally, at many levels, there are radicular arteries that run along nerve roots and supply anterior spinal arteries. The anterior spinal artery gives rise to the central arteries that supply the anterior horns and anterior parts of lateral columns of both sides. The pial plexus surrounds the spinal cord.

## 1.4 Imaging Technique and Recommended Protocol

The radiologist plays an important part of diagnostic cascade in these conditions, which can mimic non-vascular pathology both clinically and radiologically. Non-contrast computed tomography (CT) and spinal CT angiography (CTA) are generally not very helpful in the imaging of spinal cord infarction. However, in older patients, detection of atherosclerosis or vascular lesions after surgery can indirectly aid to the diagnosis.

MRI is the imaging modality of choice for the diagnosis of the spinal cord ischemia and differential diagnoses, revealing acute lesions in up to

70% of patients with suspected diagnosis (Harringan and Deveikis 2013). The proposed protocol should include the following:

1. T1-weighted sagittal spin-echo.
2. T2-weighted sagittal spin-echo,
3. short-tau inversion recovery (STIR) sagittal,
4. T2-weighted gradient-echo axial sequences.

Diffusion-weighted imaging (DWI) is not routinely performed in majority of the centers, but aids to the diagnosis. DWI can be acquired in sagittal or axial plane. Sagittal plane has the advantage of a larger coverage in shorter time, while axial acquisition allows visualization of restricted diffusion on both sides of the spinal cord and is useful in differentiation of this entity from similar conditions.

Contrast study aids to the diagnosis since enhancement is usually absent in the acute stage. T1-weighted postcontrast study contributes to the differential diagnosis in indefinite cases. Additional diagnostic studies might include magnetic resonance angiography, CTA, and digital subtraction angiography (especially in cases of suspected thrombus in the abdominal aorta, or Adamkiewicz artery).

MRI findings that are required for diagnosis of SCI are as follows:

1. no findings of spinal cord compression,
2. specific finding of DWI restriction, associated vertebral body infarction, or arterial occlusion/dissection adjacent to the lesion,
3. supportive: intramedullary T2-hyperintense lesions (Zalewski et al. 2019).

It is important to support the diagnosis with analysis of cerebrospinal fluid, primarily in order to exclude inflammatory etiology (cell count, IgG index, oligoclonal bands).

## 1.5 MRI Findings

Findings on MRI can be normal in up to one fourth of patients. Usually, the most informative findings are identified on T2W sequence, with hyperintensity in the central cord more than in the peripheral, and usually in longer than one vertebral section. A common finding is associated T2W/STIR hyperintensity in the vertebral bodies (medullary bone) due to vertebral body infarct (Fig. 1). There are six different spinal stroke syndromes identified on MR imaging.

The anterior spinal artery infarction represents the most common SCI syndrome and is limited to the anterior horns and the surrounding white matter (classic "owl's eyes" or "snake eyes" sign, Fig. 2). The anterior unilateral infarct unilateraly affects anterior horn. Posterior spinal artery infarct is limited to the posterior columns, but may extend to the posterior parts of lateral columns. Posterior unilateral infarct is restricted to one posterior horn and sometimes extends into the posterior part of ipsilateral lateral column/posterolateral region. Central infarct is located around the anterior sulcus, in the shape of crescent. Transverse infarct involves anterior and posterior columns and extends to both anteo- and posterolateral regions.

Diffusion restriction is present, following the similar pattern as in the cerebral stroke. Restriction is demonstrated approximately hours after the onset of symptoms, with pseudo-normalization after approximately 1 week (Peckham and Hutchins 2019). Typical contrast enhancement in SCI is linear craniocaudal strip of enhancement, reflecting the predominant ischemic area, usually in the grey matter and confirmed to a specific arterial territory. During the subacute phase, the patchy contrast enhancement is observed, usually after 5 days and lasting for approximately 3 weeks. In general, contrast enhancement is suggestive of alternative diagnoses, at first transverse myelitis. However, in up to one half of periprocedural SCIs and in around 40% of spontaneous SCIs contrast enhancement is observed.

If the SCI is not confirmed after initial imaging and the clinical suspicion remains the same, a follow-up imaging is recommended (days later).

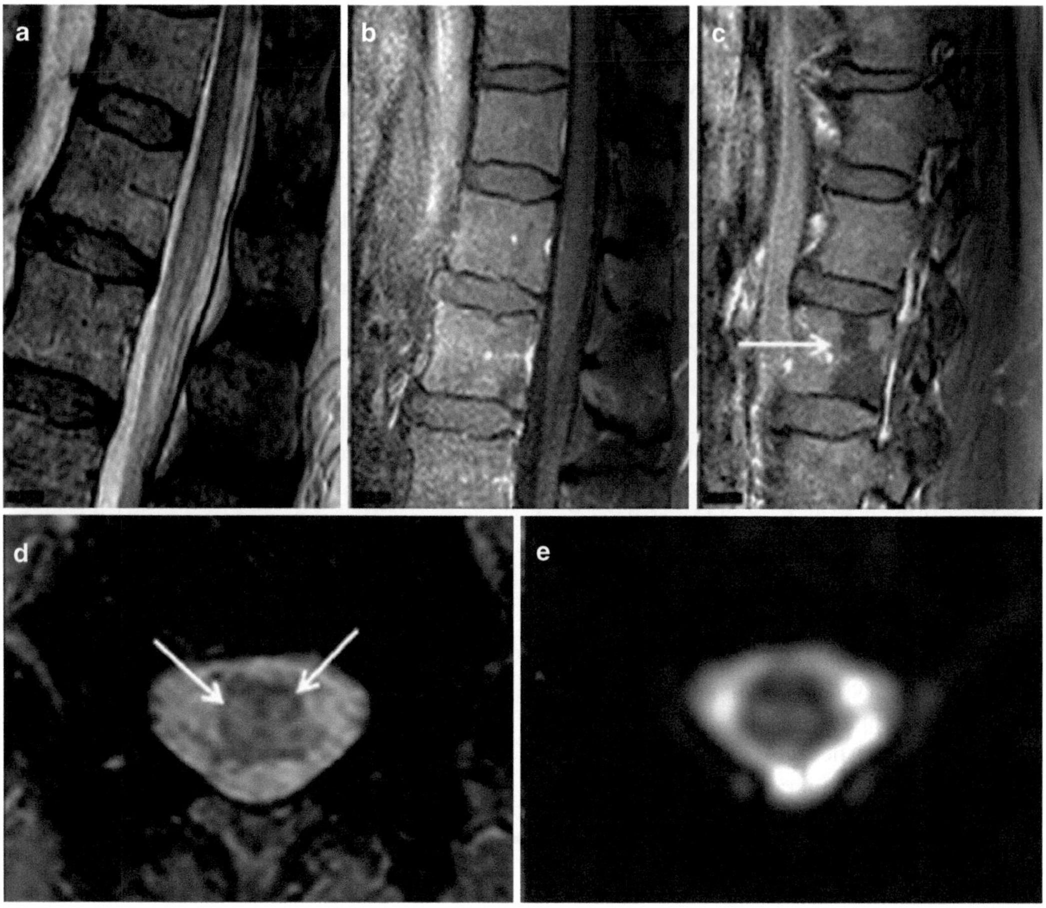


**Fig. 1** Conus medullaris infarction followed by infarction of the vertebral body. Conus medullaris is enlarged and swollen (**a** – T2W sagittal image), with no contrast enhancement (**b** – T1W FS postcontrast image). Clearly defined geographic area of the lack of contrast enhancement is observed in the posterior part of L1 vertebral body (**c** T1W FS sagittal image), corresponding with vertebral body infarction. On cross-sectional area of the spinal cord, "owl-s eyes" sign is evident on T2W axial image (**d**), followed by diffusion restriction (**e**), reflecting anterior spinal artery infarction

## 1.6 Differential Diagnosis and Pitfalls

The differential diagnosis of the spinal cord infarction is actually wide, given this is a rather rare entity. The main differentials include multiple sclerosis (MS), neoplastic lesions, idiopathic transverse myelitis, and venous congestive myelopathy.

Multiple sclerosis lesions are usually located in the peripheral white matter and comprise not more than three segments in craniocaudal direction and not more than a half of cross-sectional area. Additionally, they are commonly associated with brain lesions and have a different and relatively distinct clinical presentation.

Spinal cord neoplastic lesions present with characteristic expansion of the cord associated with nodular or diffuse enhancement after contrast. Also, cystic degeneration is common. Clinical onset is slow.

Idiopathic transverse myelitis can have similar clinical presentation, but not as acute (SCI occurs in several minutes!). The lesion is long (usually over three segments) and occupies more than two thirds of cross-sectional area.

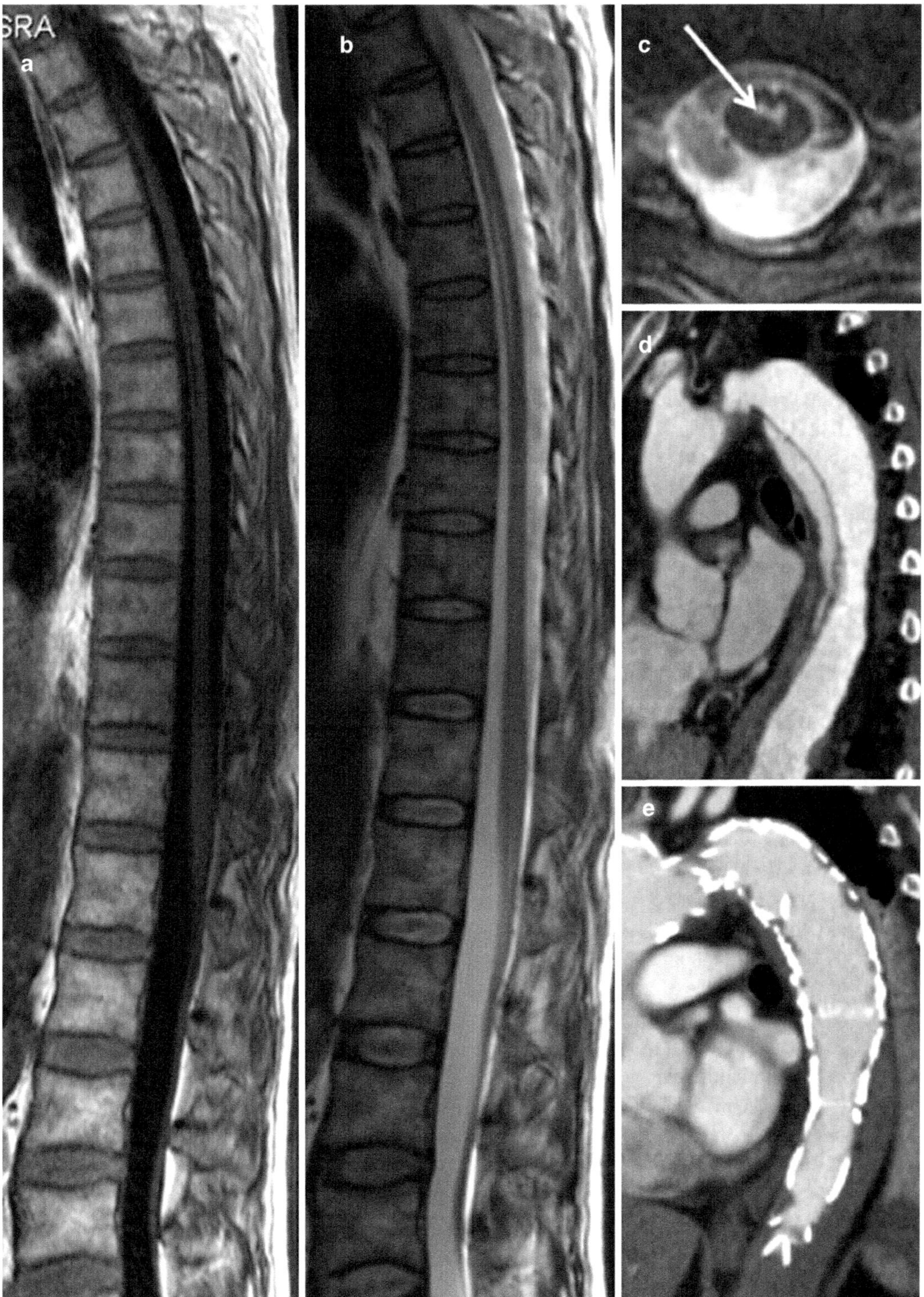


**Fig. 2** Anterior spinal artery infarction. A "pencil-like" T1 hypointense (**a**), T2-hyperintense (**b**) lesion is observed in the anterior aspect of the spinal cord on T4–7 level, with corresponding "owl's eyes" sign on the axial image (**c**), reflecting typical artery of Adamkiewitz infarction, after stent graft repair of thoracic aorta (**e**) due to dissection (**d**)

Venous congestive myelopathy is characterized by the presence of engorged pial veins associated with T2W/STIR-hyperintense signal in the central and peripheral white matter.

## 2 Spinal Arteriovenous Shunts

### 2.1 Definition of Entity and Clinical Highlights

Spinal arteriovenous (AV) shunts are rare lesions.

Numerous classification systems exist for these lesions, based on different features of the lesions (Da Costa et al. 2009). The Anson-Spetzler classificiation is based on the flow pattern and angio-architecture and therefore compatible with the imaging patterns.

1. Type I: dural AV fistula (dAVF) represents the most common type of shunt lesion, accounting for 60–80% of these lesions. This is a low flow lesion found typically in lower thoracic or lumbar spine, with a rather small probability to produce hemorrhage or to generate aneurysmatic dilatation of the vessel wall (Rodesch et al. 2004).
2. Type II: intramedullary glomus AV malformations (glomus type), representing an intradural spinal AV shunt lesion, accounting for 10–15% of the lesions. Sometimes they are referred to as pial AVMs. These high flow lesions occur throughout spinal cord and are characterized with plexiform nidus of multiple AV shunts, with feeding arteries often raising from the anterior or posterior spinal arteries and draining veins going to perimedullary veins. The incidence of associated anurysms is up to 10%.
3. Type III: Juvenile AVMs (spinal AV metameric syndrome, Cobb's syndrome) are extremely rare (up to 5% of all spinal AV shunt lesions). This is a developmental syndrome, representing a combined high flow intramedullary and extramedullary lesion due to dysfunction of vasculogenic embryionic tissues. They are usually located in cervical and upper thoracic spine and can be associated with both arterial and venous aneurysms (Gros & Du, 2014).
4. Type IV: intradural perimedullary AV fistula, accounting for 15–25% of all spinal AV shunts. These lesions are high flow but low pressure lesions, located anteriorly in the region of conus, fed by the anterior spinal artery. Arterial aneurysms and venous ectasias are common.

Clinical presentation is variable and can point to the specific type of the lesion. dAVFs usually present with radicular or non-radicular pain and slowly progressive neurological deficits (over months). Glomus type lesions present usually with acute spinal cord hemorrhage followed by severe pain described as "dagger stab". Progression of myelopathy occurs secondary to repeated hemorrhages (due to aneurysms or subarachnoid hemorrhage from the nidus). However, this is in general a condition with good prognosis and up to 80% of patients are independent in 5 year period. Type III lesions (metameric syndrome lesions) occur in children and young patients, presenting with progressive myelopathy and associated with poor prognosis. Intradural perimedullary AVFs present with progressive neurologic deficits due to venous congestion. Sometimes, subarachnoid hemorrhages occur in up to 1/5 of patients. The outcome is poor, with a complete loss of spinal cord function in 10–20 years after the onset (Fugate et al, 2021, Rosenblum et al. 1987).

### 2.2 Epidemiology/Demographics

dAVF has a strong male predominance, occurring mostly in middle aged men (40–70 years of age). Glomus type AV shunts are typically found in younger patients below the age of 40 (50% patients are younger than 25), with no sex predilection. However, up to ¼ is associated with neurocutaneous syndromes (hereditary hemorrhagic teleangiectasia—Osler-Weber-Rendu). Intradural perimedullary AV fistulae occur most frequently in younger patients, age 20–50, with no sex predilection. Like glomus type, type IV lesions present a rather strong association with neurocutaneous syndromes.

## 2.3 Pathophysiology

Symptoms of dAVFs present secondary to the medullary venous hypertension and congestion. These conditions are worsened by bending coughing, exercise, and pregnancy.

## 2.4 Imaging Technique and Recommended Protocol

Non-contrast CT is generally not used for the initial diagnosis, nor for the follow-up. The most common imaging modality used is contrast-enhanced MRI, usually followed by an angiographic examination, such as CTA or DSA.

The recommended protocol includes the following:

1. T1-weighted sagittal spin-echo.
2. T2-weighted sagittal spin-echo,
3. short-tau inversion recovery (STIR) sagittal,
4. T2-weighted gradient-echo axial sequences.
5. T1-weighted contrast-enhanced sagittal and axial tomograms.

Steady state sequences (CISS, FIESTA) are extremely useful due to heavy T2 contrast that increases sensitivity in detection of flow voids.

Susceptibility weighted imaging is a promising toll in the evaluation of hemosiderin deposits in the spinal cord, but has not yet fully entered clinical practice. However, there are some reports on the signs that can be observed in cases of chronic myleopathy caused by dAVFs (Enokizono et al. 2017).

## 2.5 MR Imaging

dAVFs have a typical presentation on MRI with prominent perimedullary vascular flow voids (especially on steady state sequences). Spinal cord is usually expanded due to edema (venous congestion and hypertension) with T2 hyperintensity in the central parts and sparing of the most peripheral parts (Fig. 3). Peripheral parts of the cord sometimes show T2 hypointensity, suggesting susceptibility changes in relation to venous deoxygenation. Small pial vessels often show enhancement, but this sign sometimes can also be absent (Krings et al, 2005). Enokizono et al. demonstrated the presence of "black butterfly sign" in the dorsal aspect of medulla and the central grey matter, probably representing hemorrhage, best observed on T2* and SWI images, although detectable on T2W also. The presumed mechanism of this finding was the prolonged venous congestion (Enokizono et al. 2017). CTA shows ectatic perimedullary veins, dilated transdural draining vein, and plexiform nidus at the level of neural foramen. DSA remains the gold standard for fistula localization and is used as a diganostic modality of choice for preoperative planning. DSA presents the pathognomonic finding of retrograde flow in transdural vein with dilated transdural radicular vein that fills tortuous perimedullary veins retrogradely (Fig. 4).

Glomus type fistulas show intramedullary nidus with expanded cord due to parenchymal edema and intramedullary blood products. Feeding vessels are usually derived from the anterior and posterior circulations, while the drainage is to large perimedullary veins (Krings et al. 2007). They are usually found in the thoracolumbar spine. Sometimes they can have associated aneurysms and consequent subarachnoid hemorrhage. DSA is essential for diagnosis of these lesions, with clear delineation of the nidus itself, feeding vessels, and draining veins. MRI is not a reliable imaging modality in preoperative planning (Rubin and Rabinstein 2013).

Type III fistulas present with tortous and ectatic vessels within the spinal cord, associated with subarachnoid and epidural spaces arranged in metameric distribution. Numerous high flow AV shunts are observed on DSA, and AVMs and spinal cord share the same blood supply. Bone, muscle, and skin are often involved in the abnormality.

Type IV fistulas show anterior perimedullary flow voids, often with displacement of the spinal

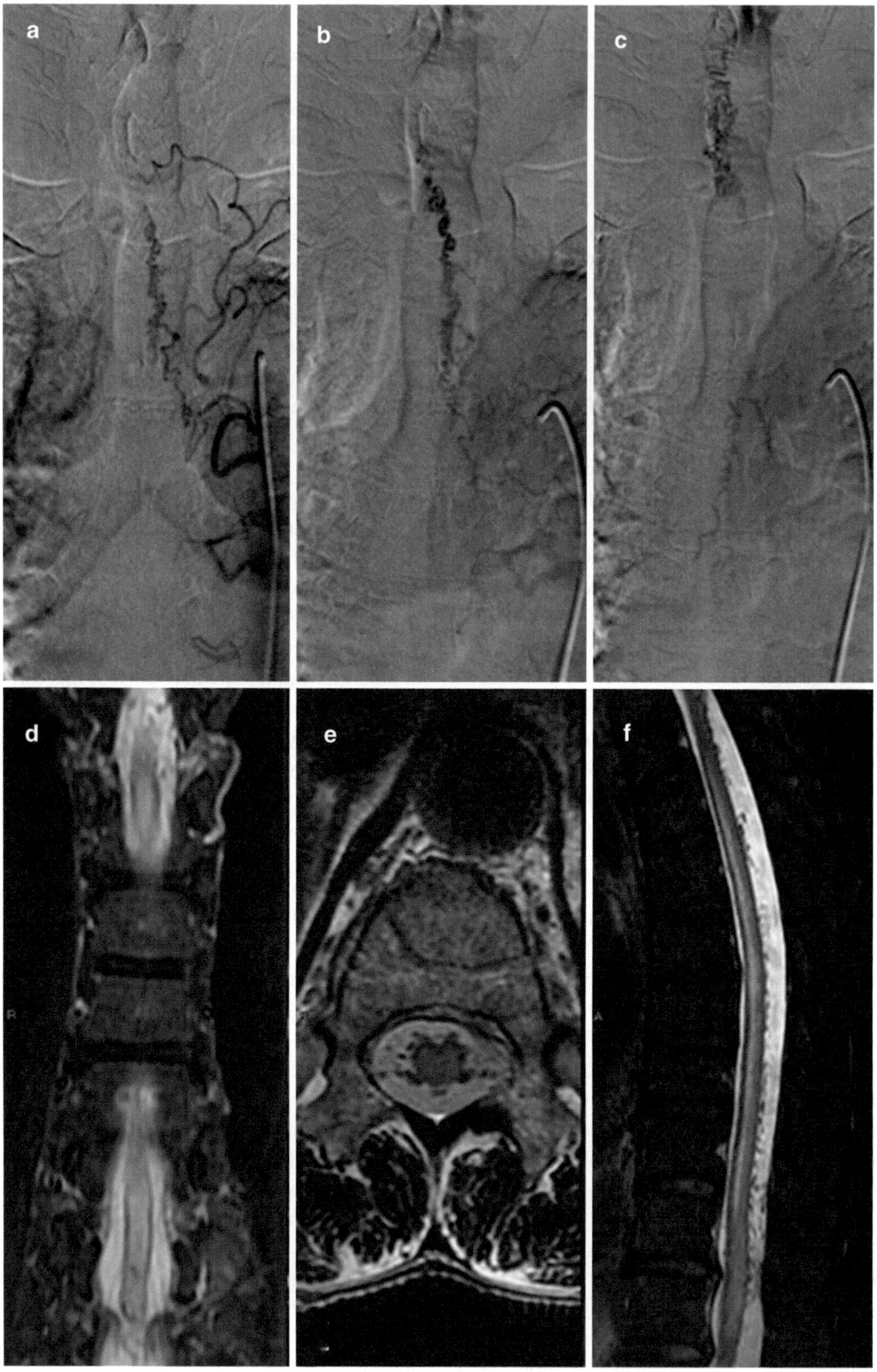


**Fig. 3** Spinal dural arteriovenous fistula. The thoracic part of the spinal cord is swollen (**a**, T2W coronal image), due to spinal dural AVF at the level of T5, with evident tortous dilated perimedullary veins around the whole circumference of the spinal cord on the cross-sectional area (**e**, axial image), although most conspicuous on the posterior surface (**f**, STIR sagittal image). DSA shows slow filling of the dilated perimedullary veins (**a**–**c**)

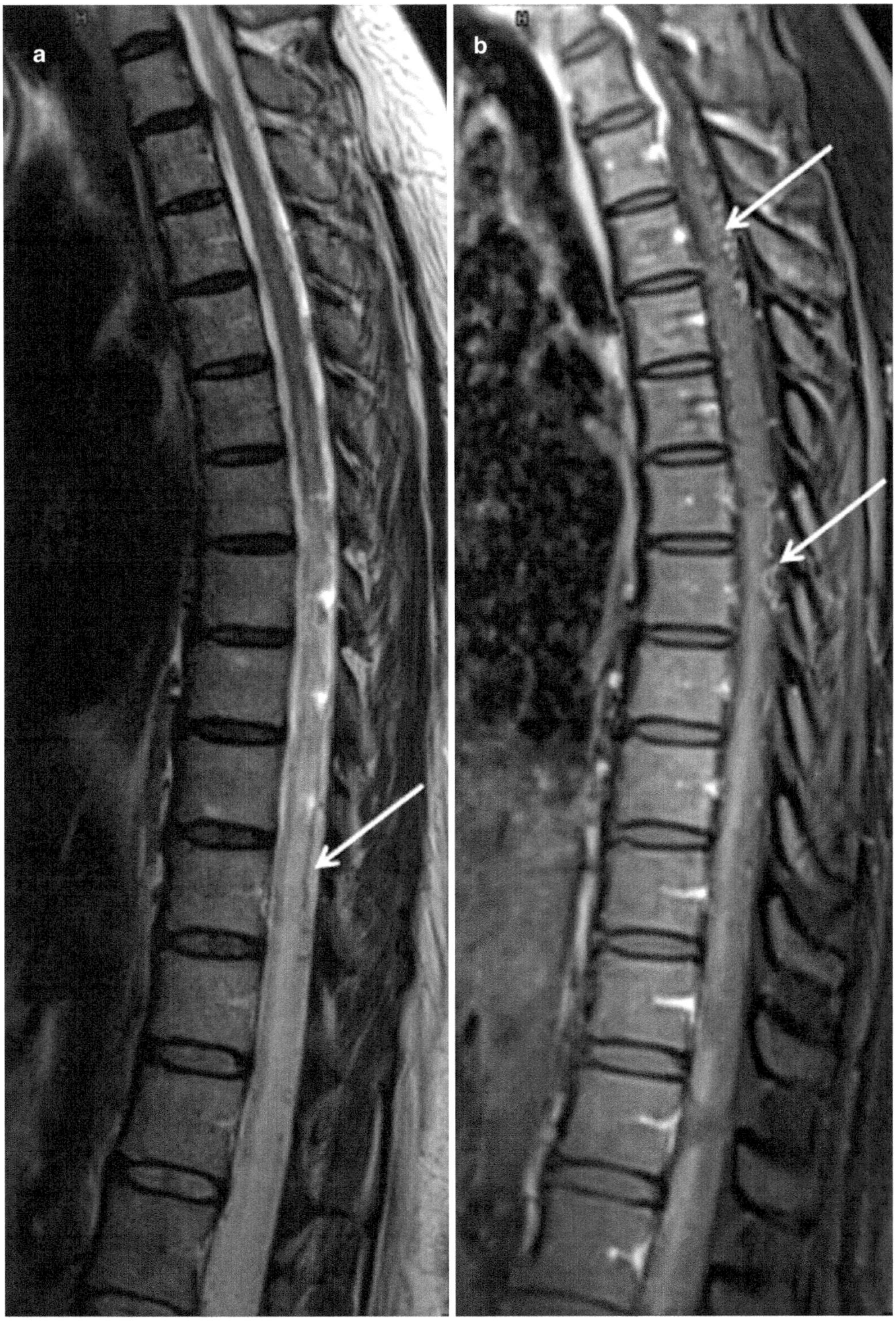


**Fig. 4** Spinal dural arteriovenous fistula. Spinal cord is enlarged and swollen in the lower thoracic part (**a** – T2W sagittal image), with evident tortous and dilated perimedullary veins on the posterior surface (**b** – postcontrast T1W FS sagittal image), representing dural arteriovenous fistula. In the lower part of thoracic medulla, one can observe "The missing piece" sign, focal geographic area with the lack of contrast enhancement within a long segment of intense holocord contrast enhancement (Zalewski et al. 2018)

cord posteriorly due to ectatic subarachnoid varices. Often, there are signs of medullary edema and expansion. DSA might show a superficial extra-axially localized nidus with arterialized perimedullary vein.

### 2.6 Differential Diagnosis and Pitfalls

The key problem in the MRI of the AV shunt lesions is the fact that often only abnormality within the spinal cord is observed, limited to the abnormally high T2 signal and expansion of the cord due to edema. The main differential diagnosis in this case is venous congestive myelopathy. Other differential diagnoses include infarction, demyelination, infection, and neoplasms.

Heavily weighted T2 sequences are helpful in accentuating enlarged and tortuous vascular structures on the dorsal or ventral surface of the cord, which are suggestive of diagnosis. Additional aid can be obtained by T1 contrast-enhanced tomograms that enable visualization of the abnormal leptomeningeal vessels. However, prominent perimedullary vessels are not specific for AV shunts. The same finding can be observed in some tumors, such as hemangioblastomas, or hypervascular schwanommas.

## 3 Spinal Hemorrhage

### 3.1 Definition of Entity and Clinical Highlights

Spinal hemorrhage is a rare but important clinical entity, classified according to the anatomical space that is involved in the pathological process. Most of the cases are due to trauma, second most common forms (up to 35%) are idiopathic; most common nontraumatic causes are coagulopathies and vascular malformations (Novy et al. 2006; Baaj 2012).

Spinal hemorrhage manifests with acute, painful myelopathy, neck or back pain. Signs and symptoms usually reflect the level of injury, the extension of the bleeding, and the acuity (Shaban et al. 2018). Symptoms may also develop subacutely (in weeks). It is important to know that slowly progressive course is very rare, seen in less than 5% of patients (Kreppel et al. 2003). SAH in the spine presents similarly like intracranial SAH, with acute headache, meningismus, or other meningeal signs (Swann et al. 1984). In addition, in spinal SAH, cranial symptoms such as headache, seizure, altered mental state, and nausea can be found (Kreppel et al. 2003). Smaller hematomas may be managed conservatively. However, since neurologic deficits can be reversible, surgical decompression is often considered (Pierce et al. 2018).

Neck or back pain is usually the leading symptom, observed at the level of hemorrhage, sometimes radiating to extremities. The hallmark of SAH is so-called "le coup de pignard" or "dagger's stab". Progressive neurological symptoms including sensory loss, bowel or bladder disturbances are usually result of venous congestion in progressive forms of myelopathies.

### 3.2 Epidemiology/Demographics

Spinal epidural hematoma (EDH) occurs in approximately 0.1/10,000 people annually and represents the most common form of spinal hemorrhage. Meta-analysis showed that 75% of all spinal hematomas are epidural (Kreppel et al. 2003). SAH in the spine is the second most common form of spinal hemorrhage. Nevertheless, this condition is extremely rare and occurs in approximately 6/100,000 people annually. Spinal subdural hematoma (SDH) and intramedullary hematoma (IMH) are two least common forms of spinal hemorrhage. SDH occurs in about 4% of cases with spinal hematomas. Hematomas occupying multiple compartments account for 2.1% of all spinal hematomas (Moriarty et al. 2019). The etiology of spinal cord hemorrhage is listed in Table 1.

**Table 1** Etiology of spinal cord hemorrhage

| | |
|---|---|
| Epidural hemorrhage/ hematoma | Iatrogenic (spinal procedure, antiplatelet, anticoagulant therapy)<br>Trauma<br>Vascular diatheses |
| Subdural hemorrhage/ hematoma | Iatrogenic<br>Trauma<br>Coagulopathy |
| Subarachnoid hemorrhage | AVM<br>Spinal aneurysm, AVF<br>Trauma<br>Iatrogenic<br>Rare: metastases, vasculitis, hemangioblastoma, ependymoma |
| Hematomyelia | Trauma<br>AVM, cavernoma, AVF<br>Anticoagulant therapy<br>Bleeding diatheses<br>Primary or secondary tumors<br>Rarely: aneurysms, irradiation |

## 3.3 Pathophysiology

EDHs represent the most common form of spinal hmorrhage (Kreppel et al. 2003). Most frequently, they are caused by epidural venous plexus hemorrhage due to minor trauma, coagulopathy, or disc extrusion. Sponatenous EDH has an incidence of 0.1/100,000 person-year. SDH is caused by iatrogenic factors in up to 70% of cases; less commonly, it is caused by trauma, surgical procedure, coagulopathy, neoplasm, or AVMs. The pathogenesis is associated with collapse of the microvasculature between dura and arachnoidea due to minor trauma. Approximately 1% of all SAHs are caused by primary spinal cord pathology, usually spinal AVMs, dAVFs, spinal aneurysms, and hemorrhagic tumors (Shaban et al. 2018). Commonly, SAH in the spine occurs as a secondary phenomenon, associated with intracranial aneurysm rupture. Spinal SAH also can happen as a result of spinal artery aneurysms (type I aneurysms are related to lesions that increase arterial blood flow, while type II are isolated forms). Spinal aneurysms have predilection for the anterior spinal artery and cervical spine (50%). They are usually fusiform, without the neck, and result from intimal dissection (Vuong et al. 2016). IMH or hematomyelia are described rarely, most commonly related to anticoagulant treatment, or trauma, neoplasms (Novy et al. 2006; Agarwal et al. 2014). Trauma represents the most common cause of hematomyelia, usually seen in the cervical cord (Pillai et al. 2008). The source of bleeding is microcirculation, creating mass effect that later results in local infarction caused by hypoxia and ischemia (Dumont et al. 2001). Vascular malformations associated with hematomyelia are AVMs and cavernomas; however, AVM usually leads to spinal SAH (Allen et al. 1979). AVFs can also sometimes cause hematomyelia, usually associated with hemorrhagic transformation of venous infarction (Mascalchi et al. 1998). Old-fashioned anticoagulant therapy has been associated with hematomyelia; however, there are no cases reported with new anticoagulants.

## 3.4 Imaging Technique and Recommended Protocol

MRI with contrast injection is the preferred diagnostic modality in evaluation of spinal cord hemorrhage. The recommended protocol consists of T1W, T2W, gradient-echo imaging or SWI, and DWI. Additional imaging usually refers to dedicated imaging of the vessel pathology, such as MRA, CTA, or DSA. DSA remains the gold standard for identification of vascular pathology (Shaban et al. 2018). Location of the hemorrhage source remains extremely challenging, even with spinal angiography, especially in the cases of isolated aneurysms.

Evaluation of the spinal hemorrhage requires the understanding of blood products' presentation on MRI, which is time-dependent. The principles of five stages of hemorrhage, described already for decades on MRI of the intracranial hemorrhage, can be applied to spinal hemorrhage as well (Table 2).

It is important to identify the precise localization of hemorrhage before the surgical exploration. The position of hematoma in relation to dura is the key feature for differentiation between subdural and epidural hematomas. This position can be best identified on MRI, using both axial and

**Table 2** Evolution of the hemmorhage on MRI

| Stage | Time period | Blood component | T1W | T2W | T2W*/SWI |
|---|---|---|---|---|---|
| Hyperacute | <24 h | Oxyhemoglobin | Hypo | Hyper | Variable/Negative |
| Acute | 1–3 days | Deoxyhemoglobin | Iso | Hypo | Hypo rim |
| Early subacute | 3–7 days | Intracellular methemoglobin | Hyper | Hypo | Hypo |
| Late subacute | 1–2 weeks | Extracellular methemoglobin | Hyper | Hyper | Hypo |
| Chronic | >2 weeks | Hemosiderin | Hypo | Hypo | Hypo |

sagittal imaged, by identifiying the fat, which is basically never affected by SDH (Kobayashi et al. 2017). Classic star-like appearance of filum terminale and cauda equina roots that are affected by SDH is called the inverted Mercedes-Benz sing (Hausmann et al. 2001).

MRI features of the spinal hemorrhage evolve with time (Table 2). On CT and MRI, spinal artery aneurysm presents as a focal fusiform dilatation of an intradural spinal vessel (usually radiculomedullary artery). They are usually very small.

EDH can be recognized in the posterior, anterior part or diffuse around the dural sac, with a specific loss of epidural fat signal and smooth contour towards the spinal canal (Figure). Seventy-five percent of the cases present with EDH dorsally or dorsolaterally within the spinal canal. This is the result of dura being more tightly attached to the posterior longitudinal ligament than yellow ligaments.

SDH occurs in the potential space between dura and arachnoidea and can be identified as separated from the epidural fat with prominent black line that represents dura. It is always contained within the wall of thecal sac. Key feature in differential diagnosis from EDH is the presence of epidural fat without inward displacement of the hypointense dura mater (Moriarty et al. 2019). The inner contour of SDH is concave but usually irregular, not smooth like in EDH. SDH generates mass effect on the cord, which is one of the important characteristics of this hematoma in differential diagnosis (Mashiko et al. 2006). Blood in the thecal sac compresses nerve roots and cord and produces the inverted Mercedes-Benz sign. Contrary to EDH, SDH does not extend into neural foramina and also does not make direct contact with the bone.

SAH usually extends in a longitudinal direction, as layering blood in the CSF space, without producing a focalized abnormality (Flanders et al. 1999). Sometimes, it can present as non-enhancing intradural extramedullary clot with mass effect on the spinal cord and nerve roots (Pierce et al. 2018). Distinguishing feature of SAH is the presence of sedimentation and fluid-fluid levels typically observed in the dependent lower lumbar region, and also the presence of epidural fat signal. Mass-like blood clot is observed rarely, with variable signal intensity on T1W and T2W images, but always with CSF signal intensity surrounding the hematoma, and thus allowing differentiation from other types of spinal hematomas.

Intramedullary hemorrhage (hematomyelia) represents blood products within the spinal cord parenchyma or syrinx (Fig. 5). It usually occurs at the point of maximal impact in trauma, most often confined to the central grey matter in the form of hemorrhagic necrosis (Looby and Flander 2011). T2* or SWI images are recommended for the proper delineation of blood products. Often, associated finding is rather extensive medullary edema, extending both cranially and caudally from the hemorrhagic lesion (Moriarty et al. 2019). Spinal hemorrhage can affect multiple compartments, thus causing diagnostic challenge. In these cases, systematic analysis of each compartment is essential for understanding the extent of the disorder.

### 3.5 Differential Diagnosis and Pitfalls

Careful evaluation of the signs for each compartmental hemorrhage is necessary, especially in cases of multicompartmental hemorrhage.

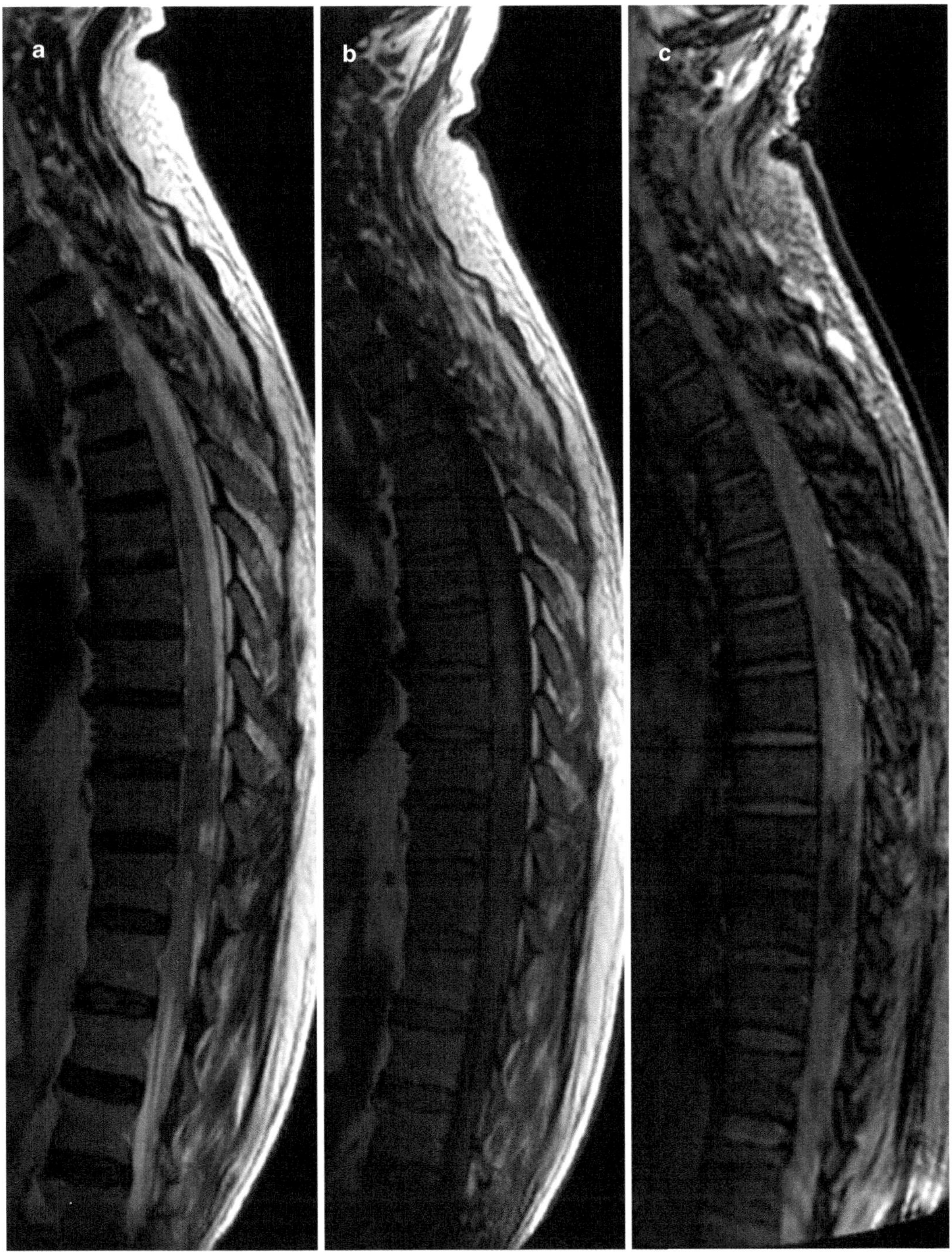


**Fig. 5** Hematomyelia. In the lower thoracic part of the spinal cord, heterogenous signal intensity can be observed, with T2 hypointense (**a**) and T1-hyperintense (**b**) areas, corresponding to SWI hypointensities (**c**), representing areas of subacute hemorrhage

Differentiating spinal hematoma from inflammation and neoplasm can be challenging. Neoplastic process shows contrast enhancement, at least marginal. Marginal enhancement can seldom be observed in the hyperacute phase of spinal hematoma (Chang et al. 2003). However, clinical history is different. Clinical history is also an important key to the diagnosis in inflammatory process, such as abscess or spondylodiscitis.

EDH should be distinguished from epidural tumor spread or metastasis (breast, lung, and prostate cancer). Epidural tumor is usually T1 hypointense, with more solid contrast enhancement. Identification of concomitant vertebral body infiltrative lesions helps in establishing the right diagnosis. Epidural abscess is an epidurally located fluid collection with heterogenous signal intensity, but shows the same mass effect as EDH. However, it typically occurs with discitis/osteomyelitis, as well as with destruction of the bone or paraspinal muscle fluid collections and inflammatory reaction. Rarely, differential diagnosis includes epidural disc sequestra, fibrosis due to postsurgical state, and facet synovial cysts (Pierce et al. 2018).

Differential diagnosis of SDH includes subdural abscess and hygroma, generally aided by clinical findings and history. Spinal subdural abscess is an extremely rare entity, presenting with fever and back pain. On the imaging, it has a complex signal intensity with peripheral enhancement, with no abnormalities on gradient-echo imaging. Subdural hygroma is observed in patients with recent trauma or intervention. They usually present with signal intensity similar to CSF space. Intradural extramedullary masses (meningeomas and nerve sheath tumors) typically enhance avidly and homogenously. Arachnoiditis can also be included in differential diagnosis, resulting in the grouping of cauda equina nerve roots.

It is important to differentiate the presence of subarachnoid spinal hematoma from the flow voids of cerebrospinal fluid (CSF). CSF does not generate mass effect and compression on the cord, as SDH. In addition, spinal hematoma is identifiable on all MR sequences, while CSF flow voids are usually most prominent on T1W/T2W sequences, but disappear on gradient-echo sequences. In addition, there is no compressive effect on the spinal cord and nerve roots. Sometimes it is hard to differentiate SDH from SAH, but the latter lacks fluid-fluid levels, which can be a helpful hint.

IMH should be differentiated from intramedullary neoplasm, especially in the cases of nontraumatic etiology (when clinical history is not helpful). In these cases, neoplasm should be considered a potential underlying cause of IMH. Both primary (hemangioblastoma and ependymoma) and secondary tumors (metastases, most commonly from renal cell, breast, and lung carcinoma) can produce hemorrhage. Ependymomas may present with peripheral rim or hypointense foci of T2 hypointensity, termed “cap sign”, and enhance avidly. Hemangioblastoma is usually in the form of a cystic lesion with an intensively enhancing nodule. Metastases have variable presentation, but most commonly, they have homogenous ehncancement with great amount of surrounding edema. Spinal AVMs are also a common cause of hematomyelia, but usually have a typical MR presentation.

## 4 Fibrocartilaginous Embolism

### 4.1 Definition of Entity and Clinical Highlights

Fibrocartilaginous embolism (FCE) represents a rare condition that occurs due to migration of fibrocartilagionous nucleus pulposus through the vasculature into the spinal cord vessels (AbdelRazek et al. 2016). Up to date, no more than 200 cases nave been described in the literature (Mateen et al. 2011). However, many authors feel that this condition is actually underestimated and often overlooked cause of the spinal cord infarction (Manara et al. 2010).

Clinical picture is that of a spinal cord infarction, with the transient back or neck pain, followed by progressive myelopathy. There is always a sensory level present, with bladder and/or bowel dysfunction. Typically, paraplegia or quadriplegia (with or without respiratory compromise) occurs, dependent on the level of lesion (thoracolumbar region vs. cervical spinal cord). Symptoms occur promptly and develop over hours, which helps in distinguishing from inflammatory or neoplastic disease. Also typically, there is temporal relationship to an event that served as a trigger for FCE (bending, minor trauma, heavy lifting) measured in hours to days. The typical clinical finding in anterior spinal infarction is the sparing of proprioception and vibration sensation below the sensory level.

The diagnosis of FCE is based on the following criteria:

1. severe acute back/neck pain followed by rapid onset of progressive paraplegia/quadriplegia with sphincter dysfunction and/or abolishment of reflexes,
2. close temporal relationship with Valsalva maneveur or a minor trauma,
3. negative CSG examination; absence of systemic embolic sources and prothrombotic conditions,
4. concordant MRI findings of a spinal cord infarction (cord edema) with signal intensity changes in the intervertebral disc or body adjacent to the level of the cord lesion or Schmorl's nodules (Spengos et al. 2006; Raghavan et al. 2004; Davis and Klug 2000).

## 4.2 Epidemiology/Demographics

FCE occurs slightly more commonly in females (63.5%), with the average age around 40. However, more than a half of reported cases occurred in patients younger than 40. In recent literature, the period between the trigger and FCE symptoms was average 2.4 days (usually within 24 h). Symptoms of neck or back pain were observed in more than ¾ of cases. Mortality due to this condition was most commonly associated with pulmonary embolism, pneumonia, and aspiration (AbdelRazek et al. 2006; Mateen et al. 2011).

## 4.3 Pathophysiology

Although intervertebral disc represents an avascular structure, it is the source of embolic material in this rare condition. Intervertebal disc consisted of two compartments: mesodermally derived annulus fibrosus and endodermally derived, centrally located nucleus pulposus. In the neonatal period, disc is supplied by rich vasculature, which regresses at the age of 2 months and the disc becomes completely avascular by the end of the first decade of life. In the normal adult, neovascularization appears at the age of 50, and in cases with developed degenerative disease, even earlier (Boos et al. 2002). Shared arterial supply between vertebral bodies and the spinal cord (spinal branches of radicular arteries supply the posterior parts of vertebral bodies and reinforce the longitudinal spinal arteries to the spinal cord) is the postulated pathophysiologic basis for the occurrence of FCE (AbdelRazek et al. 2016). Additionally, Schmorl's nodes represent *loci minoris resistentiae,* because fibrocartilaginous masses are in the close proximity to the vasculature of vertebral body. It is suggested that the initial trigger is increased intradiscal or intravertebral body pressure by axial forces during Valsalva maneuvers (heavy lifting, straining, or minor trauma to the back or neck). The fibrocartilaginous mass, after entering vasculature, travels through either arterial or venous route to reach the spinal cord. If it enters arterial route, it travels through radicular artery and causes spinal cord infarction (Yousef et al. 1998). If it, on the other hand, enters the venous route, it goes through vena cava to the Batson's plexus and spinal cord. Some cases showed the presence of both arterial and venous FCE in cases of concomitatnt arterial and venous embolizations or due to presence of normally present AV shunts in the epidural space (Vuia and Alexianu 1969).

## 4.4 Imaging Technique and Recommended Protocol

Imaging modality of choice is MRI, since CT is not sensitive for depiction of parenchymal lesions in the spinal cord. Recommended protocol is basically the same as for the spinal cord infarction:

1. T1-weighted sagittal spin-echo.
2. T2-weighted sagittal spin-echo,
3. short-tau inversion recovery (STIR) sagittal,
4. T2-weighted gradient-echo axial sequences.

Diffusion-weighted imaging (DWI) and contrast study are optional, but can aid to the diagnosis, especially DWI, that can also be of prognostic value.

Typical findings are that of the spinal cord infarction, with T2 hyperinetnse lesions in a vascular distribution, most commonly with no contrast enhancement (typically observed in inflammatory or neoplastic lesions). However, in the subacute phase, patchy gadolinium enhancement can be observed, as well as hemorrhagic transformation of infarction. Additional important imaging feature are T2 signal intensity changes in the vertebral body or intervertebral disc adjacent to the cord lesion (Fig. 6).

Standard, conventional MRI (without DWI) can be unremarkable, especially in the early stages. DWI might have a key role in establishing

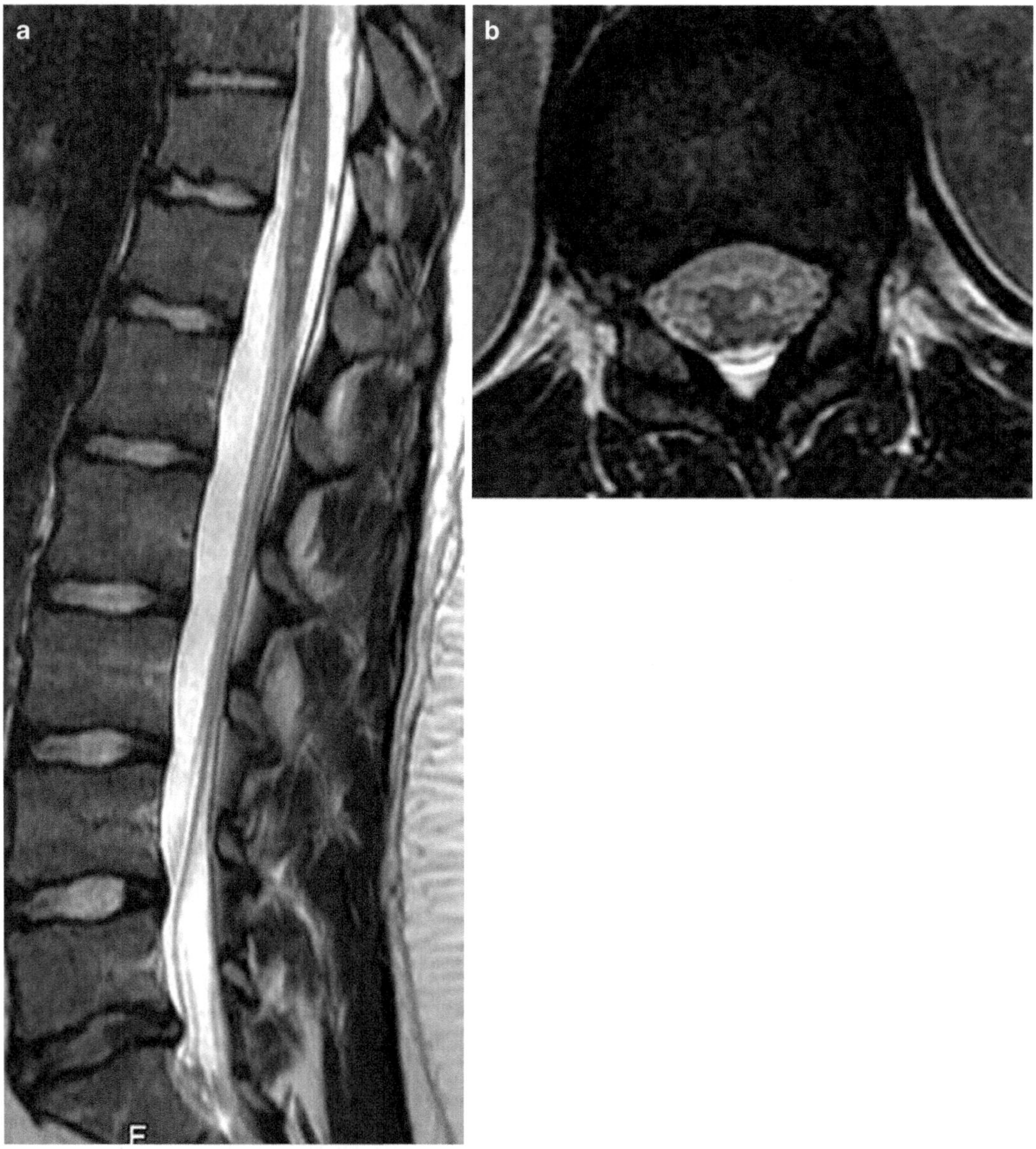


**Fig. 6** Fibrocartilaginous embolism. On T2W sagittal image, lesions in the anterior part of the conus are evident (**a**), consistent with infarction of the left anterior horn (**b**). Bulging of L5-S1 intervertebral disc is observed and represents the potential source of embolism

the accurate diagnosis, since it can differentiate vasogenic (present in inflammatory myelitis) from cytotoxic edema (present in ischemia). Changes observed on DWI predate signal changes on T2 and can be observed within a few hours after the onset of ischemia (Manara et al. 2010).

### 4.5 Differential Diagnosis and Pitfalls

FCE remains an uncommon diagnosis and is often mistaken for the inflammatory cord lesions, based solely on imaging features. However, the likelihood of FCE raises with typical clinical presentation, the presence of a trigger in close past, along with suggestive CSF findings and MRI features of a spinal cord infarction. CSF analysis is usually normal or with slightly elevated protein level. However, pleocytosis or increased IgG levels, typical for inflammatory lesions, are never observed (Frohman and Wingerchuk 2010).

DWI is an extremely useful sequence for differentiating inflammatory myelitis from spinal cord ischemia. Ischemic lesion is first observed as diffusion-restricted area in the spinal cord in the vascular distribution, predating signal changes on T2. To the contrary, in the inflammatory lesions, signal intensity changes are well-observed on T2, while there are no concordant abnormalities on DWI (insensitive), or there can be signs of facilitated diffusion consistent with vasogenic edema. Therefore, DWI should be included in the standard protocol for evaluation of the spinal cord lesions, since it proves the ischemic nature of the lesion very early in the course of disease.

## References

AbdelRazek MA, Mowla A, Farooq S, Silvestri N, Sawyer R, Wolfe G (2016) Fibrocartilaginous embolism: a comprehensive review of an under-studied cause of spinal cord infarction and proposed diagnostic criteria. J Spinal Cord Med 39(2):146–154

Agarwal A, Kanekar S, Thamburaj K, Vijay K (2014) Radiation-induced spinal cord hemorrhage (hematomyelia). Neuro Int 6(4):5553

Allen JP, McDonald JV, Horner FA (1979) Hematomyelia with arteriovenous malformation of the cord: successful surgical treatment. Arch Neurol 36:455

Baaj A (2012) Spinal emergencies. In: Handbook of spine surgery. Thieme, New York, pp 190–191

Barreras P, Fitzgerald KC, Mealy MA et al (2018) Clinical biomarkers differentiate myelitis from vascular and other causes of myelopathy. Neurology 90(1):e12–e21

Boos N, Weissbach S, Rohrbach H, Weiler C, Spratt KF, Nerlich AG (2002) Classification of age-related changes in lumbar intervertebral discs. Spine 27(23):2631–2644

Chang F, Lirng J, Chen S et al (2003) Contrast enhancement patterns of acute spinal epidural hematomas: a report of two cases. AJNR Am J Neuroradiol 24(3):366–369

Da Costa L, Dehdashti AR, terBrugge KG (2009) Spinal cord vascular shunts: spinal cord vascular malformations and dural arteriovenous fistulas. Neurosurg Focus 26(1):E26

Davis GA, Klug GL (2000) Acute-onset nontraumatic paraplegia in childhood: fibrocartilaginous embolism in acute myelitis? Childs Nerv Syst 16:551–554

Dumont RJ, Okonkwo DO, Verma S et al (2001) Acute spinal cord injury. Part I: pathophysiologic mechanisms. Clin Neuropharmacol 24:254–264

Enokizono M, Sato N, Morikawa M et al (2017) "Black butterfly" sign on T2*-weighted and susceptibility-weighted imaging: a novel finding of chronic venous congestion of the brain stem and spinal cord associated with dural arteriovenous fistulas. J Neurol Sci 379:64–68

Flanders AE, Settell CM, Friedman DP, Marino RJ, Herbison GJ (1999) The relationship between the functional abilities of patients with cervical spinal cord injury and the severity of damage revealed by MR imaging. AJNR Am J Neuroradiol 20:926–934

Frohman EM, Wingerchuk DM (2010) Clinical practice. Transverse myelitis. N Engl J Med 363(6):564–572

Fugate JE, Lanzino G, Rabinstein AA (2012) Clinical presentation and prognostic facotrs of spinal dural arteriovenous fistulas: an overview. Neurosurg Focus 32(5):E17

Ghandehari K, Gerami Sarabi MR, Maarufi P (2010) Clinical evaluation of patients with spinal cord infarction in Mashad, Iran. Stroke Res Treat 2010:942417

Gross BA, Du R (2014) Spinal juvenile (Type III) extradural-intradural arteriovenous malformations. J Neurosurg Spine 20(4):452–458

Hanson SR, Romi F, Rekand T, Naess H (2015) Long-term outcome after spinal cord infarctions. Acta Neurol Scand 131:253–257

Harringan M, Deveikis J (2013) Handbook of cerebrovascular disease and neurointerventional technique, 2nd edn. Humana Press, New York

Hausmann O, Kirsch E, Radu E et al (2001) Coagulopathy induced spinal intradural extramedullary haematoma: report of thre cases and review of the literature. Acta Neurochir 143:135–140

Jorgensen HS, Nakayama H, Raaschou HO, Olsen TS (1994) Effect of blood pressure and diabetes on stroke in progression. Lancet 344:156–159
Kobayashi K, Imagama S, Ando K et al (2017) Acute non-traumatic idiopathic spinal subdural hematoma: radiographic findings and surgical results with a literature review. Eur Spine J 26:2739–2743
Kreppel D, Antoniadis G, Seeling W (2003) Spinal hematoma: a literature survey with meta-analysis of 613 patients. Neurosurg Rev 26:1–49
Krings T, Mull M, Gilsbach JM et al (2005) Spinal vascular malformations. Eur Radiol 15:267–278
Krings T, Lasjaunias PL, Hans FJ et al (2007) Imaging in spinal vascular disease. Neuroimaging Clin N Am 17(1):57–72
Looby S, Flander A (2011) Spina trauma. Radiol Clin N Am 49(1):129–163
Manara R, Calderone M, Severino MS et al (2010) Spinal cord nfarction due to fibrocartilaginous embolization: the role of diffusion weighted imaging and short-tau inversion recovery sequences. J Child Neurol 25(8):1024–1028
Mascalchi M, Mangiafico S, Marn E (1998) Hematomyelia complicating a spinal dural arteriovenous fistula. Report of a case. J Neuroradiol 25:140–143
Mashiko R, Noguchi S, Uemura K, Takada T, Matsumura A (2006) Lumbosacral subdural hematoma. Neurol Med Chir (Tokyo) 46:258–261
Mateen FJ, Monrad PA, Hunderfund AN, Robertson CE, Sorenson EJ (2011) Clinically suspected fibrocartilaginous embolism : clinical characteristics, treatments, and outcomes. Eur J Neurol 18(2):218–225
Moriarty HK, O'Cearbhail R, Moriarty PD, Stanley ER, Lawler LP, Kavanagh EC (2019) MR imaging of spinal haematoma. Br J Radiol 92(1095):20180532
Naess H, Romi F (2011) Comparing patients with spinal cord infarction and cerebral infarction: clinical characteristics, and short-term outcome. Vasc Health Risk Manag 7:497–502
Naess H, Nyland HI, Thomassen L, Aarseth J, Myhr KM (2005) Fatigue at long-term follow-up in young adults with cerebral infarction. Cerebrovasc Dis 20:245–250
Nedeltchev K, Loher TJ, Stepper F, Arnold M, Schroth G, Mattle HP et al (2004) Long-term outcome of acute spinal ischemia syndrome. Stroke 35:560–565
Novy J, Carruzzo A, Maeder P, Bogousslavsky J (2006) Spinal cord ischemia: clinical and imaging patterns, pathogenesis, and putcomes in 27 patients. Arch Neurol 63(8):1113–1120
Peckham ME, Hutchins TA (2019) Imaging of vascular disorders of the spine. Radiol Clin N Am 57(2):307–318
Pierce JL, Donahue JH, Nacey NC et al (2018) Spinal hematomas: what a radiologist needs to know. Radiographics 38:1516–1535
Pillai A, Crane E, Chappell A et al (2008) Traumatic cervical hematomyelia: report of a rare spinal cord injury without radiographic abnormality. J Trauma 65:938–941
Raghavan A, Onikul E, Ryan MM et al (2004) Anterior spinal cord infarction owing to possible fibrocartilaginous embolism. Pediatr Radiol 28:44–47
Robertson CE, Brown RD, Wijdicks EF, Rabinstein AA (2012) Recovery after spinal cord infarcts: long-term outcome in 115 patients. Neurology 78:114–121
Rodesch G, Hurth M, Alvarez H et al (2004) Angioarchitecture of spinal cord aretriovenous shunts at presentation. Clinical correlations in adults in children. The Bicentre experience on 155 consecutive patients seen between 1981-1999. Acta Neurochir 146(3):217–226
Romi F, Naess H (2011) Characteristics of spinal cord stroke in clinical neurology. Eur Neurol 66:305–309
Romi F, Naess H (2016) Spinal cord infarction in clinical neurology: a review of characteristics and long-term prognosis in comparison to cerebral infarction. Eur Neurol 76:95–98
Rosenblum B, Oldfield EH, Doppman JL et al (1987) Spinal arteriovenous malformations: a comparison of dural arteriovenous fistulas and intradural AVMs in 81 patients. J Neurosurg 67:795–802
Rubin MN, Rabinstein AA (2013) Vascular diseases of the spinal cord. Neurol Clin 31(1):153–181
Shaban A, Moritani T, Al Kasab S, Sheharyar A, Limaye KS, Adams HP (2018) Spinal cord hemorrhage. J Stroke Cerebrovasc Dis 27(6):1435–1446
Spengos K, Tsivgoulis G, Toulas P et al (2006) Spinal cord stroke in a baller dancer. J Neurol Sci 15:159–161
Sullivan TM, Sundt TM (2006) Complications of thoracic aortic endograft: spinal cord ischemia and stroke. J Vasc Surg 43(Suppl A):85A–88A
Swann KW, Ropper EH, New PF et al (1984) Spontaneous spinal subarachnoid hemorrhage and subdural hematoma. Report of two cases. J Neurosurg 61:975–980
Vargas MI, Gariani J, Sztajzel R, Barnaure-Nachbar I, Delattre BM, Lovblad KO, Dietermann JL (2015) Spinal cord ischemia: practical imaging tips, pearls and pitfalls. AJNR Am J Neuroradiol 36:825–830
Vuia O, Alexianu M (1969) Arteriovenous shunt in the spinal cord circulation. Acta Neurol Scand 45(2):216–223
Vuong MD, Jeong WJ, Morales H, Abruzzo TA (2016) Vascular diseases of the spinal cord: infarction, hemorrhage and venous congestive myelopathy. Semin Ultrasound CT MR 37(5):466–481
Yousef OM, Appenzeller P, Kornfeld M (1998) Fibrocartilaginous embolism: an unusual case of spinal cord infarction. Am J Forensic Med Pathol 19(4):395–399
Zalewski NL, Flanagan EP, Keegan BM (2018) Evaluation of idiopathic transverse myelitis revealing specific myelopathy diagnoses. Neurology 90(2):e96–e102
Zalewski NL, Rabinstein AA, Krecke KN, Brown RD, Wijdicks EFM, Weinshenker BG et al (2019) Characteristics of spontaneous spinal cord infarction and proposed diagnostic criteria. JAMA Neurol 76(1):56–63

# Emergent Tumors and Infections of the Spinal Cord

Zulejha Merhemic, Martina Spero, Jasmina Boban, and Majda M. Thurnher

## Contents




Z. Merhemic (✉)
Department of Radiology, General Hospital Sarajevo, Sarajevo, Bosnia and Herzegovina

M. Spero
Department of Diagnostic and Interventional Radiology, University Hospital – Dubrava, Zagreb, Croatia

J. Boban
Department of Radiology, Faculty of Medicine Novi Sad, University of Novi Sad, Novi Sad, Serbia

M. M. Thurnher
Department for Biomedical Imaging and Image-guided Therapy, Medical University of Vienna, Vienna, Austria


## 1 Introduction

Spinal tumors broadly fall into two divisions, extradural tumors and intradural tumors, which can be either intra- or extramedullary in location. Intradural spinal tumors are rare tumors with long duration of nonspecific symptoms prior to diagnosis. Intramedullary spinal tumors are rare, representing 20% of all intraspinal tumors in adults and 35% of all intraspinal tumors in children, while intradural extramedullary tumors account for 80% of all intradural spinal tumors (Duong et al. 2012).




M. Scaglione et al. (eds.), *Emergency Radiology of the Head and Spine*,
Medical Radiology Diagnostic Imaging, https://doi.org/10.1007/978-3-030-91047-1_18

## 2 Clinics

Spinal cord compression (SCC) due to spinal tumor is an emergency that requires prompt diagnosis and treatment if permanent neurologic damage is to be prevented. In spinal tumors, SCC could be secondary to vertebral fracture due to a tumor involving bony elements of the spine or due to a spinal tumor itself compressing the cord. The pain produced by spinal tumor is caused by either spine instability or compression of the spinal structures and roots. Other symptoms include weakness and autonomic or sensory symptoms. Progression of symptoms is more rapid with metastatic tumors in comparison to primary spinal cord tumors. As a first step in patients with back pain in identifying spinal neoplastic lesions as a possible cause, the guidelines recommend assessing the clinical "red flags": a previous history of cancer, unexplained weight loss, age greater than 50 years, no improvement in symptoms after 1 month, insidious onset, no relief with bed rest, and fever (Henschke et al. 2013). The spine is more frequently the site of metastatic disease than primary tumors. Emergency decompressive surgery is often necessary, either alone or in combination with other treatments, especially radiation (Arce et al. 2001). Pretreatment high-dose corticosteroid therapy may be initiated to reduce cord edema (Flounders and Ott 2003).

## 3 Imaging

Magnetic resonance imaging (MRI) is the method of choice for detection and evaluation of intradural spinal lesions. Standard imaging protocol should include sagittal and axial T1-weighted and T2-weighted sequences without contrast and short time inversion recovery (STIR). Further, contrast-enhanced T1-weighted sequences in the sagittal, axial, and coronal planes should be performed. Diffusion-weighted imaging (DWI) and diffusion tensor imaging (DTI), as advanced techniques, are increasingly used in the evaluation of spinal lesions as well. DTI and fiber tractography are novel techniques that provide more details about the white matter tracts in relation to space-occupying lesions (Landi et al. 2016). Angiography will be necessary to demonstrate the vascularization of some tumors, such as hemangioblastomas, as well as for presurgical interventions, such as the embolization of hypervascular lesions (Krings et al. 2007). Positron emission tomography/computed tomography (PET/CT) using fludeoxyglucose or 11(C) methionine has been used to evaluate intramedullary lesions, particularly for tumors with high-grade malignancy (Naito et al. 2015).

## 4 Spinal Tumors

### 4.1 Intramedullary Tumors

#### 4.1.1 Ependymoma

Ependymomas are the most common intramedullary tumors in adults with a peak incidence in the fourth decade. Ependymoma is a slow-growing tumor developing from ependymal cells, the epithelial-like cells lining the ventricles of the brain and the central canal of the spinal cord. It compresses adjacent spinal cord tissue rather than infiltrate it, leaving a plane between the tumor and normal spinal cord tissue, and thus, gross total resection is possible in many cases (Kim et al. 2016). The World Health Organization (WHO) classifies them into three histological grades (Louis et al. 2016). Myxopapillary ependymoma and subependymoma are grade I lesions, the most benign in histologic appearance. Grade II lesions include papillary, clear cell, and tanycytic subtypes, grouped together for their lack of anaplastic features and similar biologic behavior (Perry et al. 2012). Anaplastic ependymomas are grade III and have the most malignant behavior. Ependymoma RELA fusion-positive, recently accepted molecular variant of ependymoma, is not found in the spinal cord (Louis et al. 2016). Ependymoma may be associated with neurofibromatosis type 2 (NF2). In NF2, most ependymomas are WHO grade II, and rarely, WHO grade III. Ependymomas can occur anywhere along the spinal cord: the cervical cord is the most common site (44%), 26% occur in the thoracic cord alone, while 23% occur within the cervical cord and extend into the upper thoracic cord. MRI features of classic ependymoma include well-circumscribed lesion involving up to four segments, occupying the central portion of the spinal cord and causing cord expansion. Those tumors have cystic presentation in 50–90% of cases: cysts usually have CSF intensity. The solid portion of the tumor is isointense or mildly hypointense on T1-weighted images (T1WI), hyperintense on T2-weighted images (T2WI) and STIR, and always enhances after contrast administration. The "cap sign" (hypointense hemosiderin rim on T2WI on cranial or caudal margin) due to hemorrhage strongly suggests cord ependymoma, but is not pathognomonic for ependymoma as it may also be seen in hemangioblastomas and paragangliomas. Syrinx, a cystic cavity lined by gliotic parenchyma that arises outside the central canal, is also a common finding (Fig. 1).

Myxopapillary ependymoma (MPE) is most common tumor of the conus medullare or filum terminale originating from ependymal cells of the filum. They present as T2-high, T1-iso, or low intensity masses with strong but inhomogeneous enhancement. Scalloping of the vertebral bodies, scoliosis, and enlargement of the neural foramina will be detected often (Merhemic et al. 2016). Although MPEs are characterized as histologically benign, slow-growing tumors, some patients demonstrate local recurrence or even distant metastasis, more likely in the pediatric age (Fig. 2). Anaplastic ependymomas are typically T1 isointense, T2 iso-, or hyperintense and have variable contrast enhancement. Infiltration into surrounding tissue may be visible, making them difficult to differentiate from an infiltrative glioma. Due to their aggressive nature, screening for CNS metastases of the entire neural axis is mandatory (Celano et al. 2016).

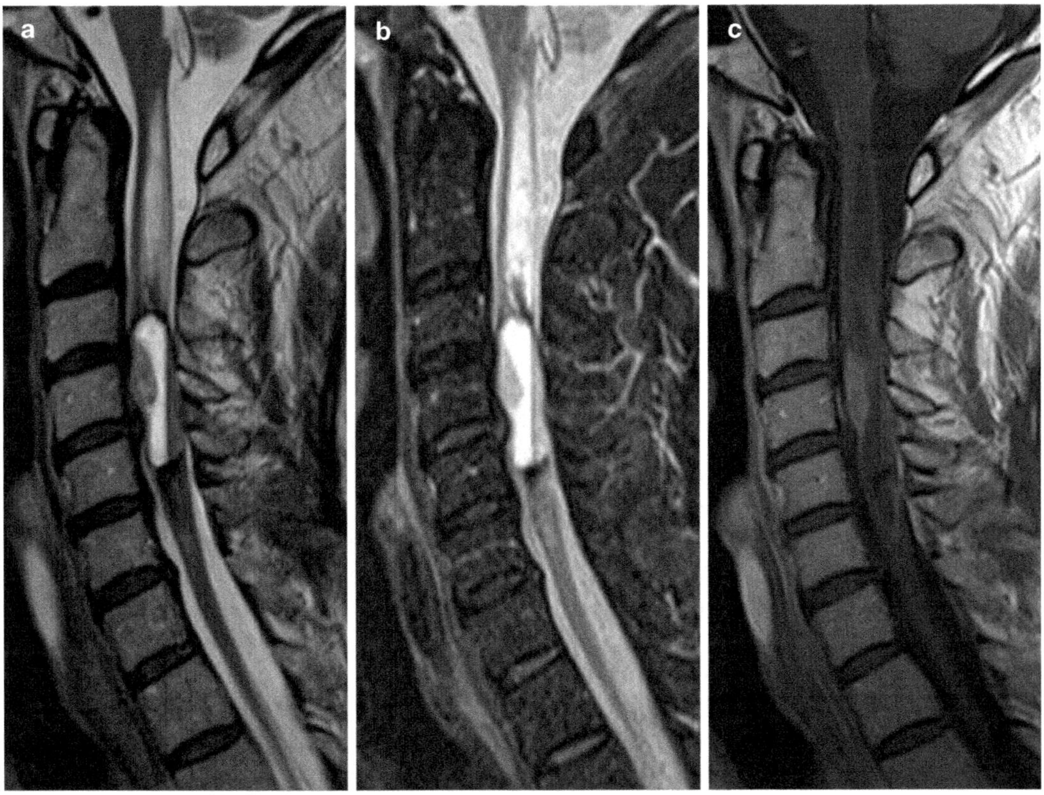


**Fig. 1** Ependymoma (WHO II). Sagittal T2WI (**a**), STIR (**b**), contrast-enhanced T1WI (**c**). Expansile cystic lesion centrally located in the cervical spinal cord: CSF signal intensity with hemorrhagic level (**a**, **b**) and enhancing solid part (**c**). Cyst walls enhance as well (**c**). "Cap sign" at cranial and caudal margin of the tumor and edema in the cord above the cranial margin of the tumor (**a**, **b**)

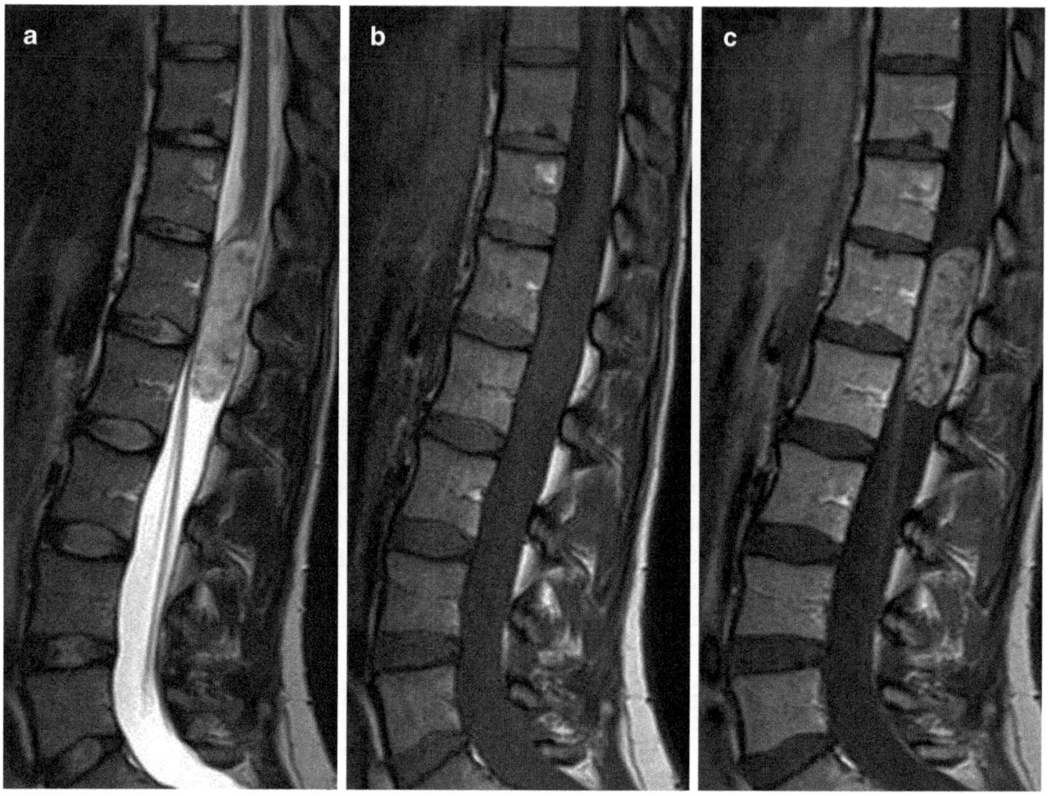


**Fig. 2** Myxopapillary ependymoma. Sagittal non-contrast T2WI (**a**), T1WI (**b**), contrast-enhanced T1WI. Oval, well-circumscribed tumor at the conus level, hyperintense on T2WI (**a**), isointense on T1WI (**b**), revealing inhomogeneous, intense contrast enhancement on contrast-enhanced T1WI (**c**)

### 4.1.2 Astrocytoma

Astrocytoma is the second most common spinal cord tumor in adults and the most common spinal cord tumor in children. These tumors are infiltrating masses composed of neoplastic transformed astrocytes, which vary from well-differentiated to anaplastic. Due to infiltrative nature of the tumor, complete surgical removal without damage to functional tissue is usually impossible (Kim et al. 2016). In almost 90% of cases, astrocytomas are low-grade neoplasms. Fibrillary astrocytoma (WHO II) is usually seen in the cervical spine, whereas pilocytic astrocytoma (WHO I) is found mostly in the conus. The glioneuronal tumor with neuropil-like islands is a newly described variant of the anaplastic astrocytoma (WHO II or III): several cases have been reported in the spinal cord, recently also with diffuse meningeal dissemination (Huisman 2009; Ruppert et al. 2011). Glioblastomas in the spinal cord are uncommon. Astrocytomas are typically intramedullary masses which diffusely expand the spinal cord having an eccentric location within the cord. They usually span spinal multiple segments in craniocaudal extent with an average length of involvement of 4 to 7 vertebral body segments, or the entire spinal cord (holocord presentation) which is more common in children than in adults. They can show areas of necrotic-cystic degeneration, can have a "cyst with a mural nodule" appearance, or can be completely solid (approximately 40% of the cases). The solid portion of the tumor is isointense or mildly hypointense on T1WI, hyperintense on T2WI, and may show mild to moderate contrast enhancement, usually patchy enhancement pattern. On DTI, long-tract fibers may be interrupted. The cystic part is usually moderately hyperintense to CSF on T2WI (Merhemic et al. 2016). Peritumoral edema could be present in up to 40%. Astrocytomas have an association with NF-1. Based on one study on intramedullary tumors in

NF-1, intramedullary spinal cord tumors associated with NF-1 tend to occur predominantly in male patients and are histopathologically likely to be an astrocytoma (Marko and Weil 2012).

### 4.1.3 Hemangioblastoma

Hemangioblastoma (HB) of the CNS is the third most common intramedullary spinal neoplasm, representing 2 to 10% of all intramedullary tumors. It is a benign vascular lesion classified as a WHO grade 1 tumor. Two thirds of HB are mostly sporadic with a peak presentation in the fourth decade, only rarely occur in children. One third of patients with HB have von Hippel-Lindau syndrome, presenting earlier in life with multiple tumors (Chung et al. 2014). HBs consist of large pale stromal cells packed between blood vessels, usually occur in the cerebellum, brainstem, and spinal cord, most common thoracic cord followed by the cervical cord. The majority of HBs consist of intramedullary component, mostly located eccentrically, and exophytic component, often along the dorsum of the cord. One quarter of HB are entirely intramedullary, while minority appear entirely extramedullary. On MRI, HBs usually appear as discrete nodules, but can cause diffuse cord expansion as well. Solid component of the HB is usually hypo- to isointense on T1WI, rarely hyperintense, iso- to hyperintense on T2WI with focal flow voids. Surrounding edema and associated syrinx are usually seen while hemosiderin "cap sign" may be present. On contrast-enhanced T1WI the tumor nodule strongly enhances. About 60–75% of HBs are disseminated or due to transudation of fluid by the tumor itself. HB are rarely the cause of subarachnoid or intramedullary hemorrhage (Koda et al. 2014). Surgery is curative in sporadic cases. The recurrence rate after surgery has been reported to be 15–27%, and diffuse spread and disseminated seeding are rarely reported.

### 4.1.4 Spinal Cord Metastases

Intramedullary spinal metastases (ISM) represent 8.5% of CNS metastases, account for 5% of all intramedullary lesions, and are less common than leptomeningeal metastases. Intramedullary metastases are most common in lung cancer (>50% of cases). Other primary malignancies include breast cancer, melanoma, lymphoma, leukemia, renal cell cancer, and colorectal cancer. According to the study of Rykken et al., the primary malignancy has not always been diagnosed at the time of ISM symptom onset or reference MR imaging, and patients can be asymptomatic with regard to the ISM, even in the case of multiple ISMs (Rykken et al. 2013a, b). The mechanism of cord infiltration of a metastatic mass is ambiguous. Proposed theories of tumor seeding are: (1) hematogenous dissemination leading to arterial embolization, (2) retrograde infiltration via the spinal cord venous system (Batson plexus), (3) spread through perforating veins in the bone, (4) metastatic antidromic cellular migration via nerve root to the spinal cord, (5) CSF dissemination through intraspinal perineural sheaths, (6) penetration of the spinal cord parenchyma via penetrating vessels within the Virchow-Robin spaces (Samartzis et al. 2015). Spinal cord metastases are well-encapsulated masses eccentrically located in the cord, causing its expansion over several segments, usually involving the thoracic cord. Cystic changes or intralesional hemorrhage is rare. On MRI, intramedullary metastases are hypointense on T1WI and hyperintense on T2WI with prominent surrounding edema. On contrast-enhanced T1WI, almost all enhance: two signs, "rim" sign (peripheral thin, complete or partial, rim of increased enhancement) and "flame" sign (ill-defined enhancement extending above and/or below the lesion) are reported useful in the differentiation of intramedullary metastases and primary spinal cord tumors (Rykken et al. 2013a, b; Fig. 3).

### 4.1.5 Spinal Cord Cavernous Malformation

Spinal cord cavernous malformations or spinal cavernomas are rare vascular malformations that occur within the spinal cord consisting of blood-filled endothelial-lined spaces lined by thickened, hyalinized walls that lack elastic fibers and smooth muscles. Most common location is thoracic cord followed by cervical spinal cord. They represent up to 5% of intramedullary lesions in adults and 1% in children (Kharkar et al. 2007). In adult age, they usually present during the fourth decade with pain, weakness,

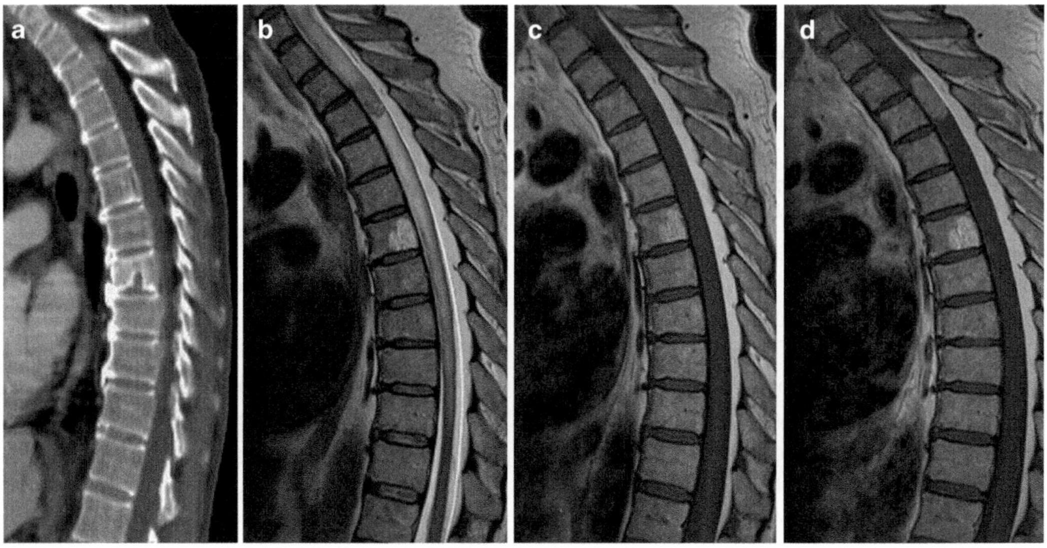


**Fig. 3** Spinal cord metastasis in male patient with disseminated lung carcinoma (one brain metastasis in precentral gyrus). Sagittal CT (**a**), non-contrast T2WI (**b**) and T1WI (**c**), contrast-enhanced T1WI (**d**). Expansile solid lesion centrally located in the thoracic spinal cord: hypointense on T2WI (**b**), isointense on T1WI (**c**), demonstrates intense homogeneous contrast enhancement on CT (**a**) and contrast-enhanced T1WI (**d**). Pronounced spinal cord edema above and below metastasis (**b**)

and paresthesias. Episodes of hemorrhage underlay acute episodes of neurological deterioration (Ogilvy et al. 1992). "Popcorn-like" appearance is a typical MRI feature of the spinal cavernomas: rounded lesions of heterogeneous signal intensity on T1WI and T2WI due to blood products of varying ages, and hypointense rim on T2WI due to hemosiderin, with minimal or no contrast enhancement on post-contrast T1WI. These tumors cause minimal cord expansion or edema unless there has been recent hemorrhage. Surgical resection should be considered for all symptomatic patients before repeated hemorrhage or enlargement occur (Ogilvy et al. 1992; Figs. 4 and 5).

## 4.2 Intradural-Extramedullary Tumors

### 4.2.1 Schwannomas

Schwannomas or neurinomas are the most common benign (WHO grade I) nerve sheath tumors of the spine arising from Schwann cells of a sensory nerve root. Males and females are equally affected, and the age of onset is usually between 25 and 50 years (Lenzi et al. 2017). They may be intradural (70–75%), extradural (15%), or combined intradural/extradural (15%) or a dumbbell tumor. They appear as a solitary, globular, well-defined, encapsulated mass, well-defined and separated from the other rootlets. Multiple schwannomas occur in children with neurofibromatosis type 2 (NF-2), an autosomal dominant genetic disorder caused by inactivation of the gene 22q, which acts as a tumor suppressor. Patients with NF-2 develop multiple central and peripheral nervous system tumors, a hallmark unilateral or bilateral vestibular schwannoma, and other cranial and spinal nerve schwannomas, as well as meningiomas and ependymomas (Evans 2009). Schwannomas are classified into two types based on distinct histological patterns: Antoni A and B types. Both types are composed of uniformly spindled Schwann cells, type A is highly cellular with cellular fascicular regions, while type B is hypocellular with myxoid stroma, and cystic or microcystic areas. It is often thought that type B represents degenerated type A tissue. Tumors develop as fusiform masses eccentrically

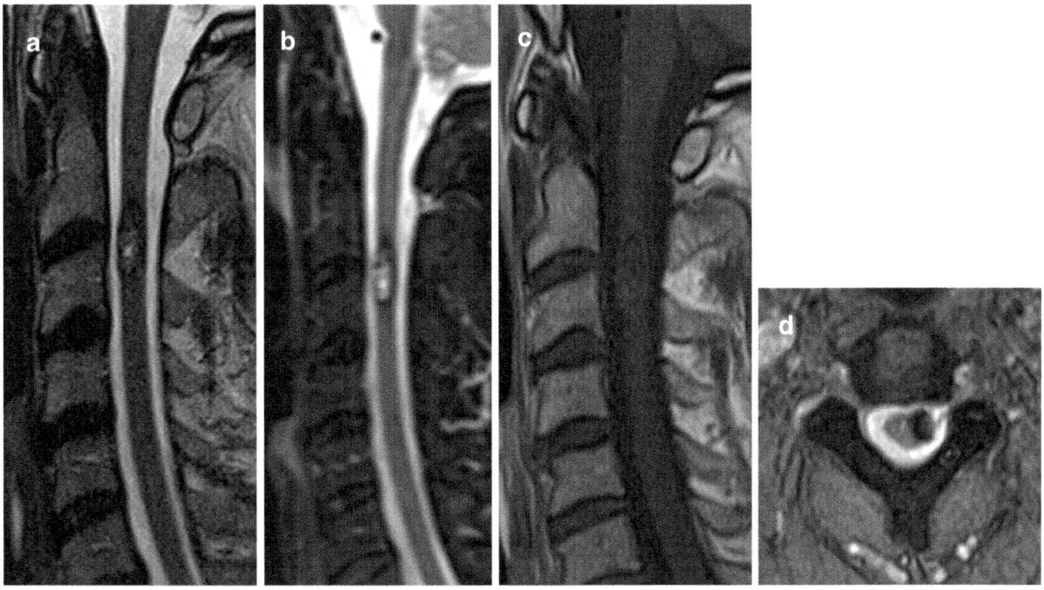


**Fig. 4** Spinal cord cavernous malformation in the cervical spinal cord. Sagittal T2WI (**a**), STIR (**b**), T1WI (**c**), axial T2WI. "Pop corn" lesion in the left lateral column with hemosiderin rim (**a**, **b**, **d**)

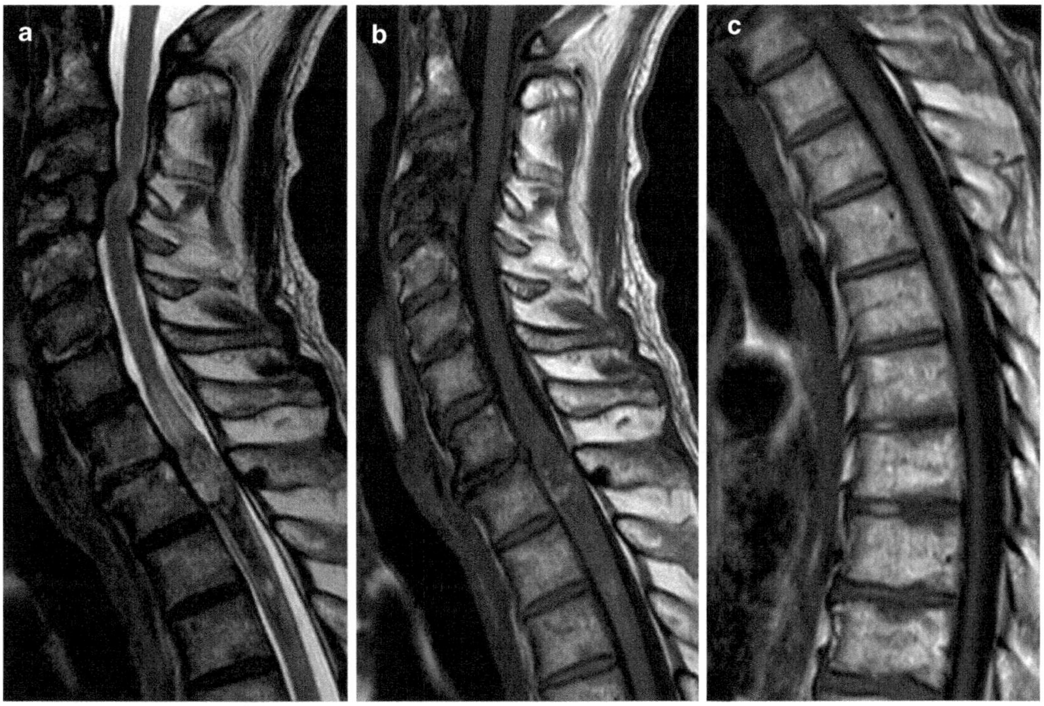


**Fig. 5** Spinal cord cavernous malformation with previous hemorrhage. Sagittal T2WI (**a**), T1WI (**b**, **c**). Cavernous malformation in the thoracic spinal cord: mild cord expansion, mild edema above the cavernoma superior margin, sign of previous hemorrhage in the central spinal cord canal below the cavernoma (**a**–**c**)

located with the involved nerve and are contained within the epineurium; on MRI, typically iso-to-hyperintense on T1WI, hyperintense on T2WI, revealing moderate to marked, usually homogenous, enhancement on contrast-enhanced T1WI. Tissue heterogeneity is relatively common, particularly cystic degeneration, and correlates histologically with a greater ratio of Antoni B tissue (Crist et al. 2017; Fig. 6).

On MRI, type A predominant tumors tend to be small and homogeneous, while heterogeneous tumors (with or without cystic degeneration) tend to have higher proportions of type B. Larger and more heterogeneous tumors also demonstrate increased hemosiderin deposits and may be referred to ancient schwannomas (Wippold 2nd et al. 2007). Malignant degeneration of schwannomas is exceedingly rare. According to a recently published study, heterogeneously enhancing schwannomas should be followed closely, as they grow more rapidly and may require surgery (Ando et al. 2016; Fig. 7).

### 4.2.2 Neurofibromas

Neurofibromas are slow-growing benign tumors (WHO grade I), composed of neoplastic Schwan cells and fibroblasts, without a true capsule developing from dorsal spinal nerve roots, peripheral nerves, and in the spinal canal (40% of patients). Neurofibromas comprise 5% of all benign soft tissue tumors, and in 90%, occur as sporadic solitary tumors. Neurofibromas are associated with NF-1, common genetic autosomal dominant syndrome characterized by a combination of clinical traits: cafe´ au lait macules, Lisch nodules (iris hamartomas), neurofibromas (cutaneous, subcutaneous, plexiform), optic pathway gliomas, and bone dysplasia. Spinal manifestations of NF-1 include bone changes such as acute kyphoscoliosis at the cervical-thoracic junction and vertebral body anomalies, soft tissue abnormalities such as dural ectasia and lateral meningocele, and various spinal tumors, including nerve sheath tumors such as neurofibromas, plexiform neurofibromas (PN), and intramedullary glial tumors. Patients with

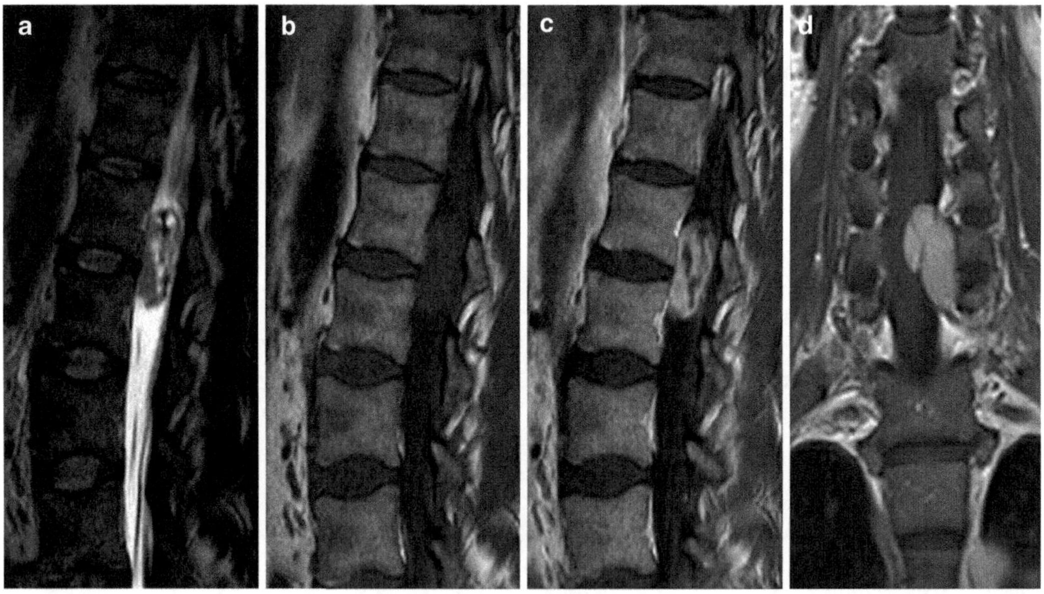


**Fig. 6** Schwannoma. Sagittal non-contrast T2WI (**a**, **e**) and T1WI (**b**, **f**), contrast-enhanced sagittal (**c**, **g**) and coronal (**d**) T1WI. Intradural extramedullary schwannoma in the lumbar spinal canal. Large, oval, well-circumscribed Schwannoma, heterogeneous in appearance with cystic areas (**a**, **c**) and a few hemosiderin deposits (**a**), demonstrates heterogeneous, intense contrast enhancement (**c**). Large, well-circumscribed dumbbell-shaped Schwannoma in the left neural foramina—thoracic spine (**d**). Small, round, well-defined Schwannoma between spinal roots in the left part of the dural sac, hypointense on T2WI (**e**), isointense on T1WI (**f**), demonstrates homogeneous contrast enhancement (**g**)

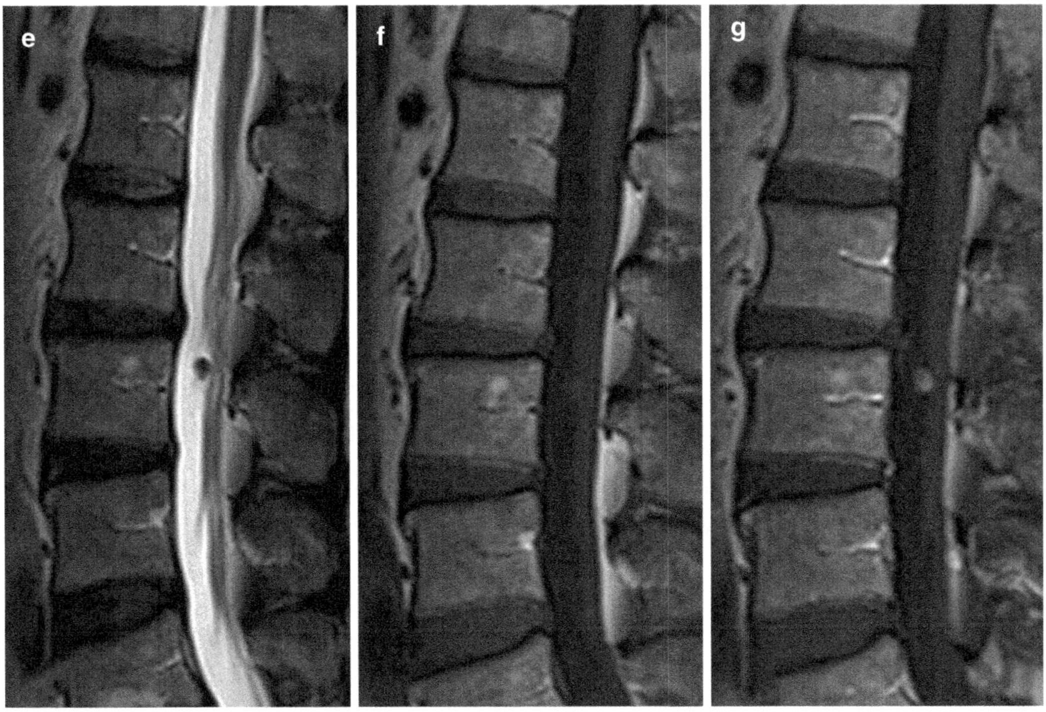

**Fig. 6** (continued)

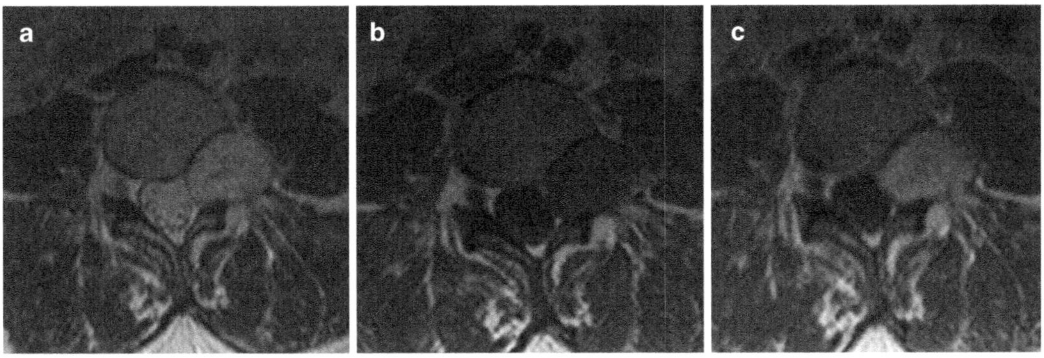

**Fig. 7** Ancient Schwannoma. Axial non-contrast T2WI (**a**) and T1WI (**b**), contrast-enhanced T1WI (**c**). Large, oval, well-circumscribed tumor in the left neural foramina at the L4-L5 level of the lumbar spine: slightly inhomogeneous, hyperintense on T2WI (**a**), hypointense on T1WI (**b**), demonstrates intense contrast enhancement (**c**)

neurofibromatosis have an increased risk of developing malignant peripheral nerve sheath tumors, which tend to be more aggressive compared with patients without neurofibromatosis (Mauda-Havakuk et al. 2017; Fig. 8). Neurofibromas are typically recognized as round or fusiform tumors, isointense on T1WI and markedly hyperintense on T2-weighted MR images, revealing intense homogeneous enhancement or, in some cases, peripheral enhancement on post-contrast T1WIs. They are difficult or impossible to categorically distinguish from Schwannomas.

### 4.2.3 Meningiomas

Meningiomas are the second most common intradural extramedullary tumor arising from the coverings of the spinal cord. They have the highest incidence in women between 45 and 74 years of

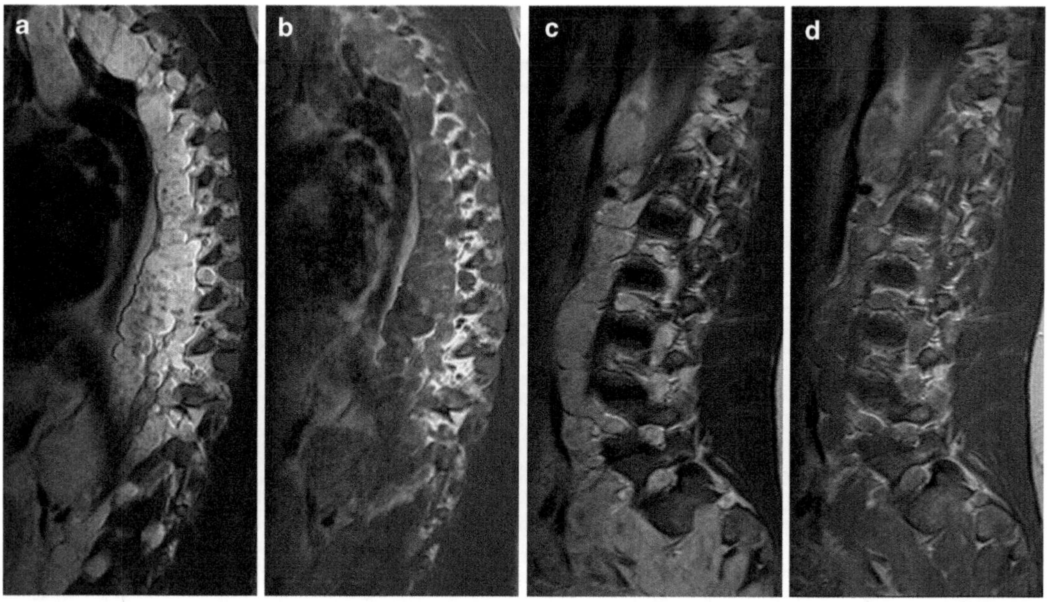


**Fig. 8** Plexiform neurofibromas in NF-1 along the thoracal and lumbosacral spine. Sagittal T2WI (**a**, **c**) and contrast-enhanced T1WI (**b**, **d**)

age and predominantly occur in the thoracic region located posterolaterally, followed by cervical and lumbosacral region (Kshettry et al. 2015). Most meningiomas are intradural and only 10% are extradural or dumbbell tumors. Meningiomas are benign tumors (WHO grade I), while grade II (intermediate) or atypical meningiomas and grade III (malignant) or anaplastic meningioma are less common, having more aggressive features, differing according to number of mitosis and several other cytologic characteristics. Grade III tumors are often solitary tumors, while rare multiple tumors are associated with NF-2 (Louis et al. 2016). MRI characteristics of spinal meningiomas are typically round, well-circumscribed broad-base masses with a "dural tail" into the adjacent dura, isointense to the spinal cord on T1WI and T2WI, revealing moderate or marked homogeneous enhancement on post-contrast T1WI (Fig. 9). Meningiomas have an excellent prognosis with complete surgical resection in more than 90% of cases.

### 4.2.4 Hemangiopericytoma

Hemangiopericytomas (HPCs) are rare vascular tumors that arise from pericytes, the contractile cells surrounding capillaries, also known as the pericytes of Zimmermann (Chew et al. 2017). HPCs share histological features and genetic alteration similar to solitary fibrous tumors (Louis et al. 2016). This tumor is classified as a WHO grade II tumor. Anaplastic HPC grade III will be diagnosed if the tumor contains infiltrative margins, high cellularity, nuclear pleomorphism, areas of tumor necrosis, and an increased mitotic index. Primary spinal HPCs are divided into extradural lesions, and intradural intramedullary or extramedullary lesions. The extradural lesions are further classified as either dural-based or primarily osseous (Ramdasi et al. 2014). HPCs' features on imaging are multilobulated "dumbbell"-shaped masses, expanding and eroding bone, hypointense on T1WI, moderately hyperintense on T2WI, revealing homogeneous enhancement on contrast-enhanced T1WI (Zhang et al. 2014). Total resection is possible, but intraoperative bleeding due to the high vascularity of this tumor may be the greatest obstruction. Therefore, preoperative embolization is recommended to facilitate surgical resection.

### 4.2.5 Paraganglioma

Paragangliomas (PGs) are neuroendocrine tumors that arise in adrenal glands or in the head

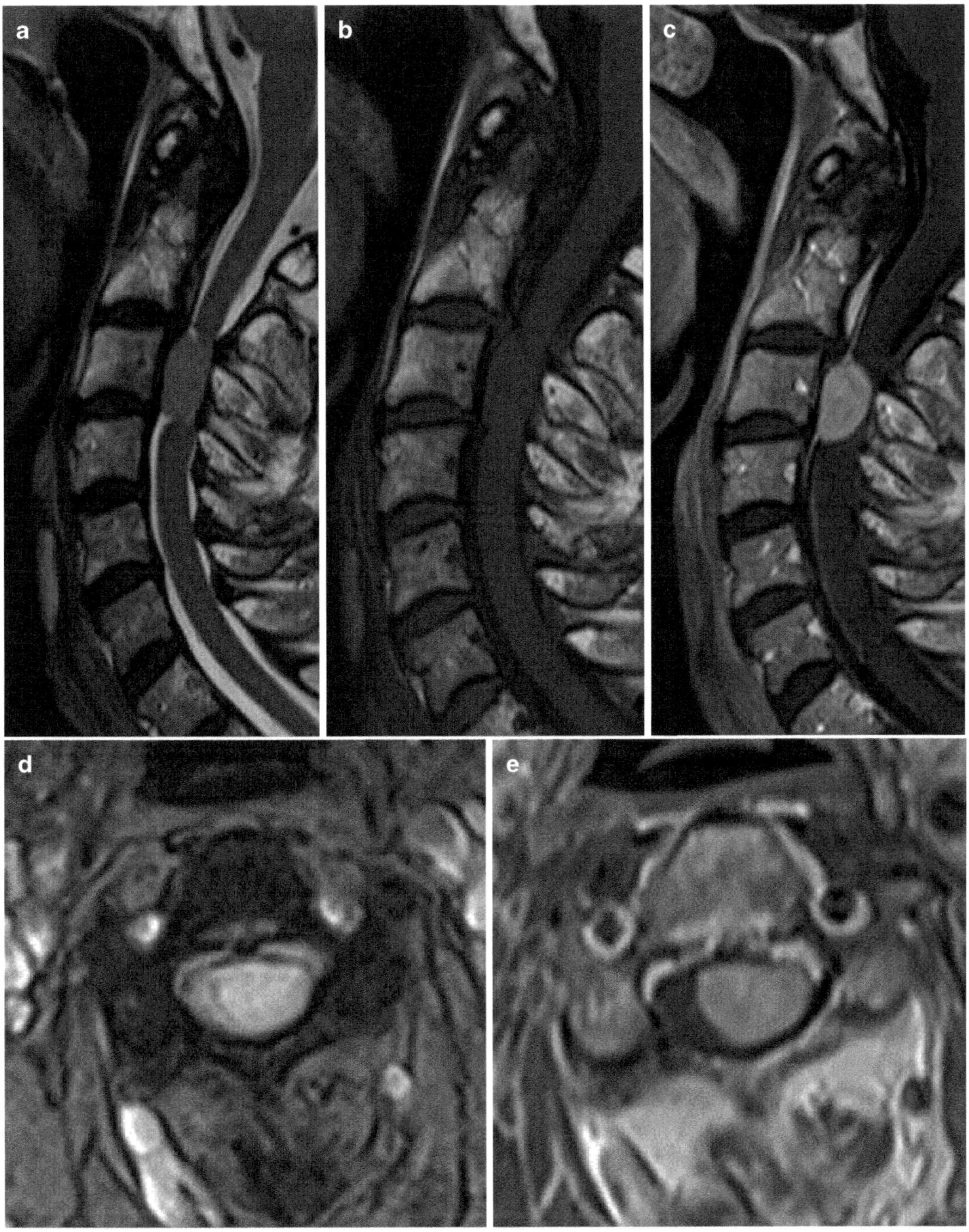


**Fig. 9** Meningioma in the cervical spinal canal. Sagittal non-contrast T2WI (**a**) and T1WI (**b**), and contrast-enhanced T1WI (**c**), axial T2WI (**d**) and contrast-enhanced T1WI (**e**). Intradural extramedullary mass in the cervical spinal canal at the C3 level, hyperintense on T2WI (**a**, **d**), isointense on non-contrast T1WI (**b**), demonstrates intense homogeneous contrast enhancement on T1WI (**c**, **e**) and a "dural tail" sign (**c**). Mass is compressing and dislocating spinal cord (**d**, **e**), without signs of compression myelopathy (**a**, **d**)

and neck: tumors of the carotid body and glomus jugulare constitute more than 90% of reported extra-adrenal PGs. Spinal PGs are rare, slow-growing benign tumors (WHO grade I) that involve filum terminale and cauda equina (Mishra et al. 2014). All PFs consists of two cell types, type I which represents lobules or nests of chief cells, called Zellballen, which are surrounded by a single layer of sustentacular cells or type II (Louis et al. 2016). Most cases of spinal PGs are diagnosed between 30 and 60 years (mean 46 years), with a slight predominance in males. The clinical presentation is either with neuroendocrine symptoms or local mass effect, like lower back pain and sciatica. On MR imaging, PG is a well-delineated mass inferior to the conus, isointense or hypointense on T1WI, hyperintense on T2WI, with a hemosiderin "cap" due to hemorrhage, and marked enhancement. Prominent flow voids and cystic areas can be present. These imaging characteristics could be found in other tumors as well, therefore the diagnosis is rarely made before surgery. Spinal PGs are well-encapsulated tumors and surgical resection is curative in most cases. Radiotherapy is reserved for incompletely resected tumors. Prolonged postoperative observation is mandatory because of the possibility of tumor relapse, even up to 30 years after surgery (Corinaldesi et al. 2015).

### 4.2.6 Melanocytoma

Meningeal melanocytomas are rare, benign, primary melanocytic tumors of the CNS derived from leptomeningeal melanocytes. They are most commonly found in the spinal canal near the foramen magnum, but can occur anywhere along the neuroaxis. Most cases are found in the intradural extramedullary compartment, whereas an intramedullary location is rare (Karikari et al. 2009). These tumors have a peak incidence in the fourth and fifth decades (O'Brien et al. 2006). Melanocytomas appear as well-circumscribed or encapsulated pigmented masses indistinguishable from pigmented meningiomas, schwannomas, and melanomas. On MRI, these tumors appear as isointense to slightly hyperintense lesions on T1-weighted MRI, isointense to hypointense on T2WI, and homogeneously enhance on post-contrast images. The optimal treatment for spinal melanocytoma is complete resection: definitive diagnosis is based solely on histopathological and immunohistochemical examination (Dorwal et al. 2014).

### 4.2.7 Leptomeningeal Metastases

More than 95% of spinal metastases occur in the extradural space, whereas intradural extramedullary and intramedullary metastases are relatively rare. Five routes for metastatic intradural spinal tumor spread have been hypothesized: (1) the rich venous plexus, (2) perineural lymphatics, (3) seeding from involved osseous structures to the CSF through the dura, (4) spreading via the subarachnoid space, and (5) hematogenous spreading via the arterial system (Perrin et al. 1982; Samartzis et al. 2015).

Drop metastasis is considered to occur as a tertiary metastasis of brain metastasis, induced by the circulation of CSF and gravity in the subarachnoid space. Leptomeningeal dissemination from CNS neoplasms occurs in younger patients, most common in medulloblastoma and ependymoma (Lee et al. 2012). Unenhanced MRI may be normal if the lesions are isointense to the spinal cord, or could reveal thickened nerve roots and nodular T2-hypointense lesions. Contrast-enhanced T1WI is mandatory to demonstrate enhancing tumor nodules, nerve roots or cauda equina, or diffuse sheet-like coating of the spinal cord or roots ("carcinomatous meningitis") and thickening of the cauda equina (Merhemic et al. 2016; Fig. 10).

## 4.3 Epidural Tumors

An epidural mass compressing the cord is considered an emergency condition. The major clinical symptoms of acute spinal cord compression are: relatively symmetric paralysis of the limbs, urinary retention/incontinence, and a circumferential boundary below which there is loss of sensation, referred to as the "sensory level" (Ropper and Ropper 2017). Spinal cord or cauda equina compression is an increasing challenge due to a higher prevalence of long-term cancer survivors. Cord compression in patients with cancer is due to spinal metastasis. In one recently published study on 230 patients with neoplastic spinal cord compression, no difference was found between extradural and intradural-extramedullary tumors (Mohme et al.

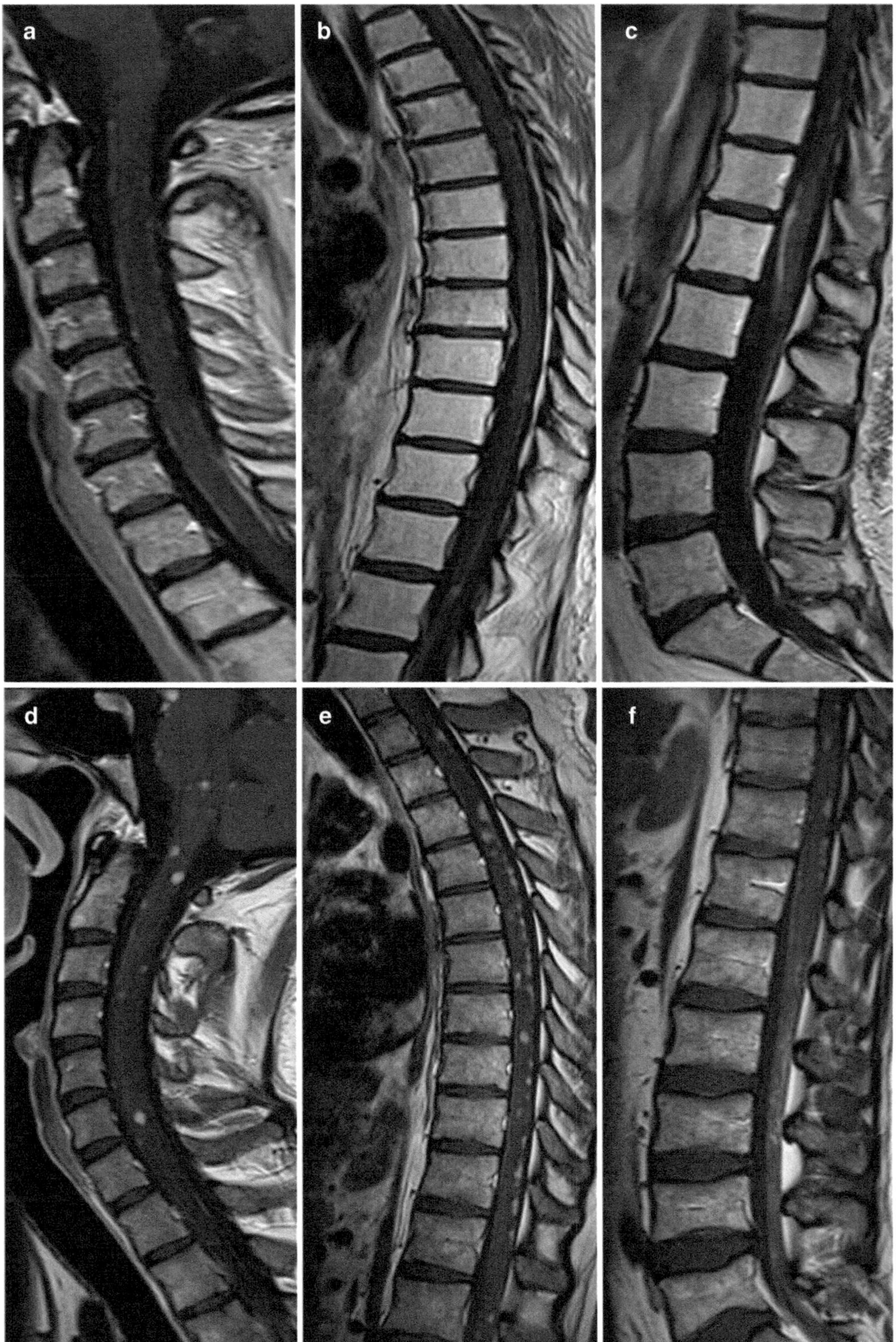


**Fig. 10** Leptomeningeal metastases. Sagittal contrast-enhanced T1WI (**a**–**c**): dissemination of breast carcinoma (**a**–**c**) demonstrates linear leptomeningeal contrast enhancement along the spinal cord. Sagittal contrast-enhanced T1WI (**d**–**f**): dissemination of non-Hodgkin lymphoma (**d**–**f**) demonstrates tumor enhancing nodules along the spinal cord

2017). Beside metastatic disease, spinal cord compression may be caused by lymphoma, myeloma, sarcoma, neuroblastoma, and chloroma. Compression occurs most commonly in thoracic (60%), followed by lumbar (25%) and cervical region (15%) (Ropper and Ropper 2017). MRI is the method of choice in detection of epidural mass compressing the cord with the sensitivity as high as 100%. Treatment of malignant spinal cord compression is palliative with radiotherapy and surgical decompression supplemented by glucocorticoids. A delay in imaging and subsequent treatment may be associated with loss of neurologic function. Imaging of the entire spine is mandatory as patients with tumors-related compression may compress the cord at multiple sites.

#### 4.3.1 Metastases

Vertebral bodies with epidural extension are common site for metastatic disease. Metastatic epidural lesions cause the displacement of the spinal cord from its normal position in the vertebral canal. It represents an oncologic emergency, and if not promptly diagnosed, can lead to a permanent neurological damage. However, recently published study indicates that there is no difference in the chance of neurological recovery if surgery is performed within or after 24 h of the admission to hospital (Pipola et al. 2018). The most commonly affected region is thoracic spine, and the most common primary tumors are lung, breast, and prostate cancer. In the early stages of compression, the spinal cord will show T2-hyperintensity consistent with edema. Later, findings consistent with spinal cord ischemia will be present. Contrast-enhanced sequences with fat-suppression are recommended for better delineation of the extent of epidural invasion.

#### 4.3.2 Lymphoma

Spinal epidural space is a rare location of primary lymphoma, whereas secondary lymphoma may be seen. In children, spinal epidural lymphoma with compressive myelopathy is a serious condition and requires urgent treatment. Common initial symptoms are back pain and low extremity weakness. Higher frequency has been reported in patients with acquired immunodeficiency syndrome (AIDS). On conventional MR sequences, epidural spinal lymphomas show T1- and T2-low signal and intense, homogeneous enhancement (Fig. 11). In immunocompromised individuals, they range from non-enhancing, inhomogeneous enhancing to marked enhancing masses (Thurnher et al. 2000). On diffusion-weighted MR imaging (DWI), they have high signal on trace images and low ADC values due to their high cellularity (Plank et al. 2007). Lymphomas can also be located in the vertebral bodies and also in the paraspinal tissues, all three locations simultaneously are very common.

#### 4.3.3 Sarcoma

Ewing Sarcoma (ES) is among the most frequented extremity osseous tumor in childhood, and spinal epidural space ES presenting with acute tetraplegia has been reported also. Extraosseous ES has a similar demographic as osseous ES, primarily affecting adolescents and young adults (Fletcher et al. 2019).

#### 4.3.4 Chloroma

Chloroma (granulocytic sarcoma) are solid masses composed of malignant myeloid blast cells outside the hematopoietic system. Patients with acute or chronic myeloid leukemia presenting with progressive neurological dysfunction should be suspected of epidural spinal chloroma (Koh et al. 2019). Chloroma will be recognized on MRI as T1- and T2-low signal intensity masses with homogeneous enhancement.

## 5 Spinal Infections

Spinal infections and inflammations carry a risk of severe morbidity and high mortality. They are challenging to diagnose and difficult to distinguish from degenerative processes, vascular injuries, and neoplasms, based only on imaging findings. Clinical symptoms of spinal infections most often include back pain, sensory motor deficits, fever, and obtundation. Fever, however, may not be prominent and body temperature can be normal in patients with chronic infection. Mechanical compression is the most common cause of functional compromise of the spinal cord, with deterioration secondary to ischemic compromise. The clinical presentation of a spon-

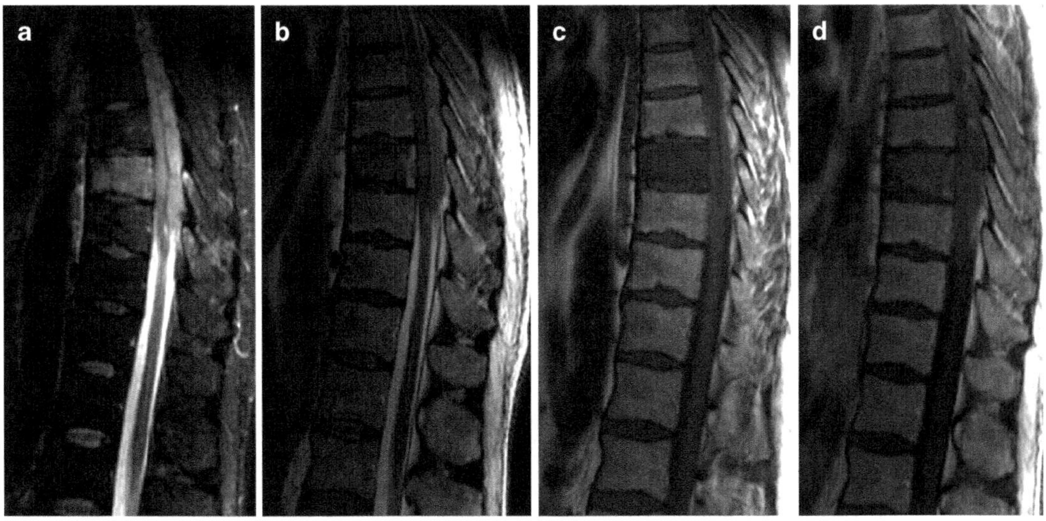


**Fig. 11** Osseous and epidural lymphoma in a 67-year-old male patient. Sagittal STIR (**a**) and T2 (**b**) demonstrate STIR-high, T2-low signal intensity of the vertebral body and T2-low signal intensity epidural mass in the posterior epidural space compressing the thoracic cord. Abnormalities show low signal on T1WI (**c**). Only faint enhancement is noted on sagittal post-contrast T1-WI (**d**)

dylodiscitis is nonspecific with back pain being the most common symptom. In patients with chronic back pain, increase in pain and change of the quality of pain should raise suspicion. Increased temperature and raised erythrocyte sedimentation rate (ESR) are more common than leukocytosis. Epidural abscesses arise with intense pain, but the neurological signs are often vague and usually not localized to a level. In delayed spinal infections after surgery or trauma, the ESR is unreliable; new onset of pain or increase level of pain is a common feature. Biopsies and blood cultures are usually performed to isolate the infectious agent; however, negative results do not exclude spinal infection. Blood cultures are reported positive in 25–50% of cases, whereas needle biopsies have higher sensitivity with positive result in 50–90% (Segreto et al. 2018).

## 5.1 Spinal Cord Abscess/Myelitis

Intramedullary spinal cord abscesses are very rare condition, which may result in serious neurological complication if the diagnosis is delayed. Patients will present with pain, motor and sensory deficits, urinary incontinence, fever, and meningismus (Dörflinger-Hejlek et al. 2010). In children, spinal cord abscesses are related to spinal dysraphism or extension of meningitis. In adults, it could be associated with direct trauma, neurosurgical procedure, and direct extension of infection. The most common bacterial agents are *Mycobacterium tuberculosis*, *Borrelia burgdorferi*, and *Treponema pallidum*. Viral myelitis can be caused by Herpes simplex virus 1 and 2 (HSV), varicella-zoster-virus (VZV), Cytomegalovirus (CMV), Epstein-Bar-Virus (EBV), West Nile Virus and enteroviruses, human immunodeficiency virus (HIV), and Poliovirus. Schistosomiasis is the most common parasitic myelitis (Flanagan and Pittock 2017). MR imaging features of a spinal cord abscess are intramedullary T1-low and T2-high signal intensity abnormality with rim-like enhancement on post-contrast T1WI (Thurnher and Olatunji 2016). DWI can be used to differentiate it from a neoplastic lesion; abscess will show high signal due to restricted diffusion (Dörflinger-Hejlek et al. 2010). Tuberculous myelitis with tuberculoma is common in endemic areas with imaging findings not different from cerebral lesions. Non-caseating tuberculomas are T1- and T2-hypointense, with homogeneous enhancement on post-contrast images. Caseating tuberculomas will show peripheral enhancement

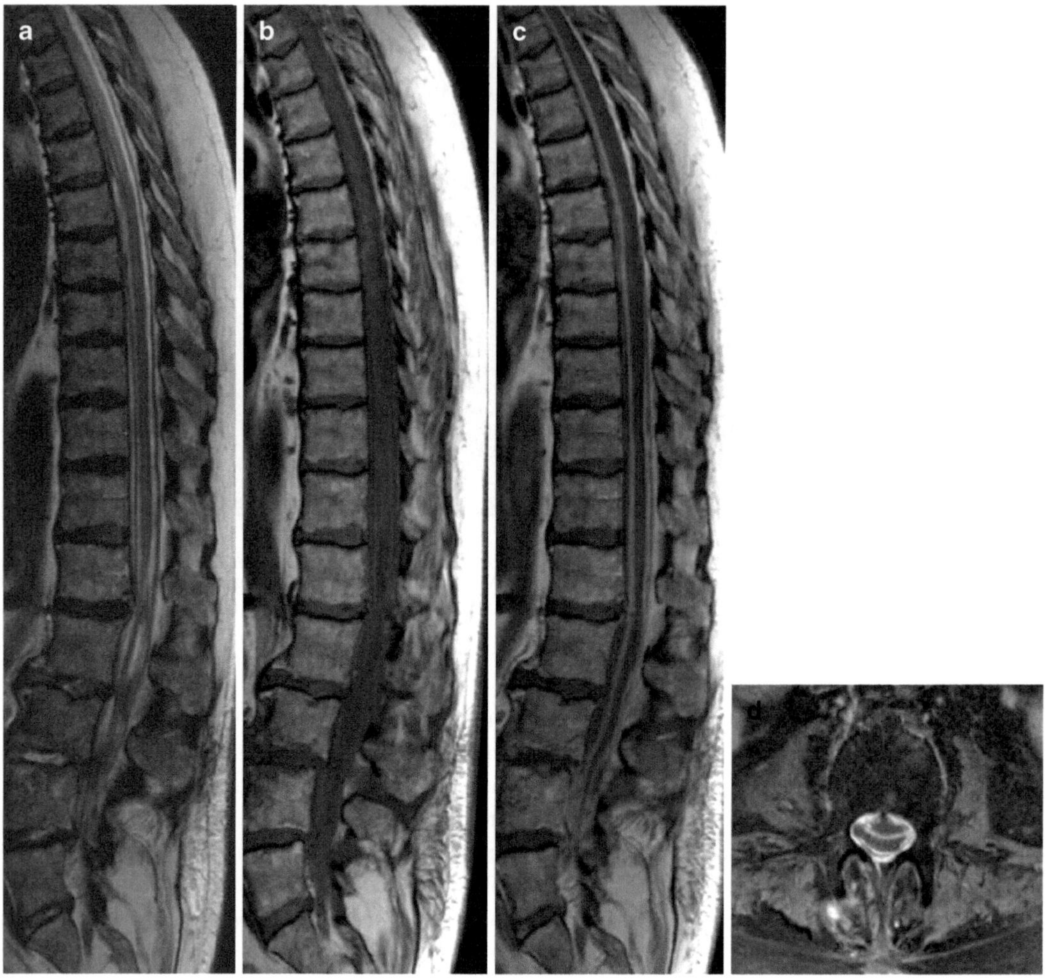


**Fig. 12** Anterior and posterior epidural abscesses extending several spinal segments. Sagittal T2 (**a**) and T1 (**b**) demonstrate T2-high signal intensity, T1-low signal intensity epidural mass in the anterior and posterior epidural space. Peripheral enhancement is detected on sagittal (**c**) and axial (**d**) post-contrast T1-WI (**d**)

(Torres et al. 2014). Viral myelitis usually shows edema of the cord with intramedullary ill-defined T2-hyerintensity with faint or no enhancement.

## 5.2 Spinal Epidural Asbcess

Patients with spinal epidural abscess will present with fever, severe back pain, and/or radicular pain. Thoracic spine is the most frequent location and usually multiple segments are involved. Panspinal epidural abscess has also been reported (Wen et al. 2019). Underlying conditions associated with bacterial spinal epidural abscesses are diabetes, immunosuppression, intravenous drug abuse, and cancer. Staphylococcus aureus is the most common causing agent; however, blood cultures of the cerebrospinal fluid (CSF) are often negative. Epidural abscess can be the only infectious lesion in the spinal canal, mostly due to hematogenus spread of the infection from a non-CNS site. More frequently, epidural abscesses are result of the direct extension of the infection from the spondylodiscitis (Fig. 12). On MRI T2-high, T1-low signal intensity epidural mass will be found with either homogeneous enhancement (phlegmon) or peripheral enhancement (abscess formation) (Figs. 12 and 13). Bacterial spinal epidural abscesses exhibit high signal on

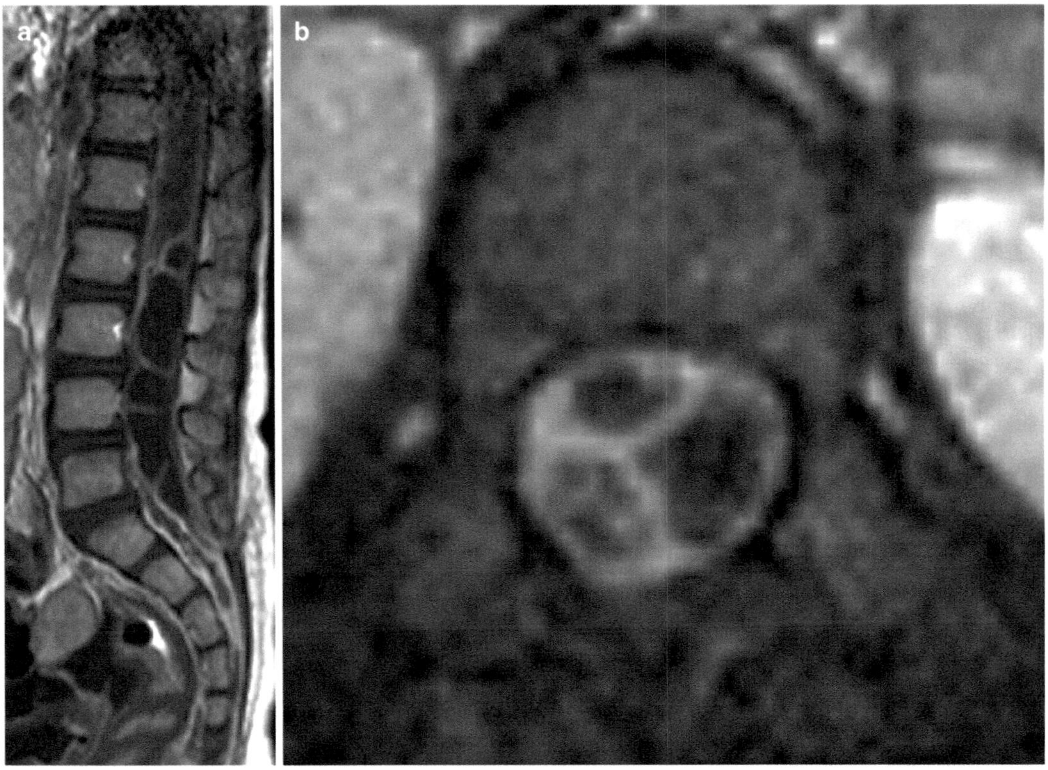


**Fig. 13** Sagittal (**a**) and axial (**b**) contrast-enhanced T1 demonstrate intraspinal multiloculated abscess formation in a 26-month-old infant

trace image with corresponding low ADC values on DWI (Plank et al. 2007). Differential diagnosis includes epidural hematoma, which demonstrates similar findings but does not show gadolinium enhancement. Heterogeneity of signal suggests anticoagulation-associated epidural hematoma. Surgical evacuation is the most successful treatment option (Spennato et al. 2020).

## References

Ando K, Imagama S, Ito Z et al (2016) How do spinal schwannomas progress? The natural progression of spinal schwannomas on MRI. J Neurosurg Spine 24(1):155–159

Arce D, Sass P, Abdul-Khoudoud H (2001) Recognizing spinal cord emergencies. Am Fam Physician 64(4):631–639

Celano E, Salehani A, Malcom J et al (2016) Spinal cord ependymoma: a review of the literature and case series of ten patients. J Neuro-Oncol 128(3):377–386

Chew LS, Han XJ, Tan KK, Bundele MM (2017) Hemangiopericxtoma of the thoracic spine: a case report. J Surg Case Rep 2017(7):rjx121. https://doi.org/10.1093/jscr/rjx121

Chung SY, Jeun SS, Park JH (2014) Disseminated hemangioblastoma of the central nervous system without Von Hippel-Lindau disease. Brain Tumor Res Treat 2(2):96–101

Corinaldesi R, Novegno F, Giovenali P et al (2015) Paraganglioma of the cauda equina region. Spine J 15(3):e1–e8

Crist J, Hodge JR, Frick M et al (2017) Magnetic resonance imaging appearance of schwannomas from head to toe: a pictorial review. J Clin Imaging Sci 7:38

Dörflinger-Hejlek E, Kirsch EC, Reiter H, Opravil M, Kaim AH (2010) Diffusion-weighted MR imaging of intramedullary spinal cord abscess. AJNR Am J Neuroradiol 31(9):1651–2

Dorwal P, Mohapatra I, Gautam D et al (2014) Intramedullary melanocytoma of thoracic spine: a rare case report. Asian J Neurosurg 9(1):36–39

Duong LM, McCarthy BJ, McLendon RE et al (2012) Descriptive epidemiology of malignant and nonmalignant primary spinal cord, spinal meninges, and cauda equina tumors, United States, 2004–2007. Cancer 118(17):4220–4227

Evans DG (2009) Neurofibromatosis type 2 (NF2): a clinical and molecular review. Orphanet J Rare Dis 4:16

Flanagan EP, Pittock SJ (2017) Diagnosis and management of spinal cord emergencies. Handbook of clinical neurology, (3rd series), Critical care neurology Part 1; p 140. Elsevier, Amsterdam

Fletcher AN, Marasigan JAM, Hiatt SV et al (2019) Primary spinal epidural/extramedullary Ewing sarcoma in young female patient. J Am Acad Orthop Glob Res Rev 27(3):e10.5435

Flounders JA, Ott BB (2003) Oncology emergency modules. Spinal cord compression. Oncol Nurs Forum 30(1):E17–E21

Henschke N, Maher CG, Ostelo RW et al (2013) Red flags to screen for malignancy in patients with low-back pain. Cochrane Database Syst Rev 28(2):CD008686

Huisman TA (2009) Pediatric tumors of the spine. Cancer Imaging 2(9):45–48

Karikari IO, Powers CJ, Bagley CA et al (2009) Primary intramedullary melanocytoma of the spinal cord: case report. Neurosurgery 64(4):E777–E778

Kharkar S, Shuck J, Conway J et al (2007) The natural history of conservatively managed symptomatic intramedullary spinal cord cavernomas. Neurosurgery 60(5):865–872

Kim DH, Kim JH, Choi S et al (2016) Differentiation between Intramedullary spinal ependymoma and astrocytoma: Comparative MRI analysis. Clin Radiol 69:29–35

Koda M, Mannoji C, Itabashi T et al (2014) Intramedullary hemorrhage caused by spinal cord hemangioblastoma: a case report. BMC Res Notes 7:823

Koh H, Baek J, Lee MS, Park HJ (2019) Epidural chloroma and spinal cord compression. Chin Med J 132(7):853–855

Krings T, Lasjaunias PL, Hans FJ et al (2007) Imaging in spinal vascular disease. Neuroimaging Clin N Am 17:57–72

Kshettry VR, Hsieh JK, Ostrom QT et al (2015) Descriptive epidemiology of spinal meningiomas in the United States. Spine (Phila Pa 1976) 40(15):886–889

Landi A, Palmarini V, D'Elia A et al (2016) Magnetic resonance diffusion tensor imaging and fibertracking diffusion tensor tractography in the management of spinal astrocytomas. World J Clin Cases 4(1):1–4

Lee CH, Kim KJ, Hyun SJ et al (2012) Intradural extramedullary metastasis of small cell lung cancer: a case report. Korean J Spine 9(3):293–296

Lenzi J, Anichini G, Landi A et al (2017) Spinal nerves schwannomas: experience on 367 cases – historic overview on how clinical, radiological, and surgical practices have changed over a course of 60 years. Neurol Res Int 2017:1–12

Louis DN, Perry A, Reifenberger G et al (2016) The 2016 World Health Organization classification of tumors of the central nervous system: a summary. Acta Neuropathol 131:803–820

Marko NF, Weil RJ (2012) The molecular biology of WHO grade I astrocytomas. Neuro-Oncology 14(12):1424–1431

Mauda-Havakuk M, Shofty B, Ben-Shachar S et al (2017) Spinal and paraspinal plexiform neurofibromas in patients with neurofibromatosis type 1: a novel scoring system for radiological-clinical correlation. AJNR Am J Neuroradiol 38:1869–1875

Merhemic Z, Stosic-Opincal T, Thurnher MM (2016) Neuroimaging of spinal tumors. Magn Reson Imaging Clin N Am 24:563–579

Mishra T, Goel NA, Goel AH (2014) Primary paraganglioma of the spine: a clinicopathological study of eight cases. J Craniovertebr Junction Spine 5(1):20–24

Mohme M, Mende KC, Krätzig T et al (2017) Impact of spinal cord compression from intradural and epidural spinal tumors on perioperative symptoms-implications for surgical decision making. Neurosurg Rev 40(3):377–387

Naito K, Yamagata T, Arima H et al (2015) Qualitative analysis of spinal intramedullary lesions using PET/CT. J Neurosurg Spine 31:1–7

O'Brien DF, Crooks D, Mallucci C et al (2006) Meningeal melanocytoma. Childs Nerv Syst 22(6):556–561

Ogilvy CS, Louis DN, Ojemann RG (1992) Intramedullary cavernous angiomas of the spinal cord: clinical presentation, pathological features, and surgical management. Neurosurgery 31(2):219–229

Perrin RG, Livingston KE, Aarabi B (1982) Intradural extramedullary spinal metastasis. A report of 10 cases. J Neurosurg 56:835–837

Perry A, Prayson RA (2012) Glial and glioneuronal tumors. In: Prayson RA (ed) Neuropathology, vol 2. Elsevier Inc, Philadelphia, pp 461–512

Pipola V, Terzi S, Tedesco G et al (2018) Metastatic epidural spinal cord compression: does timing of surgery influence the chance of neurological recovery? An observational case-control study. Support Care Cancer 26(9):3181–3186

Plank C, Koller A, Mueller-Mang C et al (2007) Diffusion-weighted MR imaging (DWI) in the evaluation of epidural spinal lesions. Neuroradiology 49(12):977–985

Ramdasi RV, Nadkarni TD, Goel NA (2014) Hemangiopericytoma of the cervical spine. J Craniovertebr Junction Spine 5(2):95–98

Ropper AE, Ropper AH (2017) Acute spinal cord compression. N Engl J Med 376:1358–1369

Ruppert B, Welsh CT, Hannah J et al (2011) Glioneuronal tumor with neuropil-like islands of the spinal cord with diffuse leptomeningeal neuraxis dissemination. J Neuro-Oncol 104(2):529–533

Rykken JB, Diehn FE, Hunt KM et al (2013a) Intramedullary spinal cord metastases: MRI and relevant clinical features from a 13-year institutional case series. AJNR Am J Neuroradiol 34(10):2043–2049

Rykken JB, Diehn FE, Hunt CH, Eckel LJ, Schwartz KM, Kaufmann TJ, Wald JT, Giannini C, Wood CP (2013b) Rim and flame signs: postgadolinium MRI findings specific for non-CNS intramedullary spinal cord metastases. AJNR Am J Neuroradiol 34(4):908–915

Samartzis D, Gillis CC, Shih P et al (2015) Intramedullary spinal cord tumors: part I-epidemiology, pathophysiology, and diagnosis. Glob Spine J 5(5):425–435
Segreto FA, Beyer GA, Grieco P et al (2018) Vertebral osteomyelitis: a comparison of associated outcomes in early versus delayed surgical treatment. Int J Spine Surg 12(6):703–712
Spennato P, Renedo D, Cascone D et al (2020) Spinal epidural abscess in children: a case-based review. Childs Nerv Syst 14. https://doi.org/10.1007/s00381-020-04609-3. Epub ahead of print
Thurnher MM, Olatunji RB (2016) Infections of the spine and spinal cord. Handbook of clinical neurology, Vol. 136 (3rd series) Neuroimaging Part II. Elsevier, Amsterdam
Thurnher MM, Post MJ, Jinkins JR (2000) MRI of infections and neoplasms of the spine and spinal cord in 55 patients with AIDS. Neuroradiology 42(8):551–563
Torres C, Riascos R, Figueroa R et al (2014) Central nervous system tuberculosis. Top Magn Reson Imaging 23:173–189
Wen D, Norman J, Dassan P, Sandhu G (2019) Resolution of group B streptococcal panspinal epidural abscess in a patient with diabetes after treatment with ceftriaxone and linezolid. BMJ Case Rep 12(11):e232243. https://doi.org/10.1136/bcr-2019-232243
Wippold FJ 2nd, Lubner M, Perrin RJ et al (2007) Neuropathology for the neuroradiologist: antoni a and antoni B tissue patterns. AJNR Am J Neuroradiol 28:1633–1638
Zhang P, Hu J, Zhou D (2014) Hemangiopericytoma of the cervicothoracic spine: a case report and literature review. Turk Neurosurg 24(6):948–953

# Myelitis and Myelopathies

Paola Crivelli and Maurizio Conti

## Contents



## 1 Introduction

The term "myelopathy" is usually used to indicate spinal cord involvement caused by some pathological conditions (Hauser 2005). Myelitis is the medical term used to define spinal cord involvement only by an inflammatory or infectious disorder. Spinal cord disorders may have a different course, and it can occur as a single event or a recurrent disease (Sánchez et al. 2011).

P. Crivelli (✉) · M. Conti
University of Sassari, Sassari, Italy
e-mail: mconti@uniss.it

Clinical presentation can vary, depending on specific tract and localization involved, as well as their extension. In particular, on axial plane, lesions may be prevalent in grey matter (segmentary syndrome, both ventral and dorsal), white matter (anterolateral or posterior columns), or both (segmentary syndrome with columns involvement), resulting in a complete or no transection (Fig. 1). We define Brown-Sequard syndrome as the clinical syndrome resulting from an injury to one lateral side of spinal cord, complete or partial. Moreover, we classify spinal syndrome on the basis of longitudinal extension in mono or poli metameric, according to numbers of



M. Scaglione et al. (eds.), *Emergency Radiology of the Head and Spine*,
Medical Radiology Diagnostic Imaging, https://doi.org/10.1007/978-3-030-91047-1_19

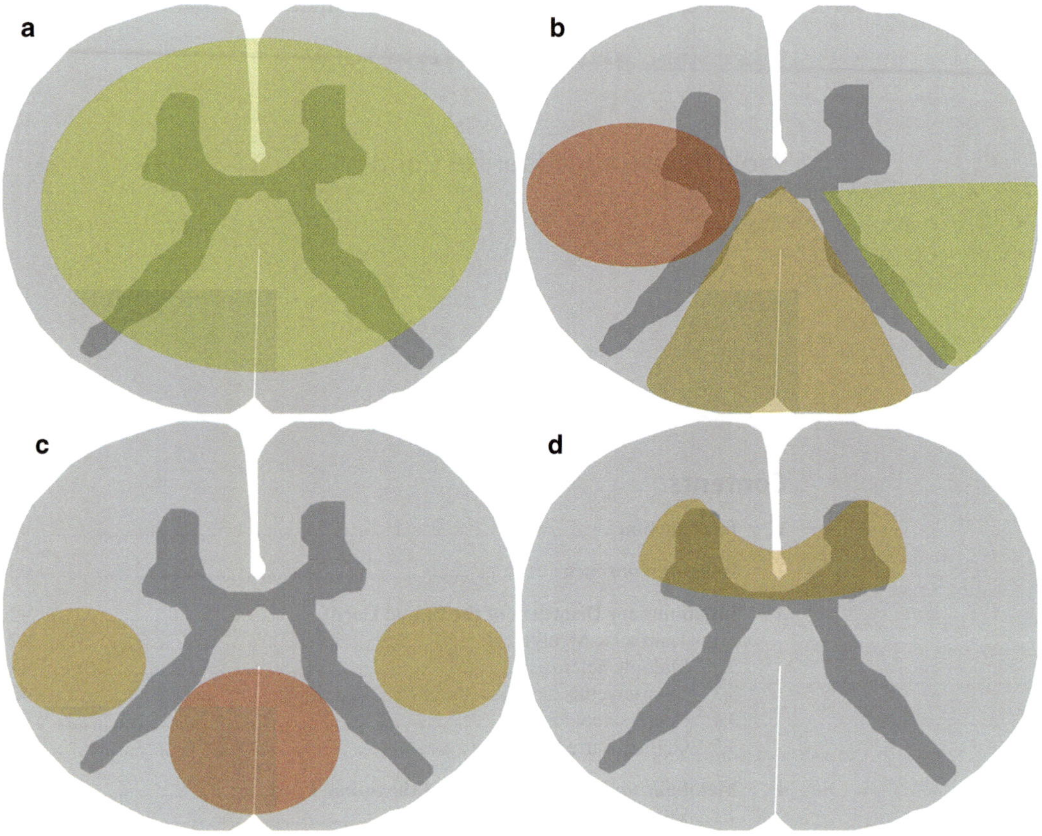


**Fig. 1** Differential diagnosis of myelopathies based on the patterns of spinal cord involvement on axial MR images. (**a**) Acute transverse myelitis. Centrally located lesion involving both halves of the cord. (**b**) Multiple sclerosis. Triangular or round in shape and mostly located dorsally or laterally, usually less than two thirds of the axial plane. (**c**) Vitamin B12 deficiency. Posterior and/or lateral columns involved. (**d**) Spinal cord infarction. Typically located in the anterior spinal artery territory (owl-eyes appearance)

metamers involved. An accurate clinical examination associated with a correct neuroimaging pathway is mandatory to lead a correct and early etiological diagnosis (Scotti and Gerevini 2001).

Myelopathy can be classified into compressive or not compressive, depending on subarachnoid space obstruction (Hauser 2005).

## 2 Imaging Approach

Magnetic Resonance Imaging (MRI) plays a pivotal role in the study of spinal cord, being extremely sensitive in detecting their signal alteration also in earlier phase. MRI was performed with high-field equipment, from 1.5 to 3 Tesla, and usually requires medium contrast administration, which enables radiologist to distinguish not just different pathological conditions, but also the activity degree of disease (Ghezzi et al. 2001). Computed tomography (CT) is useful only in case of trauma injuries, but it is inadequate to provide information about damages of nervous structures constituting spinal cord. In the past decades, myelography was utilized as alternative imaging tool to study spinal cord, in patients whose MRI was contraindicated, but nowadays their application is extremely limited (Hauser 2005).

## 3 Inflammatory Disorders of the Spinal Cord

Inflammatory noninfectious disorders of the spinal cord are represented by several different conditions, characterized by a broad spectrum of symptoms and imaging findings, nonspecific and overlapping with other diseases. Transverse myelitis is the most prevalent spinal cord disease, frequently triggered by both inflammatory and infectious disorders (Ghezzi et al. 2001). We describe neuroimaging of transverse myelitis, being a "model" of other inflammatory spinal cord injuries, and then multiple sclerosis, neuromyelitis optica, neuro-sarcoidosis, and Guillan-Barré syndrome (Schmalstieg et al. 2010).

## 3.1 Transverse Myelitis

Transverse myelitis, both idiopathic and secondary to inflammatory, infectious, or other pathological conditions, is a rare focal disorder approximately affecting 1–8 per one million people per year, without sex and race prevalence. The transverse myelitis shows a bimodal peak of incidence, between 10 to 19 years and 30 to 39; in 64% of cases, the disorder is idiopathic. Clinical presentation depends on the spinal cord level involved and their extension, the onset may be acute or subacute, resulting in signs and symptoms of motor, and autonomic disorders, variably associated with a clear sensory rostral level. Thirty-three percent of cases recover without severe deficit, 33% have a moderate grade of residual disability, and 33% are permanently disabled (Ghezzi et al. 2001). Pathogenesis differs in idiopathic or secondary transverse myelitis, and this spinal affection cannot be defined as a pure demyelinating disorder, involving neurons, axons, oligodendrocytes, and myelin. The thoracic spinal cord is the most prevalent site involved (Jacob and Weinshenker 2008). In emergency setting, neuroimaging must be performed in order to exclude compressive cause in patient with spinal syndrome; CT could be done to find a compressive cause, but MRI remains the main diagnostic instrument to study medullary alterations (Transverse Myelitis Consortium Working Group 2002). We find a different, nonspecific finding, such as increased signal on T2 sequences, involving more than two thirds of the cross-sectional area of the cord (Fig. 2) with longitudinal extension variable between three or more metamers (Choi et al. 1996). A small area, hypointense to cord, central to lesion, can be found in rare cases (Jacob and Weinshenker 2008). Gadolinium enhancement is generally strong, quite homogeneous but peripherally prevalent, and it is useful for differential diagnosis between inflammatory and neoplastic lesion (Choi et al. 1996).

## 3.2 Multiple Sclerosis

Multiple Sclerosis (MS) is an inflammatory demyelinating disease of the central nervous system, and it is the most frequent neurological degenerative cause of disability in young adult, with an incidence variable from 1 per 100,000 in equatorial region to 30 to 80 per 100,000 in the northern Europe and the United States. MS occurs more frequently in female, and the common age of presentation is between 30 and 40 years. The clinical presentation is variable, depending on lesion site (Tartaglino et al. 1995). The spinal localization of MS is responsible for a variety of symptoms, from paresthesia or weakness to sphincter dysfunctions, such as bowel and bladder disorders (i.e., constipation, urgent incontinence).

MRI is mandatory in case of suspected spinal MS lesions, but it must be completed by a brain neuroradiological study to assess encephalic involvement (McDonalds criteria, reviewed by Polman in 2010). MS lesions are typically peripheral, involving less than half of the area of spinal cord in the axial images and less than two vertebral bodies in the sagittal plane. They show a high signal on T2-weighted sequences and iso to low signal on T1-W ones (Sánchez et al. 2011). MS plaques can show a variable contrast enhancement after Gadolinium administration, and it depends on the inflammatory activity degree, being more intense in acute or subacute lesions (until 2 months). The pattern of enhancement varies, and it may be nodular, ring-like, or homogeneous (Fig. 3). In the acute and subacute stage of disease, a moderate spinal cord swelling can be associated, while in the chronic or advanced phase of MS the cord atrophy is prevalent (Polman et al. 2010). Several authors reported a

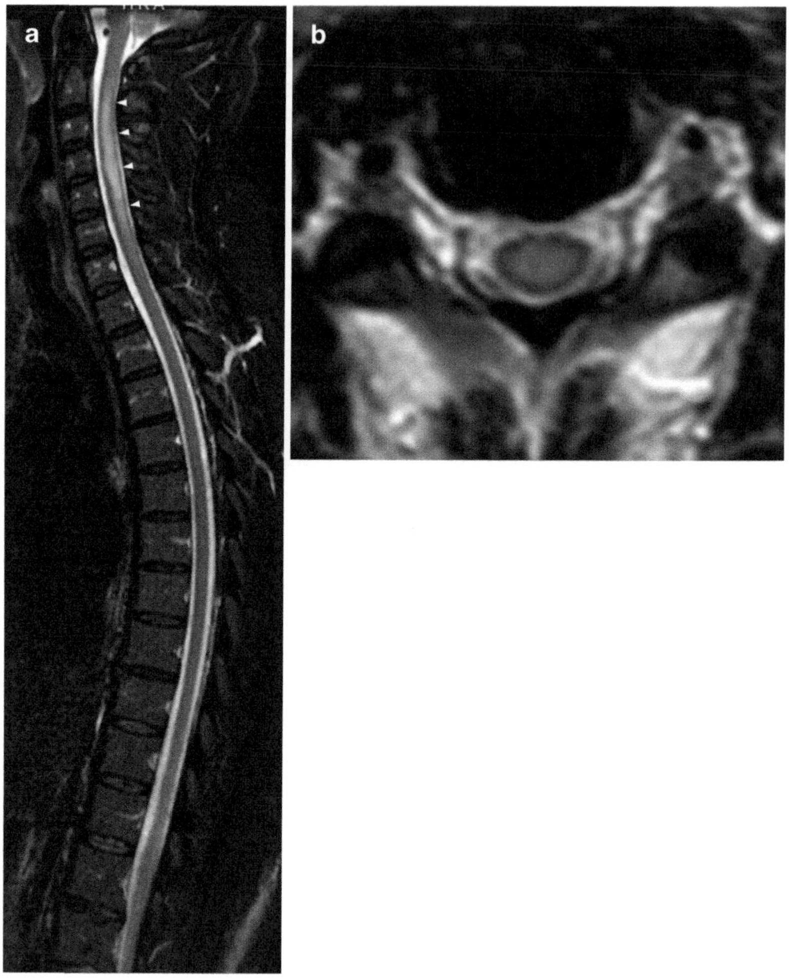


**Fig. 2** Transverse myelitis. STIR sagittal (**a**) and T2W axial (**b**) MR images show a large lesion in the cervical cord extending over a length of three-four vertebral bodies with high signal cord expansion and edema (arrowheads). On the axial image, the lesion occupies the entire cross-sectional cord area

decreased fractional anisotropy with increased mean diffusivity in MS acute spinal cord lesions, similarly to vascular injury. MRI plays a pivotal role in follow-up, being essential to monitoring evolution and therapeutical efficacy (Bot et al. 2004).

## 3.3 Neuromyelitis Optica

Neuromyelitis optica, or Devic's disease, is a demyelinating syndrome clinically characterized by the coexisting of optic neuritis, unilateral or bilateral (i.e., visual symptoms, from ocular pain to blindness), and extensive transverse myelitis (often weakness with bowel or bladder dysfunction), usually recurrent (Wingerchuk 2006).

The real incidence of this pathological condition is controversial, being higher in Asia and South America, and it affects more frequently women (female to male ratio 3:1) with mean age of 38–40 years. The symptoms are often similar to MS, but the identification of a specific serum biomarker, called aquaporina-4 antibody, makes the difference. Although optic nerve lesion is not frequently found on MRI images, the cord involvement can always be found. In particular, MRI shows a central-longitudinal lesion, extended for three or more metamers, frequently with swelling or edema (T2-high intensity), however indistinguishable from other transverse myelitis (Fig. 4) (Sánchez et al. 2011). In some cases, axial images show a typical spine aspect "snake-eyes"; gadolinium enhancement can be

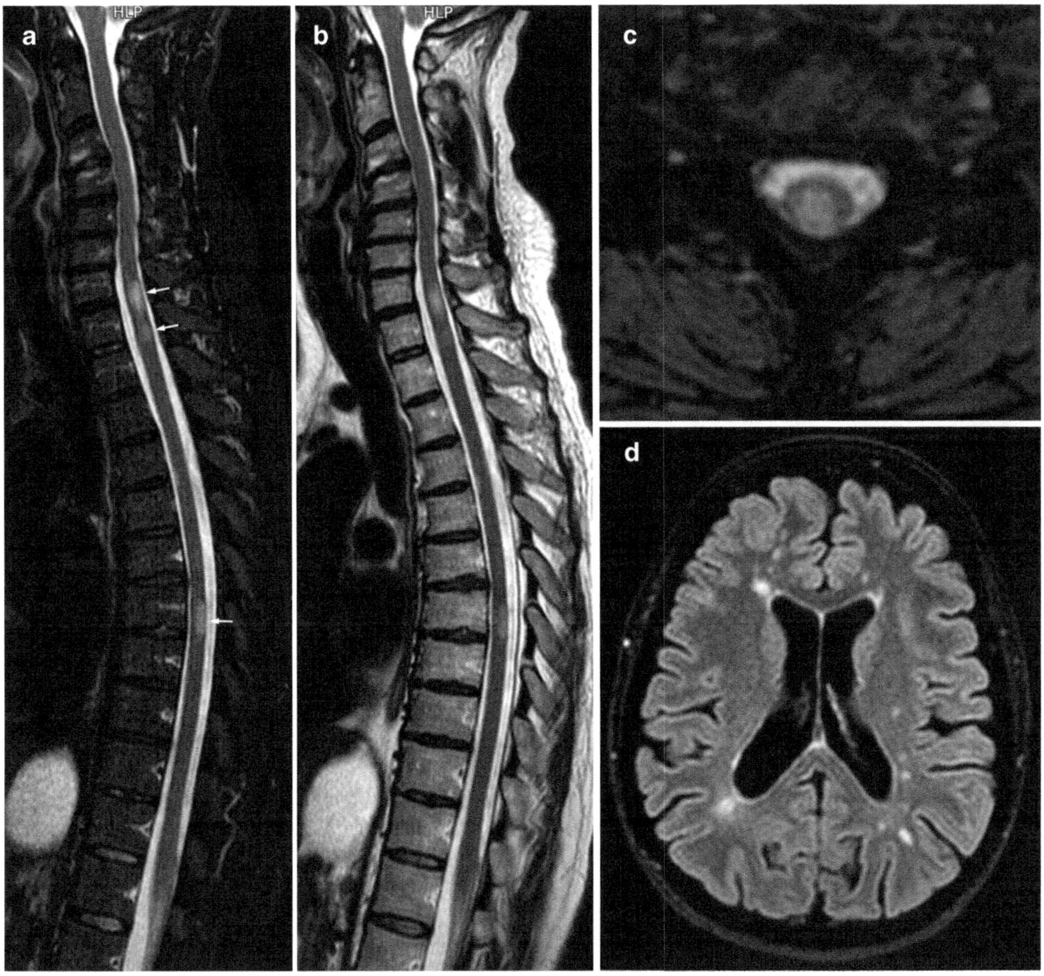


**Fig. 3** Multiple sclerosis in a 54-year-old woman. STIR (**a**) and T2-W (**b**) sagittal image shows multifocal hyperintense lesions (arrows) in spinal cord at the C7-T1 and T7 level extending longitudinally for less than two vertebral bodies. Gradient echo T2 axial image through the level of C7-T1 (**c**) shows abnormal hyperintensity located centrally and dorsally. FLAIR axial image of brain (**d**) reveals multiple patchy hyperintense lesions in deep periventricular white matter, suggestive of typical multiple sclerosis

found, especially in clinical acute phase of disease. The spinal cord atrophy can be a consequence of continuous recurrences (Wingerchuk 2006).

## 3.4 Neuro-sarcoidosis

Sarcoidosis is an idiopathic granulomatous inflammatory disease, characterized by the presence of noncaseating granulomas potentially involving all parts of the body. The incidence of systemic form of sarcoidosis is variable, more prevalent in Northern Europe population (in Sweden about 11.5 per 100,000 per years) and in African American (17.8 per 100,000 per years), with female prevalence (Arkema and Cozier 2018). The mean age can vary, occurring early in males (45 years old vs 54). The sites typically affected are the lymph-nodes and the lung, but the central nervous system involvement is frequent, accounting about 25% of autopsy. Nevertheless, only 10% of patients of systemic sarcoidosis show images' involvement of CNS, and 5% are symptomatic (Arkema and Cozier 2018). The clinical presentation is often similar to MS, in particular

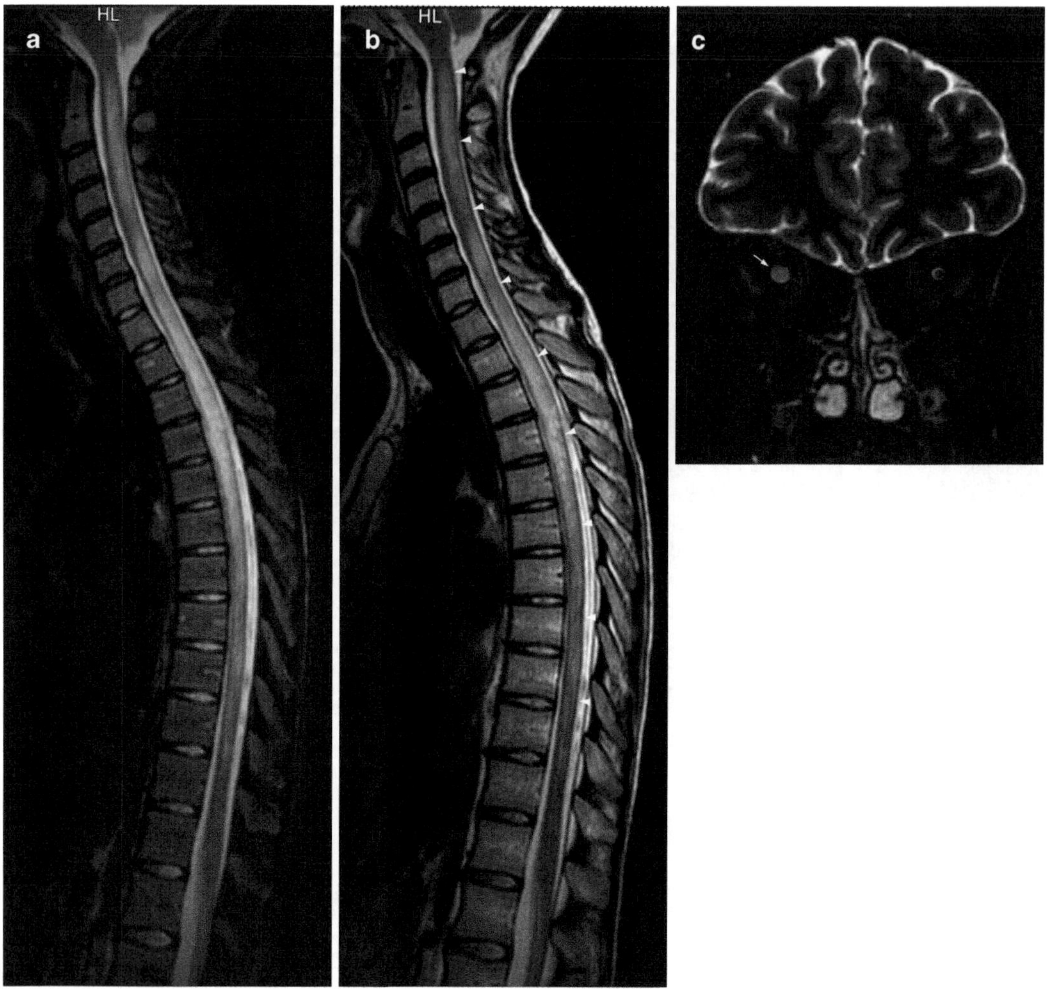


**Fig. 4** Neuromyelitis optica. T2W (**a**) and STIR (**b**) MR images of the spine show a longitudinally extensive lesion with high signal cord expansion and edema (arrowheads). Coronal STIR MR image (**c**) through the orbits shows hyperintensity of the right optic nerve (arrow), consistent with optic neuritis in neuromyelitis optica

spinal cord lesions can present with lower limbs' weakness or not specific signs of myelopathy. Spinal cord lesions are typically localized on the cervical or upper-dorsal tract (Junger et al. 1993). MRI detects a focal fusiform enlargement of spinal cord, hyperintense in T2 images, hypointense in T1 ones, and with patchy contrast enhancement (Fig. 5) (Lury et al. 2004). Leptomeningeal or dura involvement can occur, alone or in association with medullary lesions, often in early stages, according to Junger classification (Junger et al. 1993). Spinal atrophy occurs in late stage of disease. Imaging is mandatory to diagnosis; early treatment of spinal symptomatic lesions can reduce the complications, although the radiological improvement seems not to correlate with clinical resolution (Koike et al. 2000).

## 3.5 Guillan-Barré Syndrome

Guillan-Barré syndrome (GBS) is the most common cause of acute flaccid paralysis, racing from 1,2–3 per 100,000 cases per years in the United Stated of America. GBS can occur equally in males and females, and their incidence increases with age, but it can be found also in young people; a genetic susceptibility has been hypnotized

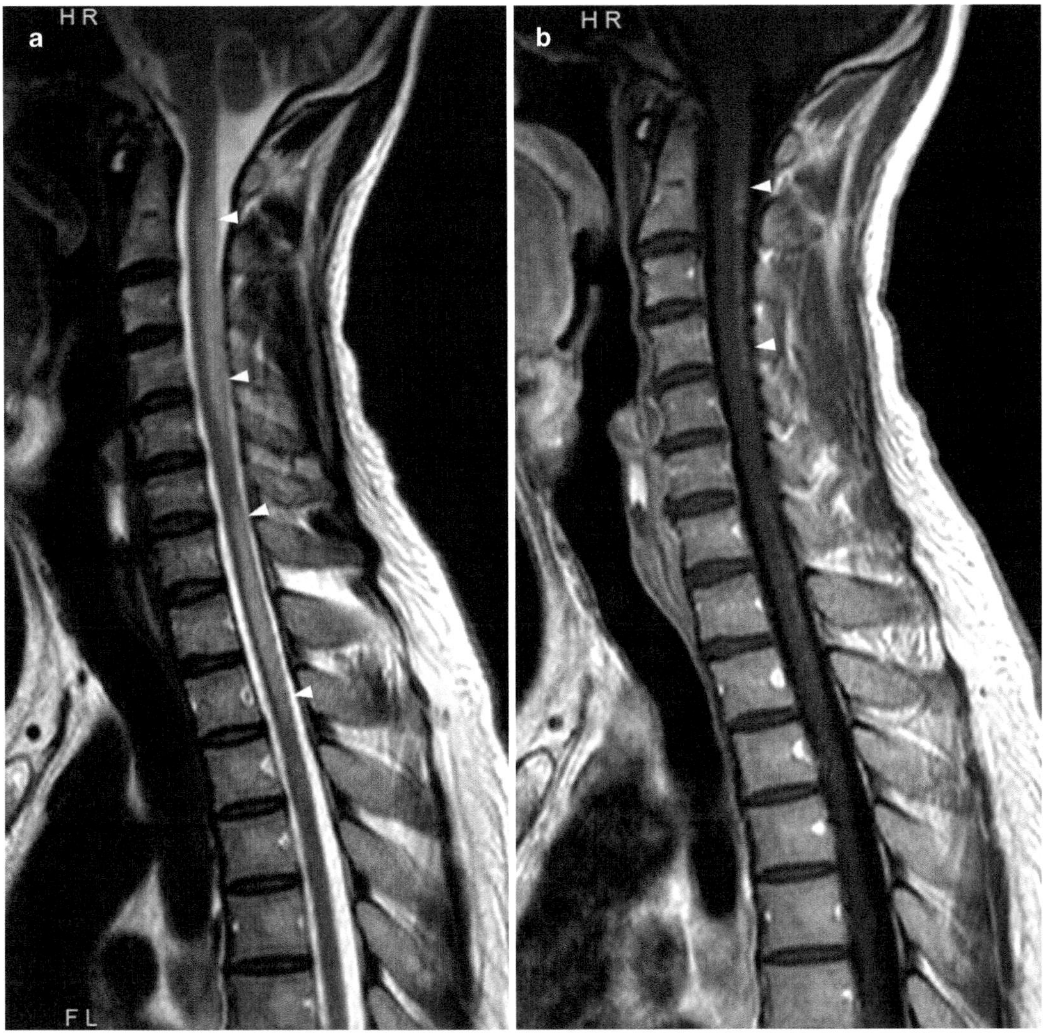


**Fig. 5** Neuro-sarcoidosis myelitis. T2W (**a**) and T1W post-contrast sagittal (**b**) MR images show fusiform enlargement of the spinal cord in the cervical and upper thoracic level in craniocaudal dimension, with high signal on T2W image (arrowheads) and enhancement along the posterior spinal surface after gadolinium administration (arrowheads)

(Andari et al. 2020). Despite their idiopathic nature, several viral or bacterial infections and vaccinations have been described to precede the clinical onset, probably responsible of an immune-mediated reaction against Schwann cells myelin sheath (Yu et al. 2006). Clinical presentation can vary; usually patients complain of a symmetric and rapidly progressive weakness of more than one limb, up to paralysis, without sensory damages (Yuki and Odaka 2005). Neurological examination reveals hypo-areflexia of affected limbs as well as cranial nerve involvement and autonomic dysfunction. In more severe cases, respiratory paralysis can occur, requiring ventilation (Kuwabara 2007).

MRI should be done in all suspected cases before the liquor examination, but often CT is preliminary performed in emergency room to exclude an acute compression cause. MRI shows a typical slight and smooth enlargement of the spinal nerve roots of the cauda equina, usually the ventral ones, often pathologically enhanced (Fig. 6). There isn't pathological signal alteration of the spinal cord (Kuwabara 2007).

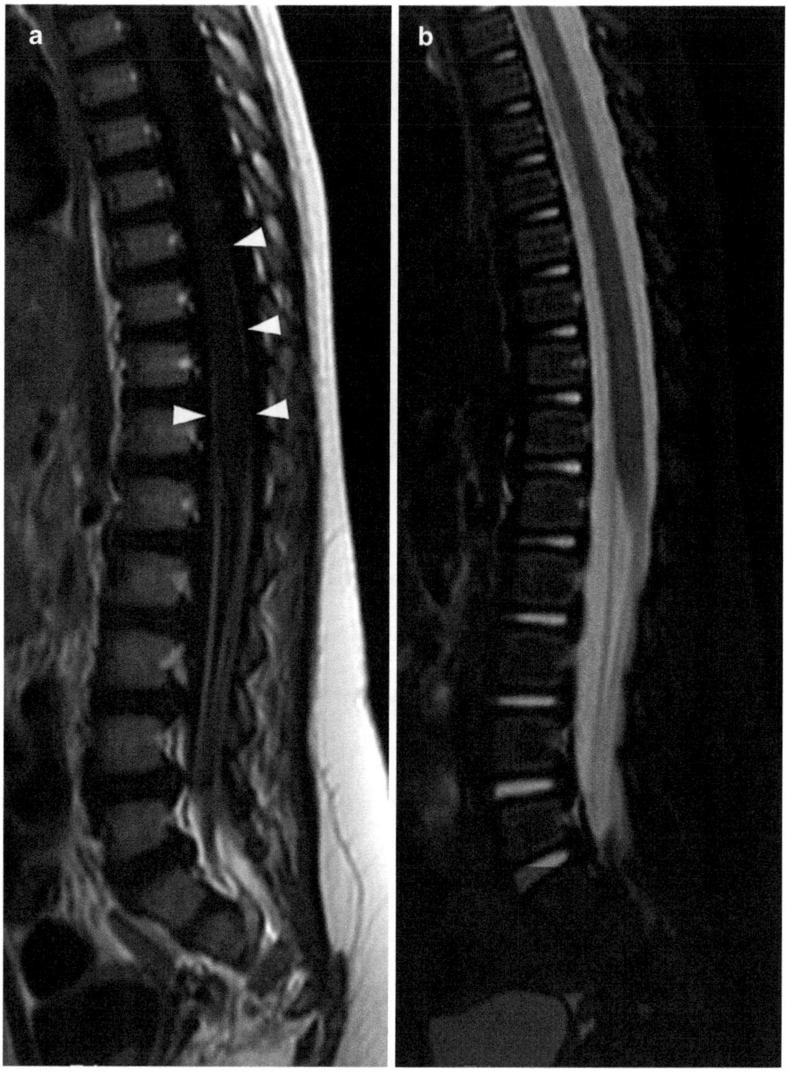


**Fig. 6** Post-vaccination, Guillain-Barré syndrome in a child. Sagittal T1W MR image (**a**) shows enlargement and contrast enhancement of the spinal nerve roots of the cauda equine and a slight pial enhancement on the distal cord surface (arrowheads). There is no signal abnormality on STIR MR image (**b**)

## 4 Metabolic and Toxic Affections of the Spinal Cord

Several metabolic affections, both nutritional deficiency and systemic disorders, involve nervous system, usually peripheral nerves or brain, but also spinal cord can be affected by these pathological conditions, although more rarely. Clinical presentation can vary on the basis of cause of spinal cord injury, and we could classify these heterogeneous groups of conditions in myelopathy secondary to identified nutritional deficit (i.e., vitamin B12, folate, or vitamin E deficiencies), to systemic metabolic conditions (i.e., diabetes mellitus, chronic hepatic diseases), to drugs or toxic agents' exposure (i.e., drugs, chemotherapeutic agents, or radiation) (Ramalho et al. 2016).

We illustrate the most frequent metabolic and toxic myelopathies, focusing on vitamin B12 deficiencies, diabetic and hepatic myelopathy, and spinal cord injury caused by toxicity, both iatrogenic (i.e., chemotherapeutical drugs or radiation) and accidental (i.e., heroine abuse or organophosphate poisoning).

### 4.1 Vitamin B12 Myelopathy

Nutrition deficit of vitamin B12 can be secondary to inadequate intake (i.e., strict vegetarian) or malabsorption (i.e., gastrectomy, intestinal infections, or ileal resection, intestinal disorders causing chronic malabsorption such as celiac disease) and it represents the most common cause of metabolic myelopathies, accounting from 4.8% to 12% of elderly population (Andres et al. 2004). The vitamin B12 deficiency determines spongy vacuolation and myelin degeneration and can cause several nervous damages, involving both peripheral and central nervous system, particularly dorsal and lateral spinal cord columns, resulting in symmetric subacute combined degeneration (Ramalho et al. 2016). Clinical presentation is heterogenous, depending on site affected, and can be characterized by paresthesia, stiffness, gait disorders, ataxia, spasticity, and sensory limbs loss especially in lower ones. Paresthesia is usually symmetric and distal, representing the early symptom; progression of disease can lead to ataxia, spastic paraparesis, and sensory loss until anesthesia. Early diagnosis and prompt treatment are essential to reduce permanent damages, and imaging plays a pivotal role identifying the cord involvement, their precise localization, and extension (Andres et al. 2004). CT is not helpful, being in the most cases normal. MRI could be performed in all suspected cases, in order to demonstrate the signal alteration (hyperintensity on T2 sequences) of dorsal and, less frequently, lateral columns, usually localized in cervical and upper thoracic cord. Sagittal T2 sequences show a long continuous hyperintensity along the dorsal cord surface, and axial T2 view can demonstrate the symmetric involvement of dorsal-lateral columns in the form of increased signal, pathognomonic of SCD (Fig. 7). MRI could be performed also in follow-up, to demonstrate decrease of signal abnormalities due to treatment (Ramalho et al. 2016).

### 4.2 Diabetic Myelopathy

Although the peripheral nervous system is more frequently involved, the spinal cord can also be involved in diabetes mellitus, probably in patient with genetic predisposition, accounting up to 41% of medullary abnormalities on autoptic study of diabetic population (Selvarajah et al. 2006). Clinical presentation can overlap with symptoms due to peripheral nerves damages, but the signs of posterior and lateral columns' involvement are helpful for differential diagnosis (Prick et al. 2001). MRI is mandatory to detect abnormalities of spinal cord, usually in the cervical tract, representing hyperintensity of lateral-posterior columns, well-demonstrated on T2 sequences, likely due to both demyelination phenomena and coexisting microvessel damages, but less extent than in B12 deficiencies myelopathy. A relative spinal atrophy can be found (Eaton et al. 2001).

### 4.3 Hepatic Myelopathy

Chronic liver disease with portal hypertension is often associated with porto-systemic encephalopathy, which is the most common neurological complication (Utku et al. 2005). In some cases, also spinal cord can be involved and this pathological condition, usually found in patient with shunting both spontaneous and surgical, is called hepatic or porto-systemic myelopathy. The abnormal concentration of nitrogenous products, such as ammonia or mercaptans, bypass the liver, causing demyelination, with a predilection of lateral corticospinal tract, prevalent in the cervical spine. In several patients, the spinal involvement can be extent to posterior columns, spinothalamic and spinocerebellar tracts, but likely due to alcohol abuse (Premkumar et al. 2012). Clinically, patients show a pure motor progressive spastic paraparesis, without other sensitive or autonomic signs. MRI demonstrates the lateral corticospinal tract involvement as an increased signal on T2 sequences, with an inconstant patchy gadolinium

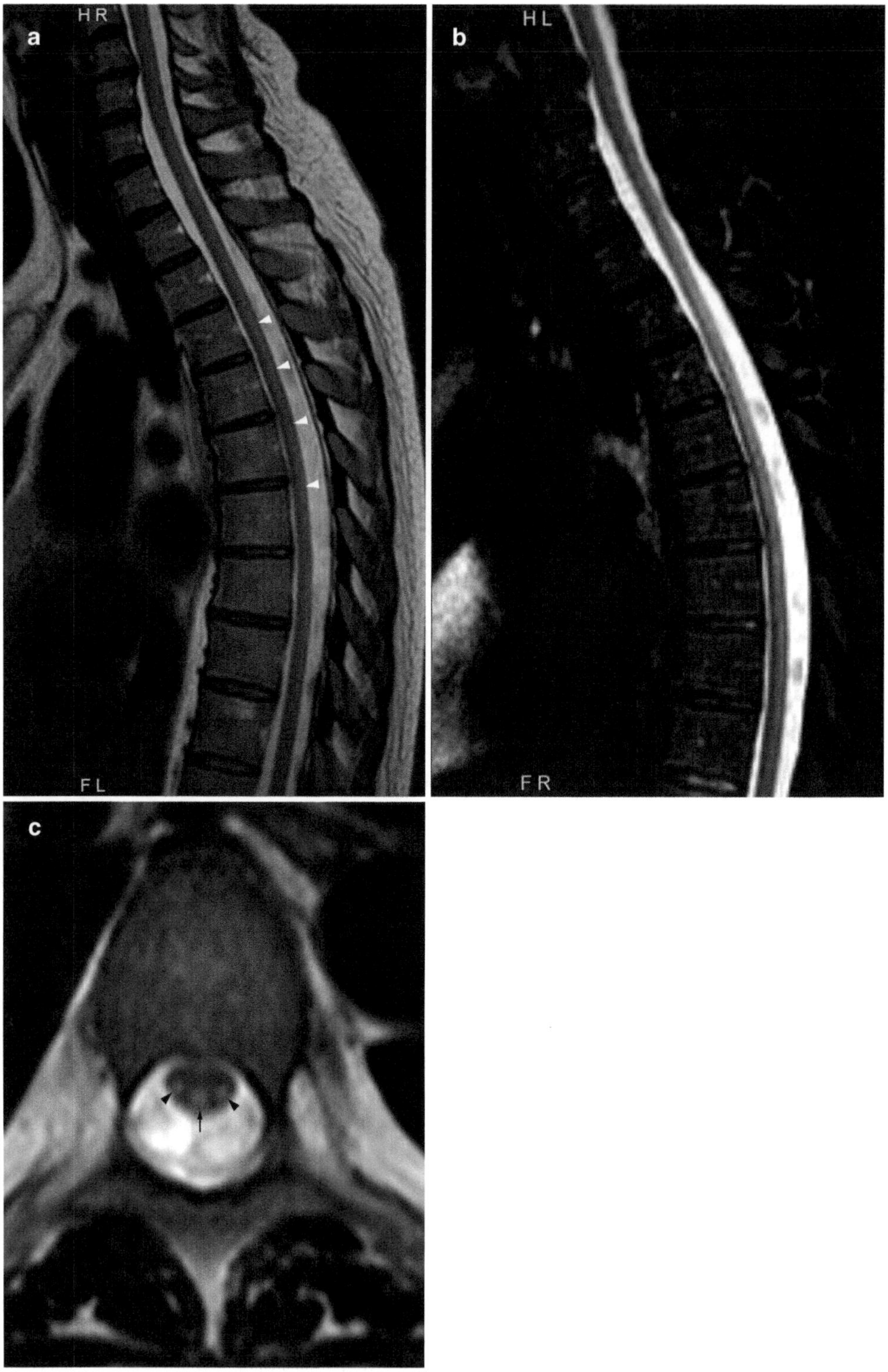


**Fig. 7** Subacute combined degeneration (vitamin B12 deficiency). Sagittal T2W (**a**) and STIR (**b**) MR images show a very thin linear hyperintensity along the posterior aspect of the cord (arrowheads). Axial T2W image (**c**) demonstrates abnormal symmetric increased signal in the posterior (arrow) and lateral columns (arrowhead) of the spinal cord. The presence of symmetric signal abnormalities confined to the posterior columns and, in some cases, also to the lateral columns, over multiple vertebral segments is suggestive of SCD

enhancement. In some cases, spinal cord could be normal (Nardone et al. 2006).

## 4.4 Iatrogenic Myelopathies

Several chemotherapeutical agents, such as methotrexate, cytarabine, doxorubicin, cisplatin, and vincristine, intrathecally or systemically administered, can cause multifactorial myelopathies, secondary to direct toxicity or metabolic mechanism, resulting in necrosis and vacuolar degeneration of withe matter, variably associated (Ramalho et al. 2016). The combination of radiation therapy can increase the spinal damages, also depending on the dose administered. Ionizing radiation causes of myelopathies are several, inducing vascular endothelial cells' damages and the vein walls lesions which determine abnormal venous drainage and demyelination phenomena (Werner-Wasik et al. 2004). It is important to know the total radiation dose, radiation dose per fraction, and time between applications in order to define the severity of myelopathy, considering the high radiosensitivity of medulla even if universally accepted threshold dose (Gocheva 2000). The cervical tract is more prone to radiation damages if compared with thoracic ones. The clinical onset of these myelopathies (both chemotherapeutical and radiation-related) can manifest with a relatively long latency, until 3–4 years after radiation treatment (Koehler et al. 1996). Chemotherapeutical agents cause two different types of paraparesis: transient, flaccid, and areflexic paraparesis, or spastic and ataxic ones; the sphincter or sensitive involvement can be associated. Radiation treatment can provoke a more different clinical scenario, from acute transient early myelopathy characterized by Lhermitte sign, to para or quadriplegia, up to a chronic progressive spinal damage, usually called delayed radiation myelopathy, irreversible and variable on the basis of spinal level involved. In both cases, MRI is done to define the spinal involvement, and in acute setting, usually shows normal findings. In chemotherapy-induced myelopathy, the damages variably occur, both as dorsal-lateral columns' hyperintensity on T2 sequences and cord swelling; cord atrophy without signal alteration is been reported on follow-up (Schlegel 2001). MRI in radiation-related myelopathy can show cord swelling, sometimes with an increased signal on T2 images and frequently gadolinium enhancement; cord atrophy is often detected (Gocheva 2000). We highlight that radiation treatment usually induces bone marrow changes, which is clearly detectable as vertebral signal alterations on MRI images, and it could be helpful to define with precision the level of spinal involvement (Werner-Wasik et al. 2004).

## 4.5 Accidental or Voluptuous Toxic-Related Myelopathies

Heroin abuse both by inhalation and intravenous can cause medullary injury, due to direct toxicity, or hypersensitivity or vascular damage, resulting in extensive necrosis of the lateral and posterior columns of the cervical-thoracic cord (Ramalho et al. 2016). Clinical presentation usually consists of sudden onset of flaccid paraparesis/paraplegia associated with sensory loss and bladder symptoms such as acute retention; more rarely, patients could manifest signs and symptoms mimicking transverse myelitis. MRI usually shows normal findings; in some cases, we can find an increased signal on T2 sequences involving posterior or lateral columns. In few cases, we found neuroradiological signs of transverse myelitis (Ramalho et al. 2016).

Acute intoxication organophosphate agents manifest itself as a cholinergic crisis; in some cases, a delayed myelopathy associated with neuropathy had been reported, called organophosphate-induced-delayed neurotoxicity (Lotti et al. 1984). Myelopathy can occur until 3 weeks after acute intoxication; in case of chronic exposure, onset latency is unclear. Patients complain about distal paresthesia, cramping pain, and progressive leg weakness, usually without sensory disturbances (Chuang et al. 2002). MRI can show a relative spinal cord atrophy, even in late phase of exposure (Ramalho et al. 2016).

## References

Andari MT et al (2020) What is the incidence of Guillain-Barre syndrome (GBS) in the US? MedScape

Andres E, Loukili NH, Noel E et al (2004) Vitamin B12 (cobalamin) deficiency in elderly patients. Can Med Assoc J 171:251–259

Arkema EV, Cozier YC (2018) Epidemiology of sarcoidosis: current findings and future directions. Ther Adv Chronic Dis 9(11):227–240

Bot JC, Blezer EL, Kamphorst W et al (2004) The spinal cord in multiple sclerosis: relationship of high-spatial-resolution quantitative MR imaging findings to histopathologic results. Radiology 233:531–540

Choi KH, Lee KS, Chung SO et al (1996) Idiopathic transverse myelitis: MR characteristics. AJNR Am J Neuroradiol 17:1151–1160

Chuang C-C, Lin T-S, Tsai M-C (2002) Delayed neuropathy and myelopathy after organophosphate intoxication. N Engl J Med 347(14):1119–1121

Eaton SE, Harris ND, Rajbhandari SM et al (2001) Spinal cord involvement in diabetic peripheral neuropathy. Lancet 358:35–36

Ghezzi A, Baldini SM, Zaffaroni M (2001) Differential diagnosis of acute myelopathies. Neurol Sci 22(Suppl 2):S60–S64

Gocheva L (2000) Radiation tolerance of the spinal cord: doctrine, dogmas, data. Arch Oncol 8(3):1–4

Hauser SL (2005) Diseases of the spinal cord. In: Harrison's principles of internal medicine, 16th edn. McGraw-Hill, New York, pp 2438–2447

Jacob A, Weinshenker BG (2008) An approach to the diagnosis of acute transverse myelitis. Semin Neurol 28:105–120

Junger SS, Stern BJ, Levine SR et al (1993) Intramedullary spinal sarcoid- osis: clinical and magnetic resonance imaging characteristics. Neurology 43:333–337

Koehler PJ, Verbiest H, Jager J, Vecht CJ (1996) Delayed radiation myelopathy: serial MR-imaging and pathology. Clin Neurol Neurosurg 98(2):197–201

Koike H, Misu K, Yasui K et al (2000) Differential response to corticosteroid therapy of MRI findings and clinical manifestations in spinal cord sarcoidosis. J Neurol 247:544–549

Kuwabara S (2007) Guillain-Barré syndrome. Curr Neurol Neurosci Rep 7:57–62

Lotti M, Becker CE, Aminoff MJ (1984) Organophosphate polyneuropathy: pathogenesis and prevention. Neurology 34(5):658–662

Lury KM, Smith JK, Matheus MG et al (2004) Neurosarcoidosis. Review of imaging findings. Semin Roentgenol 39:495–504

Nardone R, Buratti T, Oliviero A, Lochmann A, Tezzon F (2006) Corticospinal involvement in patients with a portosystemic shunt due to liver cirrhosis: a MEP study. J Neurol 253(1):81–85

Polman C, Reingold S, Banwell B et al (2011) Diagnostic criteria for Multiple Sclerosis: 2010 revisions to the McDonald criteria. Ann Neurol, 69: 292–302

Premkumar M, Bagchi A, Kapoor N, Gupta A, Maurya G, Vatsya S et al (2012) Hepatic myelopathy in a patient with decompensated alcoholic cirrhosis and portal colopathy. Case Rep Hepatol 2012(4):1–4

Prick JJ, Prevo RL, Hoogenraad TU (2001) Transient myelopathy of the cervical posterior columns in a young man with recently diagnosed diabetes mellitus. Clin Neurol Neurosurg 103:234–237

Ramalho J, Nunes RH, da Rocha AJ, Castillo M (2016) Toxic and metabolic myelopathies. Semin Ultrasound CT MR 37(5):448–465

Sánchez AMG, Lina María García Posada LM, Ortega Toscano CA, López A (2011) Diagnostic approach to myelopathies. Rev Colomb Radiol 22(3):1–2

Schlegel U (2001) Central Nervous System toxicity of Chemotherapy. Eur Assoc NeuroOncol Mag 1(1):25–29

Schmalstieg WF, Weinshenker BG (2010) Approach to acute or sub- acute myelopathy. Neurology 75(18 Suppl 1):S2–S8

Scotti G, Gerevini S (2001) Diagnosis and differential diagnosis of acute transverse myelopathy. The role of neuroradiological investigations and review of the literature. Neurol Sci 22Suppl 2:S69–S73

Selvarajah D, Wilkinson ID, Emery CJ et al (2006) Early involvement of the spinal cord in diabetic peripheral neuropathy. Diabetes Care 29:2664–2669

Tartaglino LM, Friedman DP, Flanders AE et al (1995) Multiple sclerosis in the spinal cord: MR appearance and correlation with clinical parameters. Radiology 195:725–732

Transverse Myelitis Consortium Working Group (2002) Proposed diagnostic criteria and nosology of acute transverse myelitis. Neurology 59:499–505

Utku U, Asil T, Balci K et al (2005) Hepatic myelopathy with spastic para- paresis. Clin Neurol Neurosurg 107:514–516

Werner-Wasik M, Yu X, Marks LB, Schultheiss TE (2004) Normal-tissue toxicities of thoracic radiation therapy: esophagus, lung, and spinal cord as organs at risk. Hematol Oncol Clin North Am 18(1):131–1xi

Wingerchuk DM (2006) Neuromyelitis optica. Int MS J 13:42–50

Yu RK, Usuki S, Ariga T (2006) Ganglioside molecular mimicry and its pathological roles in Guillain-Barré syndrome and related diseases. Infect Immun 74:6517–6527

Yuki N, Odaka M (2005) Ganglioside mimicry as a cause of Guillain-Barré syndrome. Curr Opin Neurol 18:557–561

# Spinal Post-operative Complications

Pia C. Sundgren and Johan W. M. Van Goethem

## Contents




**Abstract**

Complications to spinal surgery are not uncommon. The type of complications may, in part, vary depending on the surgical procedure. Some complications may occur during the intraoperative procedure, while others are considered to be delayed and occur during the post-surgical recovery phase. The present chapter will focus on the more common acute and delayed post-operative complications related to spinal surgery.



P. C. Sundgren (✉)
Institution of Clinical Sciences/Division of Radiology, Lund University, Lund, Sweden
e-mail: Pia.sundgren@med.lu.se

J. W. M. Van Goethem
Department of Radiology, University of Antwerp, Antwerp, Belgium
e-mail: Johan.vangoethem@uantwerpen.be


## 1 Introduction

The risk for complications of spinal surgery depends on many factors such as type of surgery, level of the spine involved, age of the patient, general health, possible underlying diseases, presence of osteoporosis and osteopenia, among others (Bjerke et al. 2018).

It is absolutely crucial for the radiologist to be aware of potential complications. Therefore, it is important when evaluating patients post-operatively to review all images obtained both preoperatively and those performed intraoperatively with images obtained post-surgically to evaluate for possible complications. Also, good knowledge about what to expect in the immediate post-surgical setting depending on type of intervention performed is of importance. This is




M. Scaglione et al. (eds.), *Emergency Radiology of the Head and Spine*,
Medical Radiology Diagnostic Imaging, https://doi.org/10.1007/978-3-030-91047-1_20

to avoid misdiagnosis of typical treatment-related changes in contrast to obvious complications. The most serious and feared complication from spinal surgery is neurologic injury, both in the intra- and post-operative period. The most common post-operative complications are surgical site infection, venous thromboembolism, gastrointestinal complications, and implant-related complications (Robert et al. 2016). In patients operated for scoliosis, there are also risk for ophthalmologic or peripheral nerve deficits, which may be related to positioning (Robert et al. 2016). A recent study demonstrated an increased risk for iatrogenic spondylolisthesis in patients with no preoperative instability after being operated with laminectomy for spinal stenosis, especially if the laminectomy had been performed at several levels (Ramhmdani et al. 2018). Factors like extent of decompression of the facet joints, levels of decompression and laminectomy, and preoperative disc space height might be used to assess the risk for developing iatrogenic spondylolisthesis (Ramhmdani et al. 2018).

If patients directly post-operatively complain of new neurological deficits, increased pain, or discomfort, post-operative imaging is warranted. The imaging method depends on location and symptoms and what to evaluate, so, for example, plain radiographs might be enough to evaluate the location of instrumentation/hardware, while a contrast enhanced MRI is needed for better depiction of the spinal canal and spinal cord and is often used to evaluate acute or delayed complications such as spinal infections or fluid collections (Ortiz et al. 2018).

It shall be noted that immediate post-surgical changes are often present at post-surgical imaging. Typical immediate post-operative findings are smaller or larger fluid collection at the surgical bed after laminectomy that may represent a seroma, paravertebral soft tissue oedema along the surgical tract, or post-operative and reactive changes in the adjacent vertebral body endplates; discs after discectomy or around implanted hardware are common findings after spinal surgery (Ortiz et al. 2018). These findings can be well-demonstrated on MRI as increased hyperintense T2w signal and increased contrast enhancement in the disc at the site of the discectomy. Bone marrow oedema may present as increased T2w signal and hypointense T1w signal in the vertebral body endplates. In later stage, focal muscle atrophy might be present (Ortiz et al. 2018). Another expected finding is granulation or scar tissue, especially epidural and perineural space(s) at the site of disc resection and level of surgery. This scar tissue can sometimes be difficult to distinguish from persisting or recurrent disc herniation. Normally, the scar tissue, compared to acute disc herniation, demonstrates contrast enhancement for anywhere between 6 weeks and 6 months post-surgical (Van Goethem et al. 1996). These findings should not be considered as a complication, but regarded as treatment-related changes that in most cases will resolve without further intervention.

Complications that occur in the scale of days and weeks post the surgical procedure with or without hardware placement are seroma/haematoma and infection within the post-operative site, including the hardware or superinfection of post-operative collections. Hardware loosening or hardware failure usually occurs over a period of months to years' post-surgery.

## 2 Acute Complications

These are complications that occur during or immediately after the surgical procedure.

### 2.1 Vascular Complications

Direct injury to adjacent vascular structures may result not only in small haemorrhages, but also in ischemic injury such as dissections, pseudo aneurysms, or in worst case, spinal cord ischemia with more devastating neurological consequence. Venous thromboembolism (VTE), i.e. pulmonary embolism, is another well-known complication of adult spine surgery (Yoshioka et al. 2015; Tominaga et al. 2015).

### 2.1.1 Spinal Cord Ischemia/Infarcts

Spinal surgery may be complicated by spinal cord ischemia. Spinal deformity surgery is the one spinal surgical procedure with a higher risk of spinal cord infarct and its incidence is estimated to be about 1.8% (Weidauer et al. 2015). Overall, the rate of neurological complications in spinal surgery is respectively for spinal tumour removing (around 1%), deformity spinal surgery (0.75–1.8%), and degenerative anterior approach (0.75–5.8%) or degenerative posterior approach (0.3–1.3%) (Sabrina 2016). MRI is the method of choice to evaluate and present the typical imaging findings in spinal cord ischemia, demonstrating focal cord swelling and 'pencil-like' hyperintensities on T2-weighted images. Contrast enhancement often presents within 2 days and diffusion-weighted images demonstrated focal area or restricted diffusion (Alblas et al. 2012; Weidauer et al. 2002; Thurnher and Bammer 2006).

### 2.1.2 Haematoma

It is, together with seroma, the most common complication after posterior fusion for spondylolisthesis with a frequency of 5.4% (Kalanithi et al. 2009). Small haematomas normally resolve without any intervention. However, if the patient complains of new neurological symptoms or increasing pain, an MRI is warranted to exclude for epidural haematoma that might need to be surgically removed if extensive. Most commonly, the epidural haematoma will be located posteriorly in the spinal canal and may result in compression of the spinal cord or nerve roots and cause neurological deficits and pain (Fig. 1).

## 2.2 Dural Tear

During surgery, there is always a risk of causing a rift or tear of the dura mater. If not observed or treated, there is a risk for leakage of the cerebral spinal fluid (CSF) along the surgical tract which might result in symptoms such as headache due to intracranial hypotension or large fluid collections. The best method to evaluate for CSF leak is contrast enhanced MRI that might detect the fluid collection communicating with the subarachnoid space or the leaking CSF along the surgical tract to the subcutaneous tissue. Also, CT myelogram, and in some cases, radionuclide cisternogram might be valuable for detection of minor CSF leaks (Ortiz et al. 2018).

## 2.3 Misplacement of Surgical Devices

Misplacement of the surgical implants is another complication that can be demonstrated directly after the surgery. This can be seen as misplaced implants into the spinal canal or neural foramina encroaching on nerves and spinal cord, causing the patient neurological symptoms and pain or through the vertebral body encroaching on vessels or paraspinal nerves (Hayashi et al. 2012). A typical example is misplaced screws at alignment surgery for scoliosis (Abul-Kasim et al. 2010). Plain radiographs or CT with a low-dose protocol can depict the misplacement very nicely (Abul-Kasim et al. 2009) (Fig. 2). Complications related to prosthesis in total disc replacement (including migration, subsidence, implant failure, and endplate fractures) are reported in 2 to 39.3% of patients (van den Eerenbeemt et al. 2010). Other implant misplacements are posterior or lateral displacement of fusion cage placement, as well as extravasation of acrylic bone cement into the spinal canal, neural foramina, and intervertebral disc space (Venmans et al. 2010; Lin et al. 2004).

# 3 Delayed Complications

The delayed complications after spinal surgery often occur days or weeks after the spinal surgery and can be suspected if the patient presents with recurrent pain, new pain, and neurological symptoms after a period of initial relief. Delayed complications may be due to infections, recurrent disk herniation, arachnoiditis, prolonged scar tissue formation, or paraspinal fluid collec-

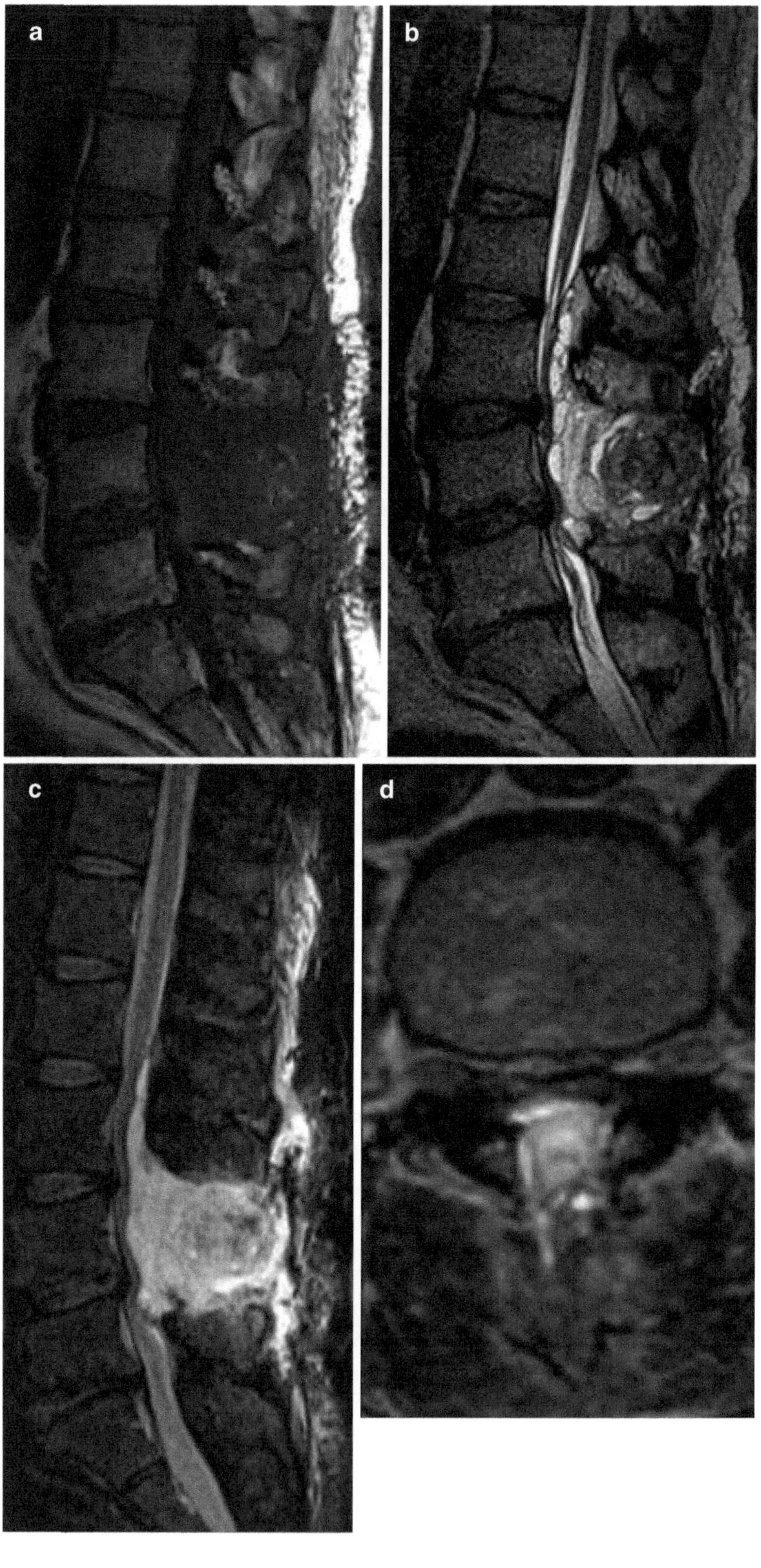


**Fig. 1** (**a–d**) Sagittal T1w (**a**), T2w (**b**), T1w post-gadolinium (**c**), and axial T1w post-gadolinium (**d**). A large haematoma at the laminectomy site in patients operated with laminectomy for spinal stenosis 4 days earlier

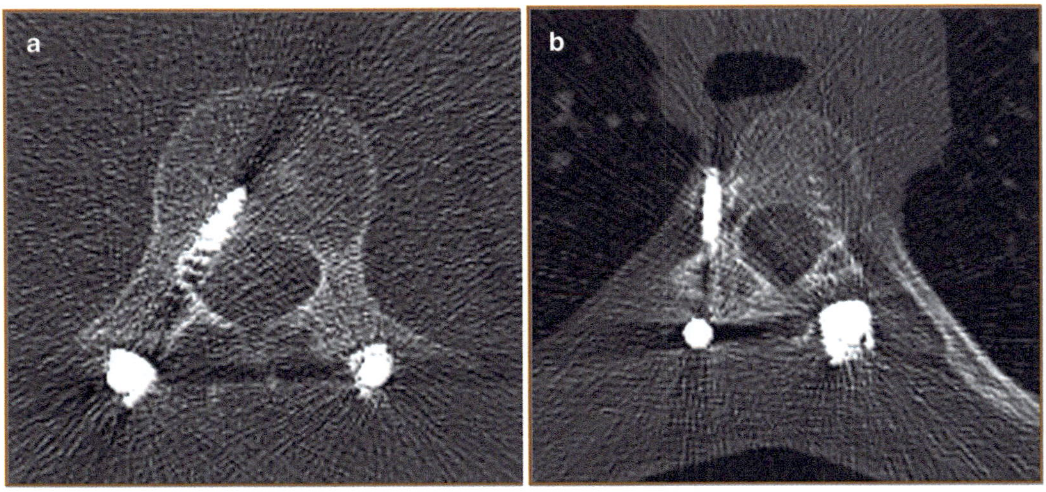


**Fig. 2** (**a**, **b**) Low-dose CT with bone windows demonstrates medial displacement of the screw (**a**), and in another case, lateral displacement of the screw (**b**) in two patients treated for scoliosis

tions, and late hardware complications; in addition, especially in the setting of spinal surgery related to spinal cord injury due to trauma development of spinal neuroarthropathy (see later in chapter).

## 3.1 Spinal Infections

The incidence of spine infection following lumbar discectomy or lumbar spine surgery is correlated to the extent of the surgery ranging from 0.1% to 3% (Van Goethem et al. 2002). Post-surgical spine infection is often a challenging clinical diagnosis and imaging is crucial. Enhancement of the posterior disc from an aseptic reaction is seen in the majority of the patients, which can mimic early infection. In addition, vertebral endplate oedema and enhancement are normal post-operative changes in asymptomatic patients (Bommireddy et al. 2007). To evaluate for more serious infection and spondylodiscitis, contrast enhanced MRI of spine is imaging method of choice. Typical MRI imaging findings of spondylodiscitis are initially strong contrast enhancement within the disk, annulus fibrosus, and bone marrow enhancement in adjacent vertebral bodies (Sanders and Truumees 2004; Malhotra et al. 2015). As the infection progresses, there is a loss of disk space height, destruction of adjacent vertebral body endplates, and vertebral body collapse. If the infection occurs in a patient with graft or implants, a displacement of these may occur. An infected fluid collection will show irregular peripheral contrast enhancement and restricted diffusion, or very hyperintense signal, on diffusion-weighted imaging (Ortiz et al. 2018) (Fig. 3).

## 3.2 Arachnoiditis

The surgical procedure may result in inflammation in and around the spinal canal. Nerve root enhancement in the early post-operative period is not a specific finding for infection and frequently represents a transient sterile radiculitis. However, enhancement persisting for more than 6 months is considered abnormal (Van Goethem et al. 1996). Arachnoiditis refers to inflammation of the nerve roots in the thecal sac or may occur in the epidural or occasionally in the perineural space and is often symptomatic with focal and/or radicular pain (Lee et al. 2009). MRI imaging demonstrated enhancing clumping of thickened nerve roots that might adhere to the wall of the dura, creating the appearance of an empty thecal sac. Intrathecal nerve root enhancement might be present initially, but should not persist more than 6–8 months after surgery (Ortiz et al. 2018) (Fig. 4).

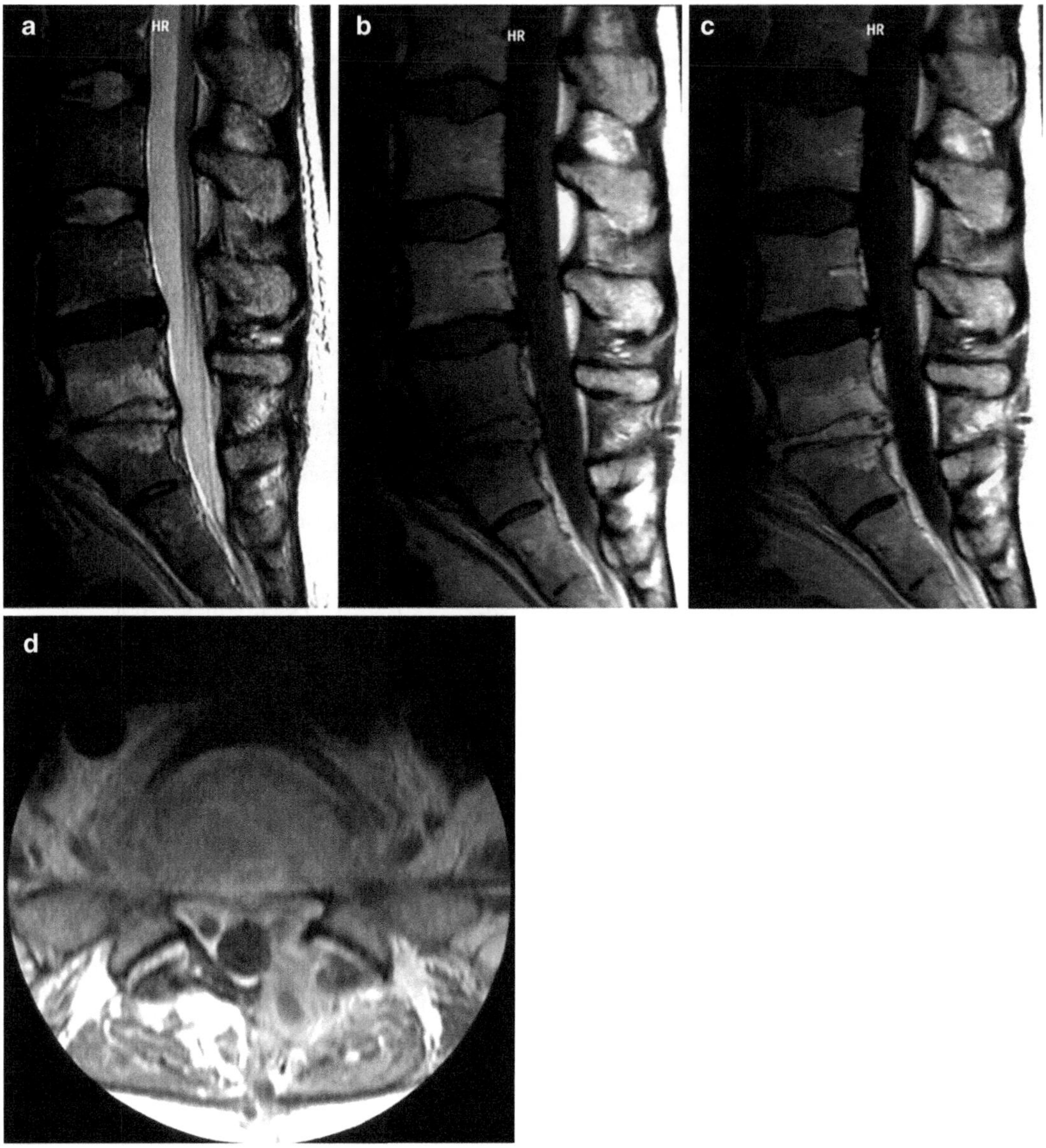


**Fig. 3** (**a–d**) Spondylodiscitis after surgery. Sagittal T2w (**a**) demonstrates signal changes in the post-operative location involving the disc and the adjacent vertebral bodies at L4-L5 level. Sagittal T1w (**b**) and sagittal and axial T1w after Gadolinium injection (**c**, **d**) demonstrate pathological contrast enhancement in the disc and contrast enhancing tissue in the left aspect of the spinal canal at the site surgery

## 3.3 Recurrent Disc Herniation

Recurrent disk herniation is not an uncommon problem following lumbar discectomy (Ambrossi et al. 2009) and often the patients are symptomatic and subsequent MRI is warranted. Clinically, recurrent disc herniation is defined as recurrence after a 6-month pain-free post-operative period. Recurrent disc herniation varies between 3% and 18% post-lumbar discectomy in previous retrospective studies (Willson and Ross 2014). A prospective imaging study over a 2-year post-operative period demonstrated recurrent disc herniation in 23%

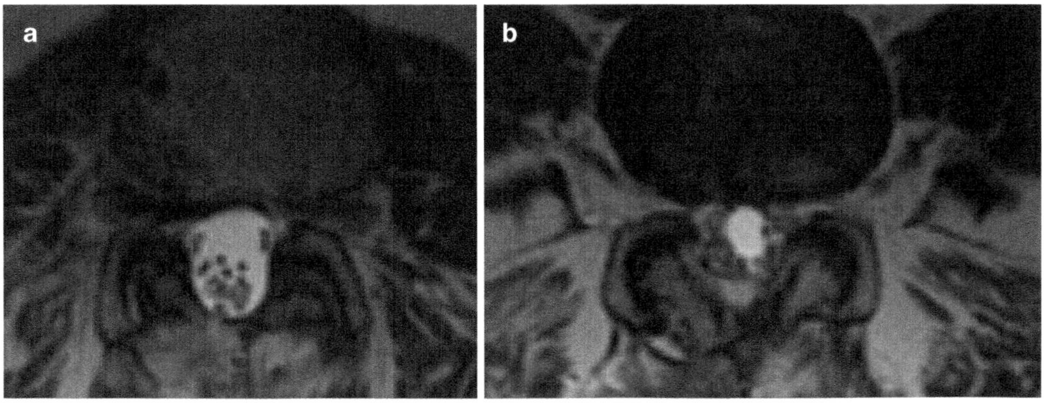


**Fig. 4** (**a**, **b**) Axial T2w images of the lumbar spine demonstrating clumping of nerve roots suggestive of arachnoiditis in a patient previously operated for recurrent disc herniation

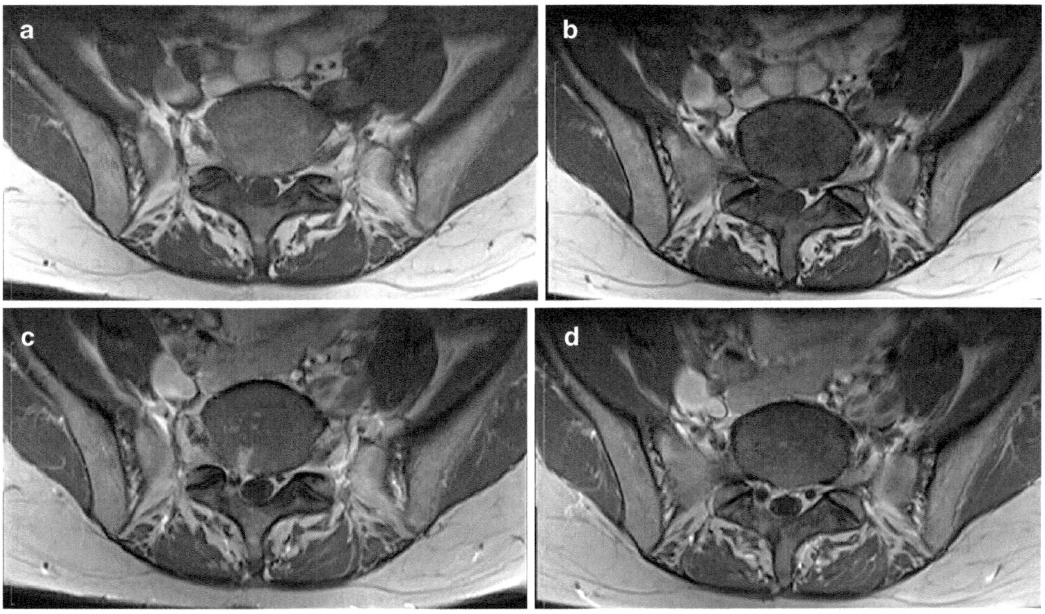


**Fig. 5** (**a**–**d**) Post-surgical scar tissue in a patient operated for a disc herniation. Axial T1w (**a**, **b**) and axial T1w after Gadolinium injection (**c**, **d**) demonstrate focal tissue in the right anterior aspect of the spinal canal that enhances after contrast injection suggestive of scar tissue/epidural fibrosis

of the patients, half being asymptomatic (Lebow et al. 2011).

Contrast enhanced MRI is key to distinguishing recurrent disc herniation from peridural fibrosis and/or scar tissue. Normally, the disc herniation demonstrates early peripheral contrast enhancement with a central non-enhanced area, whereas granulation fibrosis/scar tissue demonstrates diffuse variable enhancement. Especially, early contrast enhanced fat-suppressed T1-weighted images and contrast enhanced MR images can be used to distinguish scar tissue from a recurrent disk herniation. Typical examples of scar tissue and recurrent disc herniation are presented in Figs. 5 and 6. Additional features such as intermediate signal with irregular margins favour epidural granulation tissue and low signal with

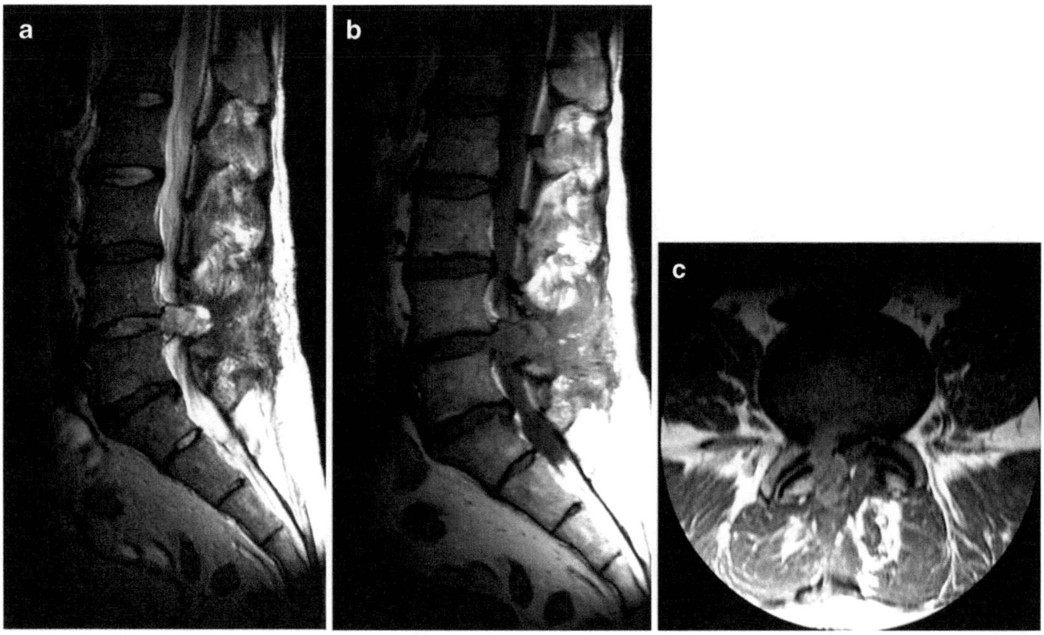



**Fig. 6** (**a–c**) Large recurrent herniated disc. Sagittal T2w (**a**), T1w (**b**), and axial T1w after Gadolinium injection (**c**) demonstrate a large recurrent disc herniation in a patient previously operated for a herniated disc

smooth margins favouring recurrent herniation. In general, delayed post-contrast imaging should be avoided in the post-operative spine as contrast may diffuse into disc material and obscure the differential diagnosis of scar tissue.

## 3.4 Complications Due to Hardware Failure

Complications related to the implant due to loosening, displacement in relation to adjacent osseous structures, migration, or direct implant fracture or damage can occur over time. This may be seen on routine post-operative surveillance radiographs or on imaging performed to assess symptomatic patients. Loosening of the implant may manifest as a lucent area or halo around the implant on plain radiographs or CT (Fig. 7). Implant failure may on imaging manifest with abnormal bending of a rod or a fracture of screw, plate, or rod (Fig. 8). A loose implant may affect stability and alignment and can cause associated spondylolisthesis at the level of surgery or at adjacent levels due to increased movement and spinal instability. A sign of appropriate spinal fusion is new bone formation within and surrounding a graft. These findings are best visualized on a CT, whereas reactive sclerosis, lucent areas around the implant, fractures of the graft or the adjacent vertebra, or a broken implant are all findings suggestive of failure of fusion. If there is an implant failure and a lack of fusion of the graft to surrounding osseous structures, there is a risk for instability, pseudo-arthrosis, and spondylolisthesis. After a fusion of a level of the spine, the level above the fusion then becomes the next mobile segment due to increased motion at this adjacent level with increased risk for spondylolisthesis and spinal stenosis. Adjacent level disease occurs at a rate of approximately 4% per year for spine fusion surgeries (Lawrence et al. 2012a, b).

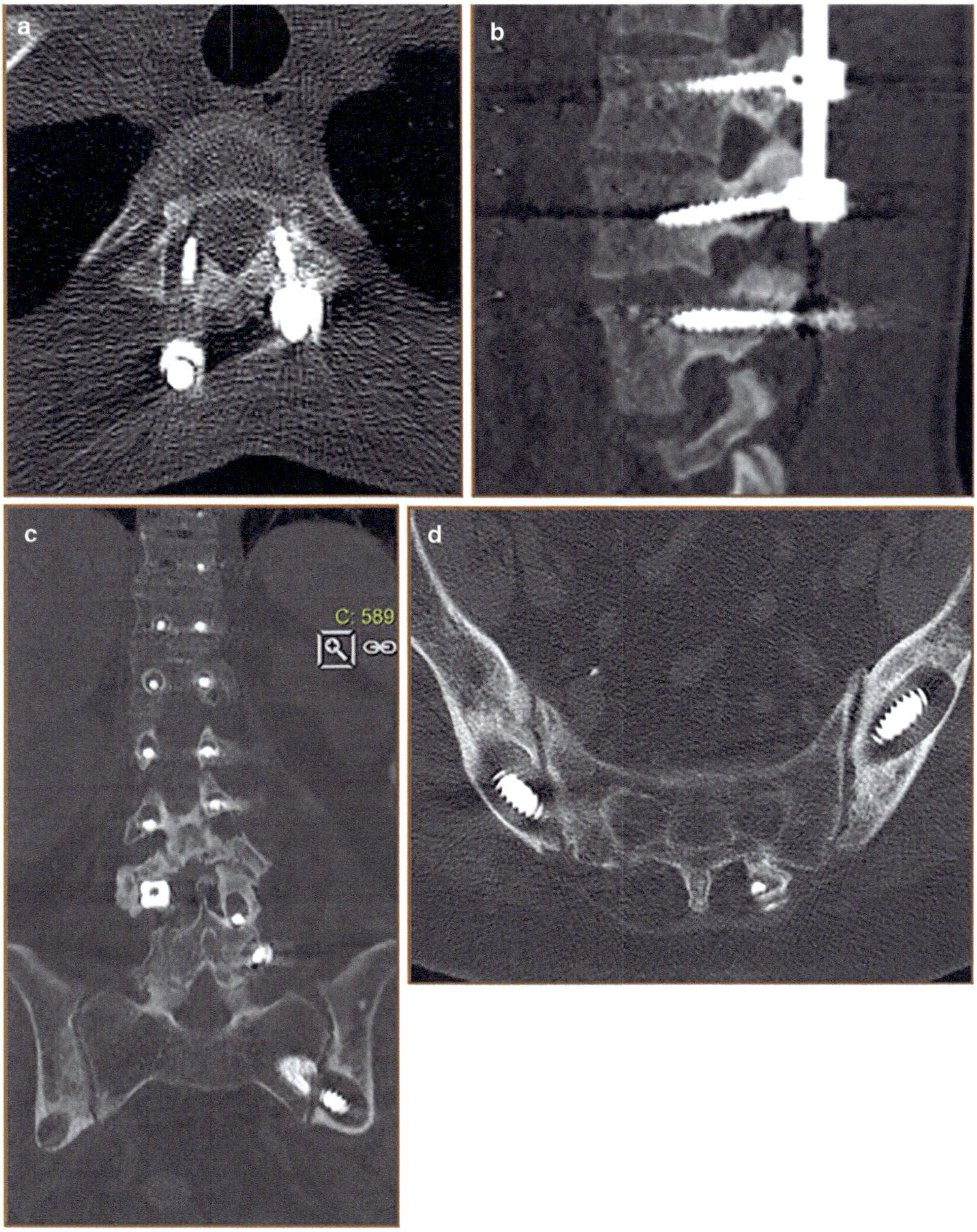


**Fig. 7** (**a**–**d**) Loss hardware. Axial (**a**) and sagittal (**b**) low-dose CT demonstrating halo around screws as a sign of loss implants. These halo zones around the screws can be gigantic (**c**, **d**) as seen in the lower lumbar and sacral spine

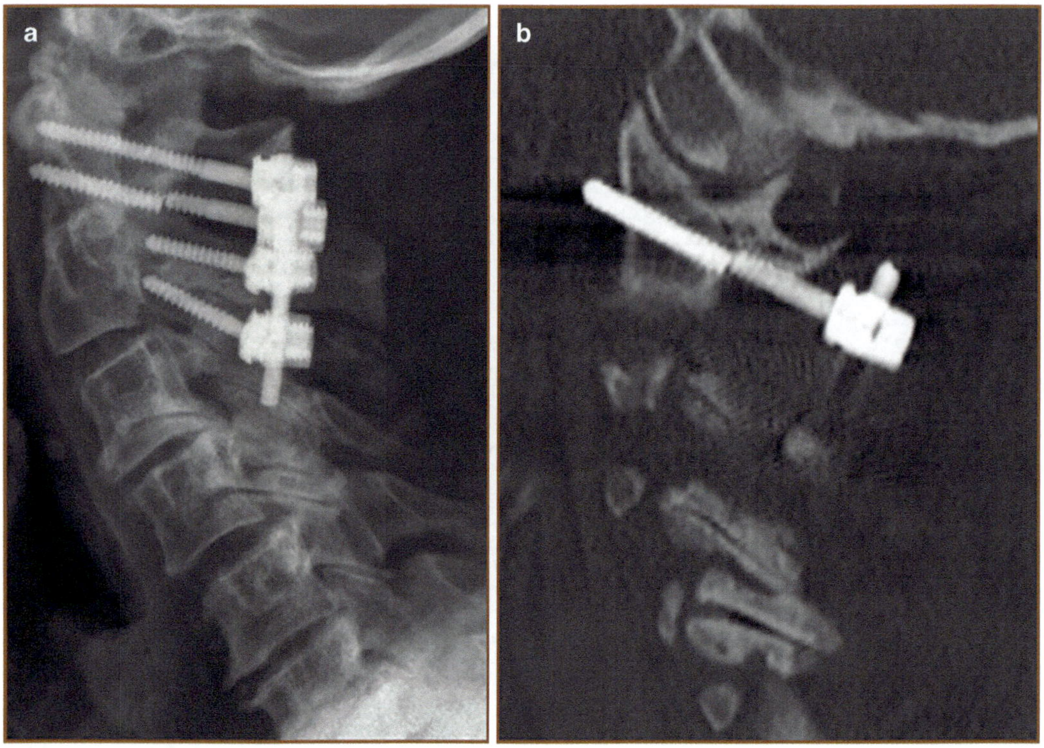


**Fig. 8** (**a**, **b**) Lateral view radiograph of the cervical spine demonstrating a fractured screw initially placed through the dens (**a**). Computed tomography of another patient demonstrates a fractured screw at C2 level (**b**)

**Acknowledgement** We will like to acknowledge the contribution by Dr. Kasim Abul-Kasim, Department for Medical Imaging and Physiology, Skåne University hospital, Malmoe, Sweden, for the support with illustrations to Figs. 1, 2, 7, and 8.

## References

Abul-Kasim K, Overgaard A, Maly P, Ohlin A, Gunnarsson M, Sundgren PC (2009) Low-dose helical computed tomography (CT) in the perioperative workup of adolescent idiopathic scoliosis. Eur Radiol 19(3):610–618

Abul-Kasim K, Ohlin A, Strömbeck A, Maly P, Sundgren PC (2010) Radiological and clinical outcome of screw placement in adolescent idiopathic scoliosis: evaluation with low-dose computed tomography. Eur Spine J 19(1):96–104

Alblas CL, Bouvy WH, Lycklama À Nijeholt GJ, Boitena J (2012) Acute spinal-cord ischemia: evolution of MRI findings. J Clin Neurol 8:218–223

Ambrossi GL, McGirt MJ, Sciubba DM et al (2009) Recurrent lumbar disc herniation after single-level lumbar discectomy: incidence and health care cost analysis. Neurosurgery 65:574–578

Bjerke BT, Mohammad Zarrabian M, Aleem IS, Fogelson JF, Currier BL, Brett A, Freedman BA, Bydon M, Nassr A (2018) Incidence of osteoporosis-related complications following posterior lumbar fusion. Glob Spine J 8(6):563–569

Bommireddy R, Kamat A, Smith ET, Nixon T, Pillay R, Pigott T et al (2007) Magnetic resonance image findings in the early postoperative period after anterior cervical discectomy. Eur Spine J 16(1):27–31

Hayashi D, Roemer FW, Mian A et al (2012) Imaging features of postoperative complications after spinal surgery and instrumentation. AJR Am J Roentgenol 199:W123–W129

Lawrence BD, Hilibrand AS, Brodt ED et al (2012a) Predicting the risk of adjacent segment pathology in the cervical spine: a systematic review. Spine 37(Suppl):S52–S64

Lawrence BD, Wang J, Arnold PM et al (2012b) Predicting the risk of adjacent segment pathology after lumbar fusion: a systematic review. Spine 37(Suppl):S123–S132

Lebow RL, Adogwa O, Parker SL, Sharma A, Cheng J, McGirt MJ (2011) Asymptomatic same-site recurrent disc herniation after lumbar discectomy: results of a prospective longitudinal study with 2-year serial imaging. Spine 36(25):2147–2151

Lee YS, Choi ES, Song CJ (2009) Symptomatic nerve root changes in contrast enhanced MR imaging after surgery for lumbar disk herniation. AJNR Am J Neuroradiol 30:1062–1067

Lin EP, Ekholm S, Hiwatashi A et al (2004) Vertebroplasty: Cement leakage into the disc increases the risk of new fracture of adjacent vertebral body. AJNR Am J Neuroradiol 25:175–180

Kalanithi PS, Patil CG, Boakye M (2009) Spine (Phila Pa 1976)

Malhotra A, Kalra VB, Wu X, Grant R, Bronen R, Abbed KA (2015) Imaging of lumbar spinal surgery complications. Insights Imaging 6:579–590

Ortiz AO, de Moura A, Johnson BJ (2018) Postsurgical spine: techniques, expected imaging findings, and complications. Semin Ultrasound CT MRI 39:630–650

Ramhmdani S, Xia Y, Xu R, Kosztowski T, Sciubba D, Witham T, Bydon A (2018) Iatrogenic spondylolisthesis following open lumbar laminectomy: case series and review of the literature. World Neurosurg 113:e383–e390

Robert F, Murphy RF, James F, Mooney JF III (2016) Complications following spine fusion for adolescent idiopathic scoliosis. Curr Rev Musculoskelet Med 9:462–469

Sabrina B (2016) The risk of spinal cord ischemia in thoraco-lumbar spine surgery: attempt to quantify predictive factor. J Surg Open Access 2(5). https://doi.org/10.16966/2470-0991.124

Sanders WP, Truumees E (2004) Imaging of the postoperative spine. Semin Ultrasound CT MR 25(6):523–535

Thurnher MM, Bammer R (2006) Diffusion-weighted MR imaging (DWI) in spinal cord ischemia. Neuroradiology 48:795–801

Tominaga H, Setoguchi T, Tanabe F et al (2015) Risk factors for venous thromboembolism after spine surgery. Medicine 94:e466

van den Eerenbeemt KD, Ostelo RW, van Royen BJ, Peul WC, van Tulder MW (2010) Total disc replacement surgery for symptomatic degenerative lumbar disc disease: a systematic review of the literature. Eur Spine. J 19(8):1262–1280

Van Goethem JW, Van de Kelft E, Biltjes IG et al (1996) MRI after successful lumbar discectomy. Neuroradiology 38:S90–S96

Van Goethem JWM, Parizel PM, Jinkins JR (2002) Review article: MRI of the postoperative lumbar spine. Neuroradiology 44:723–739

Venmans A, Klazen CAH, Lohle PNM et al (2010) Percutaneous vertebroplasty and pulmonary cement embolism: Results from VERTOS II. AJNR Am J Neuroradiol 31:1451–1453

Weidauer S, Nichtweiss M, Lanfermann H, Zanella FE (2002) Spinal cord infarction: MR imaging and clinical features in 16 cases. Neuroradiology 44:851–857

Weidauer S, Nichtweiß M, Hattingen E, Berkefeld J (2015) Spinal cord ischemia: aetiology, clinical syndromes and imaging features. Neuroradiology 57:241–257

Willson MC, Ross JS (2014) Postoperative spine complications. Neuroimaging Clin N Am 24(2): 305–326

Yoshioka K, Murakami H, Demura S, Kato S, Tsuchiya H (2015) Prevalence and risk factors for development of venous thromboembolism after degenerative spinal surgery. Spine 40:E301–E306

# Basic Neuro-Interventional Therapeutic Approaches

Francesco Briganti, Giuseppe Leone, Giuseppe Buono, Sergio Nappini, Nicola Limbucci, Dario Piccolo, Mariano Marseglia, Ferdinando Caranci, and Mario Muto

## Contents



F. Briganti · G. Leone · G. Buono · D. Piccolo
M. Marseglia
Unit of Interventional Neuroradiology, Department of Advanced Biomedical Sciences, Federico II University of Naples, Naples, Italy
e-mail: frabriga@unina.it; g.buono@sirm.org

S. Nappini · N. Limbucci
Neurovascular Interventional Unit, Careggi University Hospital, Florence, Italy

F. Caranci
Department of Medicine and Health Science "V. Tiberio", University of Molise, Campobasso, Italy
e-mail: ferdinando.caranci@unimol.it

M. Muto (✉)
Neuroradiology Department, Cardarelli Hospital, Naples, Italy

**Abstract**

The minimally invasive procedures used by interventional neuroradiologists accomplish a wide variety of treatments designed to provide correct life-threatening conditions, such as haemorrhagic or ischemic stroke.

Endovascular treatment strategies of haemorrhagic intracranial aneurysms include coiling, balloon-assisted coiling, intrasaccular flow-disruptors, stent-assisted coiling, and flow-diverter devices.

Interventional neuroradiology allows also minimally invasive treatments of haemorrhagic stroke, which are due to an underlying



M. Scaglione et al. (eds.), *Emergency Radiology of the Head and Spine*, Medical Radiology Diagnostic Imaging, https://doi.org/10.1007/978-3-030-91047-1_21

vascular lesion such as arteriovenous malformations or dural arterio-venous fistulas. Embolization with acrylic glues or with non-adhesive embolic materials may be used for "target" embolization in the setting of intracerebral haemorrhage.

Finally, endovascular treatment of acute ischemic stroke is now the younger field of interventional neuroradiology. It is important to recognize that modern endovascular stroke therapy focuses on direct clot removal with mechanical devices and it represents the standard of care in cases of proximal large vessel occlusion of the anterior circulation.

In this chapter, we review the current practice on neuroendovascular therapy in acute phase and we discuss the main techniques used by interventional neuroradiologists.

## Abbreviations

| | |
|---|---|
| bAVM | Brain arteriovenous malformation |
| CT | Computed Tomography |
| CTA | Computed Tomography Angiography |
| CTP | CT Perfusion |
| DVST | Dural venous sinus thrombosis |
| dAVF | Dural arteriovenous fistulas |
| FDD | Flow-Diverter Devices |
| GCS | Glasgow Coma Scale |
| GDC | Guglielmi Detachable Coil |
| HHS | Hunt-Hess scale |
| ICA | Internal carotid artery |
| ICH | Intracerebral haemorrhage |
| ISAT | International Subarachnoid Aneurysm Trial |
| MR | Magnetic resonance |
| MRA | Magnetic Resonance angiography |
| mRROC | Modified Raymond-Roy occlusion classification |
| mCTA | Multi-phase CT angiography |
| NIHSS | National Institutes of Health Stroke Scale |
| NBCA | N-butyl cyanoacrylate |
| SAH | Subarachnoid haemorrhage |
| SAC | Stent-assisted coiling |

# 1 Endovascular Treatment of Haemorrhagic Intracranial Aneurysms

## 1.1 Introduction

Non-traumatic subarachnoid haemorrhage (SAH) is an uncommon and severe subtype of stroke with high mortality and morbidity. The rupture of an intracranial aneurysm is the underlining cause in about 85% of cases (Mayer et al. 2002). The estimated incidence of SAH is around 9/100,000 people/year globally. It is a devastating event with a case fatality rate of 51% and a 50% rate of significant disability among survivors (Mayer et al. 2002).

Treatment is typically carried out urgently rather than emergently, usually within 24–72 h after the arrival of the patient to the hospital.

Therapy is influenced by the patient's general and neurological conditions, as well as by the morphology and location of the aneurysm. Theoretically, all patients should undergo surgical obliteration of the aneurysm sac, but mortality is unacceptably high if the patient is in a stupor or coma (grade IV or V on the Hunt-Hess scale [HHS] or with low Glasgow Coma Scale [GCS]). So, before any therapeutic approach, it is advisable to evaluate the patient on the basis of the Hunt & Hess scale (Tables 1 and 2) and the Computed Tomography (CT) grading scale according to Fisher classification (Table 3).

Endovascular treatment of cerebral aneurysm has been revolutionized by ISAT (International Subarachnoid Aneurysm Trial) (Molyneux et al. 2005).

**Table 1** Hunt & Hess Scale for Neurological evaluation

| | |
|---|---|
| 0. | No symptoms |
| 1. | Asymptomatic, mild headache, slight nuchal rigidity |
| 2. | Moderate to severe headache, nuchal rigidity, no neurologic deficit other than cranial nerve palsy |
| 3. | Drowsiness, confusion, mild focal neurologic deficit |
| 4. | Stupor, moderate-severe hemiparesis |
| 5. | Coma, decerebrate posturing |

**Table 2** Comparison Hunt & Hess e Glasgow Coma

| | | | |
|---|---|---|---|
| 0. HH | GCS > 8 | 4 | GCS < 8 |
| 1. HH | | 4. HH | |
| 2. HH | | 5. HH | |
| 3. HH | | | |

**Table 3** Fisher Scale for SAH at Computed tomography (CT)

| | |
|---|---|
| I. | No subarachnoid (SAH) or intraventricular haemorrhage (IVH) detected |
| II. | Diffuse thin (<1 mm) SAH |
| III. | Localized clots and/or layers of blood >1 mm in thickness |
| IV. | Diffuse SAH; intracerebral haemorrhage (ICH) or IVH |

This multi-center randomized trial has compared microsurgical and endovascular techniques in the treatment of ruptured intracranial aneurysms.

Evaluation of the results at 1 year revealed a reduction in mortality and disability from 31% in the microsurgical arm to 24% in the endovascular arm. This difference was mainly linked to the decrease in the rate of disability among survivors treated intravascularly (16%) compared to patients treated with microsurgery (22%) (Molyneux et al. 2005).

However, the study showed a slightly higher re-bleeding rate in the case of aneurysms treated endovascularly (2.9%) compared to the clip approach (0.9%).

Later studies underlined the significant incidence of aneurysm recanalization after a time, with risk of greater re-rupture after coil embolization compared with surgical clipping (3.4% versus 1.3%) (Johnston et al. 2008).

In the setting of SAH, neuro-endovascular techniques include coiling (Pierot et al. 2008) and balloon-assisted coiling (BAC).

Stent-assisted coiling (SAC) (Muto et al. 2017; Shapiro et al. 2012) and new generation stents, such as Flow-Diverter Devices (FDD) (Lozupone et al. 2018), have been proposed in the setting of SAH in limited series. They have been mainly used in patients with more complex aneurysm morphologies, fusiform, dissecting, or blister aneurysms. Despite these results, intracranial stenting in the setting of SAH is an off-label treatment because of an increased haemorrhagic risk, due to the need of dual antiplatelet therapy.

There are four objectives for the endovascular occlusion of aneurysms: Block bleeding in progress; avoid re-bleeding; determine the exclusion of the aneurysm sac from the circle; guarantee the duration of the result over time.

## 1.2 Factors Influencing Endovascular Approach

Several factors influence endovascular treatment of intracranial aneurysms. They include aneurysm shape, size, location, and thrombus inside the sac.

### 1.2.1 Aneurysm Shape

Dome-to-neck ratio: if the neck is small compared to the maximum diameter of the bag, with a ratio of 1:3 or greater, the aneurysm is susceptible to the treatment with coils. In the event that the ratio is in the order of 1:1 or 1:2, it is necessary to resort to self-expanding devices, stents or balloons, able to create an artificial neck.

### 1.2.2 Aneurysm Size

Absolute dimensions of the aneurysm: large aneurysms (ø 15–25 mm) or giant (ø>25 mm) usually present with a wide collar that incorporates a large part of the circumference of the vessel wall.

### 1.2.3 Location

Location: it is very often the determining factor in the choice of the type of treatment; excluding the posterior circulation aneurysms, which are preferentially treated with an endovascular approach, some sites, such as especially the bifurcation from the middle cerebral or the aneurysms located at the level of the terminal branches, make this type of approach difficult.

#### 1.2.4 Thrombus Inside The Sac

Presence of unstable thrombus inside the sac is not a contraindication to treatment with coils, but increases the risk of inter and peri-procedural thromboembolic phenomena; moreover, the presence of the thrombus, especially if large, could hinder the correct positioning of the coils inside the sac.

### 1.3 Endovascular Treatments and Techniques

All procedures are usually performed under general anaesthesia in the angiography suite. All patients received heparin (70 IU/kg) intravenous bolus after femoral puncture and continuous intravenous infusion throughout the procedure for a target activated clotting time of 250–300 s.

After single femoral puncture, a 6 F or 7 F guiding catheter is placed in the internal carotid artery or vertebral artery. Then a designed microcatheter is carefully navigated into the aneurysmal sac. The size and type of the coils were chosen according to measurement of the aneurysm width and height on three-dimensional gradient volume rendering reconstructions of rotational angiography in two orthogonal projections. Occlusion rate is commonly evaluated at the end of the procedure according to the modified Raymond-Roy occlusion classification (mRROC) (Table 4).

#### 1.3.1 Coiling

These flexible, soft, detachable coils could be delivered through a microcatheter that could be safely navigated into the targeted aneurysm (Pierot et al. 2008). Complex-shaped, three-dimensional coils were developed to facilitate the embolization of wide-necked aneurysms. Coils with faster detachment times were developed to speed the process of embolization and shorten procedure times (Fig. 1). As aneurysm embolization with the Guglielmi Detachable Coil (GDC, Boston Scientific Corporation, Natick, MA) became increasingly accepted and more widely performed, competitors emerged, and additional brands of embolization coils became available.

**Table 4** Modified Raymond–Roy occlusion classification (mRROC)

| | |
|---|---|
| 1. | Complete obliteration |
| 2. | Residual neck |
| 3. | Residual aneurysm |
| 3a | Contrast opacification within the coil interstices of a residual aneurysm |
| 3b | Contrast opacification outside the coil interstices, along the residual aneurysm wall |

#### 1.3.2 Balloon-Assisted Coiling

Wide neck intracranial aneurysms represent a challenge. Aneurysms with a neck >4 mm could be difficult to treat with a non-assisted endovascular coiling. In fact, migration of heterologous material or the same coils into the vessel could cause local thrombosis and thromboembolism in the intracranial circulation.

For these reasons, balloon-assisted coiling, also known as remodeling technique, was introduced by J. Moret and his collaborators. This technique consists in inflating a thin balloon into the parent vase along the aneurysm neck, during the positioning and the subsequent detachment of the coils. The balloon's aid takes into account the temporary remodeling of the wide-necked aneurysm during the release of the coils. This method requires the placement of a microcatheter with a non-detachable balloon in the artery at aneurysm origin along the aneurysm neck (Fig. 2). Another microcatheter is placed in the aneurysm sac. The balloon is inflated before releasing the coil and then, before the coil detachment, the balloon is gently deflated so that the stability of the mass of the coils can be evaluated. This procedure is repeated for each subsequent coil. The balloon serves three purposes during embolization: first, to stabilize the microcatheter into the aneurysm sac; second, to force the coil to assume the three-dimensional shape of the aneurysm; and third, to obtain haemostasis in case of intra-procedural rupture.

#### 1.3.3 Stent-Assisted Coiling

The stent-assisted coiling is another endovascular technique used for the treatment of wide-necked aneurysms, as well as for the treatment of

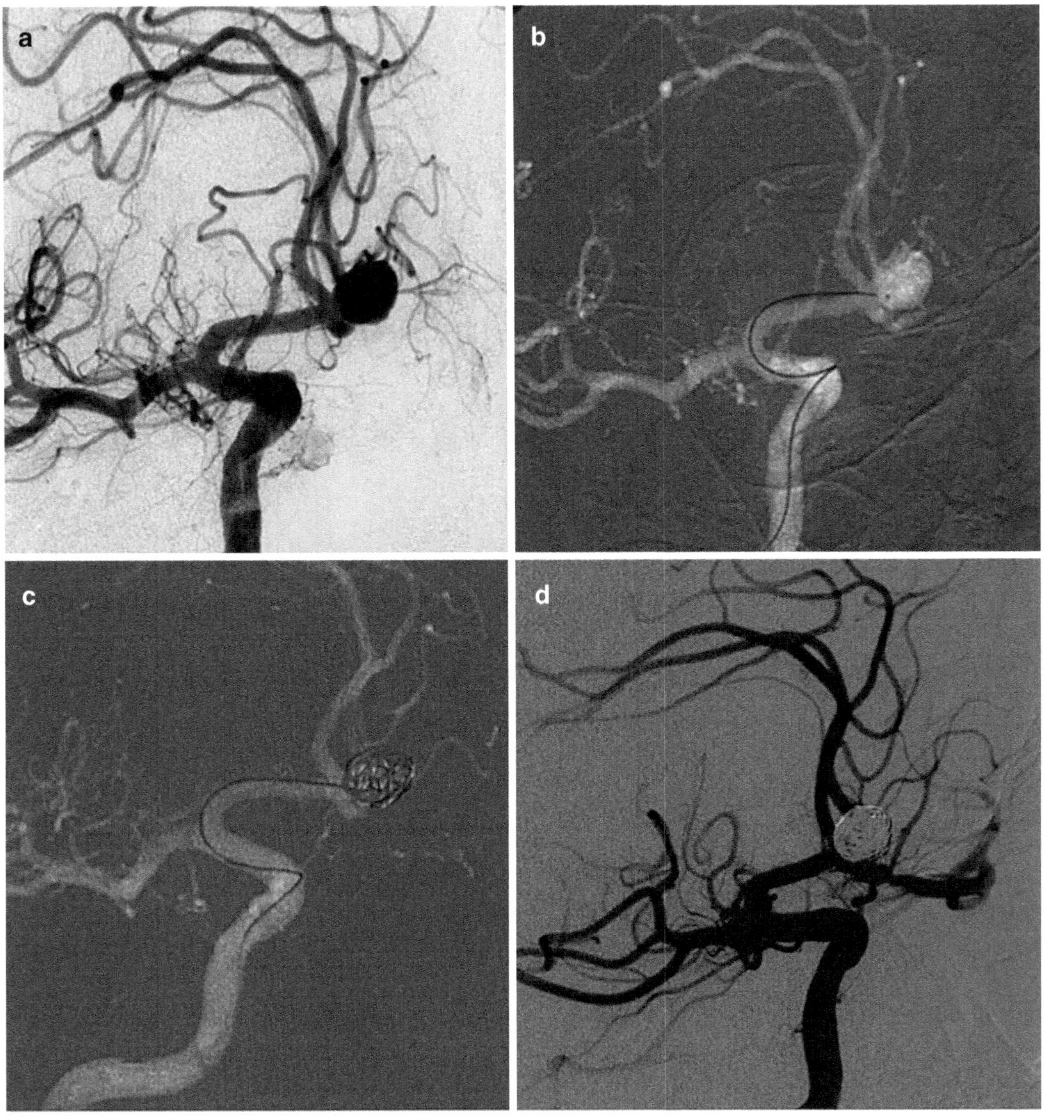


**Fig. 1** (**a**) Endovascular treatment with coiling of a small ruptured anterior communicating artery aneurysm. (**b**) Under fluoroscopic roadmap, the microcatheter is positioned into the aneurysm sac. (**c**) Deployment of the coils (**d**) Complete embolization at the end of the procedure

giant and dissecting aneurysms. The deployment of a stent at the aneurysm neck prevents the protrusion of the coils into the vessel and can help to prevent recurrence of the aneurysm (Shapiro et al. 2012) (Fig. 3).

The first stent designed for the intracranial circle was made in Nitinol (an alloy of nickel and titanium that assumes a predetermined configuration under appropriate conditions). This flexible material allows the stent to reach the tortuous vessels of the intracranial circulation. The procedure consists in positioning the stent in the parent artery along the aneurysm neck; a microcatheter is then positioned through the stent struts into the aneurysm sac, and then the coils are deployed. Alternatively, the microcatheter can be jailed into the aneurysm sac, while the stent is deployed into the parent vessel, also known as "jailing technique". With the possibility of having stents of various calibers and constructive characteristics

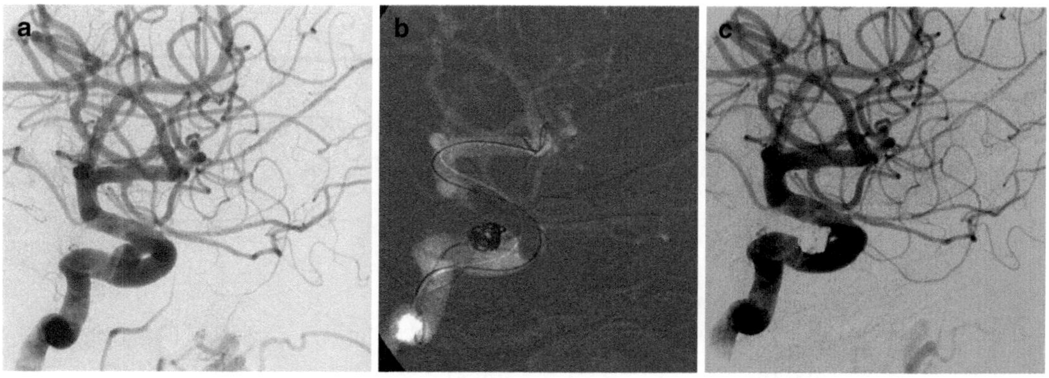


**Fig. 2** (**a**) Endovascular treatment with balloon-assisted coiling of a small ruptured carotid-cave aneurysm. (**b**) The balloon is temporary inflated during the coils' deployment (**c**) Complete embolization at the end of the procedure

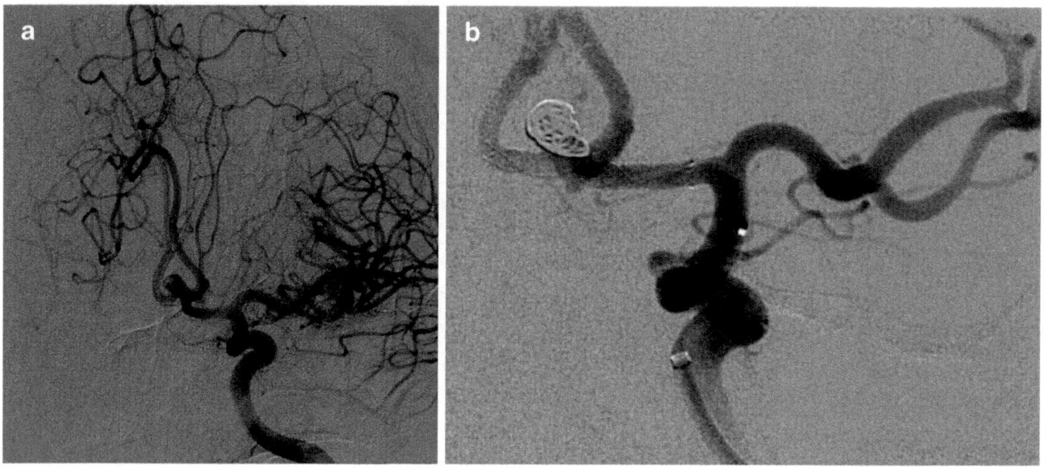


**Fig. 3** (**a**) Endovascular treatment with stent-assisted coiling of a ruptured anterior communicating artery aneurysm. (**b**) A braided stent is deployed through the anterior communicating artery; then the sac is filled with coils

(with open and closed cells, which can be recaptured and repositioned), interventional neuroradiologists have modified the technique, and with Y-stenting (Limbucci et al. 2016), all bifurcation aneurysms can be treated, allowing the reconstruction of the bifurcation.

Other newly developed devices, designed for the containment of the coils, are PulseRider® (Aguilar-Salinas et al. 2018) and pCONus® (Ulfert et al. 2018), which allow the treatment of large-bifurcation aneurysms without the need of deploying two intracranial stents.

The main drawback of this technique is the need of dual antiplatelet therapy, which represents a relative contraindication in the setting of SAH.

### 1.3.4 Intrasaccular Flow-Disruptors (WEB®)

The WEB® is a nitinol braided-wire intravascular device designed to disrupt blood flow at the aneurysmal neck.

This device has shown huge advantages in occluding difficult-to-treat aneurysms, such as wide-necked, and particularly for those located at bifurcation. These new devices consist in a high-attenuation micro-braided mesh constructed from a large number of nitinol wires (ranging from 19

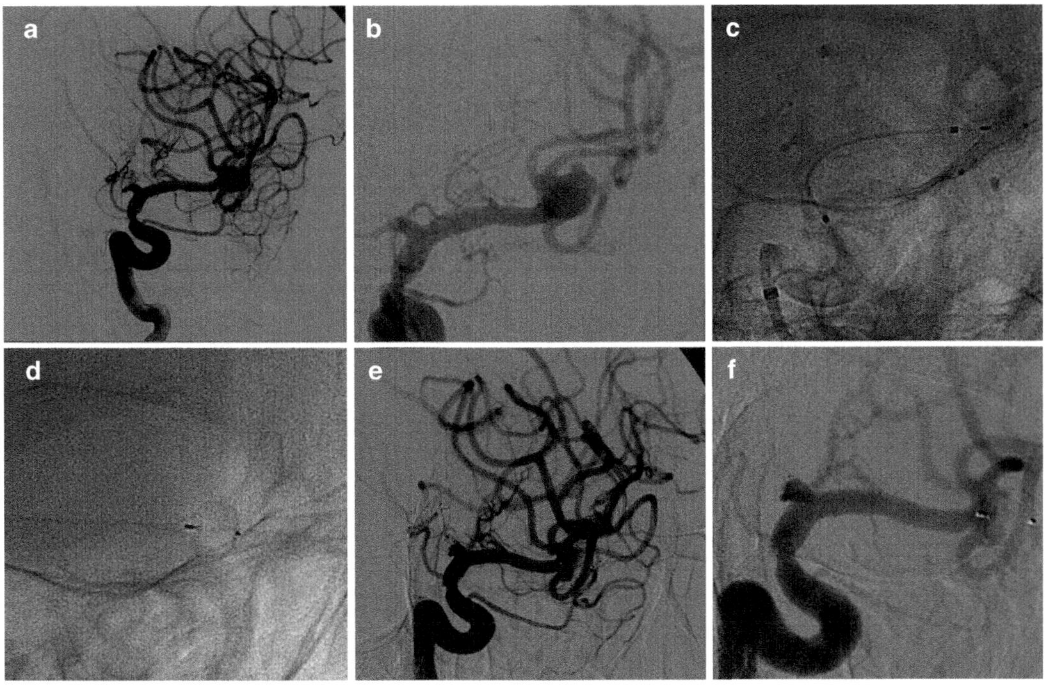


**Fig. 4** (**a**, **b**) A ruptured MCA trifurcation aneurysm; a bleb is highlighted on the superior portion of the sac. (**c**) Deployment of the WEB (**d**) Detachment of the WEB (**e**) Contrast stasis into the aneurysm sac (**f**) Complete occlusion of the aneurysm

to 38 μm) placed in the aneurysm sac to disrupt the intra-aneurysmal flow and create intra-aneurysmal thrombosis. Several studies have been focused on the treatment of unruptured cerebral aneurysms (Limbucci et al. 2018) (Fig. 4).

However, some authors have demonstrated the safety of the WEB in the treatment of ruptured intracranial aneurysms (van Rooij et al. 2016).

Particularly, the unnecessity of antiaggregation, or adjunctive stents or balloons, makes this strategy a valuable alternative to coils in the treatment of acutely ruptured aneurysms.

### 1.3.5 Flow-Diverter Devices

FDD are new and important tools in the treatment of intracranial aneurysms (Briganti et al. 2014; Briganti et al. 2015; Briganti et al. 2017). They are able to form a high-coverage mesh that induces thrombosis of the aneurysmal sac, while preserving patency of the adjacent small vessels (Kallmes et al. 2007).

Although the available data for the FDD remain extremely encouraging, there remain several theoretical limitations of the device with respect to its application in the treatment of ruptured cerebral aneurysms.

First, as with any intracranial stent-like device, a course of dual-antiplatelet medications is required for prophylaxis against thrombosis, while the construct is becoming endothelialized and incorporated into the parent artery. The optimal duration of dual-antiplatelet therapy remains uncertain, but the current recommendation is for 6 months of aspirin with clopidogrel with aspirin alone thereafter (Briganti et al. 2016). For this reason, aneurysmal subarachnoid haemorrhage represents a relative contraindication to FDD placement, given the potential for complications related to the invasive procedures frequently required during the perioperative period in these patients (i.e. ventriculostomy catheters, percutaneous gastrostomy tubes, tracheostomies, etc.).

Moreover, after FDD placement, without adjunctive coiling of the sac, the occlusion does not immediately occur and the patient is not theoretically protected by re-bleeding.

FDD are also used in ruptured aneurysms difficult to treat selectively either with the described endovascular techniques or with a microsurgical approach, such as very small aneurysms, blister-like aneurysms, dissecting aneurysms, or fusiform aneurysms (Zhu et al. 2018) (Figs. 5 and 6). However, it should be added that there are experiences of ruptured aneurysms treated with flow diverters in the acute phase, which demonstrate a rate of haemorrhagic complications not significantly different from that of other endovascular techniques and with a high percentage of complete occlusion at a distance.

On the other side, some authors have proposed staged treatment of ruptured complex and giant intracranial aneurysms with coiling in the acute phase and FDD treatment following recovery from SAH (Brinjikji et al. 2016).

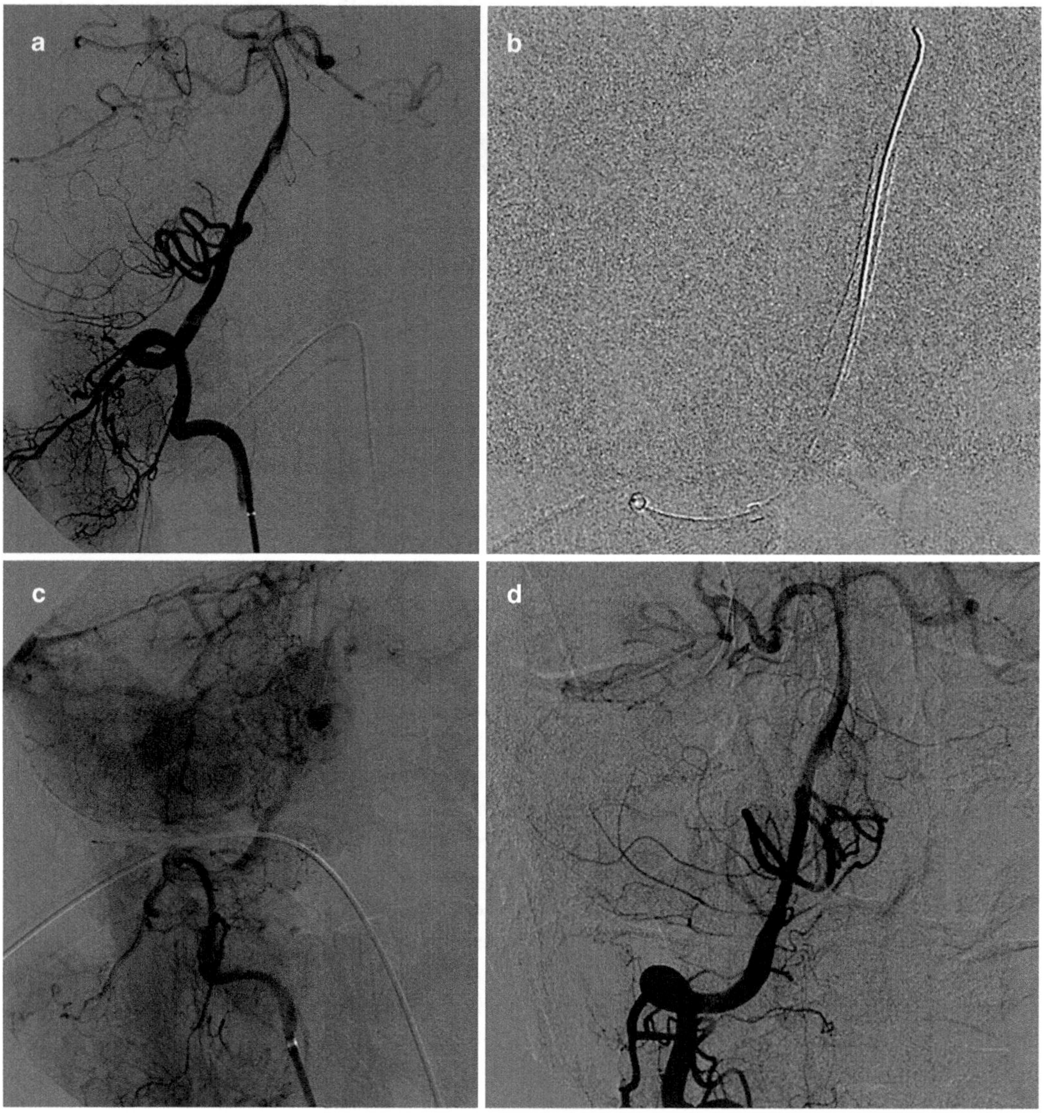


**Fig. 5** (**a**) Ruptured dissecting aneurysm of the V4 segment of the vertebral artery. (**b**) Flow-diverter device deployment. (**c**) Contrast stasis at the end of the procedure. (**d**) 3-month angiography shows complete aneurysm occlusion

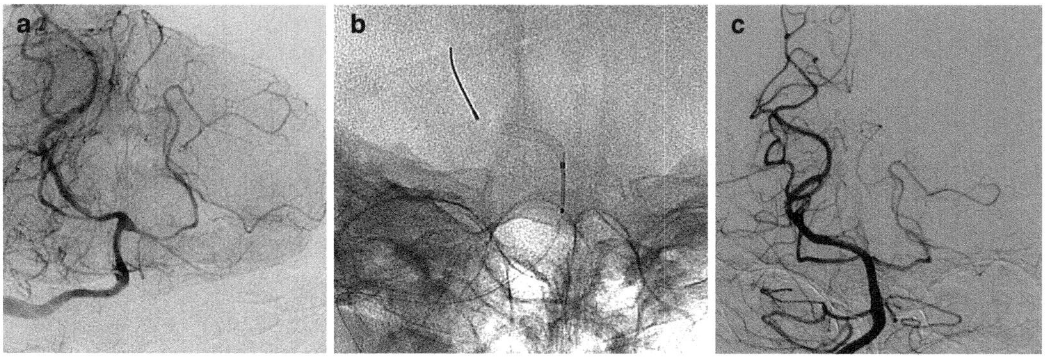


**Fig. 6** (**a**) A ruptured superior cerebellar artery aneurysm (**b**) Flow-diverter devices deployment into the basilar artery (**c**) Angiographic occlusion at 6 months

# 2 Endovascular Treatment of Haemorrhagic Intracranial Arteriovenous Malformations

## 2.1 Introduction

According to the National Stroke Association 2009 Fact Sheet, haemorrhagic stroke accounts for 13% of cases of acute stroke in the United States, with approximately 100,000 hospital admissions per year. Haemorrhagic stroke has a worse prognosis than ischemic stroke, with up to 50% 30-day mortality and very high rates of severe neurological disability among survivors (Qureshi et al. 2001).

There are two major types of haemorrhagic stroke: those that are due to an underlying vascular lesion such as a brain arteriovenous malformation (bAVM), aneurysm with intraparenchymal rupture, dural venous sinus (or cerebral vein) thrombosis (DVST), vasculitis, and Moya-Moya disease, which represent a minority of cases and are potentially treatable (secondary intracerebral haemorrhage); and those that are not due to an underlying vascular lesion (primary ICH).

The incidence of underlying vascular etiologies for an ICH varies significantly according to the patient's clinical characteristics and noncontrast CT findings, with patient age being one of the most important variables. Indeed, in recent Computed Tomography Angiography (CTA) studies, the frequency of secondary ICH has ranged from 13% to 28% in patients older than 18 years (Gazzola et al. 2008) to 65% in patients of 40 years of age (Romero et al. 2009).

## 2.2 Brain Arteriovenous Malformations

A bAVM is an abnormal connection between arteries and veins with a characteristic nidus. In patients who present with a haemorrhage, the incidence of AVM re-bleeding is increased from 2–4%/year to 6–18%/year for at least a year following the initial haemorrhage.

The ideal treatment of a bAVM is complete obliteration of the lesion which removes the risk of further haemorrhage and reduces the seizure risk.

However, an alternative approach to cure is one where endovascular intervention is directed at specific angiographic target areas in an attempt to improve symptoms and reduce the associated morbidity.

As bAVM haemorrhage rate is significantly increased after a bleed, treatment of any weakness responsible for haemorrhage also offers an opportunity to lower this bleed rate to baseline or below (Sun et al. 2017).

Under general anaesthesia, a guiding catheter is commonly placed in the internal carotid artery or in the vertebral artery. Then a microcatheter is navigated in the nidus and a microangiography is usually performed.

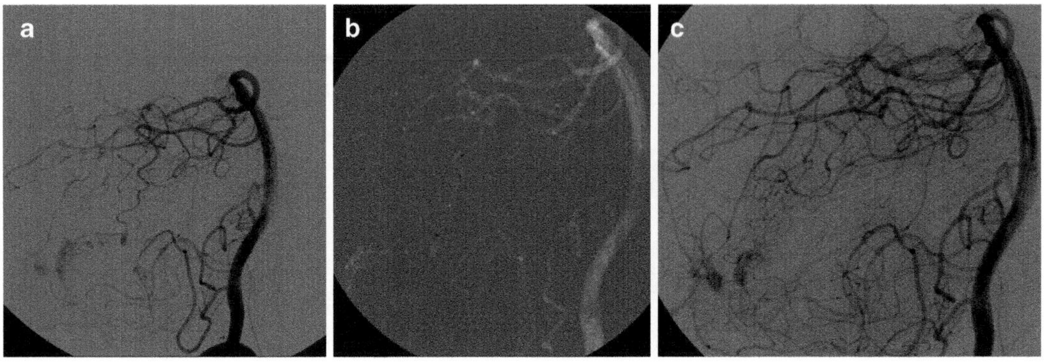


**Fig. 7** (**a**) Haemorrhagic cerebellar arteriovenous malformation fed by the right superior cerebellar artery. A pseudoaneurysm is highlighted on the feeders. (**b**) Microcatheterization of the feeder (**c**) Occlusion of the pseudoaneurysm with glue

The bleeding point is usually identified by looking for the presence of an intranidal or flow-related aneurysm. A flow-related aneurysm is defined as a saccular aneurysm in a vessel supplying the nidus, while an intranidal false aneurysm is identified as a defect with a smooth wall that was larger than the nidus channels with contrast often lingering within the defect.

In all of these case targets, endovascular embolization is usually performed (Fig. 7).

Embolization with N-butyl cyanoacrylate (NBCA), i.e. acrylic glue, is faster in injection times and requires, with the same rates of occlusion, more access for session, and more sessions. Acrylic embolization is the first option in the case of high-flow arteriovenous fistulas within the nidus or in the case of deep feeders (lenticolostriate arteries) or functional "en passage" arteries. Flow-related aneurysm or intranidal aneurysm can be occluded also with coils or with the use of nonadhesive embolic agent like, Onyx® (Medtronic), Squid® (Emboflu), and Phil® (Microvention).

## 2.3 Dural Arteriovenous Fistulas (dAVF)

Intracranial dural arteriovenous fistulas (dAVF) are pathologic shunts between dural arteries and dural venous sinuses, meningeal veins, or cortical veins, which account for 10–15% of intracranial arteriovenous malformations (Kwon et al. 2005).

Intracranial DAVFs presenting with haemorrhage require early treatment aimed at complete and definitive fistula obliteration, considering the substantial risks of re-bleeding after the first haemorrhage (Duffau et al. 1999).

The choice of endovascular treatment depends on the angioarchitecture of each dAVF and, in this regard, each individual case requires a detailed angiographic study.

The general principle of endovascular treatment is the complete obliteration of the fistula drainage and the multiple arterial feeders.

The endovascular treatment should be realized by both arterial or venous routes using two types of liquid embolic agents: adhesive (NBCA) and not adhesive (Onyx®, Squid®, Phil®).

NBCA has been used as an adhesive embolic agent with relatively good results, but it requires quick and continuous injection technique to avoid catheter tip occlusion due to high thrombogenicity of the glue. The advent of new non-adhesive liquid embolic agent has changed the treatment strategy for DAVFs because of its greater safety and efficacy compared with NBCA in endovascular embolization (Sadeh-Gonike et al. 2018).

In the endovascular treatment, it is necessary to reach with the microcatheter a point as close as possible to the fistula (Fig. 8). The main target is the closure of the vein foot or the pathological tract of the dural sinus: a too proximal injection could not favour the penetration of the embolic agent at the fistula point, with the additional inconvenience to occlude the feeder, preventing any future treatments.

The improvement of the microcatheters, however, has facilitated navigation of the meningeal

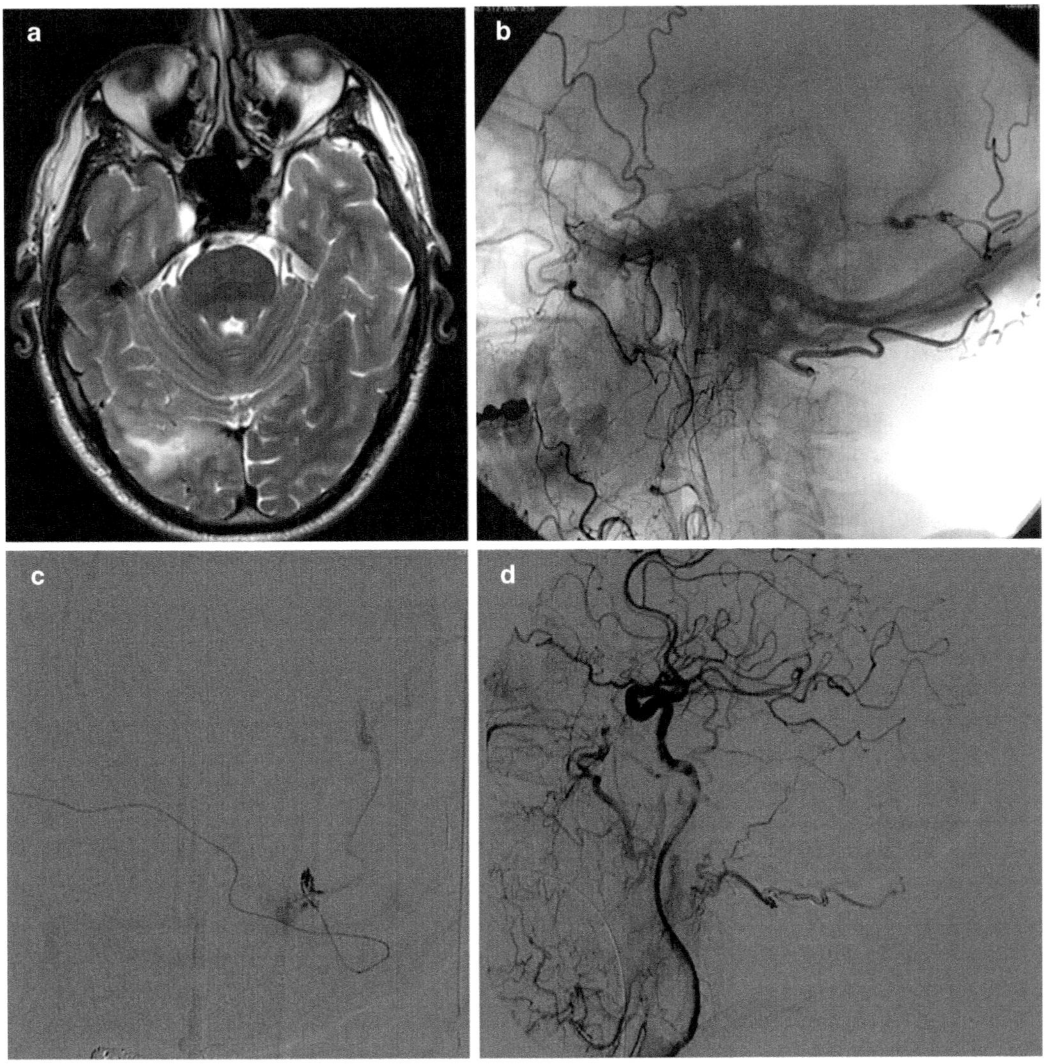

**Fig. 8** (**a**) MR of haemorrhagic dural arteriovenous fistula (DAVF) of the right occipital lobe. (**b**) The DAVF is fed by the transosseous branches of the right occipital artery and by posterior branch of the ipsilateral middle meningeal artery; the drainage occurs directly into an occipital vein (**c**, **d**) Occlusion of the fistula point with Onyx 18

vessels, almost always allowing a satisfactory injection point. A sure progress, in this sense, has been achieved with the introduction of detachable tip microcatheters, thanks to which an intermixed and prolonged injection technique of the chosen embolizing material could be implemented, avoiding the inconvenience of "gluing" of the distal end of the microcatheter, which force to leave the entire device in situ, cutting it at the level of the femoral access.

## 3 Endovascular Treatment of Acute Ischemic Stroke

### 3.1 Introduction

The efficacy of endovascular treatment in patients with acute ischemic stroke has been finally demonstrated in 2015 by 5 trials (ESCAPE, EXTEND-IA, SWIFT-PRIME, REVASCAT, and MR CLEAN) (Berkhemer et al. 2015; Campbell et al. 2016; Demchuk et al. 2014; Jovin et al. 2015; Saver et al. 2015), which have definitively established the usefulness of this type of reperfusion therapy after negative results obtained in previous published trial (MR RESCUE and SYNTHESIS) (Kidwell et al. 2013; Ciccone et al. 2013). The success of these studies is due not only to the use of new and more efficient endovascular devices, but also to the use of innovative neuroradiological techniques of computerized tomography (CT) and magnetic resonance (MR) between the inclusion and/or exclusion criteria: with the exception of MR CLEAN, in fact, in all the remaining trials, these advanced methods, represented above all by multi-phase CT angiography (multi-phase CT Angiography, mCTA), perfusion CT (CT Perfusion, CTP), and MR diffusion and perfusion, have been adopted instead of conventional CT scans without intravenous contrast medium and single-phase CTA in identifying patients for endovascular treatment. This approach has therefore shed new light on the strategies to be followed to achieve a more appropriate selection of patient candidates for endovascular therapy.

The importance of advanced neuroimaging in selecting for thrombectomy has been further demonstrated by two recent trials. In fact, according to the DAWN (Nogueira et al. 2018) (DWI or CTP Assessment with Clinical Mismatch in the Triage of Wake-Up and Late Presenting Strokes Undergoing Neurointervention with Trevo) and the DEFUSE 3 (Sheinberg et al. 2018) (Endovascular Therapy Following Imaging Evaluation for Ischaemic Stroke) trials, the therapeutic window has been extended up to 24 h in carefully selected patients.

## 3.2 Selection Criteria

Since endovascular intervention is indicated only in the cases of a primary intracranial artery occlusion, it is necessary to identify the patients to be investigated (Powers et al. 2018).

The selection is primarily made with reference to the clinical severity, according to National Institutes of Health Stroke Scale (NIHSS) clinical score.

Studies on the use of multimodal MR, which includes at least sequences in diffusion and perfusion and MR angiography (MRA), or multimodal CT, which includes perfusion study and CTA, however, have proved to be useful in defining the "salvable" brain tissue, particularly to better guide the indication to the endovascular intervention.

The use of multimodal imaging is particularly useful when the time interval from the onset of the symptoms is >4.5 h, when the endovascular treatment is performed at or above the time window, or when the stroke onset is unknown (stroke at the awakening).

The preliminary study before endovascular treatment with CTA or MRA can be very important in the planning of endovascular treatment. Careful evaluation of the angle between the aortic arch and the supra-aortic trunks and the caliber and tortuosity of the carotid artery, subclavian, and vertebral arteries make it possible to choose between a femoral or brachial/radial approach.

## 3.3 Endovascular Treatments and Techniques

All procedures are usually performed under conscious sedation in the angiography suite. No systemic heparinization is usually administered.

Femoral route is usually performed in almost cases.

The brachial/radial approach on the right should be considered in cases with marked tortuosity of the anonymous trunk (for vertebral and right internal carotid artery [ICA]) and with the origin of the left ICA from the anonymous trunk (for left ICA), while left brachial/radial approach in case of marked tortuosity of the left subclavian artery (for left vertebral artery).

Guiding catheters ranging from 6 to 9 Fr can be used depending on the caliber of carotid-vertebral arteries; it is important to obtain a stable position of the guiding catheter, trying not to block the flow if the catheterized artery supplies cerebral arteries or contribute to collateral circulation to the suffering brain region.

In the anterior circulation, it is possible to use an 8 F guiding catheter (or 9 in case of occlusion of the ICA at the origin) with a balloon to perform flow blockage and aspiration during the recovery of the stent-retriever in the ICA. It is advisable to use a coaxial system with a 5 Fr diagnostic intermediate catheter 125 cm long inside the 8 Fr catheter and 0.035 guide within the 5 Fr catheter.

### 3.3.1 Stent-retriever Thrombectomy

In the technique of thrombectomy with stent-retriever, the catheterization of the occluded artery is performed using the microwire. The occlusion point is passed with a "blind" navigation; in some cases, a wide loop at the microwire tip allows better recanalization of the vessel and reduces the engagement of collateral branches. Once the occlusion has been overcome, the microcatheter is advanced. This is followed by injection of the contrast medium from the microcatheter to confirm the position downstream of the occlusion.

Then a stent-retriever is deployed at the occlusion level; a control angiography is performed to verify the presence of the flow inside the stent-retriever. Then, the stent-retriever can be left in place for 5 min (Fig. 9).

It is advisable to remove the stent-retriever with flow block and in continuous aspiration, using a 60 cc syringe or an automatic pump; according to this technique, the balloon placed at the end of the guiding catheter is inflated by injection of contrast medium before starting the recovery of the stent-retriever which is slowly withdrawn together with the microcatheter, while the second operator carries out the aspiration of blood from the guiding catheter.

A variant of the stent-retriever retraction technique within the guiding catheter involves capture of the thrombus at the end of a large-caliber intermediate catheter, navigated in contact with the stent-retriever (Epic technique).

In cases where there is a significant vascular tortuosity, the vascular access is made by using an intermediate catheter of particular flexibility and softness that, if of appropriate caliber (5 or 6 Fr), allows the distal thromboaspiration during the concomitant maneuver of thrombectomy (Solumbra technique); in this case, thromboaspiration and stent-retriever work together (Fig. 10).

### 3.3.2 Thromboaspiration

As an alternative to the technique with stent-retriever, it can also be used as a primary aspiration (ADAPT) with a 5 or 6 Fr catheter with a wide internal lumen (between 0.056 and 0.072 in.); this catheter must be taken immediately proximal to the thrombus using a microcatheter and microguide inside, keeping the

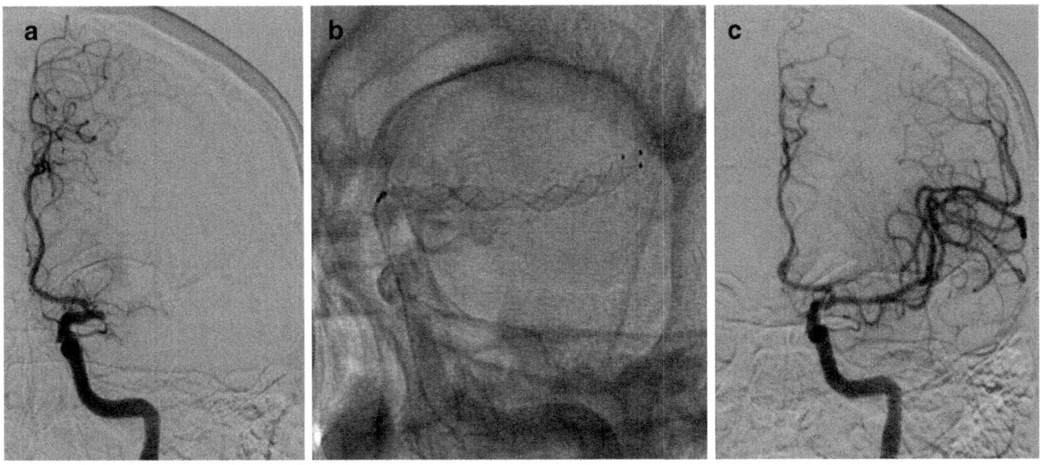


**Fig. 9** (**a**) Embolic occlusion of the proximal M1 segment of the middle cerebral artery (MCA); (**b**) Deployment of a stent-retriever (**c**) After one thrombectomy attempt, complete flow restoration

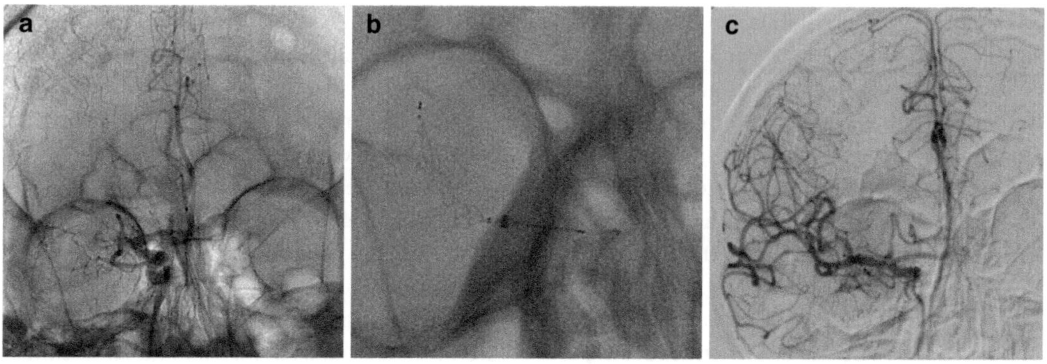


**Fig. 10** (**a**) Embolic occlusion of the proximal M1 segment of the middle cerebral artery (MCA); (**b**) Deployment of a stent-retriever into the M1-M2 segment of the MCA, while an aspiration catheter is placed in the M1, under continuous aspiration. (**c**) Complete flow restoration after the thrombectomy

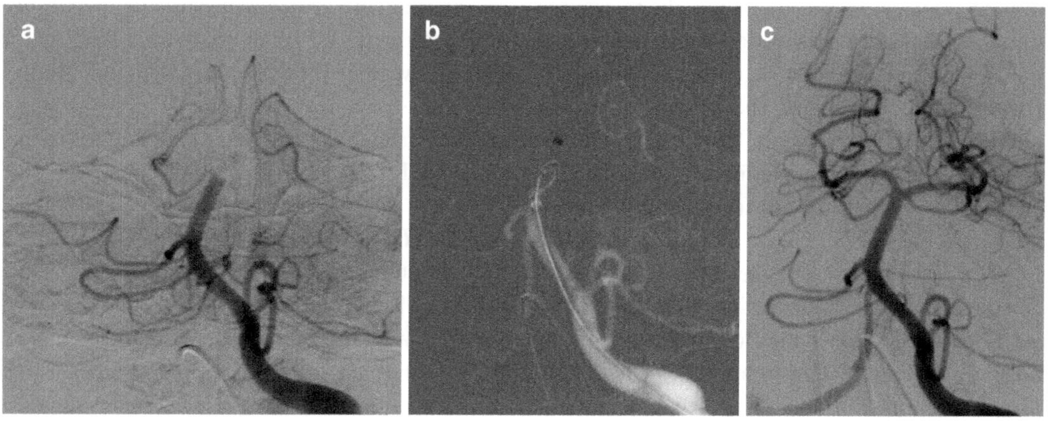


**Fig. 11** (**a**) Embolic occlusion of the mid-basilar artery. (**b**) An aspiration catheter is positioned in contact to the clot. (**c**) After one thromboaspiration maneuver, complete recanalization of the basilar artery

system in continuous suction during the recovery maneuver.

This technique can also be used as a first intention (ADAPT), in some cases recanalizing the thrombectomy without using the stent-retriever (Fig. 11).

In 2017, ASTER trial compared efficacy and adverse events using the contact aspiration technique vs the standard stent-retriever technique as a first-line endovascular treatment for successful revascularization among patients with acute ischemic stroke and large vessel occlusion (Lapergue et al. 2017).

However, among patients with ischemic stroke in the anterior circulation undergoing thrombectomy, first-line thrombectomy with contact aspiration compared with stent-retriever did not result in an increased successful revascularization rate at the end of the procedure.

Extra-cranial carotid artery occlusion associated to intracranial occlusion (Tandem occlusion).

In case of carotid artery occlusion because of atherothrombotic or occlusive dissection (between 9% and 20% in the cases of the 5 recent trials), in most cases, after passing the occlusion by the 0.014 microwire, a stent is advanced and released at the cervical carotid occlusion, proceeding later to mechanical thrombectomy or thromboaspiration.

In the cases of stent-retriever use, it is necessary to pass the carotid stent with the guiding catheter (or with intermediate catheter 5 or 6 Fr with a large internal lumen) to prevent that stent-retriever get jailed with the carotid stent during the thrombectomy maneuver.

In the case of stent placement, antiaggregation therapy (double antiaggregation with clopidogrel loading, if the patient was not already on double antiaggregation therapy) is indicated even if fibrinolytic therapy is in progress or has just been completed.

## 4 Conclusion

The minimally invasive procedures used by interventional neuroradiologists accomplish a wide variety of treatments designed to provide correct life-threatening conditions, such as haemorrhagic or ischemic stroke. As alternatives to invasive surgery, these forms of therapy are often advantageous because they can lower the risk to patients, shorten hospital stays, and hasten recovery.

Some treatments, including emergency stroke care, are not feasible using an open surgery approach and can only be performed using a neurointervention procedure to increase patient outcomes.

Continuing improvement in imaging technology is also expected to enhance the therapeutic possibilities of this fascinating field.

## References

Aguilar-Salinas P, Brasiliense LBC, Walter CM et al (2018) Current status of the PulseRider in the treatment of bifurcation aneurysms: a systematic review. World Neurosurg 115:288–294. https://doi.org/10.1016/j.wneu.2018.04.102. Epub 2018 Apr 24

Berkhemer OA, Fransen PS, Beumer D et al (2015) A randomized trial of intraarterial treatment for acute ischemic stroke. N Engl J Med 372:11–20. [Erratum, N Engl J Med 2015;372:394]

Briganti F, Napoli M, Leone G et al (2014) Treatment of intracranial aneurysms by flow diverter devices: long term results from a single center. Eur J Radiol 83:1683–1690

Briganti F, Leone G, Marseglia M et al (2015) Endovascular treatment of cerebral aneurysms using flow-diverter devices: a systematic review. Neuroradiol J 28:365–375

Briganti F, Delehaye L, Leone G et al (2016) Flow diverter device for the treatment of small middle cerebral artery aneurysms. J Neurointerv Surg 8:287–294

Briganti F, Leone G, Ugga L et al (2017) Mid-term and long-term follow-up of intracranial aneurysms treated by the p64 flow modulation device: a multicenter experience. J Neurointerv Surg 9:70–76

Brinjikji W, Piano M, Fang S et al (2016) Treatment of ruptured complex and large/giant ruptured cerebral aneurysms by acute coiling followed by staged flow diversion. J Neurosurg 125:120–127

Campbell BC, Hill MD, Rubiera M et al (2016) Safety and efficacy of solitaire stent thrombectomy: individual patient data meta-analysis of randomized trials. Stroke 47:798–806. https://doi.org/10.1161/STROKEAHA.115.012360

Ciccone A, Valvassori L, Nichelatti M, SYNTHESIS Expansion Investigators et al (2013) Endovascular treatment for acute ischemic stroke. N Engl J Med 368:904–913

Demchuk AM, Goyal M, Menon BK et al (2014) ESCAPE Trial Investigators Endovascular treatment for Small Core and Anterior circulation Proximal occlusion with Emphasis on minimizing CT to recanalization times (ESCAPE) trial: methodology. Int J Stroke. https://doi.org/10.1111/ijs.12424

Duffau H, Lopes M, Janosevic V et al (1999) Early rebleeding from intracranial dural arteriovenous fistulas: report of 20 cases and re- view of the literature. J Neurosurg 90:78–84

Gazzola S, Aviv RI, Gladstone DJ et al (2008) Vascular and nonvascular mimics of the CT angiography "spot sign" in patients with secondary intracerebral hemorrhage. Stroke 39:1177–1183

Johnston SC, Dowd CF, Higashida RT, CARAT Investigators et al (2008) Predictors of rehemorrhage after treatment of ruptured intracranial aneurysms: the Cerebral Aneurysm Rerupture After Treatment (CARAT) study. Stroke 39:120–125. Epub 2007 Nov 29

Jovin TG, Chamorro A, Cobo E et al (2015) Thrombectomy within 8 hours after symptom onset in ischemic stroke. N Engl J Med 372:2296–2306. https://doi.org/10.1056/NEJMoa1503780

Kallmes D, Ding YH, Daying D et al (2007) A new endoluminal, flow-disrupting device for the treatment of saccular aneurysms. Stroke 38:2346–2352

Kidwell CS, Jahan R, Gornbein J, MR RESCUE Investigators et al (2013) A trial of imaging selection and endovascular treatment for ischemic stroke. N Engl J Med 368:914–923. https://doi.org/10.1056/NEJMoa1212793

Kwon BJ, Han MH, Kang HS et al (2005) MR imaging findings of intracranial dural arteriovenous fistulas: relations with venous drainage patterns. AJNR Am J Neuroradiol 26:2500–2507

Lapergue B, Blanc R, Gory B, ASTER Trial Investigators et al (2017) Effect of endovascular contact aspiration vs stent retriever on revascularization in patients with acute ischemic stroke and large vessel occlusion: the ASTER randomized clinical trial. JAMA 318:443–452. https://doi.org/10.1001/jama.2017.9644

Limbucci N, Renieri L, Nappini S et al (2016) Y-stent assisted coiling of bifurcation aneurysms with Enterprise stent: long-term follow-up. J Neurointerv Surg 8:158–162. https://doi.org/10.1136/neurintsurg-2014-011483

Limbucci N, Leone G, Rosi A et al (2018) Endovascular treatment of unruptured intracranial aneurysms by the woven EndoBridge device (WEB): are there any aspects influencing aneurysm occlusion? World Neurosurg 109:e183–e193. https://doi.org/10.1016/j.wneu.2017.09.136

Lozupone E, Piano M, Valvassori L et al (2018) Flow diverter devices in ruptured intracranial aneurysms: a single-center experience. J Neurosurg 128:1037–1043

Mayer SA, Kreiter KT, Copeland D et al (2002) Global and domain-specific cognitive impairment and outcome after subarachnoid hemorrhage. Neurology 59:1750–1758

Molyneux AJ, Kerr RS, Yu LM, International Subarachnoid Aneurysm Trial (ISAT) Collaborative Group et al (2005) International subarachnoid aneurysm trial (ISAT) of neurosurgical clipping versus endovascular coiling in 2143 patients with ruptured intracranial aneurysms: a randomised comparison of effects on survival, dependency, seizures, rebleeding, subgroups, and aneurysm occlusion. Lancet 366:809–817

Muto M, Giurazza F, Ambrosanio G et al (2017) Stent-assisted coiling in ruptured cerebral aneurysms: multi-center experience in acute phase. Radiol Med 122:43–52

Nogueira RG, Jadhav AP, Haussen DC, DAWN Trial Investigators et al (2018) Thrombectomy 6 to 24 hours after stroke with a mismatch between deficit and infarct. N Engl J Med 378:11–21. https://doi.org/10.1056/NEJMoa1706442

Pierot L, Spelle L, Vitry F, for the ATENA investigators (2008) Immediate clinical outcome of patients harbouring unruptured intracranial aneurysms treated by endovascular approach: results of the ATENA trial. Stroke 39:2497–2504

Powers WJ, Rabinstein AA, Ackerson T, American Heart Association Stroke Council et al (2018) 2018 Guidelines for the early management of patients with acute ischemic stroke: a guideline for healthcare professionals from the American Heart Association/American Stroke Association. Stroke 49:e46–e110. https://doi.org/10.1161/STR.0000000000000158. Epub 2018 Jan 24. Review. Erratum in: Stroke. 2018;49:e138. Stroke. 2018 Apr 18

Qureshi AI, Tuhrim S, Broderick JP et al (2001) Spontaneous intracerebral hemorrhage. N Engl J Med 344:1450–1460

Romero JM, Artunduaga M, Forero NP et al (2009) Accuracy of CT angiography for the diagnosis of vascular abnormalities causing intraparenchymal hemorrhage in young patients. Emerg Radiol 16:195–201

Sadeh-Gonike U, Magand N, Armoiry X et al (2018) Transarterial onyx embolization of intracranial dural fistulas: a prospective cohort, systematic review, and meta-analysis. Neurosurgery 82:854–863

Saver JL, Goyal M, Bonafe A et al (2015) Stent-retriever thrombectomy after intravenous t-PA vs. t-PA alone in stroke. N Engl J Med 372(24):2285–2295. https://doi.org/10.1056/NEJMoa1415061

Shapiro M, Becske T, Sahlein D et al (2012) Stent-supported aneurysm coiling: a literature survey of treatment and follow-up. AJNR Am J Neuroradiol 33:159–163

Sheinberg DL, McCarthy DJ, Peterson EC, DEFUSE-3 Trial et al (2018) Reinforcing evidence for extended endovascular intervention time window for ischemic stroke. World Neurosurg 112:275–276. https://doi.org/10.1016/j.wneu.2018.02.064

Sun Y, Jin H, Li Y et al (2017) Target embolization of associated aneurysms in ruptured arteriovenous malformations. World Neurosurg 101:26–32. https://doi.org/10.1016/j.wneu.2017.01.081

Ulfert C, Pfaff J, Schönenberger S et al (2018) The pCONus device in treatment of wide-necked aneurysms: technical and midterm clinical and angiographic results. Clin Neuroradiol 28(1):47–54. https://doi.org/10.1007/s00062-016-0542-z

van Rooij WJ, Peluso JP, Bechan RS et al (2016) WEB treatment of ruptured intracranial aneurysms. AJNR Am J Neuroradiol 37:1679–1683. https://doi.org/10.3174/ajnr.A4811

Zhu D, Yan Y, Zhao P et al (2018) Safety and efficacy of flow diverter treatment for blood blister-like aneurysm: a systematic review and meta-analysis. World Neurosurg. https://doi.org/10.1016/j.wneu.2018.06.123. pii: S1878-8750(18)31339-1

# Emergency Paediatric Head and Neck

Hewitt Peter, Nanapragasam Andrew, Raghavan Ashok, and Senasi Ramdas

## Contents




**Abstract**

Imaging in the emergency setting is a distinct entity from other types of radiology practice, with its own challenges and pitfalls. There are unique imaging features in emergency paediatric head and neck imaging, of which radiologists ought to be aware to ensure timely and accurate reporting of these diseases. In this chapter, we will discuss these specific features and provide the reader with useful advice.



H. Peter · N. Andrew
Department of Radiology, Royal Victoria Infirmary, Newcastle-Upon-Tyne, UK

R. Ashok
Department of Radiology, Sheffield Children's Hospital, Sheffield, UK

S. Ramdas (✉)
Department of Radiology, South Tyneside and Sunderland NHS Trust, Sunderland, UK
e-mail: drsenasi@doctors.org.uk





M. Scaglione et al. (eds.), *Emergency Radiology of the Head and Spine*, Medical Radiology Diagnostic Imaging, https://doi.org/10.1007/978-3-030-91047-1_22

## Abbreviation

| | |
|---|---|
| CCJ | Craniocervical junction |
| CSF | Cerebrospinal fluid |
| CT | Computed tomography |
| DWI | Diffusion weighted imaging |
| GMH | Germinal matrix haemorrhage |
| HIE | Hypoxic ischaemic encephalopathy |
| MCA | Middle cerebral artery |
| MRI | Magnetic resonance imaging |
| MRS | MR-spectroscopy |
| NAI | Non-accidental injury |
| SWI | Susceptibility weighted imaging |

## 1 Imaging Modalities in Paediatrics

### 1.1 Plain Film

Outside of non-accidental injury (NAI) (see chapter "Acute Stroke: Management"), plain film plays a limited role in the assessment of non-traumatic paediatric emergency imaging (Culotta et al. 2016).

### 1.2 CT/CTA

For definitive diagnosis of the various presentations discussed in this chapter, CT and MRI are the investigations of choice. The recommended protocol for adequate assessment of the paediatric head is multiplanar 0.5 mm slice acquisition with 3D reformats if skull lesions are under assessment.

### 1.3 MRI

MRI assessment is a powerful tool for initial presentation or further characterisation of lesions within the head. It is recommended that local protocol is followed regarding the specific sequences to acquire.

### 1.4 Points for Consideration

- Pathology of the paediatric head and neck, especially in trauma, can be very subtle and difficult to assess. Without using the appropriate imaging modality and, with regards to CT, the appropriate reconstruction algorithms, it can be impossible to see certain pathologies.
- Plain radiographs—every effort should be made to make this patient group feel comfortable and settled to ensure adequate images without the need for repeat imaging, with its associated dose penalty (Halliday et al. 2016).
- Good communication with paediatricians will provide a wealth of knowledge and clinical expertise. Often, the information on a request card will be limited and insufficient to provide useful, diagnostic report; contact with the referring clinician can make a substantial difference.
- "Children are not little adults". This is common knowledge in paediatrics, and it is just as relevant in paediatric radiology.

## 2 Traumatic Pathology

### 2.1 Head

CT is the modality of choice for traumatic head pathology. The authors of this chapter feel it is essential to obtain thin slice (0.5 mm) acquisitions with 3D bone reformats to reduce the possibility of missing subtle pathology, or mistaking them for normal anatomy or variants.

Fractures, sutures, and wormian bones are the most common causes of a cortical 'defect' in a child's skull seen on CT (Sanchez et al. 2010). Excellent knowledge of the paediatric cranial sutures, as seen in Fig. 1, is essential to differentiate between fracture and normal anatomy.

Sutures will show ossification along their length and will have a complex 'zig-zag' serrated edge. Viewing the soft tissue windows helps to highlight any extracranial subcutaneous collection/haematoma to help direct your assessment to the adjacent skull in search of a fracture.

Wormian bones are often small and sometimes numerous bones are seen within normal cranial sutures, for example, mostly commonly along the lambdoid suture. They may also be seen centrally within the fontanelles as bony islands. Wormian bones can be a normal anatomical variant, but sometimes associated with con-

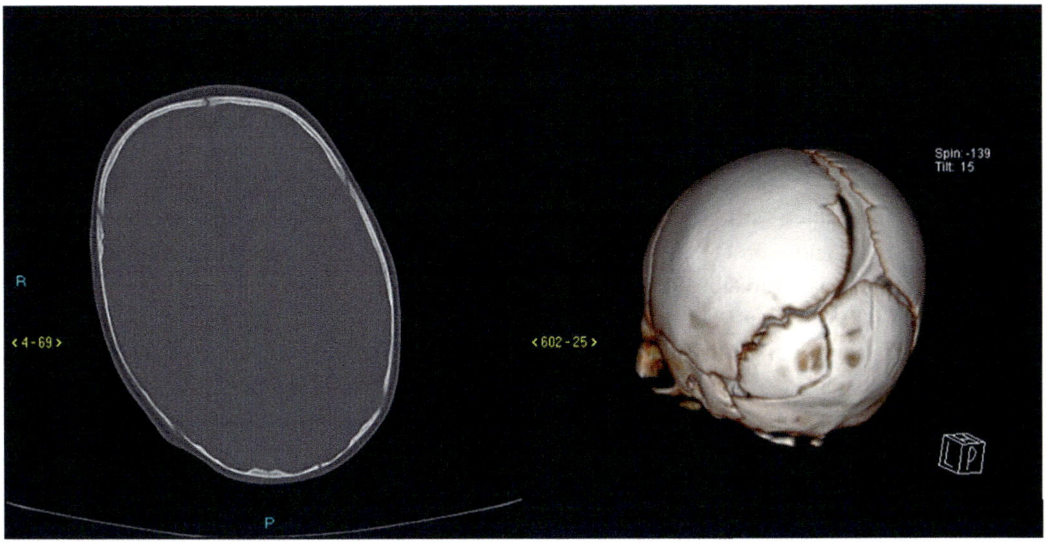


**Fig. 1** Left: Thin slice CT head (bone reformat) showing an asymmetrical defect in the left occipital bone. Right: 3D reconstruction demonstrates an accessory left occipital suture

ditions such as osteogenesis imperfecta and Down syndrome; however, it is usually considered normal if less than 10 are present up to the age of 6 months (Marti et al. 2013).

Traumatic intracranial haemorrhage follows similar principles to imaging adult head trauma; however, clinical signs and symptoms may differ and neurological assessment may be less reliable. It is important to have a low threshold to image children who have suffered traumatic head injury. Extra-axial haematoma is less common in children due to the shallow position of the middle meningeal artery and the adherent strength of the dura mater to the inner skull. Although not as common, it should not be disregarded that an extra-axial arterial haematoma can be life-threatening. Subdural haematoma is more common (Araki et al. 2017), especially in NAI cases as discussed previously. Other consequences of traumatic brain injury include brain parenchymal contusions, subarachnoid haemorrhage, and intraventricular haemorrhage, which should be evaluated in a similar way to adult imaging.

## 2.2 Cervical Spine

In this section, we will focus on the key features of traumatic injury that are unique to children (Lustrin et al. 2003). First, children suffer more from craniocervical junction (CCJ) injuries and more upper cervical injuries than adults. In fact, 90% of cervical fractures below age 8 are located between the CCJ and the fourth cervical vertebra (McAllister et al. 2019). However, in the adult population, there is a rough equal distribution of injury in the upper and lower cervical spine.

The relative prevalence of soft tissue injury/dislocation and fractures represents another important distinction between adult and paediatric cervical injuries. For patients under the age of 8, soft tissue injuries and dislocations constitute the majority of traumatic injuries (McAllister et al. 2019). However, in the adult population, this is reversed, with fractures being vastly more common than soft tissue injuries or dislocations.

The reason for the difference between injury pattern is due to the following key mechanical differences in the growing child:

- Large head:body ratio results in translation of momentum-related injury to the upper cervical vertebra.
- The fulcrum of movement in the paediatric c-spine is at C2-C3, whereas in adults it is C5-C6.
- The ligaments in children have great laxity, which is useful for growth, but it can predispose to dislocation.

- The cervical articular facets and the CCJ have a noticeable more horizontal orientation in children, which again predisposes to dislocation.

Atlanto-occipital dislocation is an injury worthy of particular attention as it is often fatal, and often difficult to diagnose on CT imaging, especially when an associated fracture is not present (Riascos et al. 2015). The Powers Ratio, the Basion-Axis Interval, and the Dens-Basion Interval have been considered as means of identifying an atlanto-occipital dislocation; however, their sensitivity is not sufficiently high to reliably exclude this serious finding. In our experience, the occipital condyle to C1 interval distance of more than 3 mm is the optimal means of identifying atlanto-occipital dislocation (Bertozzi et al. 2009). Care should be taken when making this measurement. In the unfused skeleton of young children, the medial and lateral aspects of the occipital condyle to C1 have notably different intervals. Taking measurements at the medial aspect will falsely overestimate the interval as there is non-ossified hyaline cartilage in this space that cannot be appreciated on CT imaging. Therefore, in order to avoid false positives, measurements should be taken at the lateral aspect of the occipital condyle to C1 interval (Figs. 2 and 3).

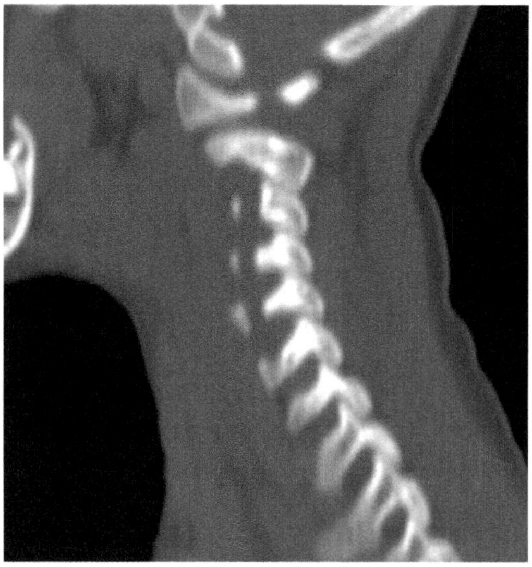

**Fig. 2** Normal occipital condyle to atlas distance

Specific attention should be paid to the predental space. The predental space is anatomical compartment between the odontoid peg and the anterior arch of the C1 vertebra. It should measure less than 5 mm in patients 8 years or under and should be less than 3 mm in patients over 8 years. If the described interval is increased, disruption of the transverse ligament and/or a fractured C1 vertebra should be suspected (Fig. 4).

Having covered these specific differences between paediatric and adult cervical spine imaging, it is important to also remember that many of the principles from adult imaging also apply. Assessment of cervical alignment using the anterior vertebral line, posterior vertebral line, spinolaminar line, and posterior spinous line is a useful way of identifying dislocations and fractures (Guarnieri et al. 2016). Evaluating the prevertebral soft tissue for thickening is an important clue for occult fractures. Radiologists should also pay close attention to the airway as foreign bodies causing airway obstruction are a rare, but important finding.

## 3 Non-traumatic Pathology

### 3.1 Cerebrovascular Disease and Stroke

Although much more commonly a disease of adults, stroke is becoming increasingly common in the paediatric population, possibly due to the increased sensitivity of imaging modalities, with incidences up to 3/100,000. Children often present slightly later than adults (over 24 h) with non-specific lethargy, coma, irritability often obscuring more subtle focal neurological deficits (Clinical Standards and Quality Improvement team 2017).

Childhood stroke is differentiated into ischaemic and haemorrhagic aetiologies shown in Box 1 (Tables 1 and 2; Figs. 5, 6, and 7).

Ultrasound is less widely used for childhood stroke in the acute setting, but a hyperechoic vascular territory may be seen in neonates with open sutures (Donahue et al. 2019). Ultrasound is

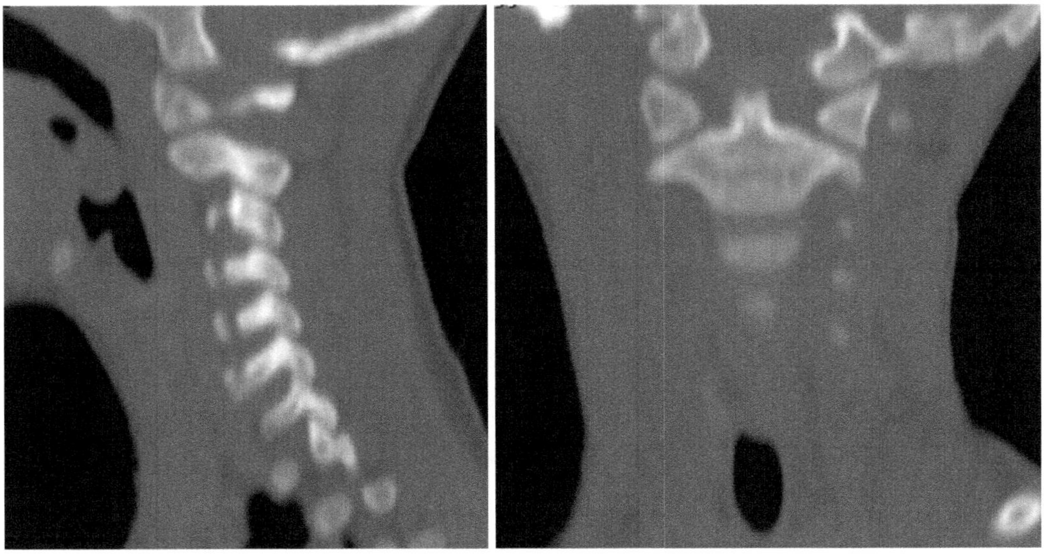

**Fig. 3** Sagittal and coronal CT reformats showing a widened occipital condyle to atlas distance

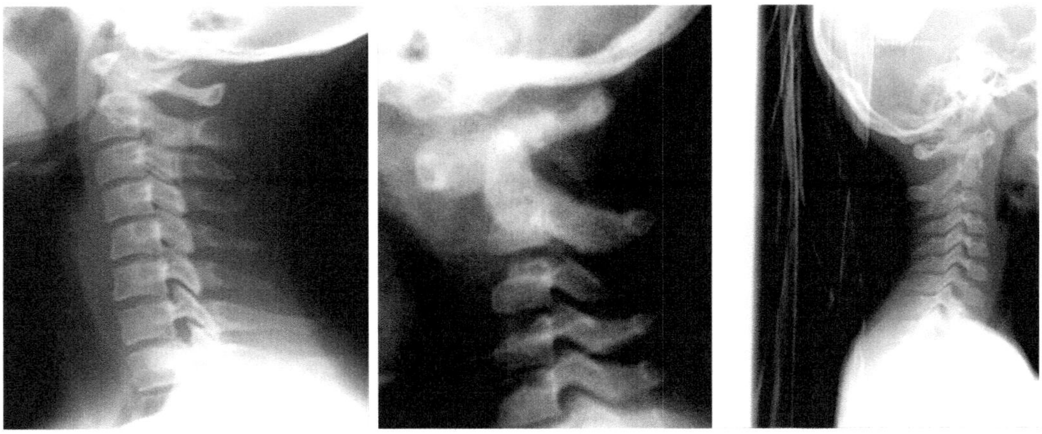

**Fig. 4** Left: lateral C-spine X-ray showing predental space. Middle: lateral c-spine X-ray showing a widened predental space. Right: lateral c-spine X-ray showing a fractured odontoid process

**Table 1** Ischaemic causes of childhood stroke

| |
|---|
| • Cardiac disease (50%) |
| • Infections (Varicella) |
| • Arterial dissection |
| • Moyamoya-type arteriopathy (sickle cell disease, neurofibromatosis type 1, or idiopathic) |
| • CNS vasculitis. |
| • Coagulopathy |
| • Idiopathic (~25%) |
| • Venous sinus thrombosis due to infection, fever, dehydration, coagulopathies (Dlamini et al. 2010) |

**Table 2** Haemorrhagic causes of childhood stroke

| |
|---|
| • Haemorrhagic disease of the newborn |
| • Ruptured arteriovenous malformation |
| • Ruptured cavernoma |

utilised for screening of children with sickle cell disease and Doppler assessment of the circle of Willis provides information on vascular stenosis or occlusion (Fig. 8).

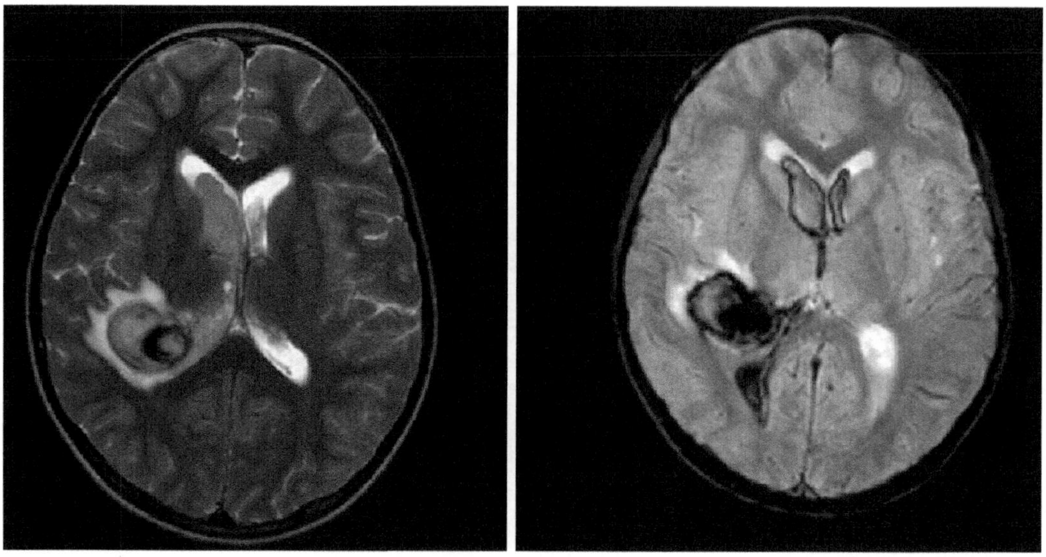

**Fig. 5** Acute intracerebral haemorrhage. Right: Axial T2 MRI showing intermediate signal haematoma with extension into the right lateral ventricle. Left: Axial T2* Gradient Echo showing low signal hemosiderin within the haematoma

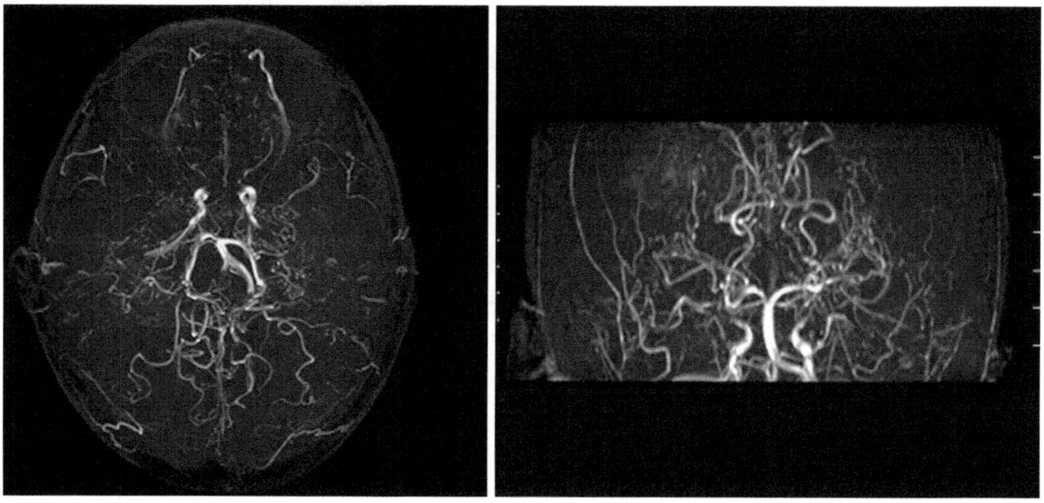

**Fig. 6** Moyamoya disease. Time of Flight 3D vessel reconstruction shows tapering of the distal internal carotid arteries and multiple small vascular collaterals

An acute presentation with the clinical features described above would prompt initial investigation with CT, much the same as the adult population, to exclude haemorrhagic causes. The imaging findings in childhood stroke are similar to those in adults including loss of grey-white matter differentiation, dense middle cerebral artery (MCA) sign, insula ribbon low attenuation (Tomandl et al. 2003), acute low T1 signal, high T2 FLAIR signal, and restricted diffusion on DWI (Allen et al. 2012).

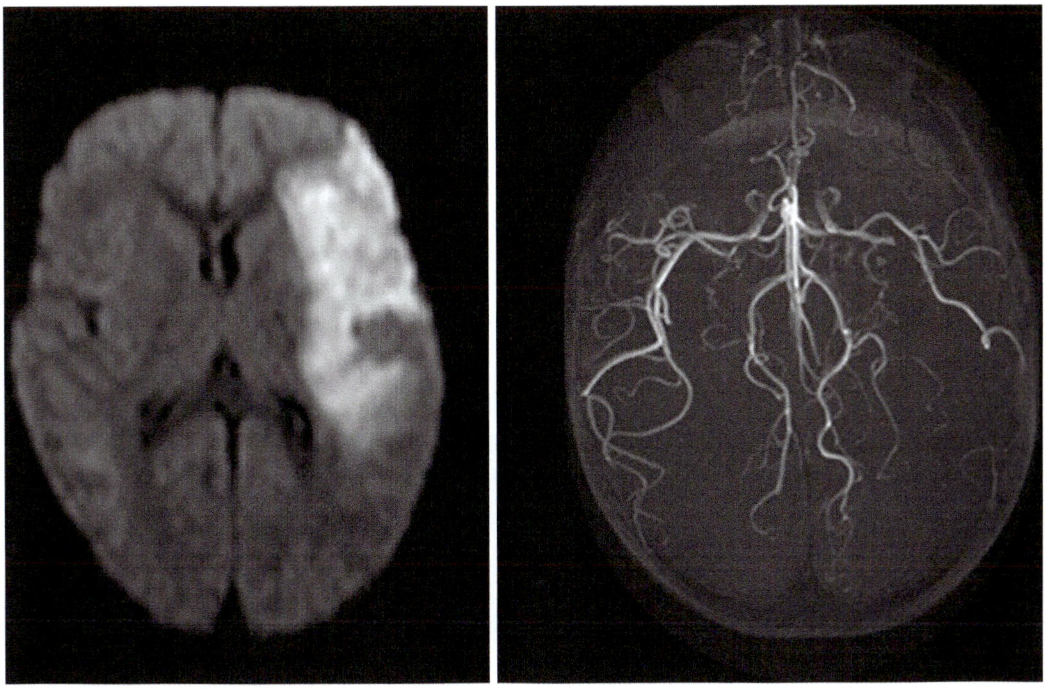

**Fig. 7** Acute Left MCA Infarct. Right: MRI diffusion weighted imaging shows restricted diffusion in the left MCA territory. Left: 3D vessel reconstruction showing an abrupt end to the left MCA, suggestive of a filling defect caused most likely by a thrombus

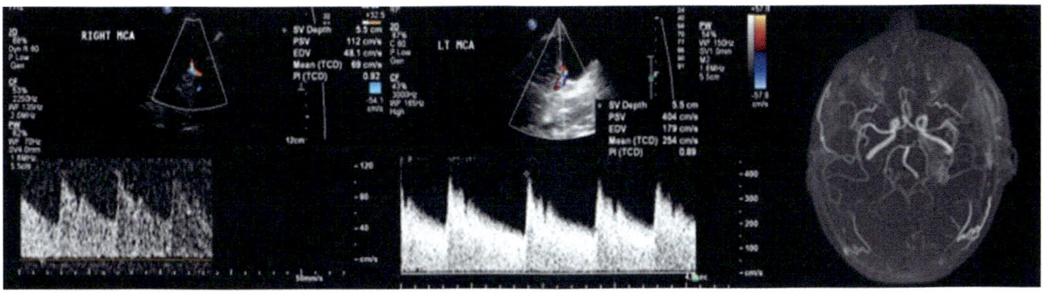


**Fig. 8** Right: normal right MCA flow. Middle: stenotic flow in the left MCA. Left: 3D vessel reconstruction showing a narrowed left MCA

## 4 Non-traumatic Intracranial Haemorrhage

Trauma is the most common cause of paediatric intracranial haemorrhage; however, there are a few important non-traumatic aetiologies which could lead to similar emergency presentations.

### 4.1 Germinal Matrix Haemorrhage (GMH)

GMH is the most common non-traumatic cause of intracranial haemorrhage in neonates and rarely occurs beyond 32 weeks. It can be due to a number of differing conditions such as coagulopathy, increased central venous pressure, and capillary fragility.

Grading of GMH is done by sonographic assessment and split into four classifications. Grade 1 GMH is high echogenicity confined to the caudothalamic groove. Grade 2 sees extension into normal-sized ventricles up to half full. In grade 3, the ventricles dilate, and in grade 4, there is parenchymal haemorrhage (Roelants-van Rijn et al. 2001). Grade 3 GMH holds a mortality of up to 20% with grade 4 increasing up to 90% (Figs. 9, 10, 11, and 12).

## 4.2 Cavernous Malformation

Cavernous malformations, which were once known as cavernous haemangiomas or cavernomas, are dilated vascular channels that can occur in either the brain or the spinal cord. These

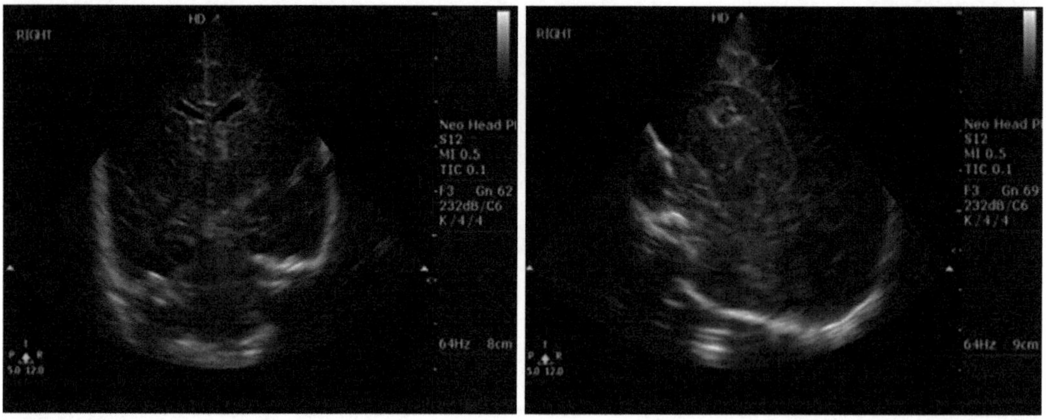


**Fig. 9** Grade I Germinal Matrix Haemorrhage. Intracranial ultrasound, coronal (left) and sagittal (right) views, showing high echogenicity haemorrhagic material at the caudothalamic groove

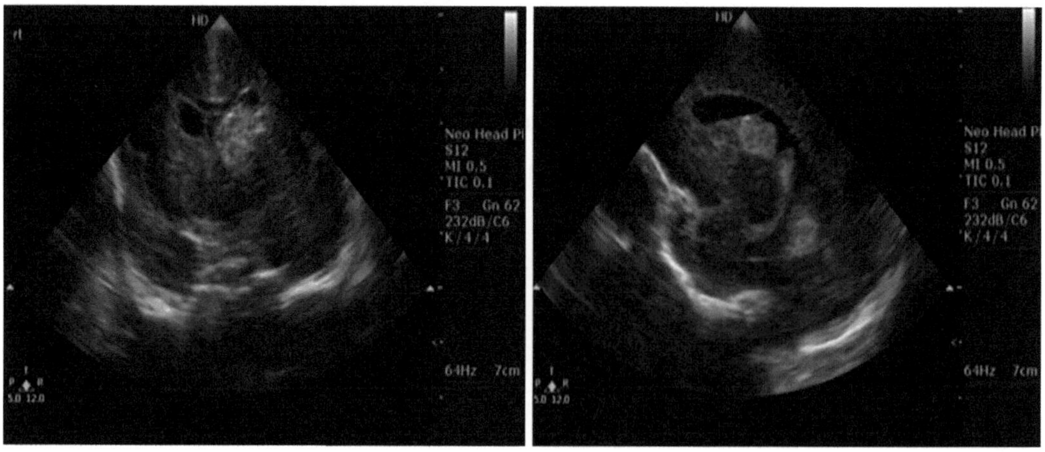


**Fig. 10** Grade II Germinal Matrix Haemorrhage. Haemorrhagic material is seen extending from the caudothalamic groove into the left lateral ventricle, without dilation of the ventricles

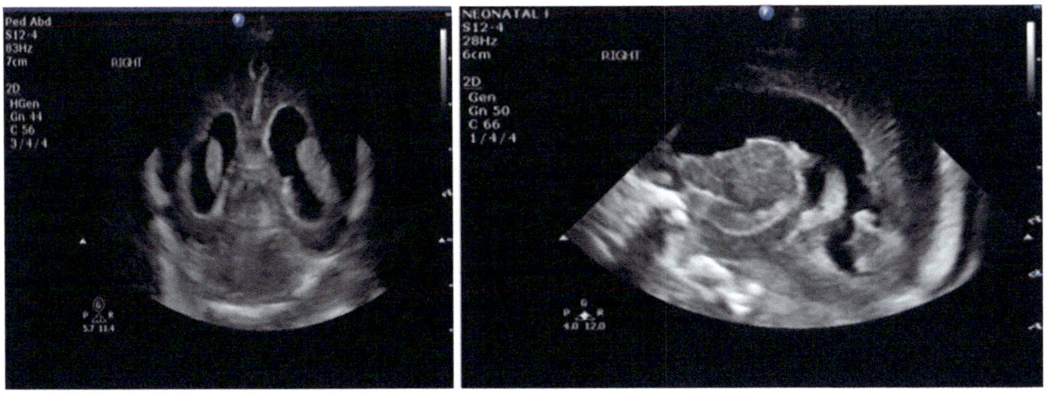


**Fig. 11** Grade III Germinal Matrix Haemorrhage. Haemorrhagic material extending from the caudothalamic groove into both lateral ventricles with associated bilateral ventricular dilation

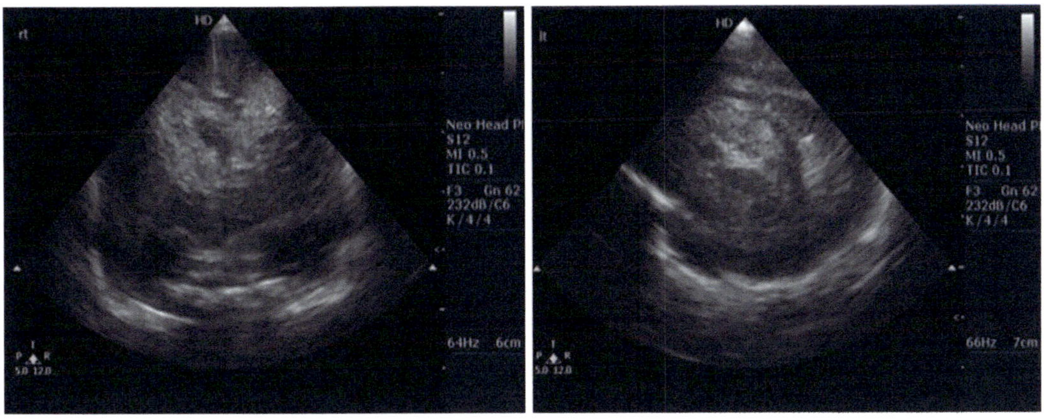


**Fig. 12** Grade IV Germinal Matrix Haemorrhage. High echogenicity haemorrhagic material seen to completely opacify the bilateral dilated ventricular system, with periventricular intra-parenchymal haemorrhage

dilated vascular channels are partially thrombosed and surrounded by blood products (haemosiderin). Cavernous malformations typically arise sporadically, but can be inherited. In cases of familial inheritance, there is a greater likelihood that these lesions will be multiple as opposed to solitary. The clinical concern associated with cavernous malformations is their predilection to haemorrhage, which ranges from microscopic subclinical bleeding to life-threatened haemorrhage.

Cavernous malformations are associated with developmental venous anomalies. These are a collection of abnormal cerebral veins, which increase the risk of haemorrhage beyond that of an isolated cavernous malformation.

A rounded hyperdense lesion on CT is consistent with a cavernous malformation; however, this imaging modality does not show the characteristic features of this finding. MR imaging is the modality of choice for cavernous malformations. The characteristic findings include a "popcorn" appearance on T1 weighted imaging indicating blood of different ages, with a low signal rim on T2 due to the haemosiderin, and signal drop out on either susceptibility weighted imaging or gradient echo sequences (Wang et al. 2017). The above describes the appearance of

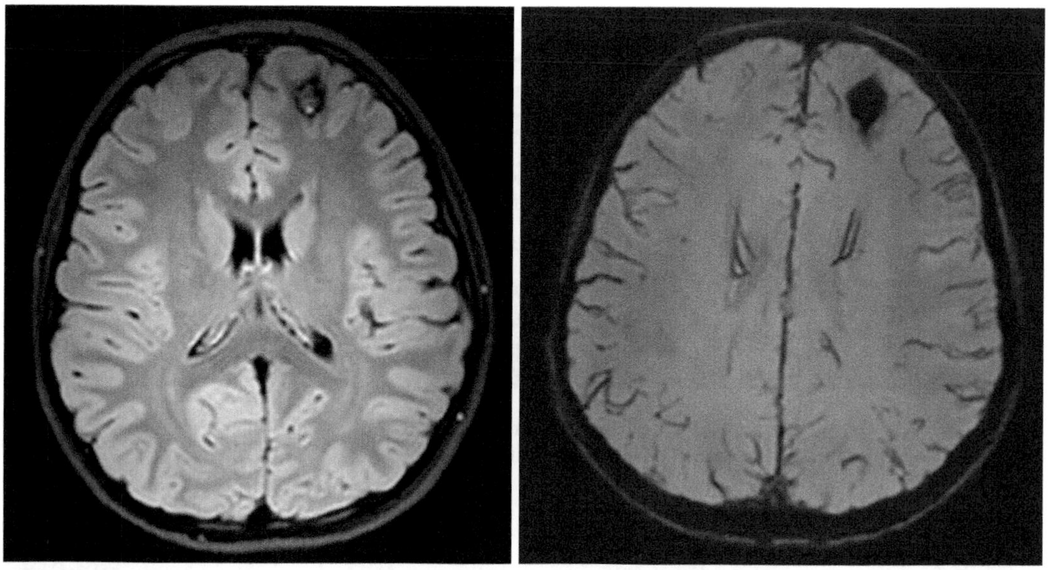

**Fig. 13** Cerebral cavernous malformation. Left: Axial susceptibility weighted image (SWI) showing striking hypointense "blooming" artefact surrounding "popcorn" mixed signal core. Right: SWI showing uniform blooming artefact throughout the lesion

cavernous malformations in their non-pathological state. In the emergency setting, the presentation will include a haemorrhage accompanying the lesion (Fig. 13).

## 4.3 Hypoxic Ischaemic Encephalopathy (HIE)

Hypoxic ischaemic insult can lead to brain injury in neonates in up to 2 in 1000 live births. The two patterns of disease (central and peripheral) are dependent on the severity and duration of hypoxia.

Central HIE is associated with severe hypoxia of short duration, leading to injury within the hippocampus, basal ganglia, thalamus, and perirolandic region. Peripheral HIE occurs more insidiously with less obvious aetiologies, primarily affecting the less metabolically active watershed regions.

CT features of HIE include early loss of grey-white differentiation and low density within the deep grey nuclei with late features of encephalomalacia/volume loss (Shahina et al. 2017).

The best imaging modality is MRI with DWI and MR-spectroscopy (MRS) after the first 24 h: T1 and T2 will return normal signal in the acute setting (1–2 days), but then both increase from day 3; DWI shows restricted diffusion in the first week and MRS shows low N-acetyl aspartate (NAA) and high lactate in affected areas (Shahina et al. 2017) (Fig. 14).

## 4.4 Hydrocephalus

Hydrocephalus is a term used to describe a clinical finding that has various aetiologies. Hydrocephalus refers to an excessive volume of cerebrospinal fluid (CSF) contained within the ventricular spaces. The majority of causes can be divided into non-obstructive and obstructive aetiologies (Cinalli et al. 2005):

- Non-obstructive hydrocephalus is also known as communicating hydrocephalus. This collection of diseases are caused by an irritant-inducing fibrosis and therefore occlusion of the subarachnoid drainage mechanism. The "irritant" is most commonly haemorrhage, but can also be suppurative meningitis, or neoplastic exudates.

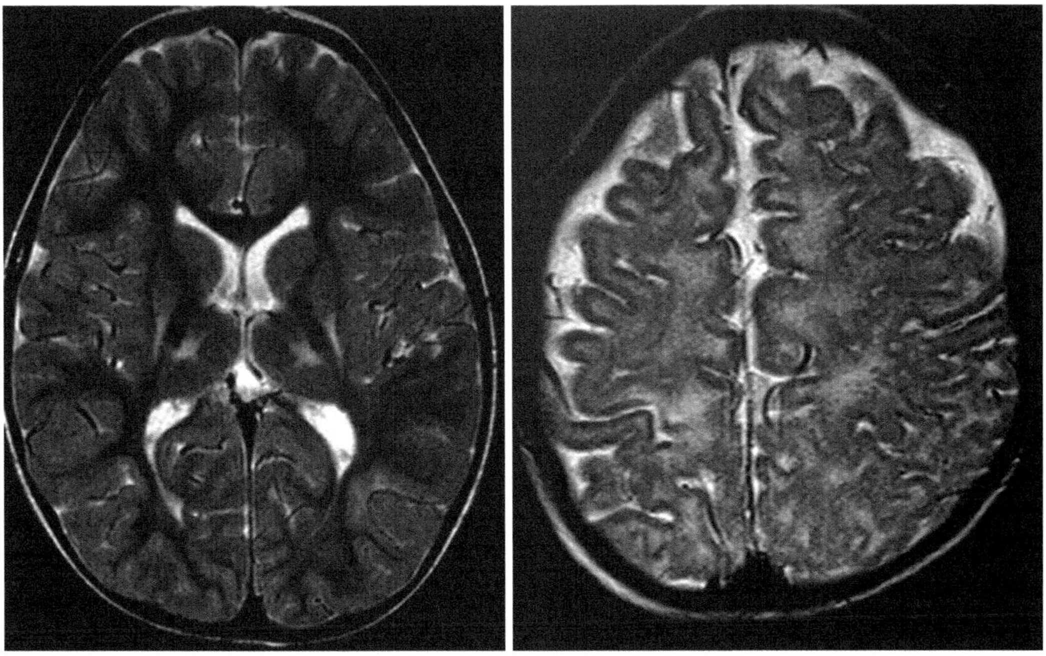

**Fig. 14** Previous perinatal hypoxic ischemic injury. Bilateral volume loss with gliosis involving the antero-lateral thalamus and the posteromedial lentiform nucleus with gliosis in the perirolandic subcortical white mater

- Obstructive hydrocephalus, which is also referred to as non-communicating hydrocephalus, describes a collection of diseases with a differing pathophysiological mechanism, but the same end result of dilated CSF spaces. As the name suggests, an obstructive or compressive mass causes occlusion of the draining CSF pathway and therefore dilation of the proximal chambers. Congenital hydrocephalus may arise from aqueductal stenosis, or from various posterior fossa malformations. The spectrum of Arnold-Chiari malformations and Dandy-Walker malformations are especially relevant in the paediatric setting. An obstructive tumour or a colloid cyst is another cause of relevance in the child/young adult.

Although rare, a choroid plexus tumour is an important differential to exclude in the paediatric setting (Jaiswal et al. 2009). A choroid plexus tumour is an overgrowth of the CSF producing tissues, as such it causes hydrocephalus because it excessively produces CSF, at a rate beyond which it can be excreted.

Choroid plexus tumours are the most common brain tumour in a child under 1 year of age. On imaging, they appear as a lobulated mass in the ventricle (most commonly the lateral ventricle).

Dilatation of the subarachnoid spaces may be a normal finding in the neonate. The underlying physiology is not well-understood; however, the widely accepted theory is that the developing drainage pathways cannot promptly divert the CSF during the first year of life, leading to CSF accumulation in the subarachnoid space. This is an incidental and self-limiting finding, for which no treatment is necessary.

**Acknowledgement** All images are anonymised having been acquired at Sheffield Children's Hospital as part of clinical care.

## References

Allen LM, Hasso AN, Handwerker J, Farid H (2012) Sequence-specific MR imaging findings that are useful in dating ischemic stroke. Radiographics 32(5):1285–1297

Araki T, Yokota H, Morita A (2017) Pediatric traumatic brain injury: characteristic features, diagnosis, and management. Neurol Med Chir 57(2):82–93

Bertozzi JC, Rojas CA, Martinez CR (2009) Evaluation of the pediatric craniocervical junction on MDCT. Am J Roentgenol 192(1):26–31

Cinalli G, Sainte-Rose C, Maixner WJ (eds) (2005) Pediatric hydrocephalus. Springer, New York

Clinical Standards and Quality Improvement team (2017) Paediatric Stroke Working Group. Stroke in childhood – clinical guideline for diagnosis, management and rehabilitation. https://www.rcpch.ac.uk/resources/stroke-childhood-clinical-guideline-diagnosis-management-rehabilitation

Culotta PA, Crowe JE, Tran Q-A, Jones JY, Mehollin-Ray AR, Tran HB, Donaruma-Kwoh M, Dodge CT, Camp EA, Cruz AT (2016) Performance of computed tomography of the head to evaluate for skull fractures in infants with suspected non-accidental trauma. Pediatr Radiol 47(1):74–81

Dlamini N, Billinghurst L, Kirkham FJ (2010) Cerebral venous sinus (Sinovenous) thrombosis in children. Neurosurg Clin N Am 21(3):511–527

Donahue MJ, Dlamini N, Bhatia A, Jordan LC (2019) Neuroimaging advances in pediatric stroke. Stroke. https://doi.org/10.1161/STROKEAHA.118.020478

Guarnieri G, Izzo R, Muto M (2016) The role of emergency radiology in spinal trauma. Br J Radiol 89(1061):20150833

Halliday K, Drinkwater K, Howlett DC (2016) Evaluation of paediatric radiology services in hospitals in the UK. Clin Radiol 71(12):1263–1267

Jaiswal AK, Jaiswal S, Sahu RN, Das KB, Jain VK, Behari S (2009) Choroid plexus papilloma in children: diagnostic and surgical considerations. J Pediatr Neurosci 4(1):10–16

Lustrin ES, Karakas SP, Ortiz AO, Cinnamon J, Castillo M, Vaheesan K, Singh S (2003) Pediatric cervical spine: normal anatomy, variants, and trauma. Radiographics 23(3):539–560

Marti B, Sirinelli D, Maurin L, Carpentier E (2013) Wormian bones in a general paediatric population. Diagn Interv Imaging 94(4):428–432

McAllister AS, Nagaraj U, Radhakrishnan R (2019) Emergent imaging of pediatric cervical spine trauma. Radiographics 39(4):1126–1142

Riascos R, Bonfante E, Cotes C et al (2015) Imaging of 980 atlanto-occipital and atlantoaxial traumatic injuries: what the radiologist needs to know. Radiographics 35(7):2121–2134

Roelants-van Rijn AM, Groenendaal F, Beek FJA, Eken P, van Haastert IC, de Vries LS (2001) Parenchymal brain injury in the preterm infant: comparison of cranial ultrasound, MRI and neurodevelopmental outcome. Neuropediatrics 32(2):80–89

Sanchez T, Stewart D, Walvick M, Swischuk L (2010) Skull fracture vs. accessory sutures: how can we tell the difference? Emerg Radiol 17(5):413–418

Shahina B, Chaudhary V, Garga UC (2017) Neonatal hypoxic-ischemic encephalopathy: a radiological review. J Pediatr Neurosci 12(1):1–6

Tomandl BF, Klotz E, Handschu R, Stemper B, Reinhardt F, Huk WJ, Fateh-Moghadam S (2003) Comprehensive imaging of ischemic stroke with multisection CT. Radiographics 23(3):565–592

Wang KY, Idowu OR, Lin DDM (2017) Radiology and imaging for cavernous malformations. Review Handb Clin Neurol 143:249–266

# Part V

# Emergencies of the Face and Neck (E. Dick, UK, M. Scaglione, IT)

# Neck Space Anatomy

Elizabeth L. Loney

## Contents



**Abstract**

Neck anatomy is often described as complex and difficult to understand. While it is true that there are many structures contained within it, separating these into compartments defined by layers of deep cervical fascia makes it far simpler to understand, not only the anatomy, but also pathology arising within them.

The concept of dividing the neck into naso-, oro-, and hypopharynx suggests discrete regions, separated from one another. In reality, there are no horizontal boundaries preventing disease spreading from one to another. Rather, anatomical structures are organized by fascial layers into craniocaudal 'tubes' along which infection, etc. can spread. By

E. L. Loney (✉)
Calderdale and Huddersfield NHS FT, Halifax, UK
e-mail: elizabeth.loney@cht.nhs.uk


M. Scaglione et al. (eds.), *Emergency Radiology of the Head and Spine*, Medical Radiology Diagnostic Imaging, https://doi.org/10.1007/978-3-030-91047-1_23

understanding this concept, one can predict disease patterns and correctly image the patient.

This chapter aims to provide the reader with simple concepts on which to build their knowledge. It is not a comprehensive list of every muscle and nerve in the head and neck. There are plenty of excellent books that do this. It is easy to read and understand with lots of pictures (as I know how much Radiologists love images!). Enjoy....

## Abbreviations

| | |
|---|---|
| ABD | Anterior belly of digastric |
| ACS | Anterior cervical space |
| CN | Cranial nerve |
| DCF | Deep cervical fascia |
| SLDCF | Superficial layer of the deep cervical fascia |
| MLDCF | Middle layer of the deep cervical fascia |
| DLDCF | Deep layer of the deep cervical fascia |
| PCS | Posterior cervical space |
| PMS | Pharyngeal mucosal space |
| PPS | Parapharyngeal space |
| PVS | Perivertebral space |
| SCC | Squamous cell carcinoma |
| SCF | Superficial cervical fascia |
| SCM | Sternocleidomastoid |
| VS | Visceral space |

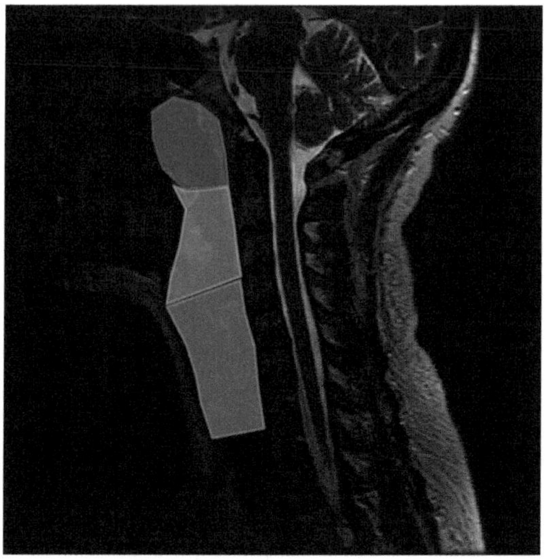

**Fig. 1** Conventional anatomical regions. Nasopharynx (red): skull base to soft palate. Oropharynx (yellow): soft palate to hyoid. Hypopharynx (green): hyoid to inferior border of the cricoid cartilage (C6)

## 1 Introduction

Head and neck anatomy is conventionally divided into the naso-, oro-, and hypopharynx (Fig. 1), along with the oral cavity. While this approach has its merits, particularly with regard to preferred patterns of metastatic nodal spread from primary head and neck squamous cell carcinoma (SCC), it erroneously suggests that they are discrete areas when if fact they form one continuous naso-digestive ‘tube’. In addition, the landmarks used to separate one from another are mobile; the soft palate differentiating the naso- and oropharynx, and the hyoid bone separating the oro- and hypopharynx. Depending on the exact position of these structures on imaging, one might label lesions inconsistently. Disease processes are free to spread craniocaudally, unhampered by fascial planes, and tend to follow the ‘path of least resistance’, travelling up and down tubular ‘elevators’ in the neck in preference to crossing between fascial compartments.

Surgeons like to think in ‘triangles’; for example, anterior, posterior, and submandibular (Fig. 2). While this approach is useful when one has the patient lying in front of you on the operating or ultrasound table, it is less applicable when viewing cross-sectional imaging.

Radiologists prefer to view the neck as a series of compartments, separated from one another by layers of the deep cervical fascia (DCF), a structure in itself split into three parts; superficial, middle, and deep. This approach is

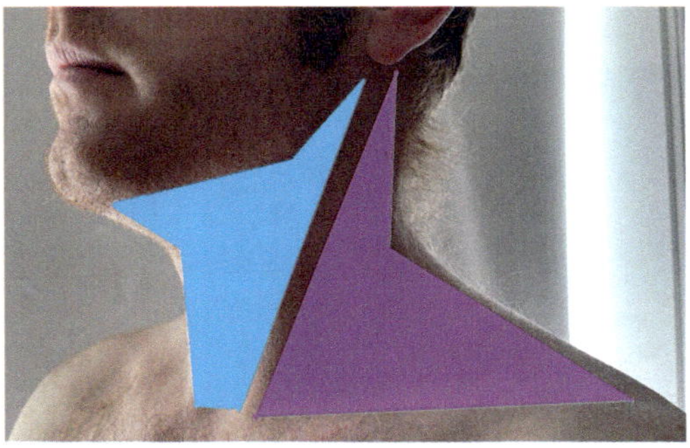

**Fig. 2** Surgical triangles. Blue: anterior triangle. Purple: posterior triangle

perfect for cross-sectional image interpretation and also more closely resembles 'real life' where, as previously mentioned, disease processes travel up and down the neck along fascial 'tubes', rather than crossing fascial planes. A compartmental system is also extremely helpful when coming up with a sensible differential diagnosis for pathology in any given space. After all, diseases tend to originate from the contents of the space and if there's no bone, for example, in a compartment you are extremely unlikely to list 'osteosarcoma' in your top three differential diagnoses! This chapter will cover anatomy of the head and neck using this system. The oral cavity will be described at the end of the chapter. Other anatomical regions lying outside fascial compartments, such as the orbit, will not be covered.

Anatomical terminology is accurate and often descriptive, albeit in Greek or Latin. Therefore, if there is a deep cervical fascia, there must be a superficial one. The superficial cervical fascia (SCF), also known as superficial subcutaneous tissue (Moore et al. 2017), forms a 'stocking' around the neck blending with platysma and the muscles of facial expression. It contains cutaneous nerves, blood vessels and lymphatics, and adipose tissue. This fascia is rarely visible on imaging and will therefore be consciously ignored in the remainder of this chapter.

Platysma (meaning 'flat plate') develops from a layer of second pharyngeal arch mesenchyme, along with facial and scalp muscles. It therefore shares a nerve supply with these (Cranial Nerve VII). It covers the anterolateral part of the neck from clavicles to mandible and blends with facial muscles superiorly. Fibres diverge inferiorly to leave a gap over the trachea and thyroid and it is of variable completeness elsewhere, depending on the individual.

As previously mentioned, the far more important DCF consists of three layers- the superficial layer of the deep cervical fascia (SLDCF), middle layer (MLDCF), and deep layer (DLDCF). In some textbooks, these are referred to as 'investing' (SLDCF), 'buccopharyngeal/'pretracheal' (MLDCF), and 'prevertebral' (DLDCF) fascia (Standring 2015). They form longitudinal tubes of differing lengths. If you look at your own (or another's) profile, you will notice that your chin protrudes anteriorly compared to your neck, conveniently splitting the face and neck into two parts; above (supra-) and below (infra-) the hyoid. As the area above the hyoid is larger in AP diameter, you might expect it to contain more compartments than the infrahyoid neck, and you'd be right. Posterior structures (the spinal column, paraspinal muscles, large neck vessels, and the pharynx) extend from the skull base to thoracic inlet and beyond, whereas anterior elements (for example, the mandible, submandibular glands, and muscles of mastication) are found only in the suprahyoid neck. Figure 3 demonstrates this concept on a sagittal T2W image, clearly showing short anterior and long posterior compartments.

Throughout this chapter, on diagrams accompanying the text, you will find that each layer of DCF has a 'colour'; red for superficial, blue for middle, and yellow for deep. If you refer to sagittal and coronal MR images (Figs. 3 and 4), you will appreciate that posterior compartments extend the full length of the neck, while those anteriorly do not.

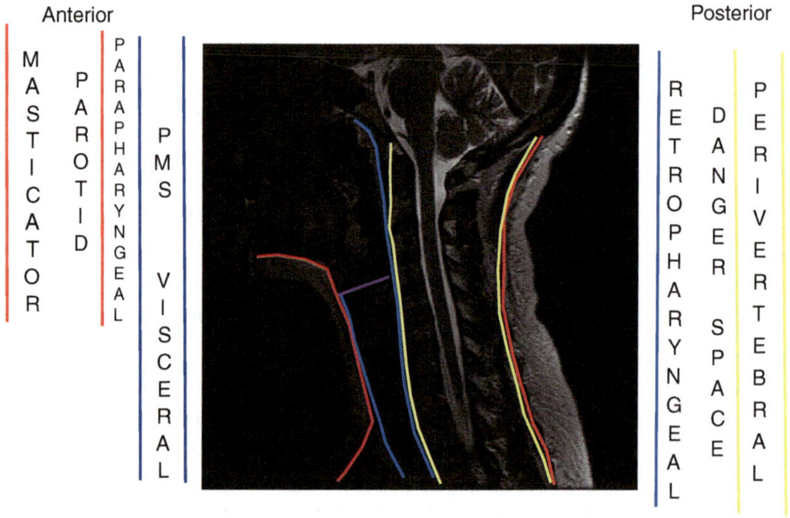


**Fig. 3** Overview of fascial spaces on sagittal T2W MRI. The purple line indicates the level of the hyoid bone, separating the neck into supra- and infrahyoid compartments. Layers of DCF are coloured as in previous figures and space names lie between lines equating to the fascial layer in which they are contained.

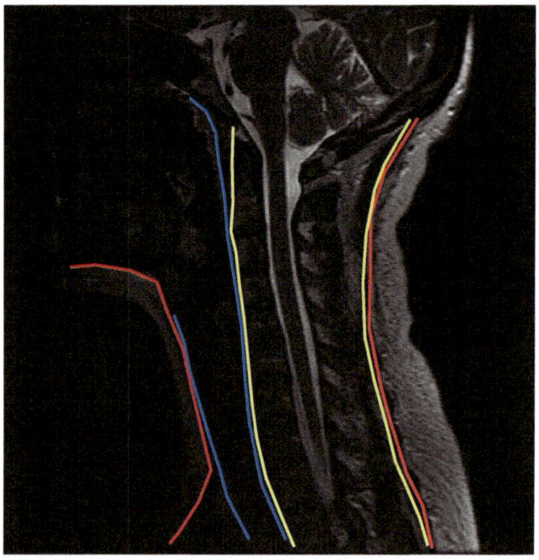

**Fig. 4** Sagittal T2W MRI of the neck. Layers of deep cervical fascia: red: superficial; blue: middle; yellow: deep

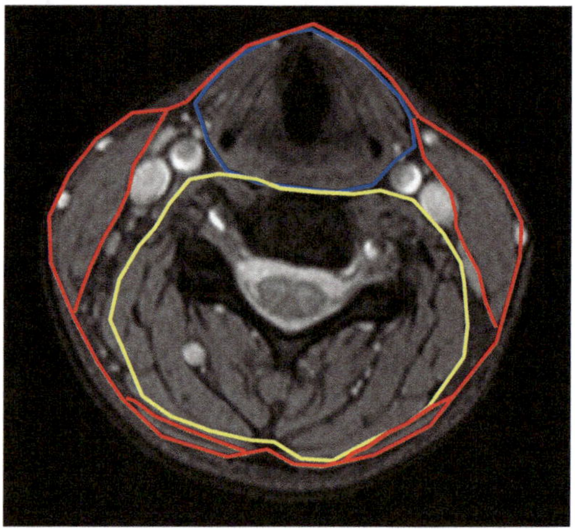

**Fig. 5** Axial T2W GrE MRI of the infrahyoid neck. Layers of deep cervical fascia: red: superficial; blue: middle; yellow: deep

## 2 Suprahyoid Compartments

### 2.1 Overview

The suprahyoid neck contains a number of compartments that extend into the infrahyoid neck, most of which maintain their name when they cross this invisible boundary, for example, carotid and perivertebral spaces. One, however, does not, and that is the pharyngeal mucosal space (PMS), demarcated by the middle layer of deep cervical fascia (MLDCF- in blue on all diagrams). Below the hyoid, it is known as the visceral space, because it contains 'viscera', including, the thyroid gland, parathyroids, and cervical oesophagus (Fig. 5).

There are other compartments confined solely to the suprahyoid neck; masticator, parotid, submandibular, submental, and parapharyngeal spaces. Most of these are concerned with salivation and eating, which (hopefully!) only occur above the hyoid bone.

The three layers of deep cervical fascia separate the suprahyoid neck into compartments. The superficial layer splits intermittently to surround muscles of mastication, the parotid glands,

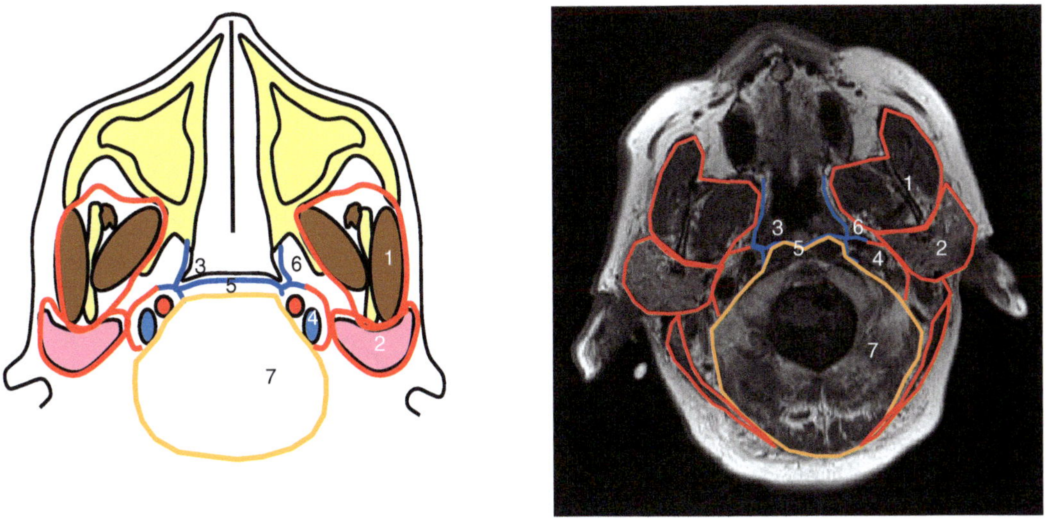


**Fig. 6** Axial T1W MRI suprahyoid neck and corresponding line diagram. (1) Masticator space, (2) parotid space, (3) PMS, (4) carotid space, (5) retropharyngeal and danger spaces (barely visible on the MR image), (6) parapharyngeal space, (7) perivertebral space

sternocleidomastoid, and trapezius. The middle layer encompasses the suprahyoid pharynx to form a 'tube' and the deep layer surrounds all things 'peri-spinal' including muscles, nerves, vertebrae, and the spinal cord. In diagrams, these layers are red (superficial), blue (middle), and yellow (deep). The spaces created by this arrangement (Fig. 6) are;

- Masticator.
- Parotid.
- Pharyngeal mucosal space.
- Carotid.
- Retropharyngeal and danger spaces.
- Parapharyngeal.
- Perivertebral.

Other suprahyoid spaces out with them include:

- Submental.
- Submandibular.

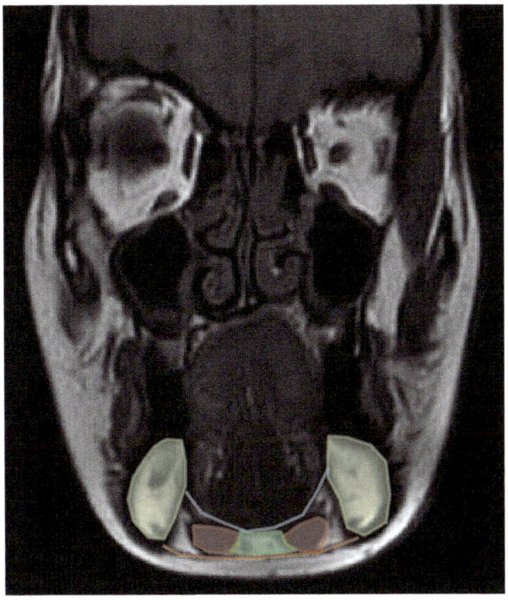

**Fig. 7** Coronal T1W MRI: submental space boundaries (one space, centrally). Superior: mylohyoid (light purple). Inferior: platysma (orange). Lateral: anterior bellies of digastric (red)

## 2.2 Submental and Submandibular Spaces

The submental and submandibular spaces are not confined by deep cervical fascial layers. As their names suggest, they lie 'sub' (under) the mentum (chin) and mandible (jaw), respectively (Figs. 7 and 8). On neck ultrasound, ultrasound platysma provides a useful landmark, forming the roof (or floor) of these spaces depending on whether you're imaging using ultrasound or cross-sectional techniques. For the sake of simplicity, the

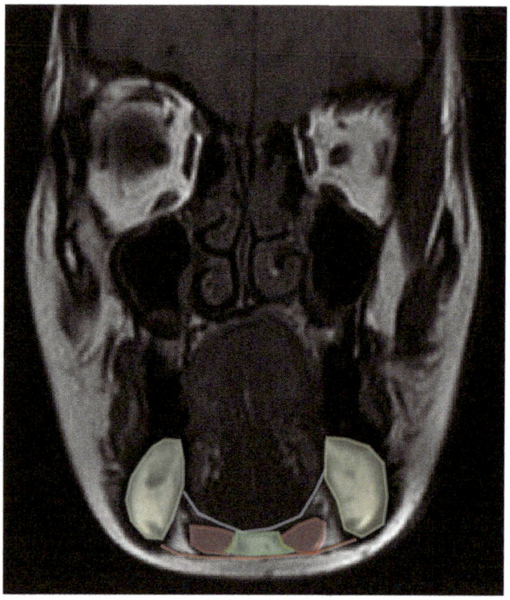

**Fig. 8** Coronal T1W MRI: submandibular space boundaries (right and left). Superior: mylohyoid (light purple). Inferior: platysma (orange). Medial: anterior bellies of digastric (red). Lateral: body of the mandible (yellow)

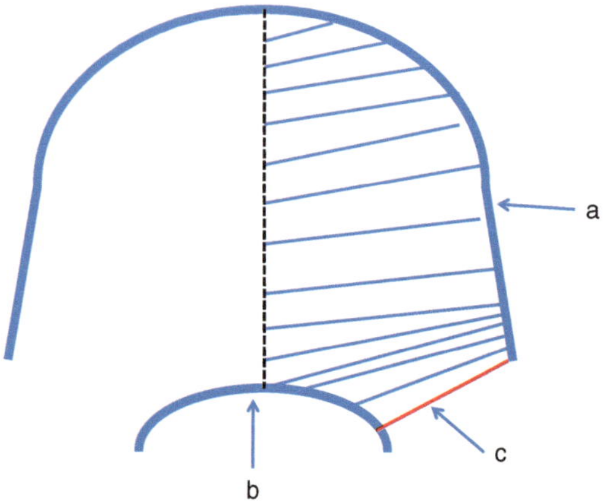


**Fig. 9** Schematic diagram showing the arc of the mandible (**a**), hyoid bone (**b**), and fibres of the left mylohyoid muscle (**c**). Red denotes the free edge of mylohyoid, bridging the gap between the posterior mandible and hyoid

rest of this description will assume you are using CT or MRI to learn your anatomy and call platysma the 'floor'.

In this case, the roof of both spaces is formed by another muscle (or really pair of muscles that interdigitate in the midline at a 'raphe') called mylohyoid. Mylohyoid is extremely useful- without it our tongue would fall out of our mouth! It forms a hammock or sling under the contents of the oral cavity and separates those structures inside the oral cavity from those outside. Like all muscles in the head and neck, it 'does what it says on the tin'- that is, it is named after its origin and insertion, making our lives so much easier. Provided you can remember the muscles' name, you can work out where it starts and stops!

Mylohyoid originates from the mylohyoid line on the inner surface of the mandible and comes together in the midline to form a raphe. As the mandible has a horseshoe shape, it is easy to visualize the muscular sling that forms as a result. 'But what about the posterior border?' I hear you say. Thinking logically, the name of the muscle is mylohyoid. The posterior edge will therefore insert into the hyoid. Well.....mostly!

Consider this- the mandible is very large compared to the size of the hyoid. We have muscles originating from a wide arc inserting into a small one. There just isn't enough space on the hyoid to fit it all in! If you look at Fig. 9 you will see what I mean. There are parts of the posterior muscle border that cannot squeeze onto the hyoid, leaving a 'free edge' on either side. Having struggled with the concept of a free border as a student, the 'not enough space on the hyoid' principle makes it clear. Around this free edge, the submandibular gland extends; the superficial lobe lying superficial to mylohyoid and the deep lobe, deep. The hilum of the gland snuggles into the free edge, which forms a useful landmark on imaging. The fact that there is no fascial boundary at the back of the submandibular space means that pathology such as infection can spread posteriorly into soft tissues of the neck, and between superficial and deep regions, around the free edge of mylohyoid. The posterior margin of the submental space is the body of the hyoid bone.

So, we have a floor (platysma) and a roof (mylohyoid). The next key structure is the anterior belly of digastric (ABD). Digastric means two (di) bellies (gastric). If there is something called 'anterior', there must be something else called 'posterior' (otherwise why bother use the word anterior at all?) and indeed there is. This muscle is extremely interesting in that it derives from two different branchial arches. In the embryo, at the stage where we resemble tadpoles, there are structures that look like gills separated by soft tissue bumps. The bumps are called branchial arches and the gills, branchial clefts. Each arch has its own cranial nerve supplying muscles originating from it. The anterior belly of digastric forms from the first branchial arch, whose nerve is the trigeminal (CN V), whereas the posterior belly forms from the second arch, whose nerve is the facial (CN VII). These muscle bellies come together at a tendinous intersection that passes through a sling connected to the hyoid. Amazing! This is the anatomical equivalent of threading a needle and it seems surprising that this process is successful almost every time. I have been looking at neck scans for many years and have never noticed an anomaly. Perhaps you have? I digress. The anterior belly of digastric arises from its own pit on the inner surface of the mandible (the digastric fossa) on each side of the symphysis. On imaging, this muscle separates the space we have created between platysma and mylohyoid into one between the muscle bellies, i.e. medial to them, and two spaces lateral to digastric. One submental and two submandibular spaces.

Their contents are limited. In the submental space, there is fat and some lymph nodes. In the submandibular space, these tissues are also present, along with the superficial lobes of the submandibular glands (we already know why the deep lobes are not included), facial artery, and vein.

The boundaries of the spaces can be summarized as:

| | Floor | Roof | Medial | Lateral |
|---|---|---|---|---|
| Submental | Platysma | Mylohyoid | N/A | ABD |
| Submandibular | Platysma | Mylohyoid | ABD | Mandible |

Disease processes in the submental space most commonly involve enlarged lymph nodes and lipomata, as is expected given the contents of the region. In the submandibular space, there is more variety, including any pathology arising from salivary tissue, and disease spread from the adjacent mandible.

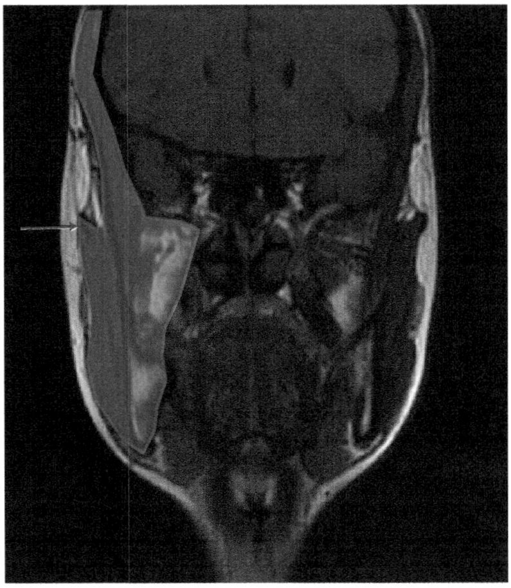

**Fig. 10** Coronal T1W MRI face/head. The red-shaded area indicates components of the right masticator space, divided into supra- and infrahyoid regions by the zygomatic arch (red arrow)

## 2.3 Masticator Space

The masticator space lies within layers of the SLDCF in the suprahyoid neck. It is more extensive than most expect, having both supra and infra zygomatic parts (Fig. 10). Superiorly, the SLDCF extends over the muscle belly of temporalis on the side of the skull, almost to the vertex. Inferiorly, it reaches the lower border of the mandible, laterally attaches to the zygomatic arch and medially to the extracranial skull base at the junction of the middle and central compartments. It contains the muscles of mastication (masseter, temporalis, medial, and lateral pterygoid), the nerve supply to these (the mandibular division of the trigeminal nerve, V3), and the mandibular condyle, neck, ramus, and posterior body. Axial imaging demonstrates the 'MMM' sandwich, formed (lateral to medial) by masseter, mandibular ramus, and medial pterygoid (Fig. 11). The masticator space can be said to centre on the mandibular ramus which divides it into medial and lateral compartments, the medial one incorporating both infratemporal and pterygopalatine fossae (Standring 2015).The

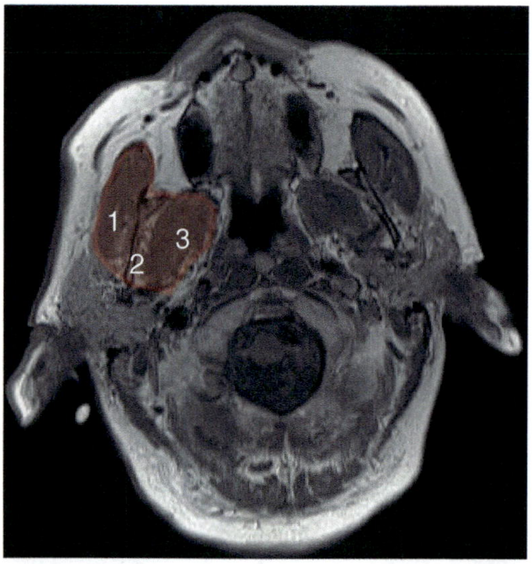


**Fig. 11** Axial T1W MRI suprahyoid neck. The red-shaded area indicates the MMM sandwich of the right masticator space: (*1*) masseter, (*2*) mandible, (*3*) medial pterygoid

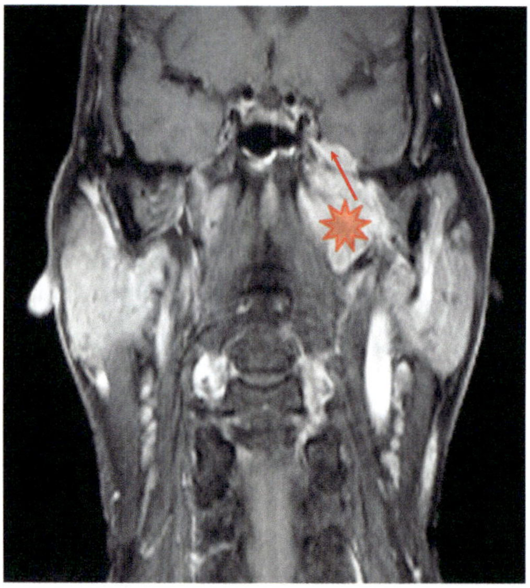

**Fig. 12** Coronal T1W fat-sat post-Gd MRI. This image demonstrates a tumour (*adenoid cystic carcinoma) in the left masticator space extending along the mandibular division of CN V into Meckel's cave to involve the trigeminal ganglion

craniocaudal extent of this compartment means that infection originating from a carious posterior molar, for example, can present on the side of the head as a lump!

Within this compartment, muscular origins and insertions are as follows:

| | Origin | Insertion |
|---|---|---|
| Temporalis | Side of the skull | Coronoid process |
| Masseter | Zygomatic arch | Angle of the mandible |
| Medial pterygoid | Medial side of the lateral pterygoid plate | Angle of the mandible (medial aspect) |
| Lateral pterygoid | Lateral side of the lateral pterygoid plate | TMJ disc (sup-head) Neck of the mandible |

Fascial attachments to the skull base need to encompass the foramen through which the nerve supplying these muscles exits the skull, namely the foramen ovale. Otherwise, the nerve would not easily be able to reach the muscles it innervates. Conversely, disease processes can travel along this route into the cranium and therefore imaging protocols of masticator space lesions must include the skull base and middle cranial fossae/Meckels caves if the pathology in question has a propensity for perineural spread or is aggressive in nature (Fig. 12).

## 2.4 Parotid Space

The parotid space also lies within the SLDCF, encasing the parotid gland and its contents. Like the submandibular gland, the parotid has superficial and deep lobes, demarcated on imaging by the neurovascular bundle (Fig. 13) comprising (from superficial to deep) the facial nerve, external carotid artery, and retromandibular vein. The facial nerve is rarely directly visible unless pathologically thickened or enhancing except if using extremely high resolution imaging techniques. However, although you can't often see it, you know where it is (one of my mantras when teaching residents anatomy!). Any lesion lateral to this bundle lies in the superficial lobe, and any medial to it within the deep lobe. Of course, lesions can cross from one lobe to another, as there is no physical boundary between them.

Ultrasound often struggles to visualize the deep lobe as high frequency probes fail to penetrate deeply enough, and also because the mandible gets

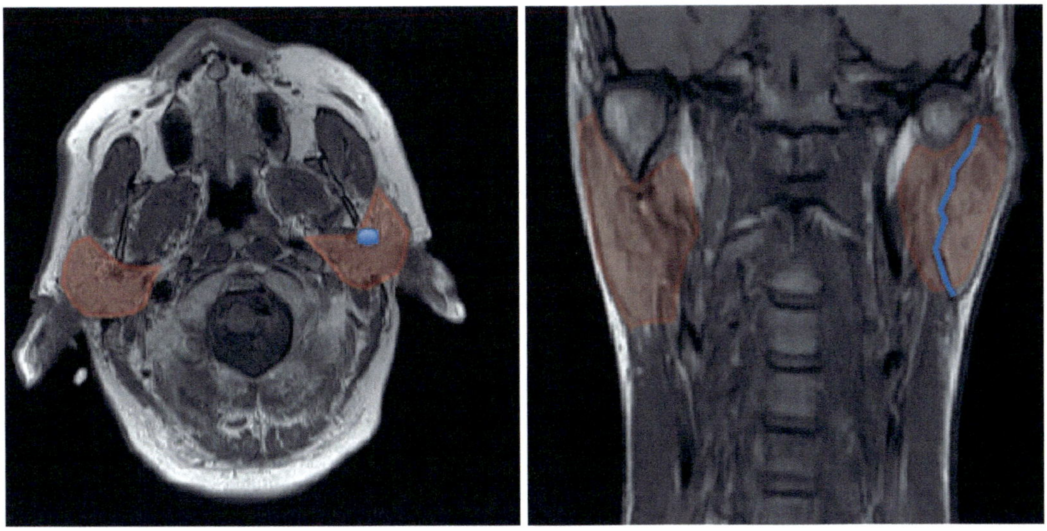

**Fig. 13** Axial and coronal T1W MRI of the parotid space. Red-shaded areas indicate the boundaries and contents of both parotid spaces. Blue dot/line show the position of the left parotid neurovascular bundle, separating superficial from deep lobes

in the way. It is therefore vital to remember to ask yourself 'what lies beneath?'. If a lesion is noted on ultrasound but the deep aspect is not visible, it is mandatory to perform cross-sectional imaging to ensure that one is not dealing with a 'dumb-bell' mass, small on the outside, and large on the inside. I have seen many large deep lobe lesions on MRI, barely visible on ultrasound. A pitfall for the unwary. However, now we have revised the anatomy we won't forget this point!

The parotid gland reaches the level of the zygomatic arch superiorly and this forms the superolateral fascial attachment for the space. Medially, the extracranial skull base attachment must, as with the masticator space, incorporate the foramen through which the nerve to this space reaches it; the stylomastoid foramen which, as its name suggest, lies between styloid and mastoid processes. Once it has emerged, it gives off a couple of small branches and then splits into 5 parts. At medical school, we had a pretty rude method of remembering them, and I'm sure you have something similar!. For the purposes of this text, however, I suggest sticking to something like 'Two zebras bashed my cat', or similar. This stands for 'Temporal, Zygomatic, Buccal, Mandibular and Cervical'. If you place your hand on the side of your face, fingers pointing forwards with your index finger along the zygomatic arch, you'll pretty much have the position of the branches, and it also helps you remember how many branches there are!

Inferiorly, the gland extends below the earlobe into the upper neck, and this part (called the tail) is visible on neck ultrasound when assessing level II structures. The tail also passes around the back of the earlobe to lie over the mastoid process. This means that a parotid lesion can present as a lump behind the ear. I like to think that the parotid gland looks like a yellow plastic bath duck (I'm sure you had one as a child!). If you took one such item and placed it next to your face (Fig. 14), you would appreciate that the duck has a body and tail. The body extends below the ear lobe and the tail behind it. The duck also has a beak that represents the hilum of the gland pointing anteriorly towards the mouth. This is where the parotid (Stensons') duct emerges. Sometimes the duck is very naughty and 'spits' (perhaps it thinks it's a swan?!) extra bits of parotid tissue along the line of the duct, known as accessory parotid glands. This additional salivary tissue can be affected by exactly the same pathologies as the main gland and therefore, if a patient presents with a lump in their cheek, always consider whether this could represent salivary disease, in accessory tissue overlying masseter.

The parotid gland contains lymph nodes, unlike the submandibular gland, which does not. This is because the submandibular gland forms earlier in the embryo and becomes completely encapsulated before lymph nodes emerge. It is therefore impossible for a lesion in the submandibular gland to represent a lymph node. There are almost always nodes on the lateral aspect of the gland which can be really difficult to separate from it on ultrasound (and they always seem to measure 6 mm in short axis….why is that!?), but lymph nodes never originate within it. Returning to the parotid, seeing lymph nodes within it is normal. Diseases affecting nodes elsewhere can occur in these also. Hyperplasia, lymphoma, metastases… the list goes on. Therefore, a lump within the parotid does not have to be salivary in origin.

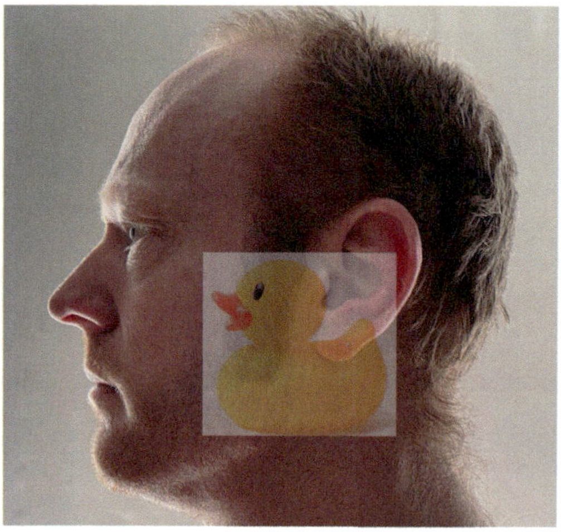

**Fig. 14** The parotid 'bath duck'! This image demonstrates the approximate shape and position of the parotid gland in relation to the pinna and zygomatic arch

When imaging the parotid gland for potential malignancy, remember perineural spread. As with the masticator space, the full extent of the parotid space and its nerve must be covered on imaging, which means protocols should include the temporal bone to exclude enhancing 'skip lesions' along the extracranial facial nerve (Fig. 15).

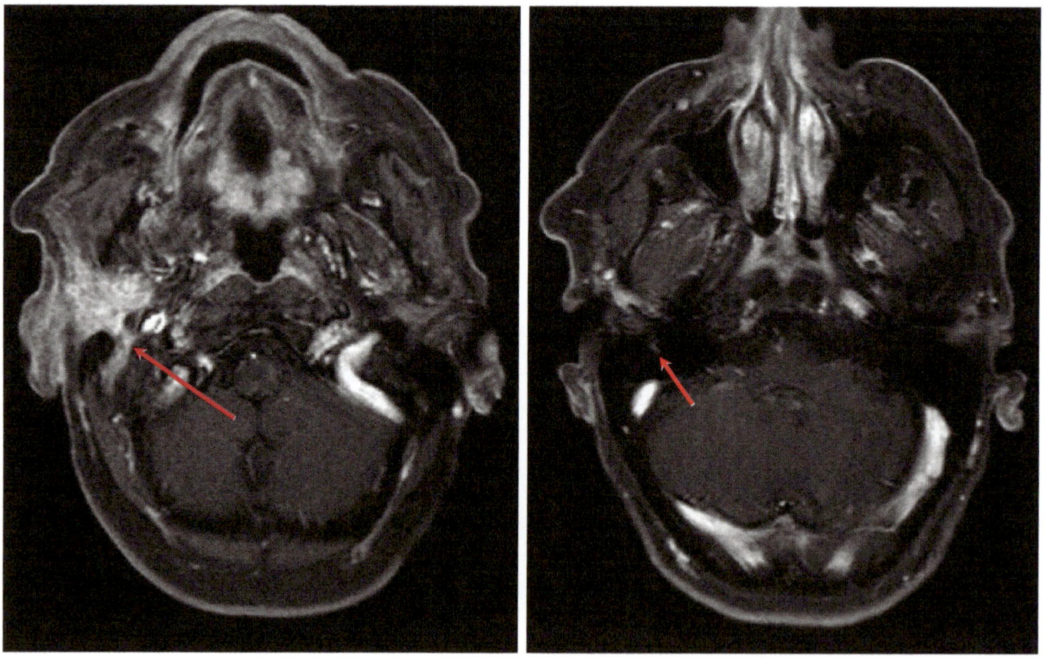

**Fig. 15** Axial T1W fat-sat post-Gd. On the right there is an enhancing parotid tumour demonstrating perineural extension along CN VII into the stylomastoid foramen and along the facial nerve canal in the temporal bone

## 2.5 Pharyngeal Mucosal Space

The pharyngeal mucosal space (PMS) is contained within the middle layer of deep cervical fascia (MLDCF) and extends from the skull base to the hyoid. As previously mentioned, this space continues inferiorly under a new name (the visceral space), but is in fact the same tube.

The principle contents of both spaces are the pharyngeal constrictor muscles; superior, middle, and inferior. I find it easiest to think of these as 'stacking cups', the one above fitting inside the one below it, with a small amount of overlap (Fig. 16). If one took three plastic cups and cut out their bases prior to stacking, one would appreciate this structure. As this stands, however, the tube formed by the cups is open only at the top and the bottom. In order to fully appreciate the structure of the PMS, one would then need to cut out one side of each cup so that, when viewed from above, each would have a 'U' shape. The sides with the opening are then aligned to face anteriorly. We now have three cups and there are three parts to the pharynx....how convenient!

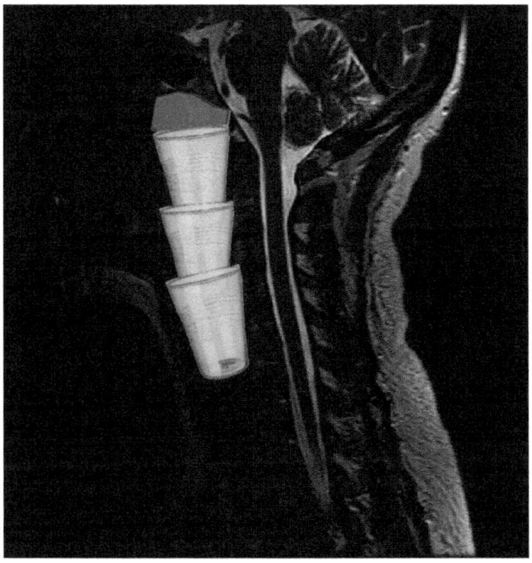

**Fig. 16** Sagittal T2W MRI demonstrating the 'stacking cups' principle. Each cup represents a pharyngeal constrictor muscle stacking inside each other: superior, middle, and inferior. The purple zone above the upper cup represents the pharyngobasilar fascia connecting superior constrictor to the skull base

Each cup roughly represents one constrictor muscle. The upper cup is the superior constrictor. The anterior opening connects the nasopharynx (the space inside the cup) with the nasal cavity. The middle cup is the middle constrictor and communicates anteriorly with the oropharynx. The lowest cup is the inferior constrictor, communicating anteriorly with the larynx. Of course, the inferior constrictor lies below the hyoid and is therefore within the visceral space, but has been included in this description for completeness.

Pharyngeal constrictors are in fact paired muscles, meeting each other posteriorly at a midline raphe (much like mylohyoid in the floor of mouth). Each has anterior origins on each side from bone, another muscles' raphe or fascial bands (Fig. 17).

Superior constrictor has three main origins anteriorly in a craniocaudal line; the medial pterygoid plate, pterygomandibular raphe, and alveolar process of the mandible. A small slip also arises from the tongue. Posteriorly, they insert into one another at the midline raphe.

Middle constrictor arises from the hyoid bone and stylohyoid ligament. Again, they meet each other posteriorly to form a muscular tube, open anteriorly.

Inferior constrictor arises from thyroid and cricoid cartilages. The inferior part, called cricopharyngeus after its origin, is horizontally oriented and forms the superior oesophageal sphincter at the junction of the pharynx and oesophagus. Thyropharyngeus sweeps obliquely upwards from its origin along the oblique line on the side of the thyroid lamina. Posteriorly, differences in fibre orientation create a gap between these muscles, called Killian's dehiscence (Fig. 18). At this point, there is a weak spot through which pharyngeal mucosa can protrude, should the inferior constrictor not relax adequately on swallowing. Over time, this mucosal sac may enlarge and become symptomatic-known as a pharyngeal pouch.

At first glance, this may all seem pretty complicated, but if you draw a line from the skull base to the cricoid cartilage along the medial pterygoid plate and look at the structures lying along this plane, all will (hopefully) become clear.

**Fig. 17** Diagram demonstrating the origins of the pharyngeal constrictor muscles

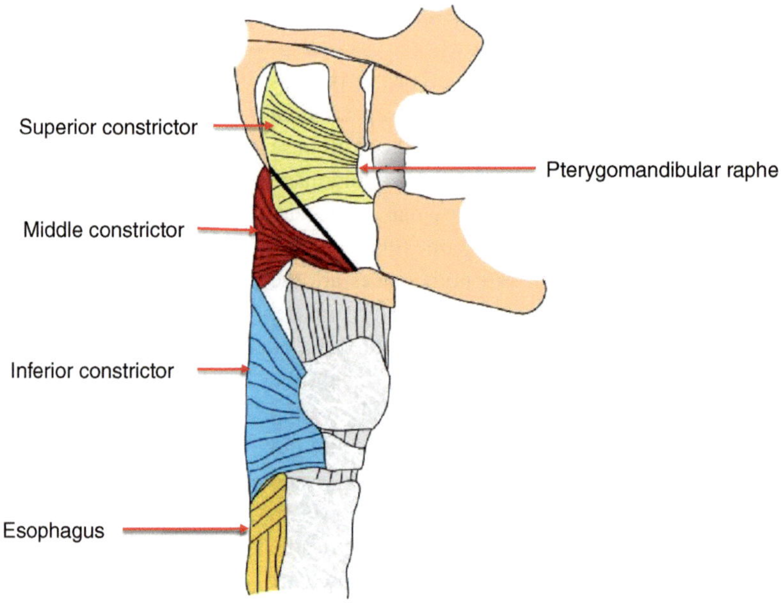


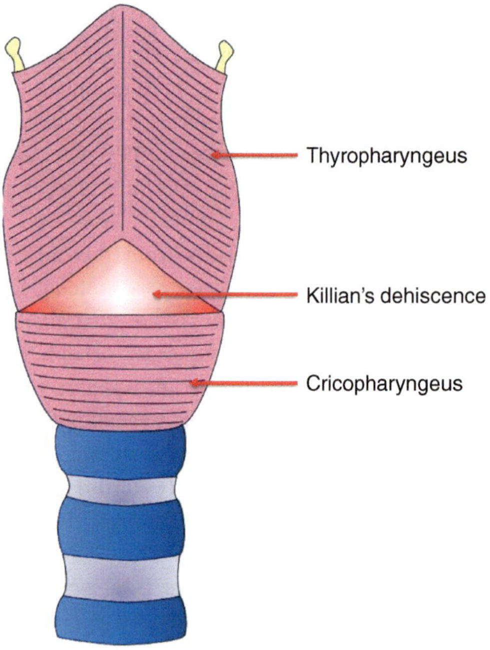


**Fig. 18** Diagram showing the posterior aspect of the inferior pharyngeal constrictor, demonstrating how different muscle fibre orientations create a gap between thyro- and cricopharyngeus, called Killian's dehiscence

If we return to the stacking cups (Fig. 16), you can see they have straight 'tops'. The upper border of the superior constrictor can be considered as such and therefore does not fit snuggly along the skull base, which is curved. There is a gap between them. Also, our tube of cups is currently floating in mid-air with no superior origin. We can therefore appreciate that there is a gap between the pharynx and the skull base and what better to bridge this than a fascia named after it….the pharyngo-basilar fascia! Our tube is now anchored securely.

An important structure passes through this fascia- the Eustachian tube. It connects the middle ear to the nasopharynx and when it opens air passes along it, equalizing pressures across the tympanic membrane. When we swallow, the tube opens and we often hear a 'click'. If the Eustachian tube passed through one of the pharyngeal constrictors would this same process happen? The answer is 'no'. Pharyngeal constrictors contract on swallowing to facilitate the movement of a food or fluid bolus. If the Eustachian tube passed through superior constrictor, every time we swallow it would close off and the rest of the time lie open. The location of the tubal orifice, in the nasopharynx, means that we do not need to worry about our lunch escaping into our middle ear on a routine basis. Closing it off on swallowing, therefore, offers no advantage, unless eating standing on one's head! Other activities would be hazardous, however- swimming would be a deafening experience and middle ear infections rife. This concept helps us remember its location. Anatomy is a very logical subject.

The Eustachian tube is formed of bony and cartilaginous parts. The latter forms a 'hook shape' as it enters the nasopharynx and contributes to a mucosal bump behind its orifice called the torus tubarius. This means 'tubal mound' which again makes sense. Muscles attaching to the tube orifice also form part of the torus, such as salpingopharyngeus. Posteriorly, there is a groove between the torus and longus colli (a 'long' muscle-longus, extending down the 'neck'- colli). This is called the Fossa of Rosenmuller and is a favourite spot for nasopharyngeal cancer to arise from. Therefore, on axial imaging, we see a groove anteriorly (the Eustachian tube orifice), then a bump (the torus tubarius) and then another groove (the Fossa of Rosenmuller) (Fig. 19).

The constrictors are not the only contents of this space. A ring of lymphoid tissue (Waldeyers' Ring) protects the upper aerodigestive tract from infection and provides a large surface area by which pathogens of all types are 'presented' to the body (Fig. 20).

Superiorly, on the posterior wall of the nasopharynx, lies the adenoid pad (pharyngeal tonsil). This is often large in children, but regresses by teenage years. It can fill the postnasal space and contribute to a persistent runny nose in childhood. As a pliable structure, its presence may cause no problems; however, when hypertrophied it can block off the Eustachian tube orifice leading to middle ear effusions. It may also enlarge in other conditions such as lymphoma, and a large adenoid pad in adults should be treated with caution. A unilateral middle ear effusion in adults is particularly suspicious and direct inspection of the postnasal space is mandatory to exclude nasopharyngeal cancer in the Fossa of Rosenmuller, as previously mentioned.

Adjacent to the Eustachian tubes lies a small amount of lymphoid tissue known as the Tubal Tonsil, separate from the adenoid pad.

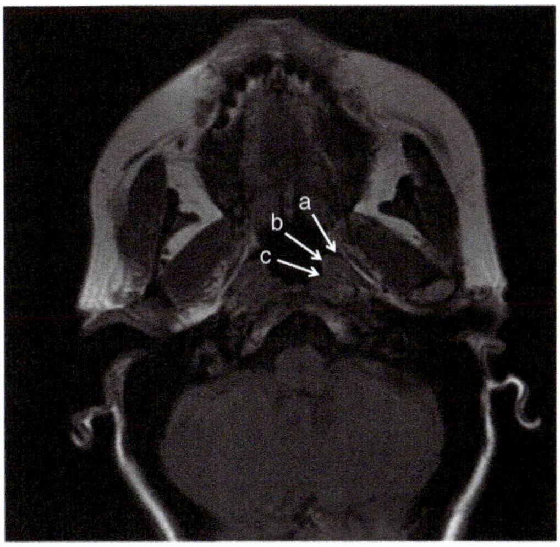


**Fig. 19** Axial T1W MRI at the level of the nasopharynx: (**a**) Eustachian tube orifice. (**b**) Torus tubarius. (**c**) Fossa of Rosenmuller

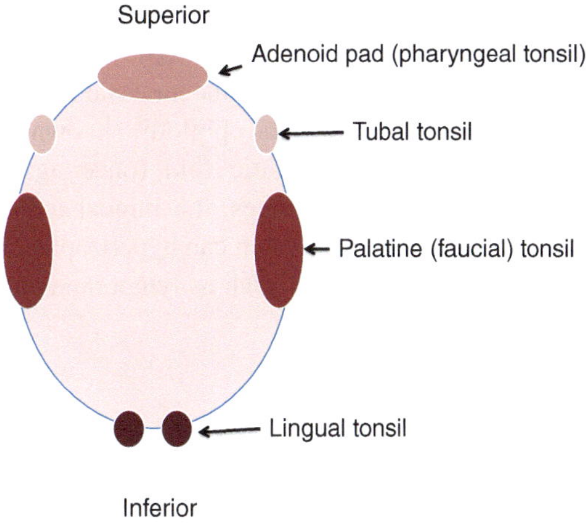


**Fig. 20** Schematic diagram of Waldeyer's ring of lymphoid tissue

On both sides, guarding the entrance to the oropharynx, lie the palatine (faucial) tonsils between two muscles- palatoglossus anteriorly and palatopharyngeus posteriorly. These form curved arches elevating overlying mucosa, on each side producing a soft tissue 'pillar'. Palatoglossus, as its name suggests, extends from the soft palate to the tongue, merging with transverse muscle fibres. It is the only extrinsic tongue muscle not supplied by the hypoglossal nerve (CN XII) and is innervated by the vagus nerve

(CN X). Palatopharyngeus also arises from the soft palate, but joins with another muscle, stylopharyngeus, to insert mainly into the posterior border of the thyroid cartilage. It is also innervated by CN X.

The palatine tonsils may become grossly hypertrophied and almost meet in the midline. They can have prominent crypts, visible on imaging, in which food debris may become trapped, leading to tonsillitis and peritonsillar abscess formation. On the lateral aspect of the palatine tonsil lies the middle constrictor and pathology is often confined to the PMS by this and overlying MLDCF. However, if these are breached the parapharyngeal space will become involved and from here infection can spread to other areas.

Inferiorly, completing the ring, lie the lingual tonsils. These sit behind the tongue base, between it and the lingual surface of the epiglottis, in a space known as the vallecula. There is one on each side, separated by a midline mucosal fold in connecting the tongue to the epiglottis- known as the median glosso-epiglottic fold (once again logic prevails!). As one ages, the lingual tonsil usually regresses. However, it can hypertrophy or be involved in pathology such as lymphoma and squamous cell carcinoma.

Mucosa lining the PMS also counts as a 'content' along with minor salivary tissue. There is a further muscle in the space called levator veli palatine which, as the name suggests, e-levates (raises) the palate. To do this, it must originate above the level of the palate, or else how could it pull it up? It therefore passes from the petrous apex/ medial lamina of the Eustachian tube cartilage to the soft palate and is again principally innervated by CN X via the pharyngeal plexus.

## 2.6 Carotid Space

The carotid space lies within the carotid sheath, formed of contributions from all three layers of deep cervical fascia (Fig. 21). This sheath passes from the skull base, through the thoracic inlet and beyond. It is therefore found in both supra- and infrahyoid compartments and keeps the same name.

Above the hyoid, like a bus, it has a lot of passengers that hop on and off. This means that there are multiple gaps in the sheath through which normal structures and pathological processes can pass. Below the hyoid, it's pretty boring with few defects, and therefore, pathology in the infrahyoid carotid sheath tends to stay within it.

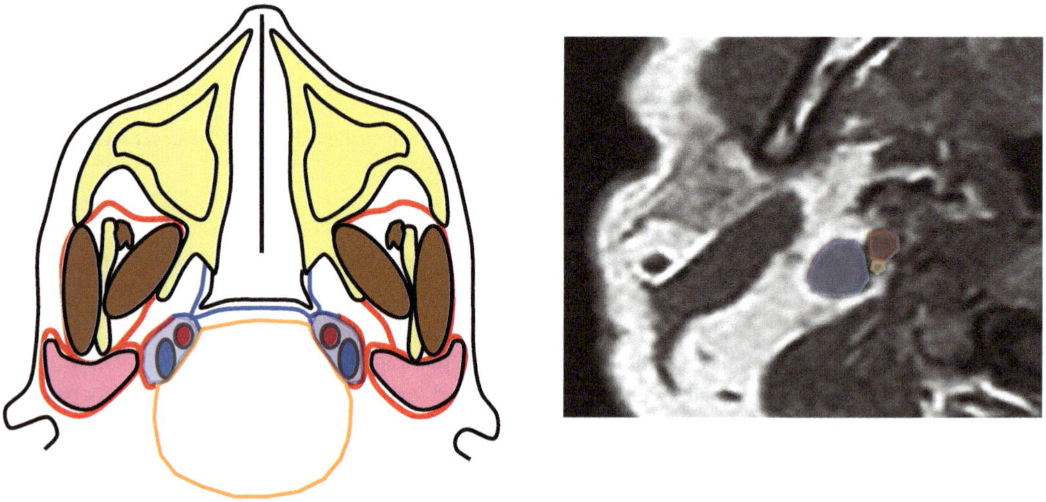

**Fig. 21** Schematic diagram highlighting (in purple) the carotid space on each side, accompanied by axial T1W MRI showing the position of the internal jugular vein (blue), internal carotid artery (red), and vagus nerve (yellow). Note the layers of DCF and how all three contribute to the carotid sheath

As the name suggests, it contains the common carotid artery below the hyoid (up to about C4 vertebral level) and the internal carotid artery cranial to this. Lateral to the arteries lie the internal jugular vein and between arteries and vein, the vagus nerve (CN X). These are constant structures, along with the peri-arterial sympathetic plexus and lymph nodes. In the suprahyoid neck, passengers include other lower cranial nerves (glossopharyngeal-IX, accessory-XI, and hypoglossal-XII) hitching a ride to the tongue and pharynx.

## 2.7 Retropharyngeal and Danger Spaces

The retropharyngeal space (RPS) lies, as the name suggests, retro (behind) the pharynx (PMS), between middle and deep layers of deep cervical fascia (Fig. 22). The alar fascia subdivides this space, creating the excitingly named "Danger Space'. In normal individuals, the RPS is extremely thin and on T1W/ T2W MRI is seen as a bright fat stripe between pharyngeal constrictors and prevertebral muscles. The danger space is almost never visible, and in reality, is a potential space containing loose areolar tissue. The RPS has few contents- fat, lymph nodes, and generally small vessels. However, tortuous carotid arteries can enter the space, and in some cases, meet in the midline (known romantically as 'kissing carotids'). This is important to mention in imaging reports, particularly if the patient is having surgery. I have seen a number of requests stating 'pulsating submucosal mass in oropharynx-? nature prior to biopsy'. This 'mass' is in fact a carotid artery and most certainly should NOT be sampled!

The RPS and the danger space extend long distances craniocaudally and disease can easily travel along them to present in other areas. The RPS passes from the skull base to the level of approximately T4 (manubriosternal joint/tracheal bifurcation) to the point at which the MLDCF and alar fascia fuse, obliterating the space (Faye et al. 2009). The Danger Space, between the alar fascia and DLDCF, continues to the level of the diaphragm. An infection in the neck can therefore easily reach the mediastinum and, if only the neck is imaged, cases of mediastinitis and abscess formation will be missed. To fully cover these spaces, one must scan to the diaphragm when pathology within them is suspected. Descending necrotising mediastinitis (first described in 1938 by Pearse), although

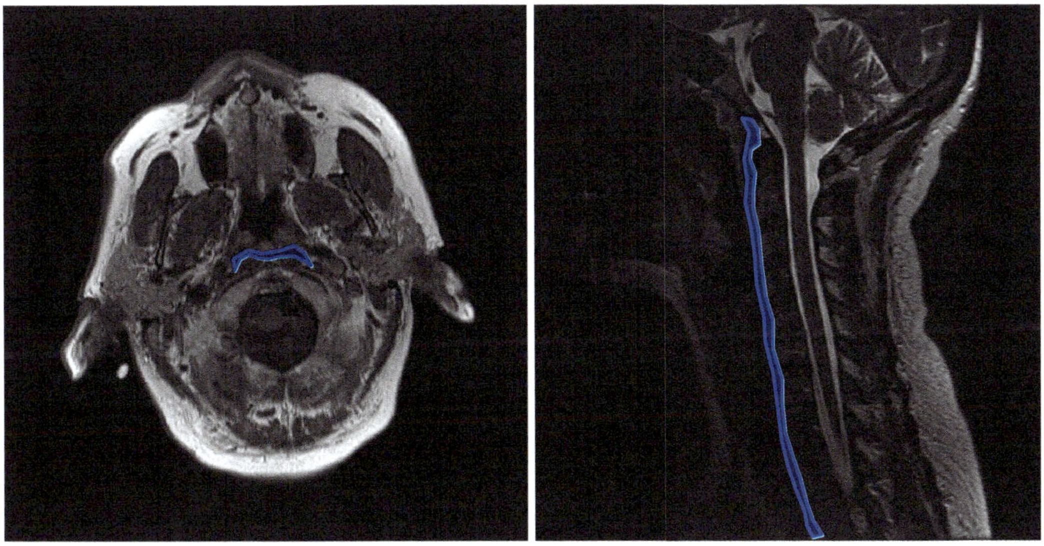

**Fig. 22** Axial T1W and sagittal T2W images highlighting the position and extent of the retropharyngeal/danger spaces in the neck

rare, has a 30–50% mortality rate and should be suspected if classical symptoms of cervical infection progress to include dyspnea or abnormal chest auscultation (Debnam and Guha-Thakurta 2012).

Retropharyngeal lymph nodes are one of a number of groups not covered by the 'Level' system used when reporting neck imaging (Kulzer and Branstetter 2017) and should be specifically looked for, along with intra-parotid, facial, and occipital nodes. They are not usually greater than 5 mm in short axis diameter, except in children when larger nodes are common. It is said that lymph nodes are only found in the suprahyoid RPS (Faye et al. 2009) and, come to think of it, I have never seen any below this level.

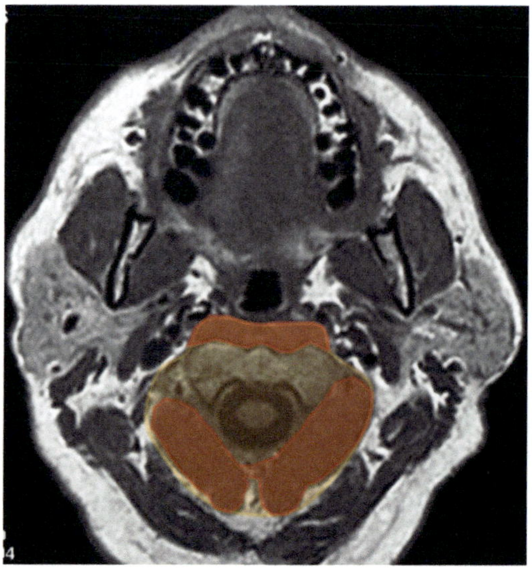

**Fig. 23** Axial T1W MRI demonstrating the position of the perivertebral space (yellow) with pre- and paravertebral muscles highlighted in orange

## 2.8 Perivertebral Space

The perivertebral space (PVS) is exactly that; peri (around) vertebral (the vertebra). It therefore has components anterior to the vertebral bodies (prevertebral) and on both sides of the vertebra (para-vertebral) (Fig. 23). As you might expect, the major tissue type within it is muscle, and this muscular tube extends from the skull base to the coccyx. Likewise, pathology within it, such as infection, can freely extend craniocaudally for any distance along it. Therefore, in theory, if there is something 'bad' going on within the space, one should image the whole tube, but in reality we are guided by symptoms and their most likely cause when deciding whether to examine the whole spine or part of it.

This space is completely surrounded by the deep layer of deep cervical fascia, (DLDCF) which forms the floor of the posterior cervical space (triangle) in the infrahyoid neck. As well as muscles, the space contains the nerves and vessels that supply them plus the vertebral column, vertebral arteries, veins and spinal cord with with exiting nerve roots. Some of these nerve roots go on to form cervical and brachial plexuses. Autonomic nerves are also present, as is the accessory nerve, which supplies sternocleidomastoid and trapezius (neither of which lie in this space by the way!). The phrenic nerve is contained within the prevertebral space from around C3 to C5 level and crosses the anterior scalene (Pinto et al. 2008). Dorsal scapular and long thoracic nerves penetrate the middle scalene muscle belly.

Muscles within the space predominantly hold one's head upright and move it around. As many span the supra and infrahyoid neck, both areas will be covered here.

In the prevertebral space, longus colli (long neck) is vertically orientated and forms a couple of subtle bumps on the posterior pharyngeal wall. Anterior to this lie the previously mentioned RPS/danger space and the PMS, separated from it by deep and middle layers of deep cervical fascia, respectively. When assessing pathology in this region, it is helpful to look at longus colli and decide whether it is truly involved or simply compressed posteriorly. If involved, it enlarges, if compressed it looks smaller. Using this simple approach, one can start to differentiate between pathology in different spaces, which in turn influences their potential inferior extent- to around

T4 in the RPS, the diaphragm in the danger space, and the coccyx in the prevertebral space.

It is beyond the scope of this chapter to go into details regarding each and every muscle within the PVS (and there are quite a few), but a couple of rules apply to all. Muscles with the name 'capitis' lie near the top (the 'capital'-head) and all insert into the occipital bone. The word before 'capitis' tells you something about them- longissimus is long, obliquus runs obliquely, rectus is straight. Those with the name 'cervicis' or 'scapulae' lie more inferiorly. The other rule is that all these muscles have to attach to cervical vertebrae (they are after all 'neck' muscles) somewhere convenient, which isn't covered up by other muscles and preferably sticks out a bit making them 'available for attachment'- i.e. transverse processes. So, if confronted in an exam with a question about the origin of cervical muscles, go for 'cervical transverse processes' as your answer, even if you can't remember the exact numbers. If the muscle is very high in the neck (a capitis muscle), it is more likely to come from the atlas and axis, which don't have true transverse processes, so modify your reply in this case and look smart.

The most important muscles in this area to a radiologist are the scalenes- anterior, middle, and posterior. Scalene means 'a triangle with sides of unequal length' and the name makes sense when you look at the muscles. Where do they originate? Cervical transverse processes of course (did you read the previous paragraph?!). Where do they insert? Into the first rib (anterior and middle scalenes) and second rib (posterior scalene).

On the superior surface of the first rib, there is a bump- the scalene tubercle- caused by the pull of the anterior scalene attachment. Behind this is a depression in which runs the subclavian artery. And behind this the middle scalene inserts. We know (I hope) that the brachial plexus surrounds the axillary artery, which is a continuation of the subclavian artery as it crosses the first rib. Therefore, nerve roots forming the plexus converge on the subclavian artery and lie between anterior and middle scalene muscles on imaging (Fig. 24). The subclavian vein passes in front of the anterior scalene, thus avoiding occlusion each time the scalenes contract. The subclavian artery is more resilient with a thicker wall and is less easily compromised. The posterior scalene doesn't have any such exciting relations and will therefore be ignored!

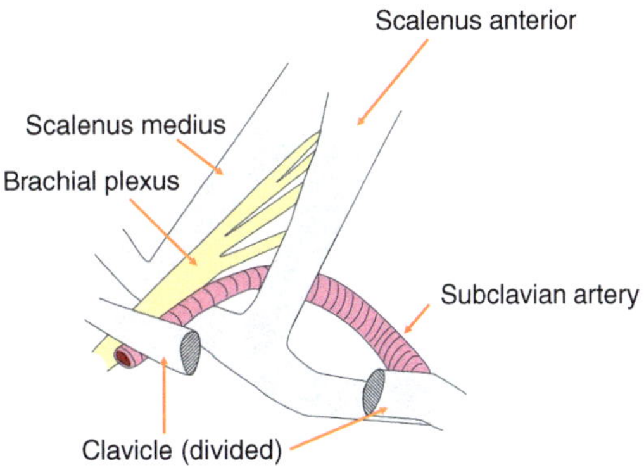


**Fig. 24** Diagram demonstrating the relationships between anterior and middle scalene muscles to the subclavian artery and brachial plexus in the root of the neck

## 2.9 Parapharyngeal Space

The parapharyngeal space (PPS) is small but mighty. At first glance, it seems to be something of a 'non-space'. After all, it doesn't have its own cervical fascial layer (boundaries come from both superficial and middle layers of DCF- Fig. 25) and there's not much in it- fat, a few lymph nodes, vessels, and some salivary gland tissue. It doesn't look impressive on imaging and is easy to overlook. However, this space holds the key to making a sensible differential diagnosis in suprahyoid soft tissue masses as it sits in the centre of the neck space universe. It is also a key conduit for the spread of infection from one neck space to another.

If you look at Fig. 26, you will see that the parapharyngeal space is a fatty island in the middle of a neck space 'sea' surrounded on all sides by regions previously discussed. Depending on

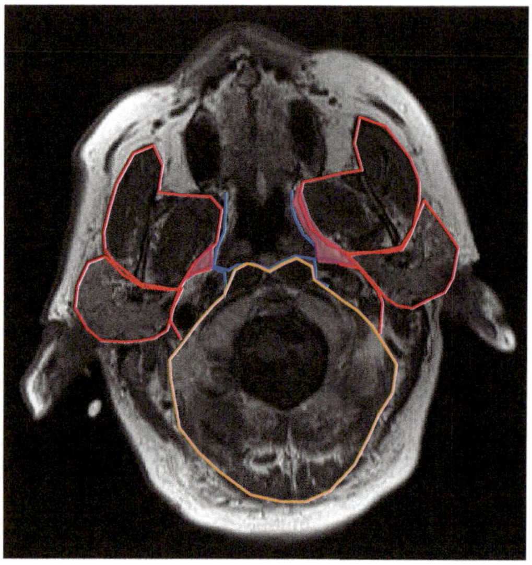

**Fig. 25** Axial T2W MRI suprahyoid neck. The components of DCF are again noted with the parapharyngeal space highlighted in pink, lying between superficial (red) and middle (blue) layers

the site of origin of a mass, parapharyngeal fat will be compressed and displaced in a particular direction.

The PPS is found only in the suprahyoid neck and extends from the skull base to the hyoid. It is open anteriorly to the back of the submandibular triangle which means that infection, etc. in this area can freely pass into it, and from here to other areas. If a peritonsillar abscess penetrates the middle constrictor, it is also into this space. Aggressive pathology can use this 'fatty elevator' to ride up and down the suprahyoid neck involving other fascial spaces as it goes.

Primary parapharyngeal pathology is rare. Fatty lesions such as lipomata occur here. Vascular malformations, pathological nodes, and salivary gland neoplasms may be present. However, the main value of the space is its displacement pattern depending on the space of origin of suprahyoid pathology (Fig. 27).

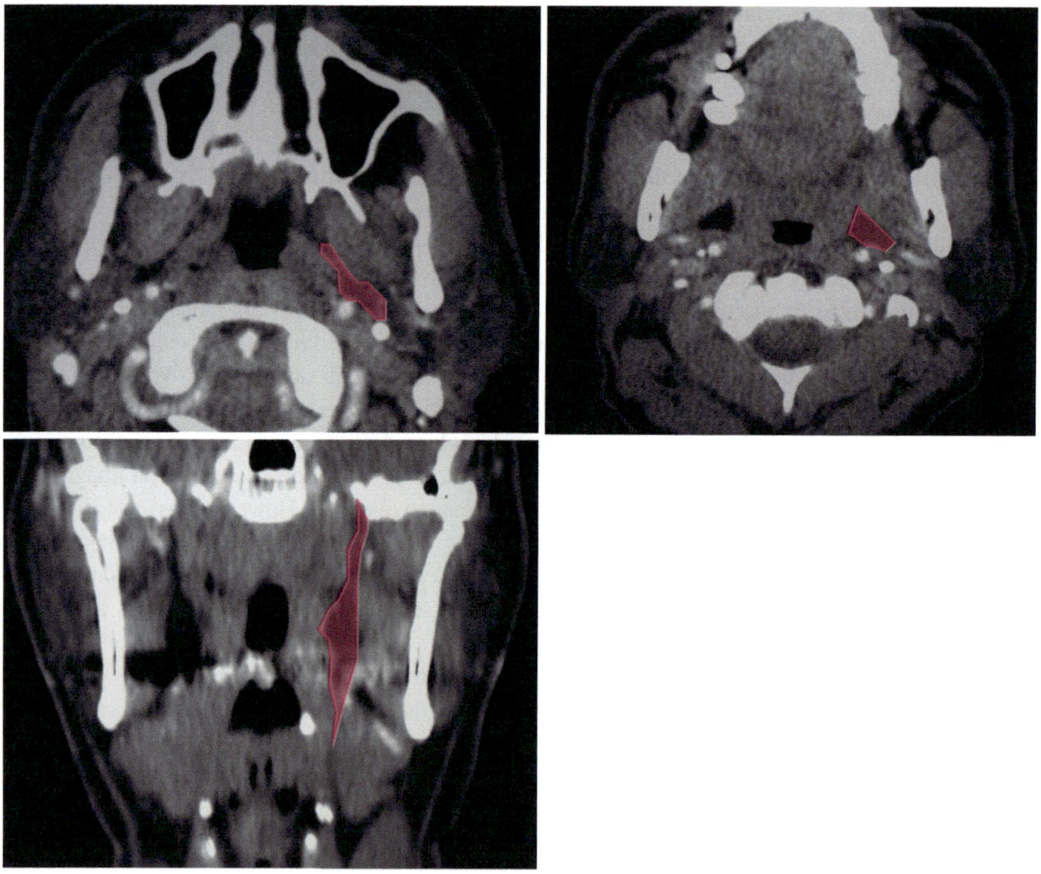

**Fig. 26** Axial and coronal CT images demonstrate the extent and location of the parapharyngeal space in pink

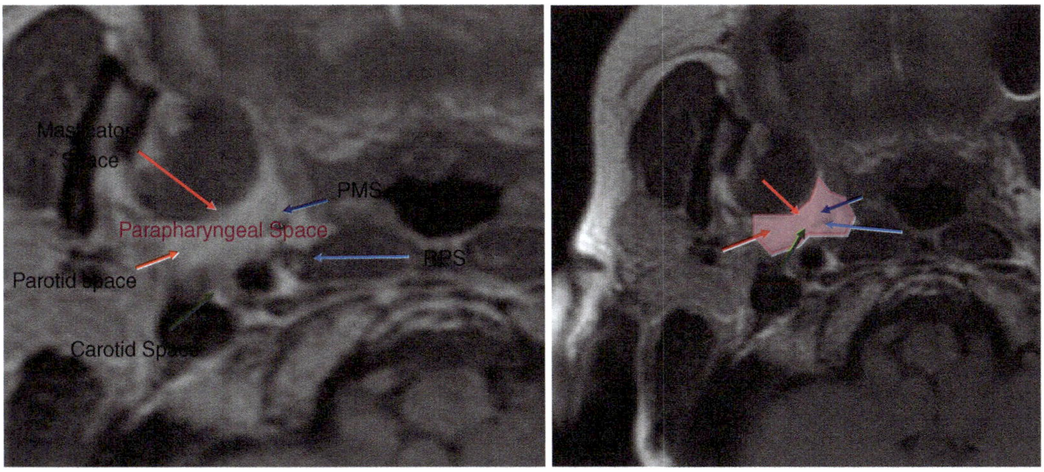


**Fig. 27** The key relationship of the PPS to surrounding suprahyoid neck spaces and the expected fat displacement pattern should a lesion arise from one of these (indicated by coloured arrows)

# 3 Infrahyoid Compartments

## 3.1 Overview

Fortunately, many of the spaces in the suprahyoid neck continue below the hyoid and change little. This means that this part of the chapter is shorter ('thank goodness' I hear you say!).

The perivertebral infrahyoid space has already been covered. The carotid space remains the same, although its sheath is continuous below the hyoid and pathology within it finds it more difficult to 'escape' unless particularly aggressive in nature. There is no parotid, parapharyngeal, or masticator space. The pharyngeal mucosal space changes its name to become the visceral space and there are a couple of new spaces, predominantly containing fat and lymph nodes, which we will now cover. Figure 28 demonstrates the infrahyoid neck spaces, highlighting those that are new or have changed their name.

## 3.2 Visceral Space

The visceral space (VS), as a continuation of the PMS, is surrounded by the middle layer of deep cervical fascia. In the infrahyoid neck, it is largely a complete tube, with an opening for the larynx at the top. It contains the inferior constrictor, the lowest stacking cup, which is continuous with the oesophagus inferiorly at cricopharyngeus.

In addition to the inferior constrictor and cervical oesophagus, this space contains the larynx, trachea, thyroid, and parathyroid glands, along with associated nerves and vessels. The anatomy of the larynx is beyond the scope of this chapter, but is extremely interesting. Suffice it to say that it can be divided into three parts; supraglottis, glottis, and infraglottis. It has supporting cartilages and mucosal folds, the latter coming together at glottic level when phonating. The epiglottis which covers the laryngeal opening like a lid protects the airway when swallowing, and the strap muscles attached to the larynx elevate and depress the whole structure to assist with swallowing and phonation.

## 3.3 Anterior Cervical Space

This space lies between superficial and middle layers of deep cervical fascia in front of the strap muscles and thyroid gland. It has few contents; mainly fat, connective tissue, veins, and lymph nodes (level VI). Pathology limited to this space is rare, but it remains important. Reflecting the anatomy, surgeons will encounter two fascial layers as they cross this space when operating on the thyroid gland.

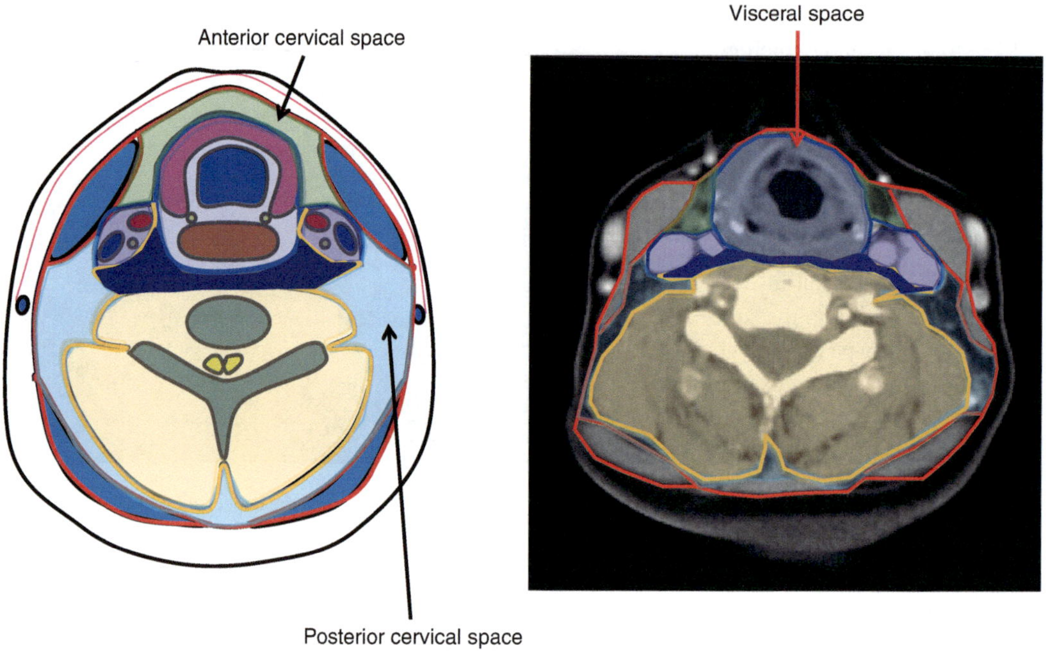


**Fig. 28** Schematic diagram and axial CT imaging of the infrahyoid neck demonstrating fascial layers and neck space compartments. Those that differ from the suprahyoid neck have been labelled

## 3.4 Posterior Cervical Space

The posterior cervical space (PCS) is likewise a thin layer predominantly composed of fatty tissues, lying on either side of the neck between superficial and deep layers of deep cervical fascia. It is more commonly known as the posterior triangle. Its anterior margin is the posterior border of sternocleidomastoid and its posterior margin is the anterior border of trapezius. It can be subdivided into occipital (superior) and subclavian (inferior) triangles by the inferior belly of omohyoid (Mills and Shah 2015), which is more easily identified on neck ultrasound than CT/MRI.

Its roof is formed by the SLDCF plus platysma, and its floor of paraspinal muscles covered by DLDCF. It contains fat, lymph nodes (level V), the external jugular vein in part, arteries, and the accessory nerve (XI) in its floor. This nerve often lies deep to the DLDCF, but occasionally ventures into the space, placing it at risk during surgery to the area.

The posterior triangle is tiny superiorly, as trapezius and sternocleidomastoid (SCM) meet on the skull base, but broad inferiorly along the clavicular margin. Pus discharging from the mastoid tip may spread within this space to present as a lump lower in the neck, often along the border of SCM (a Bezold's abscess).

# 4 Oral Cavity

The oral cavity does not comfortably sit within the spaces described so far and is not contained within layers of DCF. However, as disease can easily spread to and from spaces previously mentioned, it warrants a brief mention.

The oral cavity extends from the lips and oral aperture anteriorly to the anterior palatal arch posteriorly. Superiorly lies the hard palate and inferiorly mylohyoid. It contains the sublingual glands, submandibular duct, lingual nerve and vessels, chorda tympani, and hypoglossal nerve; also, intrinsic and extrinsic muscles of the tongue and mucosa lining the mouth. We have already heard how the posterior margin of mylohoid has a free edge, around which the submandibular gland and main duct extend. This area forms a conduit for disease in either space to spread freely to the other. Also, via this pathway, the oral cavity can connect with the parapharyngeal space and beyond. If there is a defect in mylohyoid (a boutonniere- button hole- is found in up to 40% of people), disease can also spread through the floor of the mouth into the submandibular space, without having to pass behind the free edge. This is usually the case, for example, in a plunging ranula which starts life as a small retention cyst in the sublingual region and extends, via a boutonniere, inferiorly.

Extrinsic muscles 'do what it says on the tin' and are named after their origins and insertions. Those 'above' mylohoid include geniohyoid and genioglossus which arise from the inner surface of the mandible at its anterior margin (the genu) and insert into the hyoid bone and tongue, respectively. Muscles within the tongue are named after their direction of travel and will not be mentioned further.

## 5 Summary

If all you read of this chapter is the summary, it better be good! The key points to remember are as follows:

- The neck can be split into anatomical compartments by 3 layers of deep cervical fascia- superficial, middle, and deep.
- Compartments are either supra- (above) or infra- (below) hyoid, or both.
- Posterior compartments are longer, extending into the mediastinum and beyond. Therefore, consider imaging more of the patient if you suspect infection, etc. in these areas.
- In the suprahyoid neck, the parapharyngeal space is key- if there is a mass, look at the fat displacement pattern to discern its space of origin. If there is infection, consider whether it could have utilized this 'fatty elevator' to spread beyond its original space.
- Remember- many spaces have routes via which disease can extend intracranially, generally via neural foraminae. Don't be caught out by not imaging the whole course of the nerve or considering intracranial pathology.
- Anatomy of the neck 'makes sense'- follow simple concepts to remember key facts rather than memorizing every muscle. You can always look them up!

## References


Debnam JM, Guha-Thakurta N (2012) Retropharyngeal and prevertebral spaces: anatomic imaging and diagnosis. Otolaryngol Clin N Am 45:1293–1310

Faye N, Lafitte F, Williams M et al (2009) The masticator space: from anatomy to pathology. J Neuroradiol 36:121–130

Kulzer MH, Branstetter BF (2017) Chapter 1 neck anatomy, imaging-based level nodal classification and impact of primary tumor site on patterns of nodal metastasis. Semin Ultrasound CT MRI 38:454–465

Mills MK, Shah LM (2015) Imaging of the perivertebral space. Radiol Clin N Am 53:163–180

Moore KL, Daley AF, Agur AMR (2017) Clinically oriented anatomy, 8th edn. LWW (pub), Philadelphia

Pinto A, Scaglione M, Scuderi MG et al (2008) Infections of the neck leading to descending necrotizing mediastinitis: Role of multi-detector row computed tomography. Eur J Radiol 65:389–394

Standring S (2015) Gray's anatomy: the anatomical basis of clinical practice, 41st edn. Elsevier (pub), Amsterdam

# Traumatic and Non-traumatic Head and Neck Infections

Jane A. Topple and Kunwar S. S. Bhatia

## Contents



J. A. Topple
East Sussex Healthcare Trust,
St Leonards-on-Sea, UK
e-mail: jane.topple@nhs.net

K. S. S. Bhatia (✉)
Imperial College Healthcare NHS Trust, London, UK
e-mail: kunwar.bhatia@nhs.net



M. Scaglione et al. (eds.), *Emergency Radiology of the Head and Spine*,
Medical Radiology Diagnostic Imaging, https://doi.org/10.1007/978-3-030-91047-1_24

**Abstract**

Acute infections of the head and neck region are common presenting complaints in tertiary centres and district general hospitals. Patients with neck infections can be difficult to assess clinically and they can deteriorate rapidly due to airway compromise, organ damage including visual and hearing loss, and intracranial complications. Early imaging diagnosis and treatment is pivotal to prevent significant morbidity and mortality.

Contrast enhanced multi-detector computed tomography (CECT) is the first line imaging technique for severe head and neck infections. CT scanning can assess deep neck compartments, identify collections requiring drainage, and reveal intracranial or orbital complications. Depending on availability and expertise, ultrasound may be performed initially for accessible neck swellings and has the advantage of enabling minimally invasive aspiration of any infective collections for microbiological analysis, which enables targeted treatment.

An appreciation of the subsets of acute neck infections and an understanding of the spectrum of complications of neck infections will aid image interpretation. This chapter reviews the imaging appearances and major complications of acute infections of the paranasal sinuses, middle ear and mastoid, odontogenic, pharyngeal mucosal space, orbital, salivary, facial, and other deep neck space infections. In addition, the appearances of acute suppurative lymphadenitis, tuberculous lymphadenitis (scrofula), post-traumatic and post-surgical iatrogenic infections as well as other miscellaneous infections including congenital head and neck cysts and tumours will be discussed. Paraspinal infections will not be discussed in this section as these are covered elsewhere.

## Abbreviations

| | |
|---|---|
| AOM | Acute otitis media |
| ATLS | Advanced trauma life support |
| HIV | Human Immunodeficiency Virus |
| HIV LA | HIV associated facial lipoatrophy |
| A&E | Accident and emergency |
| ATLS | Advanced trauma life support |
| CECT | Contrast enhanced CT |
| CT | Computed tomography |
| FESS | Functional endoscopic sinus surgery |
| FOM | Floor of mouth |
| IAM | Internal auditory meatus |
| MDCT | Multi-detector computed tomography |
| MRI | Magnetic resonance imaging |
| MRSA | Methicillin-resistant Staphylococcus Aureus |
| NF | Necrotising fasciitis |

| | |
|---|---|
| NOE | Necrotising otitis externa |
| OMU | Osteomeatal unit |
| OPG | Orthopantomogram |
| SSI | Surgical site infections |
| TB | Tuberculosis |
| US | Ultrasound |

# 1 Introduction

Head and neck infections can be life-threatening and organ-threatening acute emergencies. Patients with deep neck space abscesses can be difficult to assess clinically and initial symptoms may be mild due to the deep-seated nature of some infections, masking the severity of infection. Patients can deteriorate quickly; a progressive narrowed airway may collapse suddenly due to compression from pharyngeal, parapharyngeal, and floor of mouth infections. Rupture of abscesses into the airway can cause sudden laryngospasm, and intracranial extension can cause rapidly fatal neurological complications.

Early imaging plays an essential role in acute neck infections, but only should be considered after patient safety has been addressed. In this respect, supine positioning of patients with critically narrowed airways within the CT scanner may precipitate complete airway collapse and respiratory arrest. This catastrophic scenario can be prevented by pre-emptive airway assessment and management in the emergency department prior to imaging. In fact, clinical triage such as an Advanced Trauma Life Support (ATLS) approach is warranted in patients with severe neck infections, utilising a primary survey beginning with ABCD (airway, breathing, circulation, and disability) (Kool and Blickman 2007). If there is audible stridor, the patient is struggling with breathing or there is low blood oxygen saturation, an anaesthetist should be contacted to assess airway patency. Similarly, patients with severe neck infections may benefit from an early multidisciplinary team approach involving head and neck surgeons, accident and emergency clinicians, paediatricians, anaesthetists, nurses, radiographers, and radiologists.

This chapter provides a pictorial review of the radiological findings in acute head and neck infective emergencies. Paranasal sinus, middle ear and mastoid, odontogenic, pharyngeal mucosal space, orbital, salivary, facial, and other deep neck space infections will be reviewed and their complications described. The appearances of acute suppurative lymphadenitis, tuberculous lymphadenitis (scrofula), post traumatic and post-surgical iatrogenic infections as well as other miscellaneous infections including congenital head and neck cysts and tumours will be discussed.

# 2 Rhinosinusitis

The paranasal sinuses enlarge and develop throughout childhood, reaching their adult size by late adolescence (Wolf et al. 1993). Minor mucosal thickening scattered within the sinuses due to subclinical inflammatory changes is common at any age and has been identified incidentally on CT scans in approximately half of the normal adult population (Hansen et al. 2014). The severity of sinus inflammatory changes may be scored using grading systems, of which the Lund-Mackay and Kennedy grading systems are widely adopted (Lund and MacKay 1993). A plain CT is the routine investigation of choice for evaluating clinically suspected sinus inflammatory disease as it permits assessment of disease activity and is used for preoperative planning, which nowadays entails functional endoscopic sinus surgery (FESS). However, CECT is indicated if there is a suspected acute sinusitis with complications, and MRI with contrast may be employed to further characterise skull base and intracranial complications.

## 2.1 Acute Sinusitis

Most cases of acute infective sinusitis are managed in the community and resolved spontaneously without recourse to imaging. Most episodes are viral in aetiology, although acute severe infections are more frequently bacterial. Commonly implicated bacterial pathogens include Streptococcus pneumonia, Haemophilus influenza, and Staphylococcus Aureus (Momeni et al. 2007). Initial work-up for patients with sinus disease includes clinical assessment with or without a plain CT of the paranasal sinuses. On CT, infected sinuses are partially or completely opacified with low-density material, which represents inflammatory mucosal thickening and/or fluid, which may contain air bubbles (bubbly secretions) (Madani and Beale 2009, p. 17) (Fig. 1) (Momeni et al. 2007).

A sinus mucocele is an epithelium-lined cyst caused by accumulation of mucus within an obstructed sinus, which expands and remodels the sinus walls. This usually develops gradually and produces few symptoms apart from those arising from local mass effect (e.g. facial disfigurement, proptosis). However, occasionally their contents may become acutely infected and purulent, termed pyoceles, which result in rapid enlargement, pain, and septicaemia (Madani and Beale 2009).

### 2.1.1 Complications of Acute Sinusitis

Severe episodes of acute sinusitis may produce focal bony erosions of the adjacent sinus walls and inflammatory changes in the surrounding soft tissues, with or without frank abscess formation (Fig. 2). Orbital complications can develop secondary to acute sinusitis, especially if arising from the ethmoid, maxillary, or frontal sinuses. If the post-septal orbital contents are involved, this is termed orbital cellulitis (Fig. 3). Alternatively, if the inflammation is restricted to the tissues of the eyelids and adjacent face, it is termed preseptal or periorbital cellulitis (Fig. 4). The bone intervening between the infected sinus and orbit may show focal erosions, but more commonly is intact as microorganisms can traverse the bone haematogenously via microscopic vessels. Symptoms and signs of orbital involvement include reduced vision, double vision, fever, orbital pain, periorbital swelling erythema, and chemosis. In fact, orbital symptoms are often the initial presentation of an acute sinusitis, especially in children. Orbital complications are

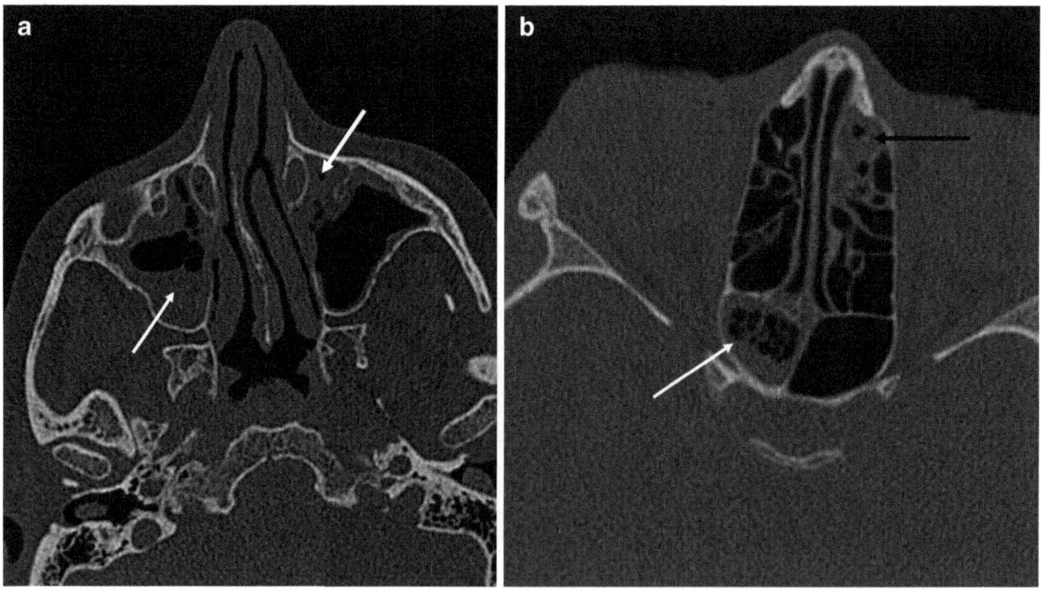


**Fig. 1** Axial CT in an adult male with acute uncomplicated sinusitis. There is partial opacification of both maxillary sinuses (white arrows in image **a**) including an air-fluid level and bubbly secretions on the right. At a higher level, (image **b**) there is partial opacification of the left anterior ethmoid (black arrow) and right sphenoid sinuses (white arrow), and the latter also contains bubbly secretions

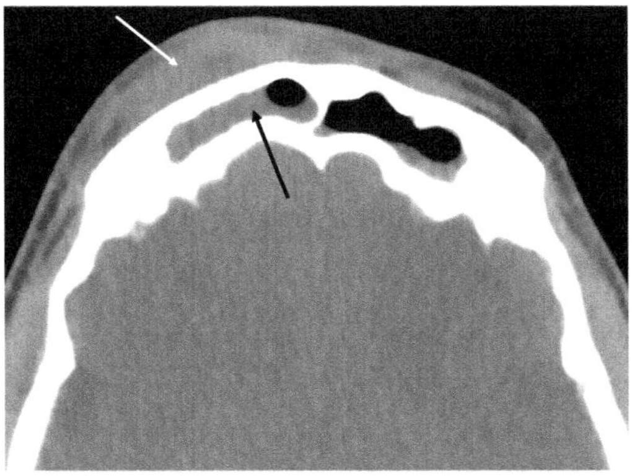

**Fig. 2** Non-contrast axial CT of the head showing bubbly secretions in the right frontal sinus (black arrow). There is fluid, subcutaneous swelling, and fat stranding anterior to the right frontal sinus in keeping a developing subgaleal abscess with overlying cellulitis (white arrow)

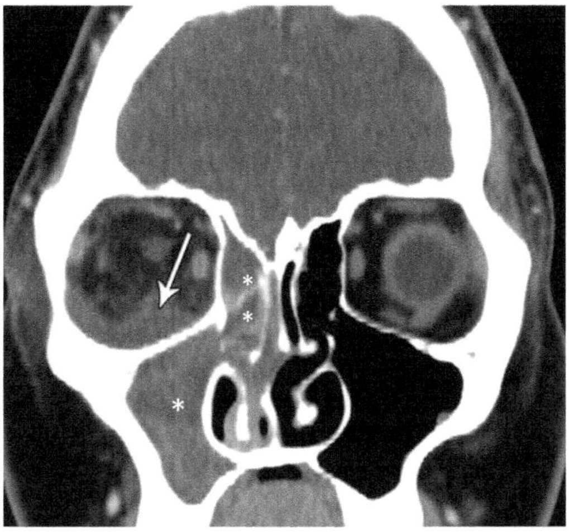

**Fig. 3** Coronal CECT soft tissue window showing fat stranding and phlegmon in the inferolateral right extraconal orbital space (white arrow). The right maxillary antrum and the ethmoid air cells are completely opacified (white asterisk ×1 and white asterisks ×2, respectively)

discussed further in Sect. 6. Intracranial complications of sinusitis are usually secondary to sphenoid, ethmoidal, or frontal sinusitis and include extra-axial abscess (Fig. 5a), intraparenchymal abscess (Fig. 6a and c), meningitis (Fig. 7), cerebritis (Fig. 8), and dural venous and cavernous sinus thrombosis. These should be suspected if symptoms include severe headache, meningism, photophobia, fever, or altered consciousness.

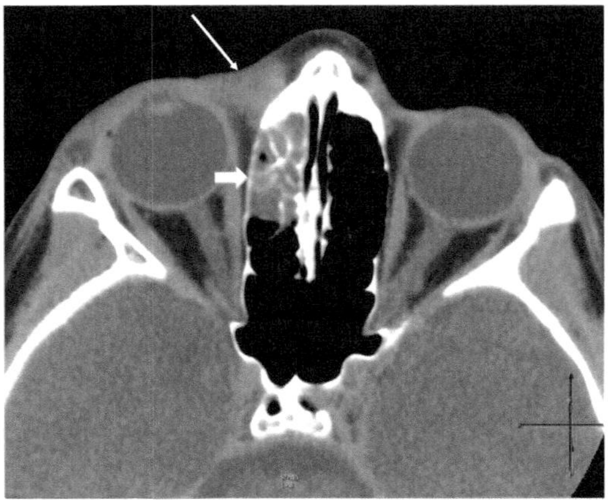

**Fig. 4** Axial CT soft tissue window showing opacification of the anterior ethmoid air cells (thick white arrow). Associated soft tissue swelling in the periorbital tissues (thin white arrow)

Immunocompromised patients and children are particularly susceptible, although complications are also encountered in immunocompetent adults who have had a protracted and untreated sinus infection.

Acute sinusitis may produce local destruction of the surrounding bone with secondary osteomyelitis, especially of the frontal bone (Fig. 5b). A subperiosteal abscess can develop in the subgaleal tissues overlying the infected sinus, which is frequently associated with marked subcutaneous induration and erythema. If occurring over the frontal sinus, this condition is eponymously called Pott's puffy tumour (Fig. 6a).

## 2.2 Fungal Sinusitis

Fungal sinus infections may be non-invasive or invasive. Chronic non-invasive colonisation with fungus can lead to development of a mycetoma (fungus ball) in a sinus cavity (Madani and Beale 2009) (Fig. 9). Invasive fungal sinusitis can be divided into acute and chronic forms and typically occurs in immunocompromised (e.g. neutropenic) or diabetic individuals. In patients with diabetic ketoacidosis, Zygomycetes, such as Rhizopus, Rhizomucor, Absidia, and Mucor, may be cultured (Aribandi et al. 2007). In contrast, Aspergillus is the most common causative

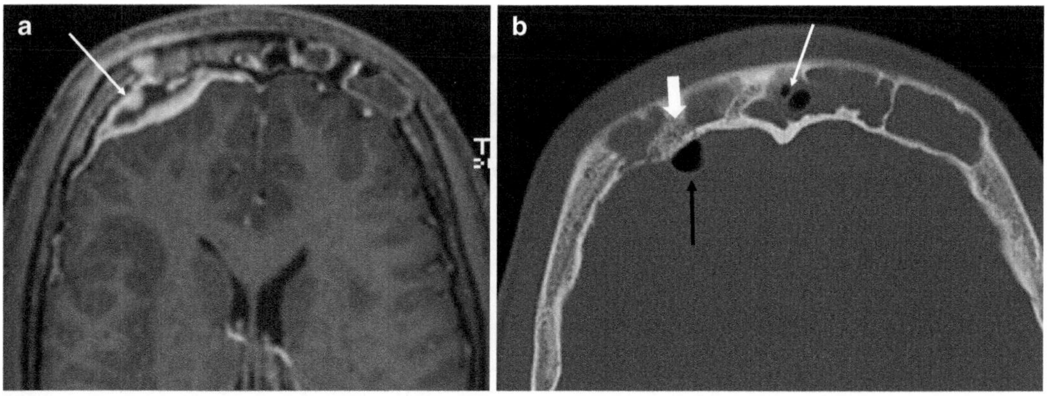


**Fig. 5** (**a**) Contrast enhanced axial T1 weighted MRI showing a rim enhancing biconvex lens-shaped extradural collection anterior to the right frontal lobe (white arrow). (**b**) Axial CT bone window reveals a locule of gas in the anterior cranial fossa (black arrow) with bubbly secretions in the adjacent frontal sinuses (thin white arrow). The inner cortex of the frontal sinus shows tiny permeative erosions in keeping with acute osteomyelitis (thick white arrow)

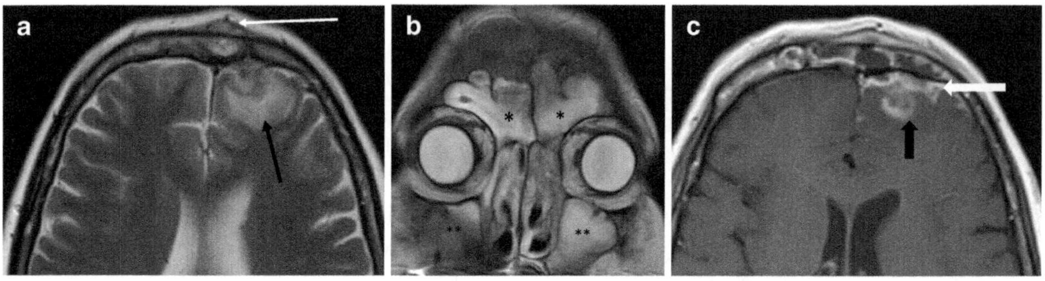


**Fig. 6** (**a**) Axial T2 weighted MRI showing a subperiosteal collection overlying the frontal bone (white arrow) and elevated parenchymal signal (oedema) in the left frontal lobe (black arrow). (**b**) Coronal T2 weighted MRI showing fluid opacification of both frontal sinuses and maxillary antra (asterisk x 1 and x 2 bilaterally). (**c**) Axial contrast enhanced T1 weighted MRI showing dural enhancement (thick white arrow) and a rim enhancing abscess in the left frontal lobe (thick black arrow)

organism in immunocompromised patients (Aribandi et al. 2007). Mortality from this condition is high, up to 80% (Aribandi et al. 2007), although reduced to around 20% in institutions that undertake close active surveillance of at-risk patients (neutropenic patients). Parikh et al. (2004) performed a retrospective review of invasive fungal sinusitis cases over a 15-year period and revealed an overall mortality of 18%. They identified greater mortality in diabetic patients, in those infected with Mucor, and in patients with intracranial extension of the infection.

Presenting symptoms and signs may include fever, facial pain, cranial nerve palsies, headaches, and visual symptoms. The fungi have a propensity for extrasinus invasion and spread along vascular channels, causing an erosive osteitis or osteomyelitis, thrombophlebitis, and infiltration of surrounding soft tissues (Fig. 10a and c). Therefore, the presence of these findings should raise the suspicion of a fungal aetiology. Cavernous sinus thrombophlebitis can occur, with secondary cranial nerve palsies (Fig. 10b). Systemic antifungal medications, with or without surgical debridement, are required to treat these life-threatening infections.

Fungal material has a relatively high protein content and contains heavy metals, which have

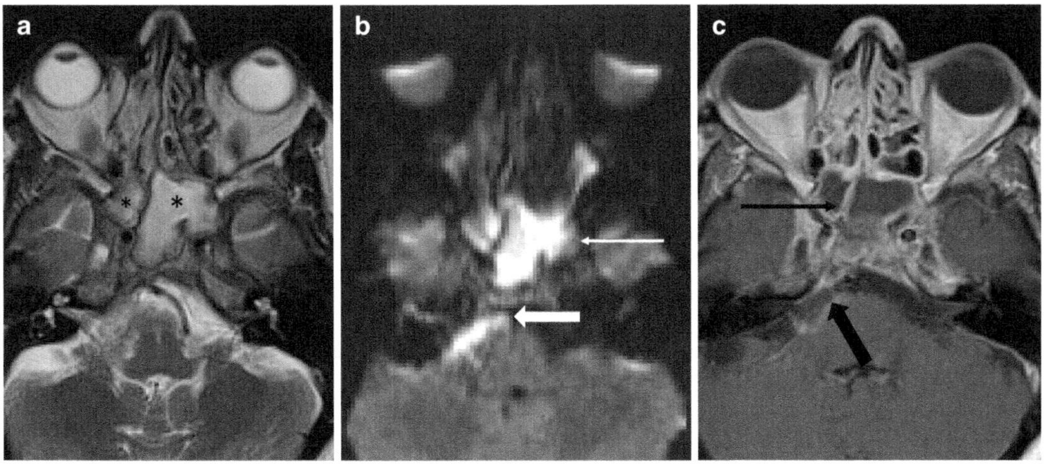


**Fig. 7** (**a**) Axial T2 weighted MRI showing complete opacification of both sphenoid sinuses (asterisk). (**b**) DWI sequence showing elevated DWI signal in the sphenoid sinuses (thin white arrow) and the prepontine cistern (thick white arrow). (**c**) Axial contrast enhanced T1 weighted MRI showing peripheral enhancement of the sphenoid sinuses (thin black arrow) and meningeal enhancement along the right pons (thick black arrow)

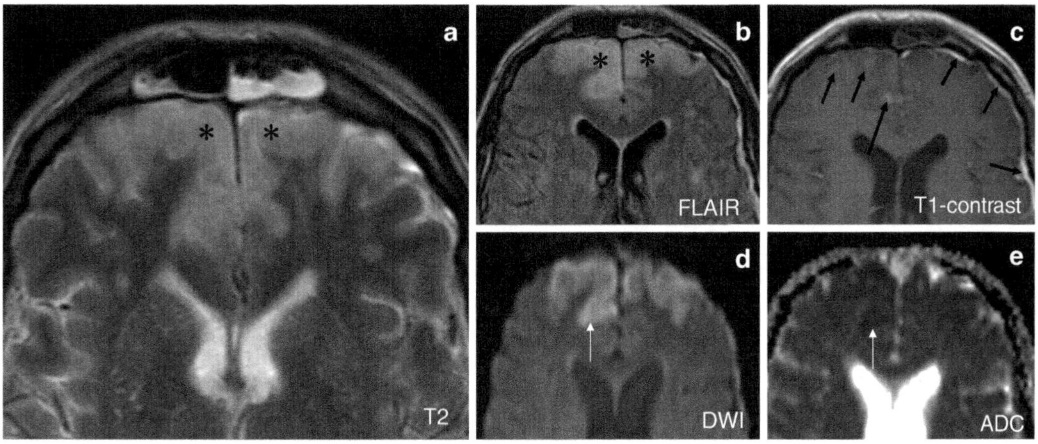


**Fig. 8** Cerebritis secondary to frontal sinusitis. Frontal cortical and subcortical swelling and high signal on FLAIR (**d**) and T2 weighted MRI (**e**, asterisks). This shows mildly restricted diffusion based on the DWI (**a**, black arrow) and ADC map (**b**). Post contrast T1 weighted MRI shows patchy dural and cortical enhancement

paramagnetic effects. This typically shows very low T2 weighted signal and variable T1 weighted signal on MRI scans (Fig. 11a and b) (Meng et al. 2019). The signal may be so low (dark) on T2 weighted sequences that it can be mistaken for an aerated sinus (pseudo air sign), although examining all available sequences can prevent this pitfall (Fig. 11b). On CT, the intra-sinus material in invasive fungal sinusitis can have a variable density, but is usually iso or hypodense. This differs from the hyperdensity and calcification of sinus contents frequently present in a non-invasive mycetoma (fungal ball).

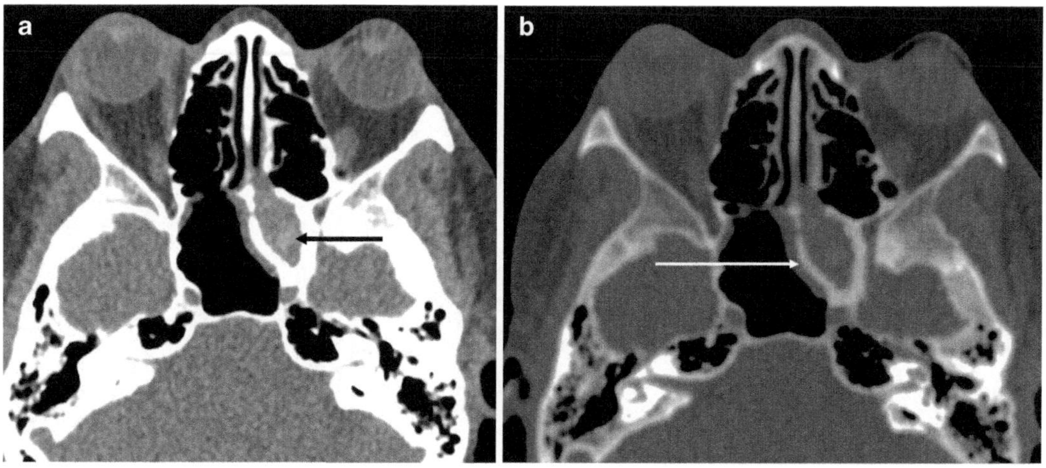


**Fig. 9** (**a** and **b**) Axial CT paranasal sinus study showing a rounded hyperdense focus in the left sphenoid sinus (black arrow). The sinus is opacified with secretions. The walls of the sinus are thickened and sclerotic in keeping with chronic sinusitis (white arrow)

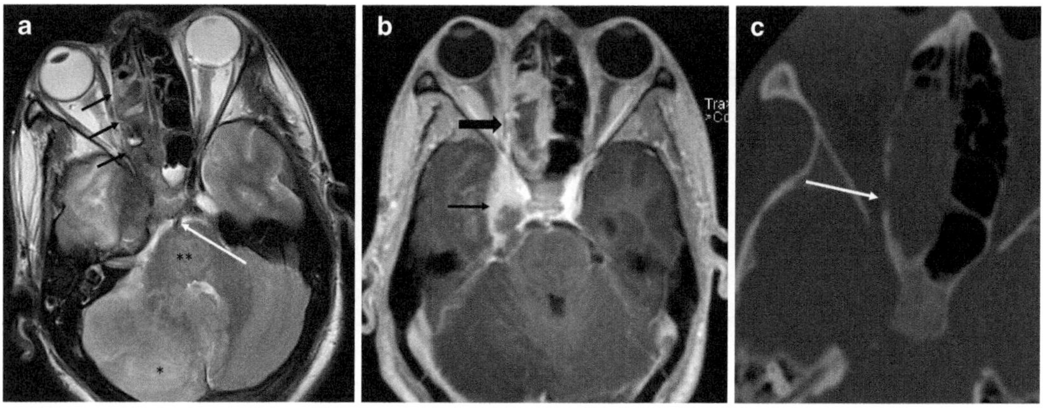


**Fig. 10** (**a**) Axial T2 weighted study showing complete opacification of the right sphenoid sinus, right posterior ethmoids (black arrows). Mural thickening of the basilar artery. Swelling pons and right cerebellar hemisphere due to infarction (asterisk x 1 and x 2). (**b**) Axial T1 weighted contrast enhanced study showing a filling defect in the expanded and enhancing right cavernous sinus (thin black arrow). The sinus collection also shows peripheral enhancement (thick black arrow). (**c**) Axial CT bone window showing a focal erosion of the right lamina papyracea (white arrow)

# 3 Otological and Skull Base Infections

## 3.1 Acute Otitis Media and Uncomplicated Mastoiditis

Acute otitis media (AOM) is common and usually secondary to viral or bacterial infections of the middle ear cavity and/or mastoid air cells. Otitis media complicated by mastoiditis can affect any age but especially children. Symptoms include fever, hearing loss, and otalgia (including ear tugging) although may be non-specific in children including vomiting, drowsiness, or irritability. Otoscopy will reveal an erythematous bulging tympanic membrane with or without perforation. AOM is a clinical diagnosis and

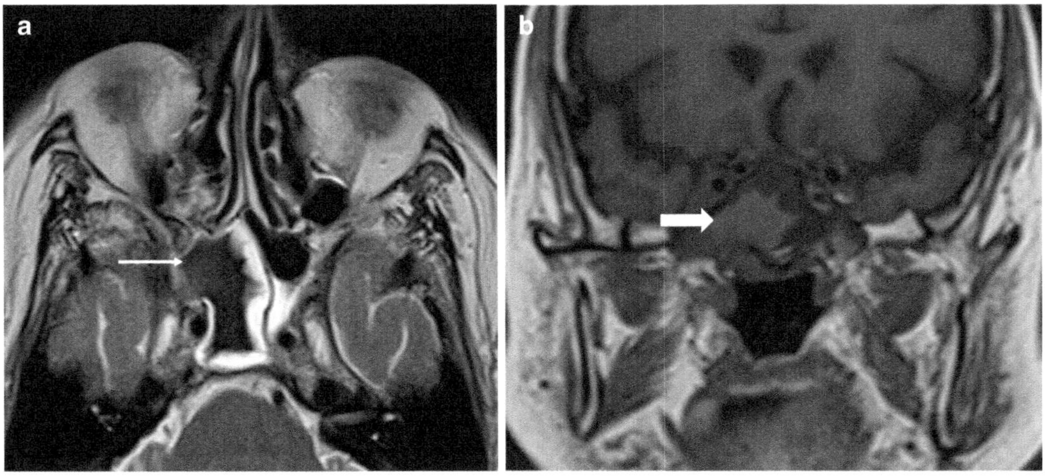


**Fig. 11** (**a**) Axial T2 weighted MRI scan showing very low signal in the right sphenoid sinus centrally (thin white arrow), similar to the signal in aerated sinus. (**b**) Coronal T1 weighted scan shows that this sinus is filled with high T1 weighted signal material, not air (thick white arrow)

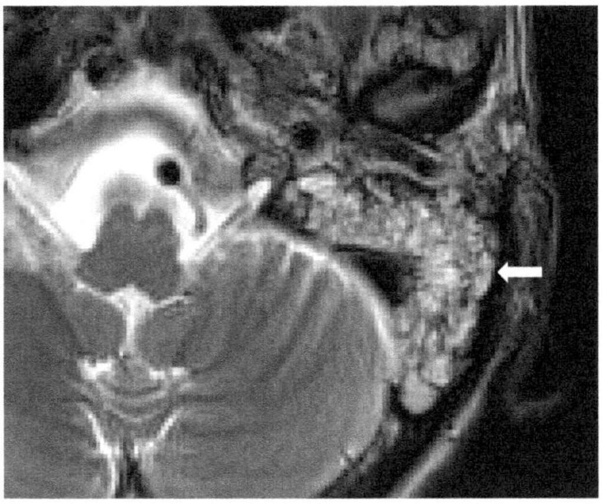

**Fig. 12** Axial T2 weighted MRI study showing a fluid signal effusion in the left mastoid and middle ear cleft (thick white arrow) with no overlying soft tissue swelling

imaging is only required if there are suspected complications. On CT, uncomplicated AOM appears as partial or complete opacification of the middle ear cavity and mastoid air cells with no associated bony erosions. Specifically, the bony septations within the mastoid appear intact (Fig. 12). The opacification reflects variable amounts of mucus, mucopurulent fluid (pus), and inflamed mucosa.

## 3.2 Acute Infective Labyrinthitis

Infectious microorganisms rarely may enter one or both inner ears as a result of either local infections (e.g. acute or chronic otitis media) or systemic infections, producing acute infective labyrinthitis. Patients present with sudden onset of vertigo and variable degree of hearing loss (Baert and Sartor 2003, p. 63). This is usually a clinical diagnosis and imaging is not required unless symptoms progress or complications are suspected. There are two classifications, serous labyrinthitis and suppurative labyrinthitis. Serous infection is caused by viral pathogens or irritation of the labyrinth by toxins or inflammatory mediators, while suppurative infection involves bacterial infiltration of the labyrinth (Chul et al. 2005). Suppurative infection can cause severe irreversible hearing loss and vertigo (Chul et al. 2005, p. 164), and may rarely progress to an aggressive otic capsular osteomyelitis (Fig. 13a–c). CT may show a halo of lucency in the bone surrounding the semicircular canals with associated canal expansion (Fig. 13b and c). MRI studies will show avid enhancement in the labyrinth acutely, followed by loss of the normal fluid signal and absent enhancement if sclerosis develops.

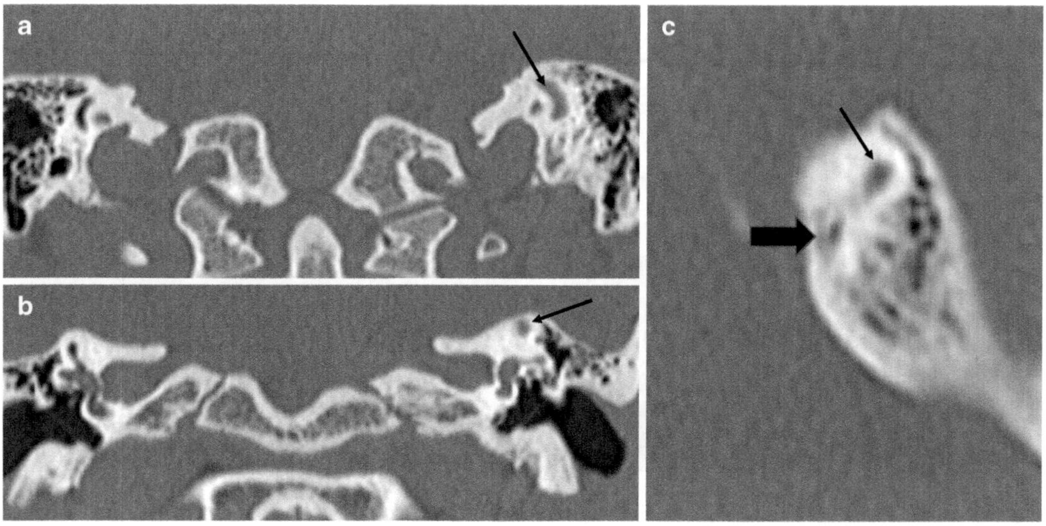


**Fig. 13** (**a**, **b**) Coronal temporal bone CT and (**c**) axial CT of the left petrous temporal bone. The left semicircular canals (thin black arrows) are expanded with a subtle surrounding halo of lucency (thick black arrow)

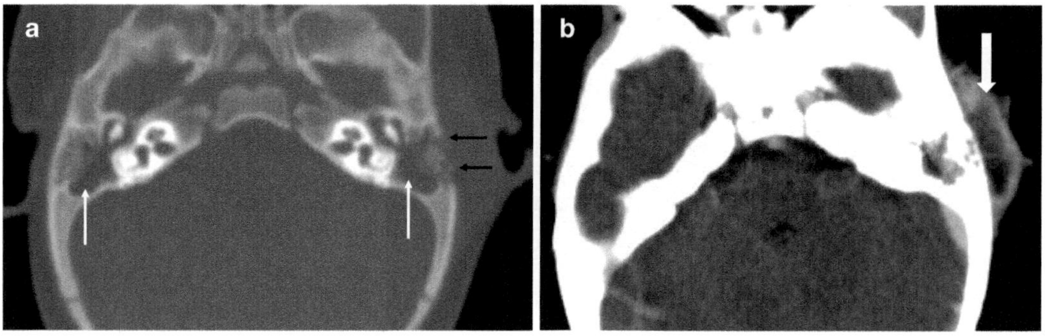


**Fig. 14** (**a**) Axial CT bone window showing bilateral mastoid opacification (white arrows) and cortical erosions of the outer cortex of left mastoid (black arrows). (**b**) Axial soft tissue window showing subperiosteal abscess overlying the left mastoid (thick white arrow)

## 3.3 Coalescent Otomastoiditis

Coalescent mastoiditis is more common in children and represents a more severe infection of the middle ear and mastoid that is associated with local or generalised destruction of adjacent osseous structures, notably of the bony septations separating the mastoid air cells (Fig. 14a). Bony scalloping and frank erosions can also develop along the cortices of the mastoid bone (Figs. 14 and 15). Besides features of AOM described above, patients may develop an ipsilateral facial palsy due to inflammation of the tympanic segment of the facial nerve. Rarefying osteitis may affect the ossicular chain (Fig. 16), typically appearing as reduced density or frank erosions of the malleus or incus, as well as erosion of the incudostapedial joint.

### 3.3.1 Complications of Otomastoiditis

Infection can spread through the mastoid bone into the subperiosteal space or the subcutaneous tissues, forming a phlegmon or frank abscess, which are optimally demonstrated on CECT. In order to identify such complications while minimising radiation exposure in children, suspected cases of acute mastoiditis should undergo a

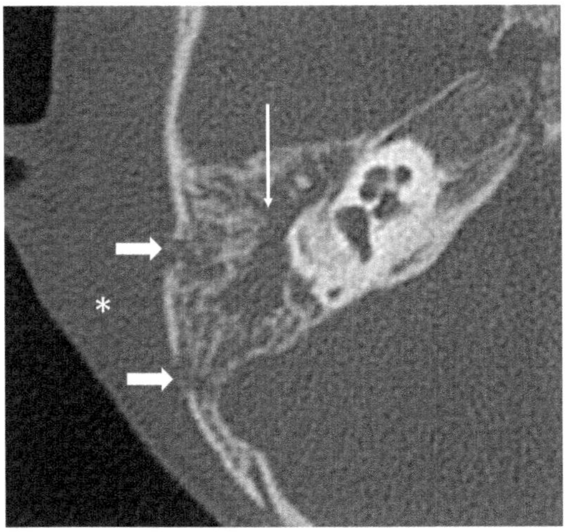

**Fig. 15** Axial CT bone window showing complete opacification of the right mastoid air cells (narrow arrow), outer cortical bony erosions (thick arrows) and overlying soft tissue swelling (asterisk)

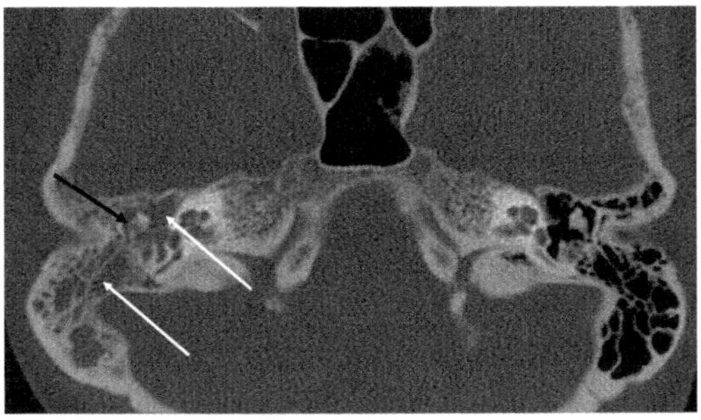

**Fig. 16** Axial CT bone window showing complete opacification of the right mastoid and middle ear cleft (white arrows). The right incus body is less dense than the opposite side, indicating demineralisation

CECT rather than a non-contrast CT initially (Fig. 14b). Less commonly, abscesses in the perimastoid tissues may spread to other sites, a few of which have eponymous names; Bezold's abscess if it surrounds the mastoid tip and extends inferiorly into the sternocleidomastoid muscle (Fig. 17), Citelli's abscess if it extends along the posterior belly of the digastric muscle (Sahoo et al. 2017), and Luc's abscess if tracking into the temporal fossa around the temporalis muscle (Scrafton et al. 2014). Abscesses can also extend into the pinna (Fig. 18).

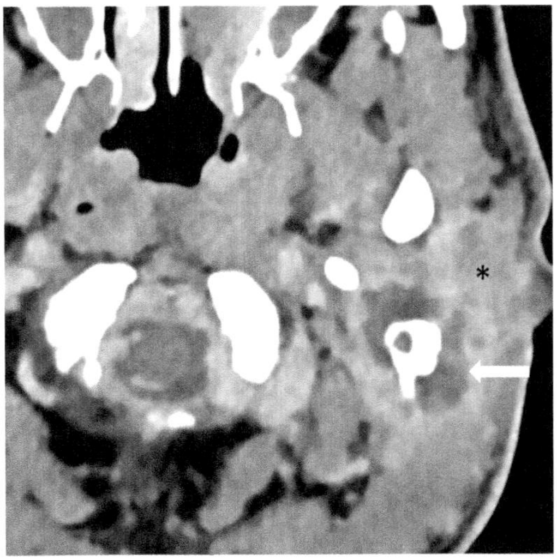

**Fig. 17** Axial CECT showing a rim enhancing collection surrounding the left mastoid process (thick white arrow) which involves into the sternocleidomastoid muscle. Inflammation extends into the left parotid gland (asterisk) and subcutaneous tissues (asterisk)

Intracranial complications are common and include otomastoiditis, subdural empyema, cerebritis, temporal lobe or cerebellar abscesses (Fig. 19b and c), sigmoid sinus thrombosis, meningitis, and cranial nerve palsies. Sigmoid sinus thrombosis appears as a hyperdense filling defect on a plain CT and as a hypodense filling defect (empty delta sign) on CECT (Fig. 20). These complications may require contrast enhanced MRI for further workup. DWI MRI is particularly useful to highlight abscesses irrespective of location, which show restricted diffusion (high signal on DWI images and low signal on ADC maps).

### 3.4 Petrous Apicitis (Gradenigo Syndrome)

Suppurative infection within a pneumatised petrous apex may occur as a complication of acute otitis media (Choi and Park 2014). Gradenigo's syndrome describes a clinical triad of suppurative otitis media, abducens nerve palsy, and retro-orbital pain. Normally, a thin layer of dura mater separates the Vth cranial nerves from the air cells of the

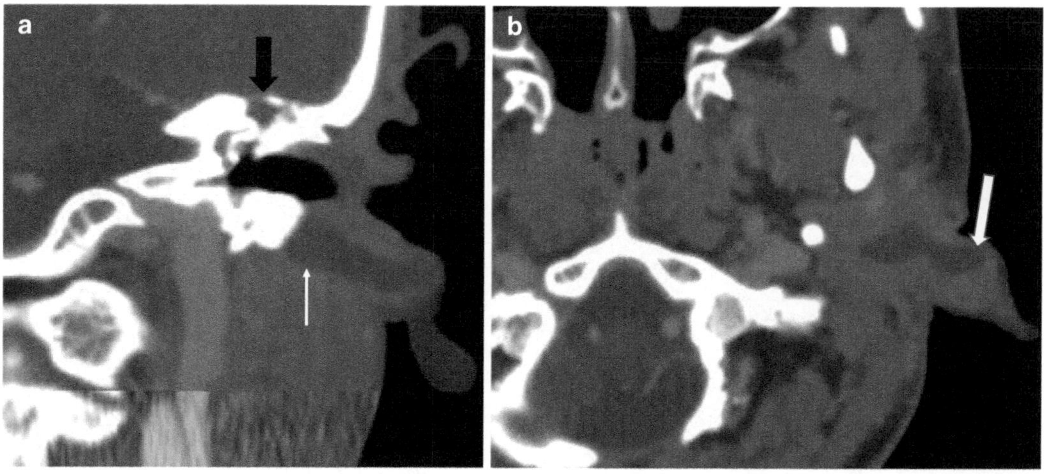


**Fig. 18** (**a** and **b**) Coronal and axial CECT showing a rim enhancing fluid collection along the floor of the left external auditory canal (thin white arrow) extending into the submucosa of the left pinna (thick white arrow). The mastoid air cells are opacified (thick black arrow)

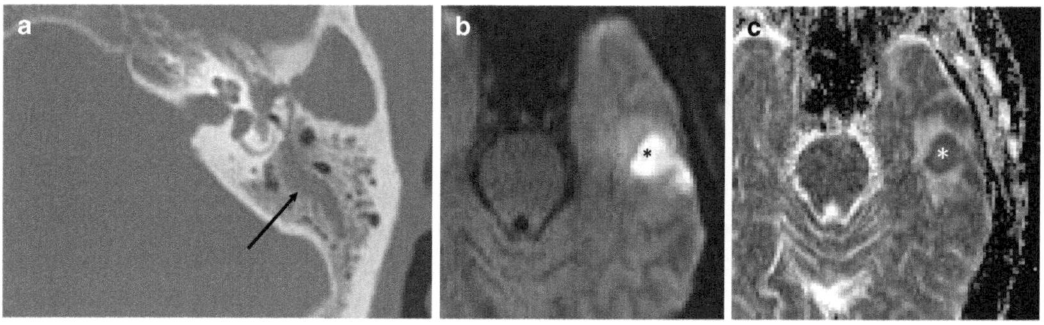


**Fig. 19** (**a**) Axial CT bone window showing a left mastoid effusion (black arrow). (**b**) Axial DWI at a higher level showing elevated signal in the left temporal lobe (black asterisk), which has low signal on the ADC image (**c**, white asterisk), and is compatible with a temporal lobe abscess

petrous apex, placing the nerve at risk in cases of coalescent apical infection (Razek and Huang 2012). The close proximity of the VIth cranial nerve within Dorello's canal beneath the petroclinoid ligament increases the risk of abducens nerve palsy. On plain CT, the air cells within the pneumatised petrous apex will be completely opacified with fluid density material, with or without erosions of the intervening bony septations (Fig. 21) or expansion of the involved air cells. On contrast enhanced MRI, there is abnormal enhancement of the affected petrous bone (Fig. 21). It should be noted that pneumatisation of the petrous apex is asymmetrical in 33% of the population (Razek and Huang 2012). Most cases are managed medically with systemic antibiotics. Surgical drainage may be required occasionally, especially as there is a risk of cavernous sinus thrombosis and meningitis in non-responsive cases (Baert and Sartor 2003, p. 63 & Choi and Park 2014).

## 3.5 Necrotising Otitis Externa

Necrotising otitis externa (NOE) occurs in diabetic or immunocompromised patients or in the geriatric population. Presenting complaints include severe otalgia and periauricular swelling. Underlying external auditory canal infection with Pseudomonas species, Staph Aureus, Aspergillus,

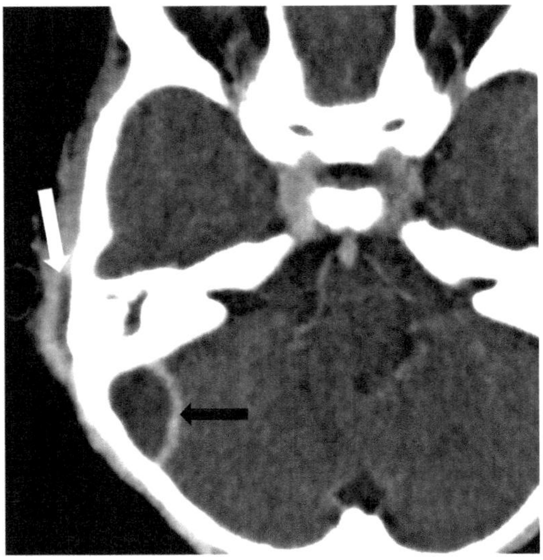

**Fig. 20** Axial CECT shows a rim enhancing subperiosteal abscess in the subcutaneous tissues overlying the right mastoid (thick white arrow). There is thrombosis in the expanded right sigmoid sinus (thick black arrow)

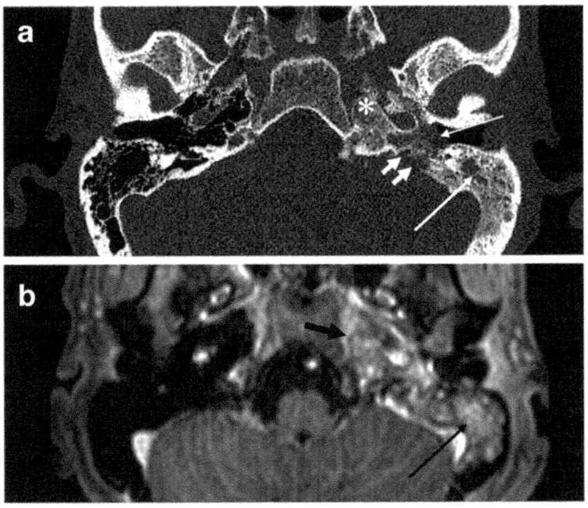


**Fig. 21** Axial CT showing opacification of a pneumatised right petrous apex, with osseus erosions of the posterior cortex (white arrows). The right mastoid and middle ear cleft are also opacified (thin black arrows)

or Proteus, leads to an aggressive osteomyelitis involving the bony external auditory canal, mastoid, and skull base. Inflammatory phlegmon or frank collections beneath the skull base lead to cranial nerve compression and cranial nerve palsies, typically the VIIth and the IXth–XIIth cranial nerves. If the petrous apex is involved, the patient may develop palsies of the Vth and VIth cranial nerves associated with facial pain.

On CT scans of the temporal bones, mucosal thickening is seen along the external auditory canal, which can occlude the canal. This will enhance if post-contrast imaging has been performed. A key feature is the presence of cortical osseous erosions along the bony canal, which can be subtle and may extend to the mastoid tip (Fig. 22). The ipsilateral mastoid air cells and middle ear cleft are invariably opacified (Fig. 22) and there is usually asymmetrical inflammatory soft tissue thickening around the mastoid process, which extends variably beneath the ipsilateral skull base. This inflammation can extend medially to the retropharynx and cause bulging

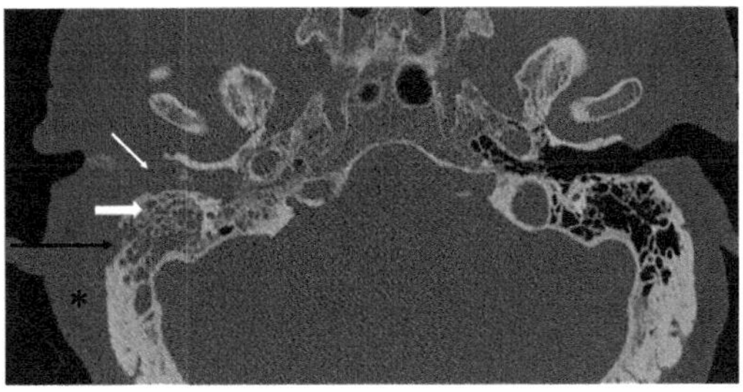

**Fig. 22** Axial CT bone window showing mucosal thickening occluding the right external auditory canal (thin white arrow) and an opacified mastoid (thick white arrow) with cortical erosion (black arrow) and overlying soft tissue swelling (asterisk)

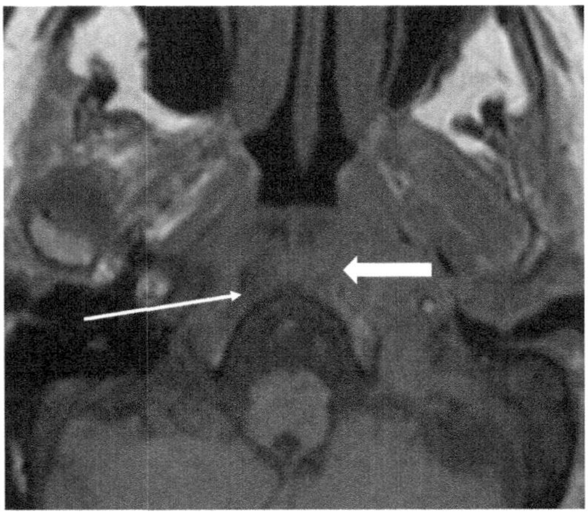

**Fig. 23** Axial T1 weighted MRI showing replacement of the normal high T1 fatty marrow signal in the clivus with low signal material (thin white arrow). The low signal clival cortex is thinned bilaterally (thick white arrow). Central skull base osteomyelitis as a complication of necrotising otitis externa

of the nasopharynx, which can be mistaken for nasopharyngeal pathology clinically.

Complications include central skull base osteomyelitis, which may be seen on CT as erosions of the clivus, hypoglossal canal, and styloid process. In patients with cranial nerve palsies, the skull base foramina should be carefully reviewed. On MRI, involved skull base will show loss of the normal fatty marrow signal (Fig. 23) and will enhance following contrast; fat saturated post-contrast MRI sequences can demonstrate this optimally. The phlegmon identified beneath the skull base tends to display low T1 and T2 weighted signal.

Other complications include vascular thromboses with secondary venous infarction and acute meningitis. This is life-threatening, necessitating swift management with admission, aural toileting, and parenteral anti-pseudomonal antibiotics. Patients may require surgical debridement. Serial imaging is necessary as resolution is protracted.

## 4 Odontogenic Infections and Their Complications

**Periapical Inflammation** There is a wide spectrum of imaging appearances for different acute dental infections, and orthopantomograms (OPG) are most often performed for these in the acute or non-acute setting. MDCT or cone beam CT can also be performed and is particularly useful for surgical planning. Acute periapical infections are extremely common and can form abscesses that appear as focal well-defined lucencies less than 10 mm at the root of a typically carious tooth, with or without surrounding sclerosis (Fig. 24a). These may expand and erode through the adjacent medullary bone and the overlying cortex (Chapman et al. 2013) (Fig. 25a). Widening of the periodontal ligament space, erosion of the lamina dura, and apical tooth resorption may also be present (Caruso et al. 2006, p. 190). Periapical or periodontal infections of the posterior maxil-

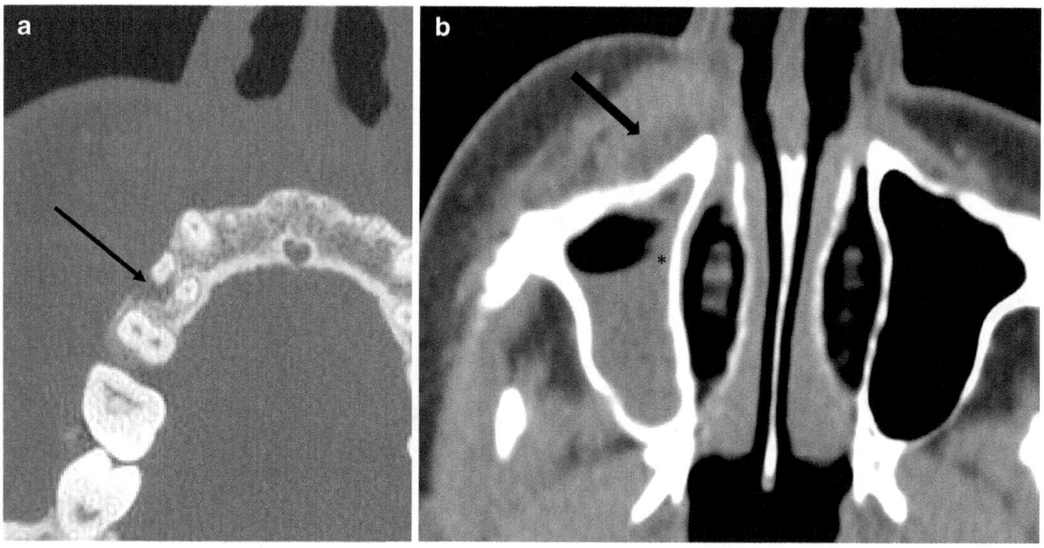


**Fig. 24** (**a**) Axial CT mandible bone window showing periapical lucency surrounding the buccal root of the right upper fourth tooth as well as buccal cortical erosion (black arrow). (**b**) Axial CECT soft tissue window showing a rim enhancing abscess (thick black arrow) and inflammatory thickening in the right premaxillary soft tissues. There is also a reactive right maxillary odontogenic sinusitis (asterisk)

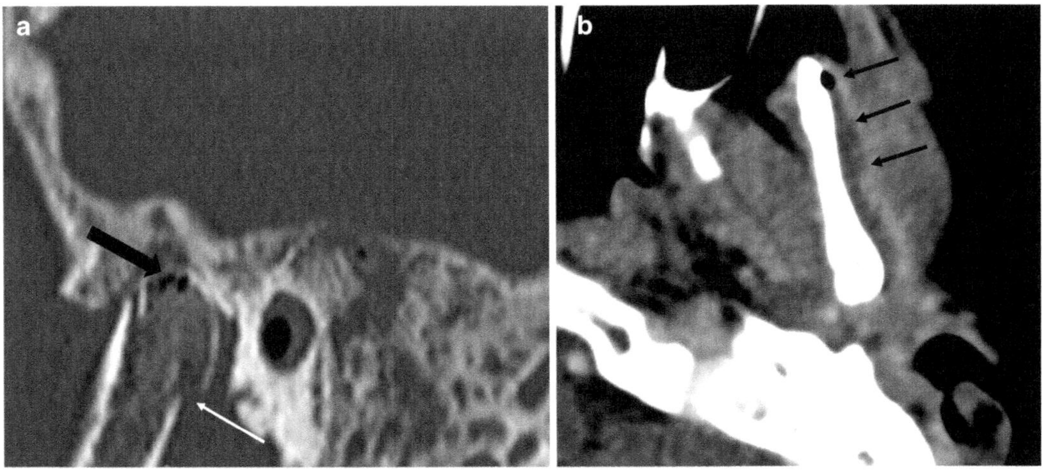


**Fig. 25** (**a**) Sagittal CT bone window showing a left mandibular condyle fracture (white arrow) and gas locules in the medullary cavity (thick black arrow). (**b**) Axial CECT soft tissue window showing a rim enhancing abscess in the masticator space overlying the left mandibular ramus (thin black arrows) reactive right maxillary odontogenic sinusitis (asterisk)

lary teeth can induce reactive mucosal thickening in the overlying maxillary antrum, which can progress to frank sinusitis, termed odontogenic sinusitis. These are responsible for around 10% of all sinusitis episodes, thus careful assessment of the dentition is important in patients with maxillary sinus opacification (Chapman et al. 2013, p. E20). A CECT of the facial bones may be performed to identify specific complications of dental infections, which are discussed subsequently.

### 4.1 Subperiosteal and Palatal Abscesses

Subperiosteal abscesses of the jaws are a frequent complication of odontogenic infections, identified as fluid density, peripherally enhancing collections closely opposed to the alveolar bone cortex (Fig. 26b).

Abscesses arising from the upper incisors or canines may also discharge into the submucosal space along the hard palate. On a coronal CT scan, this can be seen as an eccentric fluid density collection along the hard palate adjacent to the infected tooth socket.

### 4.2 Floor of Mouth and Submandibular Space Infections

Dental abscesses arising from the lower anterior teeth typically discharge into the floor of mouth (FOM) as the first to fifth teeth have roots above the level of mylohyoid muscle (Fig. 27a). By comparison, abscesses arising from the sixth to eighth molar teeth track into the submandibular space or buccal space along the buccal or lingual cortices (Scheinfeld et al. 2012, p. 1941) as the dental roots extend below the level of mylohyoid muscle (Figs. 24c and 28b).

Ludwig's angina is a severe cellulitis of the floor of mouth, which is usually a complication of dental infection, but can be caused by trauma including minor lacerations, tongue piercings, submandibular or sublingual sialadenitis, or parapharyngeal space abscesses. Immunosuppressed patients including diabetics are at greater risk. This infection produces gross floor of mouth, submandibular, and submental swelling, which displaces the tongue superiorly and posteriorly, which in turn compromises the oral and oropharyngeal airway. Prompt imaging by CECT, parenteral antiobiotics, and surgical drainage of any collections

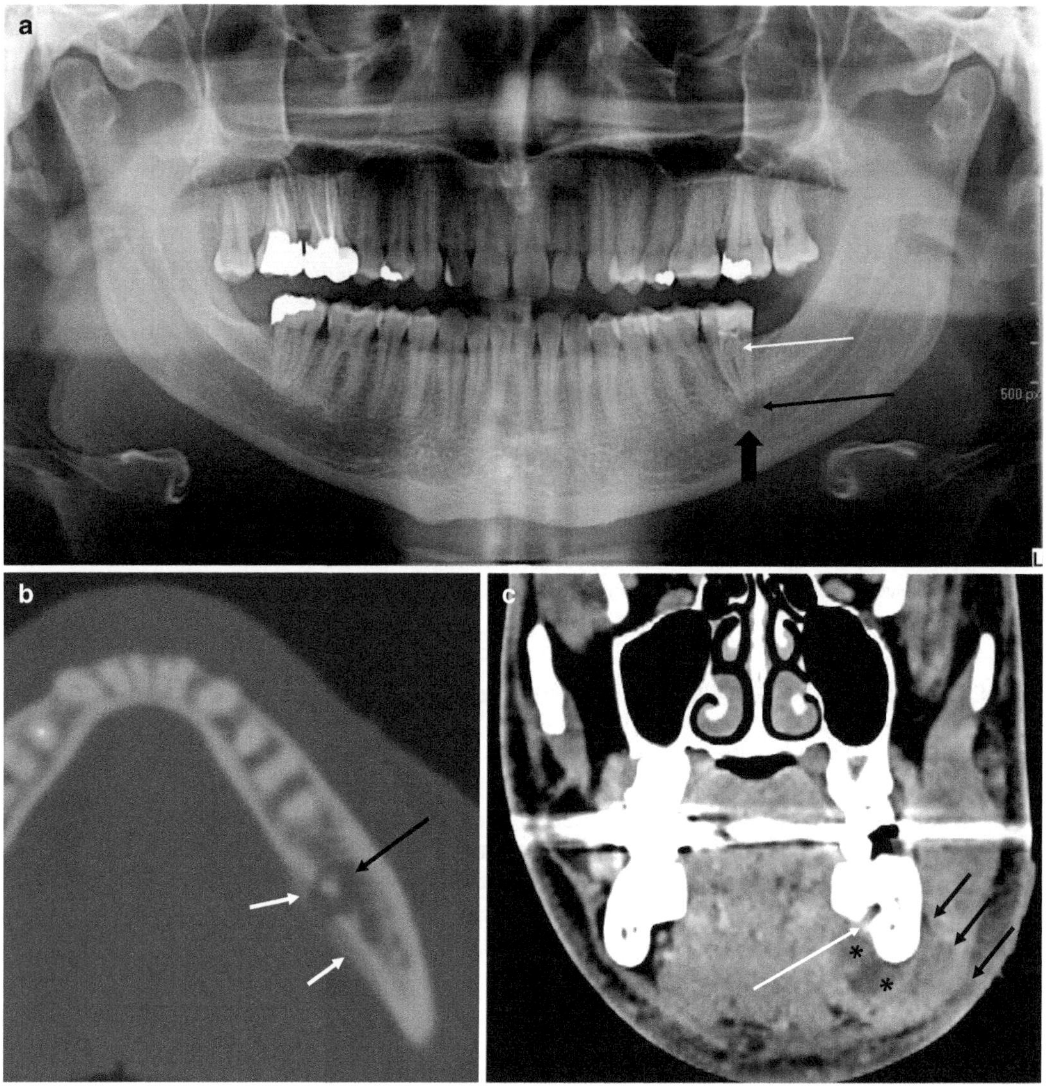


**Fig. 26** (**a**) Orthopantomogram showing a periapical abscess (thin black arrow) bordered by sclerosis (thick black arrow) surrounding the root of the lower left seventh molar tooth (white arrow). (**b**) Axial CT bone window showing periapical lucency surrounding the root of the lower left seventh molar tooth (black arrow). There is overlying periosteal reaction along the buccal cortex (white arrows). (**c**) Coronal CT soft tissue window showing a cortical defect along the lingual cortex of the left mandibular alveolus (white arrow). A fluid density tract extends from the cortical defect which communicates with a floor of mouth gutter and inferior perimandibular collection (asterisk). There is phlegmon, fat stranding, and oedema in the left buccal space (black arrows)

are required (Chapman et al. 2013, p. E22) as mortality is high without timely treatment.

## 4.3 Buccal Space or Masticator Space Infections

Patients with odontogenic infections can develop overlying facial swelling and cellulitis (Fig. 29a), as well as phlegmons and abscesses (Fig. 28b). Infections in the maxilla tend to produce buccal space collections, whereas those along the posterior body of the mandible tend to produce abscesses in the masticator space. These abscesses may partially or completely invest the mandibular ramus, often displacing but occasionally involving the overlying masticator muscles (masseter, pterygoid, and temporalis muscles), causing myositis, which can present clinically as trismus. These abscesses can track superomedially to the

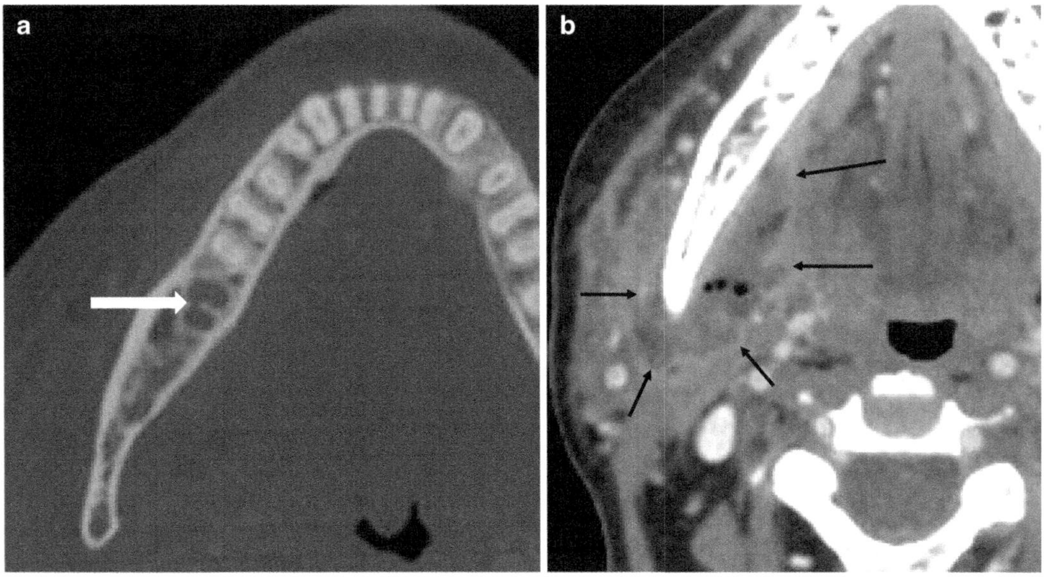


**Fig. 27** (**a**) Axial CT bone window showing alveolar lucency corresponding to the socket of a recently extracted lower right seventh molar tooth (thick white arrow). (**b**) Axial CT soft tissue window showing a rim enhancing masticator space abscess containing locules of gas surrounding the posterior body of the right mandible (thick black arrows)

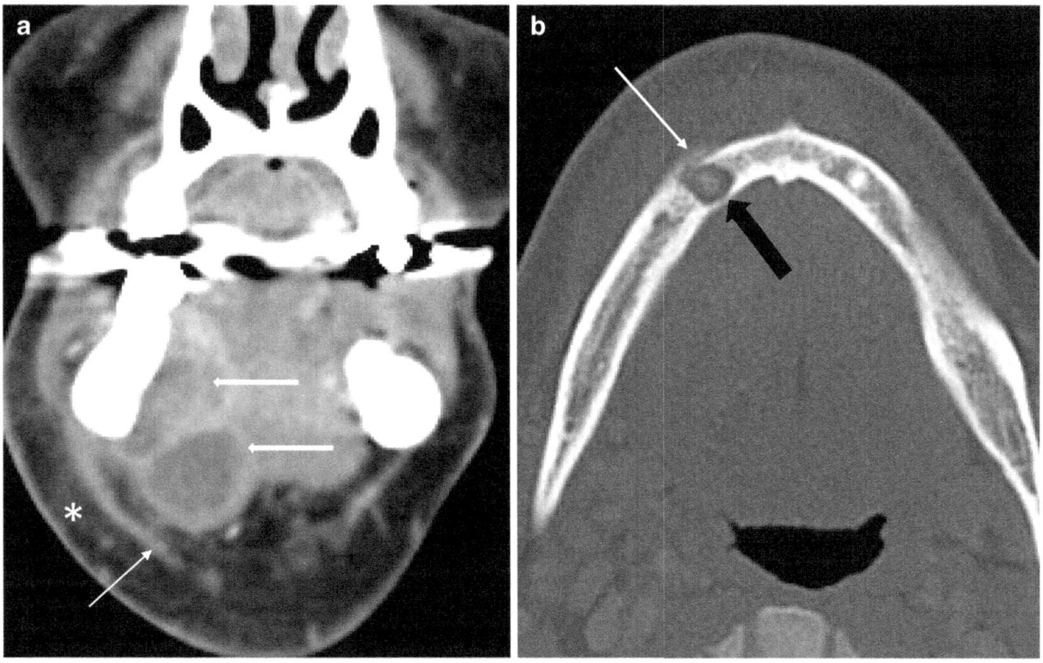


**Fig. 28** (**a**) Coronal CECT soft tissue window showing a rim enhancing abscess in the right floor of mouth (thick white arrow). Overlying thickening of the platysma (thin white arrow) and subcutaneous fat stranding (asterisk). (**b**) Axial CT bone window showing periapical lucency surrounding the root of the lower right second tooth (thick black arrow) with overlying periosteal reaction (thin white arrow)

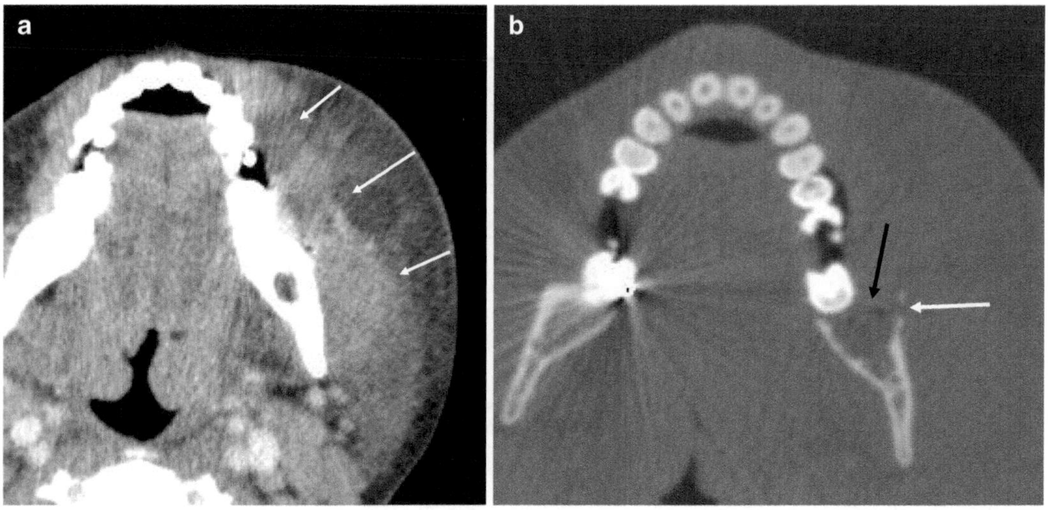


**Fig. 29** (**a**) Axial CECT soft tissue window showing phlegmon, fat stranding and soft tissue swelling overlying the body of the left hemi-mandible (white arrows). (**b**) Axial CT bone window showing medullary lucency in the posterior body and ramus of the left hemi-mandible (black arrow) as well as erosions of the outer cortex (white arrow)

foramen ovale at the skull base, or superolaterally to the temporal fossa (Figs. 26b and 28b).

### 4.4 Osteomyelitis

Maxillary and mandibular osteomyelitis may be classified as acute and suppurative or chronic and non-suppurative. Causes include dental infections and trauma including compound fractures (Fig. 26a). (Cure et al. 2012). Risk factors for osteomyelitis are listed in Table 1. Radiographic features of osteomyelitis are periosteal reaction (Fig. 24b), ill-defined medullary lucency (permeative), and/or sclerosis, endosteal scalloping, and cortical erosions. In the acute setting, gas locules can also be present within the marrow of the affected bone (Fig. 26a). Advanced or chronic infections can develop bony sequestra (bone within bone), sinuses, fistulae, or pathological fractures (Cure et al. 2012, p. 1922).

**Table 1** Risk factors for osteomyelitis of the jaw and known associations (Adapted from Cure 2012)

| Risk Factors | Causes |
|---|---|
| Immunocompromised state | Recent tooth extraction |
| Insulin-dependent diabetes | Maxillary or mandibular fractures |
| Alcoholism | Poor dentition |
| Malnutrition | |
| Sickle cell disease | |
| Collagen vascular disease | |
| Previous radiation treatment | |
| Osteopetrosis/underlying bone dysplasia | |

## 5 Pharyngeal Mucosal Space Infections and Their Complications

### 5.1 Acute Supraglottitis and Epiglottitis

Acute infections of the larynx are common in the extremes of age, namely, the paediatric population and elderly. These can be life-threatening and should be treated as a medical and airway emergency. In children with suspected acute epiglottitis, it may be practical to perform a lateral soft tissue neck radiograph, which has the added benefit of reduced radiation dose. Acute epiglottitis appears as swelling of the normally thin and sharply defined epiglottis. On CT, the epiglottis is diffusely symmetrically swollen and grossly

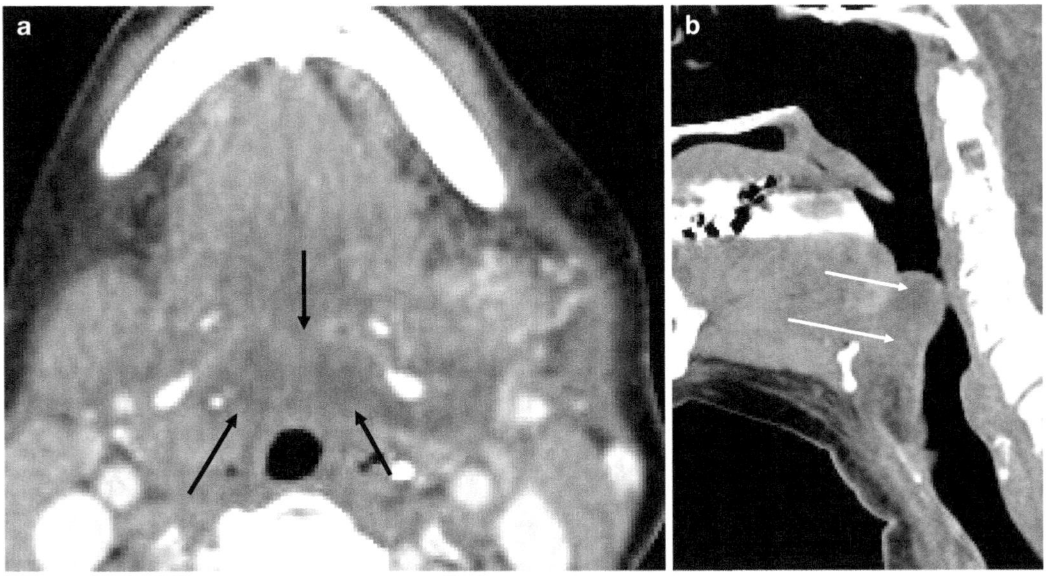


**Fig. 30** (**a** and **b**) Axial and sagittal CECT soft tissue windows showing diffuse swelling of the epiglottis (white arrows) with surrounding phlegmon in the pharyngeal mucosal space (black arrows)

oedematous, which is optimally demonstrated on a sagittal contrast enhanced CT (Fig. 30b). Acute supraglottitis is identified as diffuse swelling and oedema throughout the supraglottic laryngeal structures including the aryepiglottic folds, epiglottis, pharyngoepiglottic folds, and false cords (Fig. 31). Initially, diffuse infection of the mucosa and submucosa can progress to focal abscesses, which may spread to one or more adjacent deep neck spaces in the infrahyoid neck including the carotid, retropharyngeal, visceral, and danger spaces (Fig. 32). These can be extensive and it is vital to document all of the sites of organised collection for adequate surgical drainage.

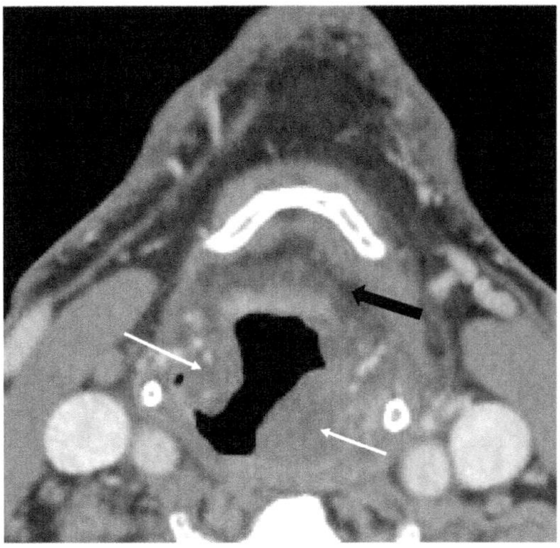

**Fig. 31** Axial CECT neck showing swelling and oedema of the aryepiglottic folds (white arrows) at the level of the supraglottic larynx. There is fat stranding in the pre-epiglottic fat (thick black arrow). No drainable collection is present

## 5.2 Tonsillitis

Tonsillitis is extremely common, resulting in numerous school and work absences per year (Warner et al. 2009). Most acute episodes are viral or bacterial in aetiology, and typical presenting complaints include odynophagia, dysphagia, pyrexia, otalgia, symmetrical tonsillar swelling with erythema, and exudates. Tonsillitis is diagnosed clinically, although imaging is indicated for suspected complications requiring surgical treatment. On CECT, uncomplicated acute tonsillitis appears as bilateral symmetrical tonsillar swelling, hyperenhancement, with non-organised phlegmon or fluid in the tonsillar crypts (Fig. 33). Mild fat stranding may be seen in the adjacent parapharyngeal and retropharyngeal

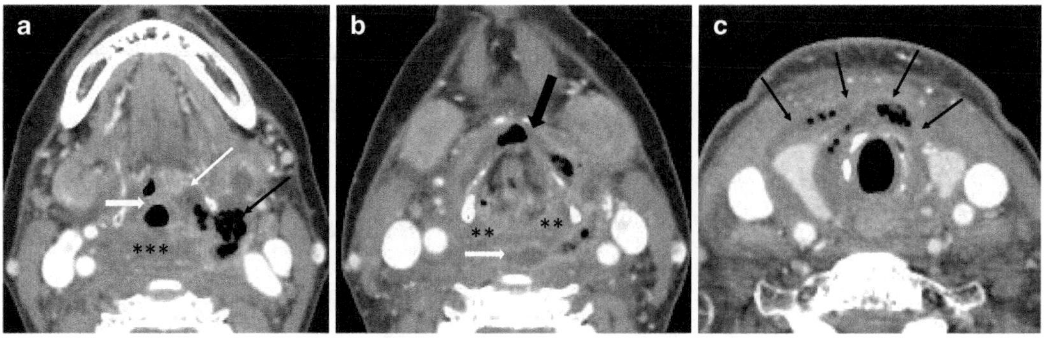


**Fig. 32** CECT neck at different levels. (**a**) Abscess containing fluid and air abscess in the left vallecula (white arrow) extending into the left parapharynx posterolateral to the left hyoid bone (black arrow). Phlegmon in the retropharyngeal space (asterisk). Epiglottic oedema (thick white arrow). (**b**) Rim enhancing retropharyngeal abscess (thick white arrow) with adjacent laryngeal oedema (asterisk). Collection in the anterior visceral space (thick black arrow) overlying the thyroid cartilage. (**c**) Collection in the visceral space anterior to the thyroid (black arrows)

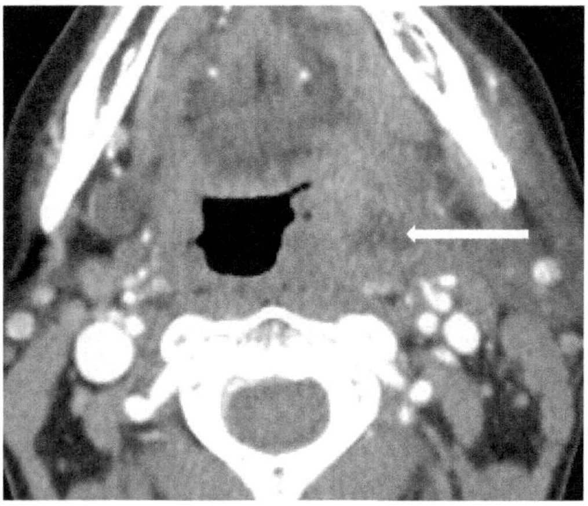

**Fig. 33** Axial CECT showing left tonsillar and peritonsillar swelling with a hypodense non rim enhancing region (phlegmon), which may develop into an abscess

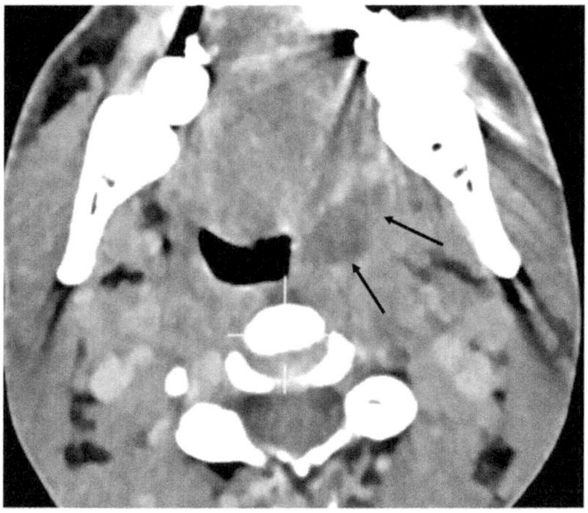

**Fig. 34** Axial CECT showing a rim enhancing left peritonsillar abscess (black arrows). This is confined to the pharynx by the overlying lateral constrictor muscle

spaces. Reactive upper cervical lymphadenopathy is frequently present.

Suppurative complications of tonsillitis include peritonsillar abscesses (quinsy), which is most common, in addition to abscesses in the extrapharyngeal deep neck spaces including the parapharynx and retropharynx/danger space. Diagnostic clues to these complications include spiking pyrexia, severe neck pain, drooling, trismus, and torticollis.

## 5.3 Peritonsillar abscess (Quinsy)

On CECT, a peritonsillar abscess appears as rim enhancing pocket or pockets of fluid (pus) superolateral to the inflamed tonsil and limited laterally by the constrictor muscle (Fig. 34). The affected tonsil may be medialised causing marked oropharyngeal airway narrowing. Treatment of quinsy involves drainage of pus, which can be performed via an intraoral approach.

## 5.4 Deep Neck Space Abscesses

Deep neck space abscesses can present late with large and extensive collections because initial symptoms may be vague and non-localising. They can be rapidly life-threatening due to extrinsic airway compression, laryngospasm, and aspiration following abscess rupture into the pharyngeal mucosal space, as well as inferior extension of danger space abscesses into the thorax causing mediastinitis. They are treated with surgical drainage (per oral or external approach) and with intravenous antibiotics.

Retropharyngeal abscesses may result from pharyngeal mucosal infections including tonsillitis, penetrating trauma including ingested foreign bodies, and suppurative lymphadenitis of retropharyngeal lymph nodes. These appear as a rim enhancing fluid collection anterior to the prevertebral muscles between C1 and C7 levels, with surrounding inflammation, oedema, and variable local mass effect including displacement of the posterior wall of the pharynx anteriorly and carotid spaces laterally (Fig. 35). It is important to differentiate true abscesses in the retropharyngeal space from oedema or phlegmon in this space as the latter does not require drainage. To this end, although oedema and phlegmon can have a low density on CT similar to fluid (due to oedema of the retropharyngeal fat) as well as pronounced mass effect, these do not show rim enhancement. The posterior wall of the retropharyngeal space abuts the danger space, although in clinical practice these spaces are indistinguishable radiologically and may communicate. Importantly, infections in these spaces may extend inferiorly into the middle mediastinum and pleural cavities (Fig. 36).

The parapharyngeal space is an important junctional space between several neck spaces including the pharyngeal mucosal, masticator, parotid, and submandibular spaces. Infections from any of these compartments may spread into the parapharyngeal space, which will appear as

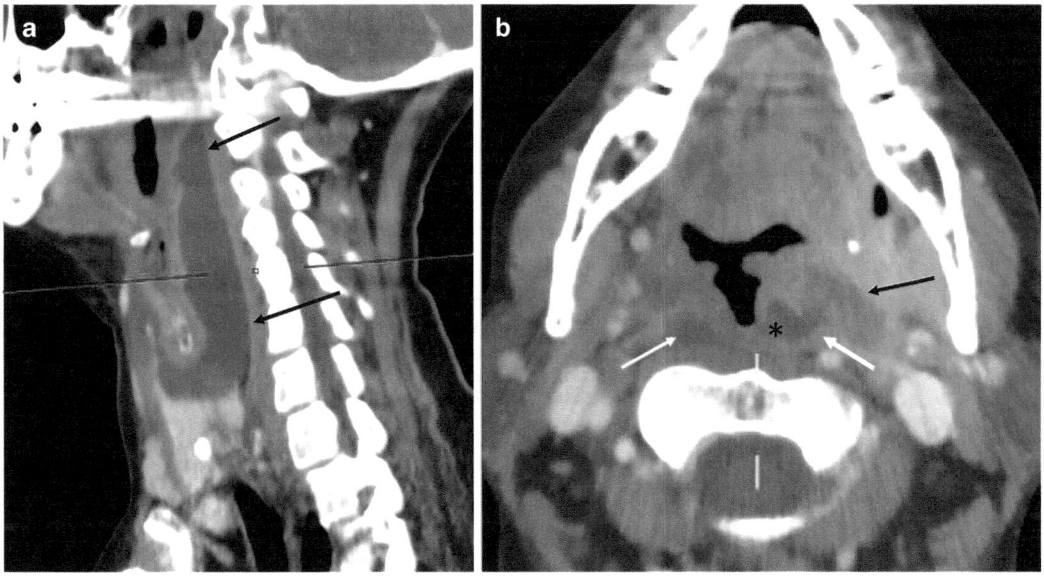


**Fig. 35** (**a**) Sagittal CECT showing a large fluid collection in the retropharyngeal space (black arrows) extending from level of hypopharynx to supraglottic larynx. (**b**) Axial CECT showing an abscess in the left faucial tonsil (asterisk) extending through the lateral constrictor muscle into the parapharyngeal (black arrow) and retropharyngeal spaces (white arrows)

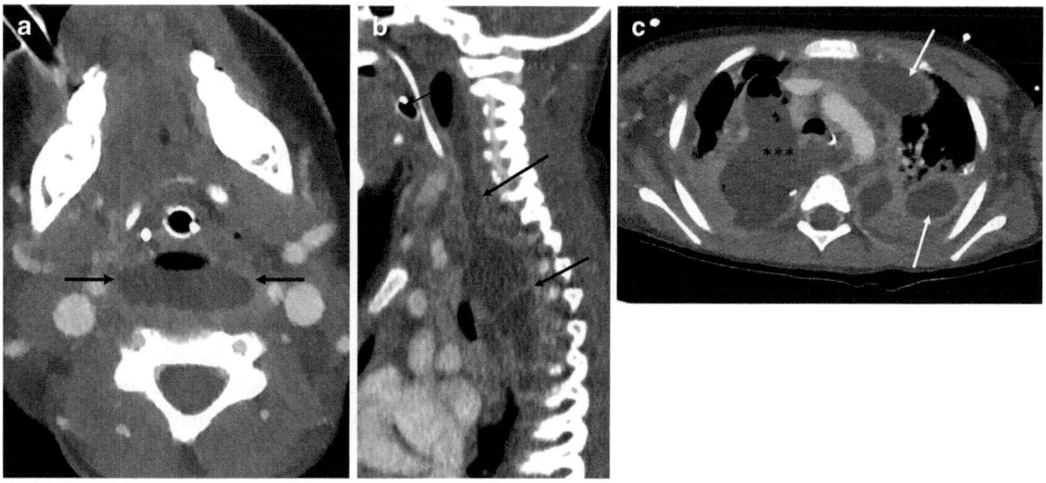


**Fig. 36** (**a**) Axial CECT neck. Endotracheal tube and nasogastric tube are visible in the oropharynx. There is a fluid and gas containing collection in the retropharyngeal/danger space (black arrows). (**b**) Sagittal contrast enhanced CT off midline showing a rim enhancing abscess in the danger space extending from the level of the oropharynx to the mediastinum (black arrows). (**c**) Axial CECT showing multiloculated collections in the mediastinum (asterisks) and pleural spaces (white arrows)

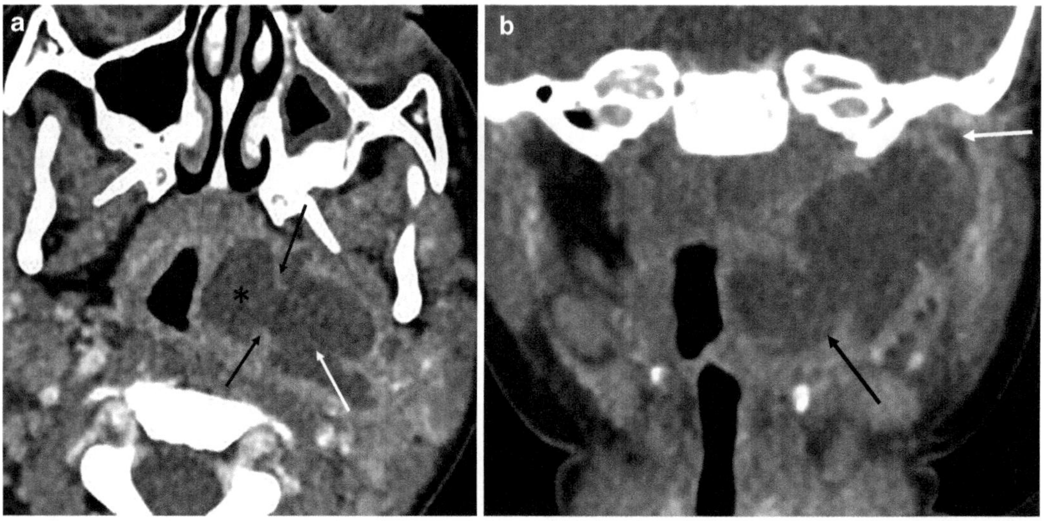


**Fig. 37** (**a**) Axial CECT showing a rim enhancing abscess in the left faucial tonsil (asterisk) extending through the constrictor muscle (black arrows) into the parapharyngeal space (white arrow). (**b**) Coronal CECT showing gross superolateral extension of the abscess from the left oropharynx (black arrow) to just below the left skull base (white arrow)

inflammatory fat stranding or rim enhancing collections replacing the normal fat plane. One of the commonest causes is lateral rupture of a peritonsillar abscess through the overlying constrictor muscle (Figs. 37 and 38). The parapharyngeal space is divided into pre-styloid (parapharyngeal space fat) and post-styloid (carotid space) compartments. Peritonsillar abscesses may also rupture posterolaterally into the carotid space and, from here, infection may spread freely between the skull base and the mediastinum. Carotid space infection may be complicated by internal jugular vein thrombosis, palsies of the IXth, Xth, XIth, XIIth cranial nerves, or the sympathetic plexus including Horner's syndrome.

## 5.5 Internal Jugular Vein Septic Thrombophlebitis (Lemierre's Syndrome)

Septic thrombophlebitis of the internal jugular vein due to anaerobic infection is called Lemierre's syndrome (Chengazi and Bhatt 2019). This is most commonly due to acute pharyngitis, especially acute tonsillitis, and the majority of cases are secondary to Fusobacterium necrophorum, anaerobic streptococci, and methicillin-resistant Staph Aureus (Brook 2003). Patients are typically septic with trismus, neck pain, and may have visible unilateral neck swelling. CECT reveals a rope-like hypodense filling defect within the internal jugular vein (Fig. 39), which is expanded and surrounded by inflammatory changes, as well as oedema within the retropharyngeal space (Chengazi and Bhatt 2019). Septic thromboemboli to distal sites can occur, especially to the lungs, which may be associated with pulmonary symptoms (e.g. haemoptysis, pleuritic chest pain) and should be actively diagnosed by CECT.

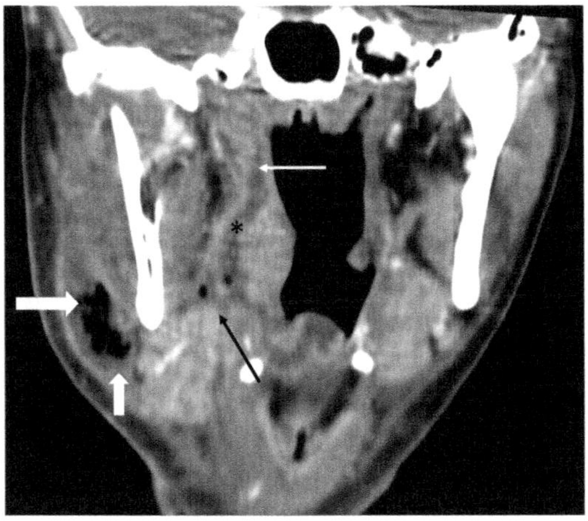

**Fig. 38** Coronal CECT showing an abscess spreading from the right faucial tonsil (white arrow) through the constrictor (asterisk), into the right parapharyngeal space fat (black arrow) and extending inferolaterally into the submandibular region (thick white arrows)

## 5.6 Traumatic Injuries of The Hypopharynx and Cervical Oesophagus

The pharyngeal mucosa can be traumatised by ingested foreign bodies as well as from iatrogenic injury such as gastroscopy-related perforation of a pharyngeal pouch. Foreign bodies typically lodge in the hypopharynx or cervical oesophagus, especially the pyriform fossa or posterior hypopharyngeal wall. These may penetrate or inoculate adjacent neck compartments including the retropharyngeal,

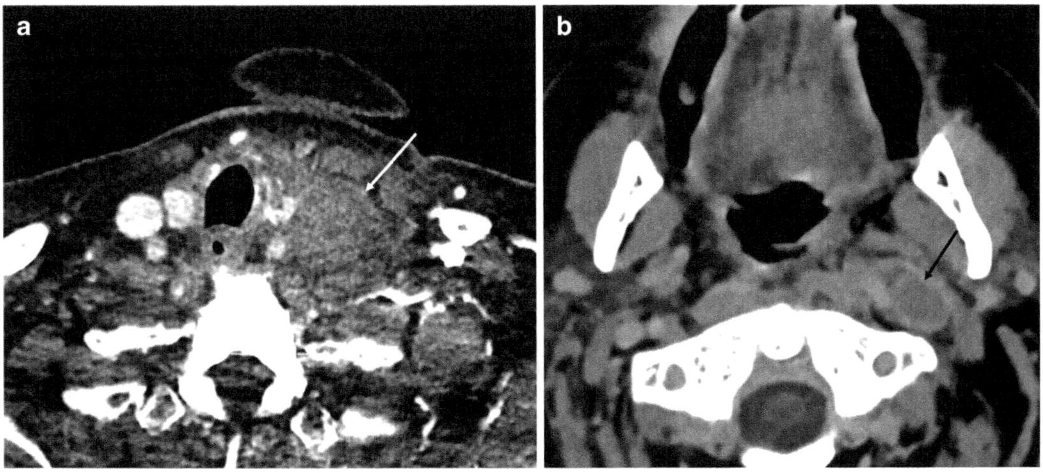


**Fig. 39** (**a**) Axial CECT showing an expanded left internal jugular vein with surrounding fat stranding (white arrow). (**b**) Axial CECT showing a filling defect (thrombus) in the expanded left internal jugular vein

parapharyngeal, and visceral spaces, thus these spaces should be inspected adjacent to any site of abnormal mucosal swelling for the presence of gas locules, oedema, rim enhancing fluid as well as the foreign bodies themselves. Fish bones are identified as curvilinear hyperdense structures and can be easily overlooked without careful inspection including using thick maximum intensity projections (MIP) (Fig. 40). Phlegmon or a frank abscess may be seen adjacent to the foreign body (Fig. 41).

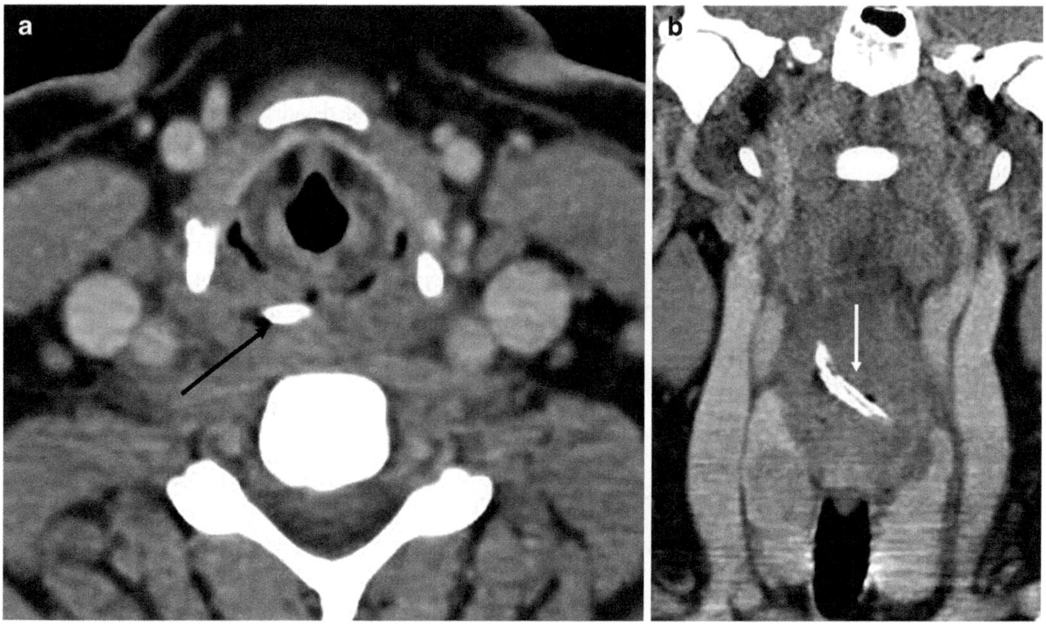


**Fig. 40** (**a**) Axial CECT showing linear hyperdense foreign body protruding through the posterior wall of the hypopharynx (black arrow). (**b**) Coronal reformat reveals a fish bone with surrounding phlegmon (white arrow)

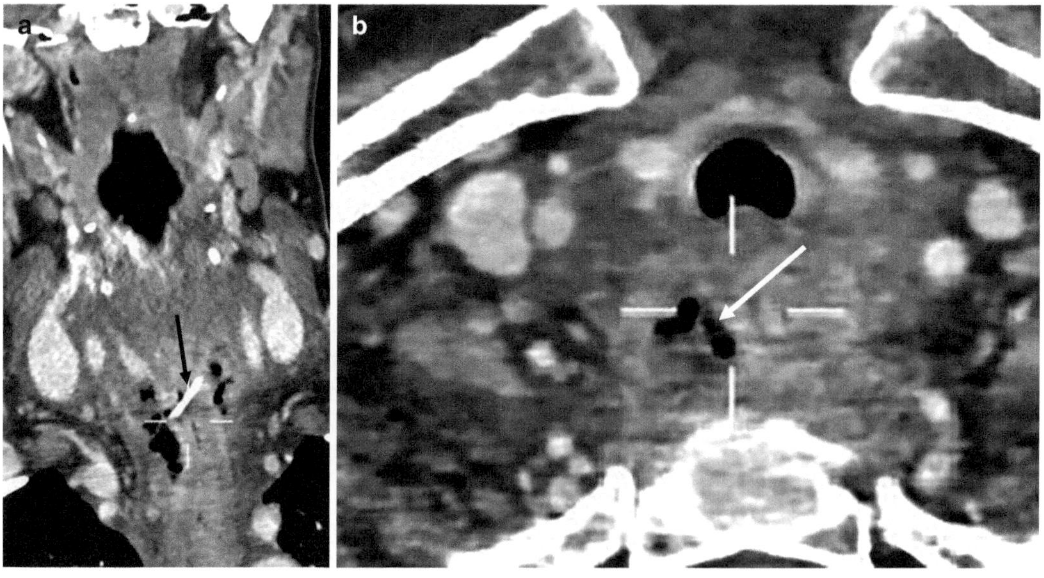


**Fig. 41** (**a** and **b**) Coronal and axial CECT showing a fish bone lodged in the upper cervical oesophagus (black arrow) with an adjacent visceral space collection containing locules of fluid and gas (white arrow)

# 6 Orbital Infections

## 6.1 Periorbital Cellulitis

Periorbital or pre-septal cellulitis involves the pre-septal tissues of the eyelids and is typically secondary to skin abrasions, styes, insect bites, or penetrating trauma Gonzalez and Durairnaj 2010), although may also result from haematogenous spread from other infections including sinusitis. Clinical features include lid and conjunctival oedema and erythema, induration, tenderness, teary eyes, and mild blurring of vision. On CT, diffuse subcutaneous swelling and fat stranding in one or both eyelids are present, which can extend onto the nose, forehead, and cheek (Nguyen et al. 2017) (Fig. 42). Rarely, abscesses can develop within the eyelid itself (Baert and Sartor 2003, p. 144). This condition does not require imaging per se, although CT may be requested if clinical features are equivocal or also suggestive of posterior extension into the orbit, i.e. concomitant orbital cellulitis.

## 6.2 Orbital Cellulitis

Orbital cellulitis affects the post-septal orbital tissues and usually occurs as a secondary infection following an episode of sinusitis or dental infection, but can have other causes including penetrating foreign bodies. Orbital complications of sinusitis have been graded with Chandler's classification (Table 2). In contradistinction to periorbital cellulitis, orbital cellulitis is associated with higher degree of proptosis, restricted eye movements, pain, fever, and impaired visual acuity (Caruso et al. 2006). Pathogens include Streptococcus Milleri, Streptococcus pneumonia, Staphylococcus Aureus, and Streptococcus Pyogenes (Gonzalez and Durairnaj 2010) as well as fungi, which are discussed separately.

Orbital cellulitis warrants urgent admission for parenteral antibiotics as well as imaging by CECT to assess for complications. On CECT, orbital cellulitis initially appears as fat stranding in the intraconal retrobulbar space or extraconal post-septal orbital space (Fig. 43). Intraorbital abscesses are an important complication, which

**Table 2** Chandler's classification system for the orbital complications of sinusitis (Baert and Sartor 2003, p. 144)

| Grade | Findings |
|---|---|
| I | Pre-septal periorbital cellulitis |
| II | Orbital cellulitis without abscess |
| III | Orbital cellulitis with subperiosteal abscess |
| IV | Orbital abscess |
| V | Cavernous sinus thrombosis |

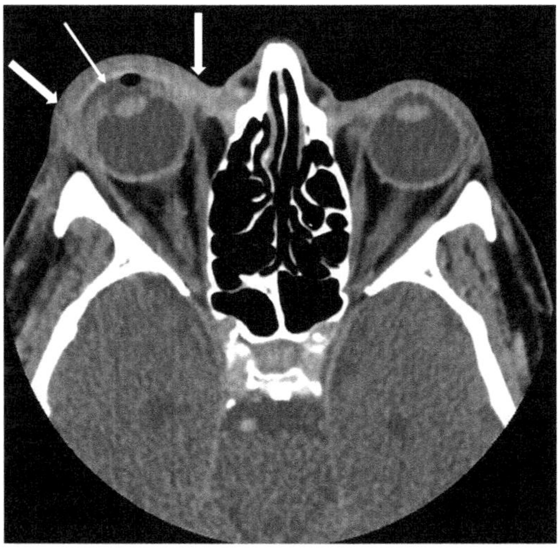

**Fig. 42** Axial CECT showing a enhancing fluid collection (thin white arrow) and pre-septal fat stranding in the right periorbital tissues (thick white arrows)

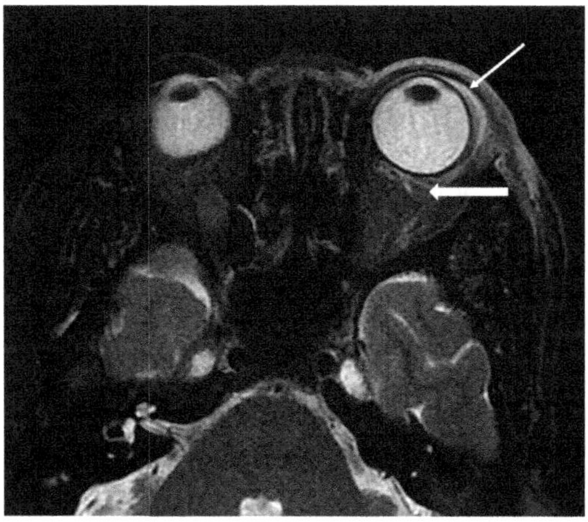

**Fig. 43** Axial fat saturated T2 weighted MRI showing fluid in the pre-septal periorbital tissues (thin white arrow) and fat stranding in the retrobulbar post-septal intraconal space (thick white arrow)

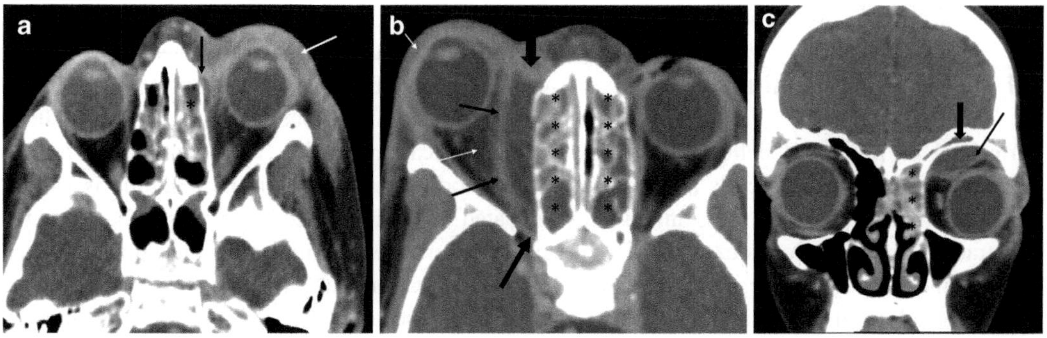


**Fig. 44** Orbital abscess in 3 different patients. (**a**) Axial CECT showing left periorbital inflammatory thickening (white arrow), opacified left ethmoid sinuses (asterisk), and a small overlying subperiosteal orbital abscess (black arrow). (**b**) Axial CECT showing is a large subperiosteal abscess extending the full length of the lamina papyracea (thin black arrows) from the medial canthus region (black arrow head) to the orbital apex (thick black arrow). This produces gross right proptosis as well as pre-septal and post-septal oedema (white arrows). The anterior and posterior ethmoid air cells are opacified bilaterally (asterisks). (**c**) Coronal CECT showing a subperiosteal abscess in the superior extraconal space of the left orbit (thin black arrow). The left globe is displaced inferolaterally. The left frontal sinus (thick black arrow) and anterior ethmoid air cells (asterisks) are opacified

require prompt surgical drainage. Subperiosteal abscesses are the most common type, which, by definition, elevate the periosteum from the bone. These usually appear as a slender rim enhancing fluid collection along the medial, superior, or inferior orbital wall and can be easily missed without intravenous contrast administration (Fig. 44a and c). These initially exert local mass effect on the extra-ocular muscles and intraconal structures, although may progress to frank abscess formation within the orbital tissues, herein termed an orbital abscess.

Infections can extend posteriorly to the relatively confined space of the orbital apex, which may cause cranial neuropathies resulting in ophthalmoplegia, proptosis, and severe visual loss, termed orbital apex syndrome (Fig. 44b). Therefore, the posterior extent of any inflammatory orbital changes should be documented carefully. Orbital cellulitis can cause elevated intraorbital pressure, with resultant vascular compression and ischaemic damage, which is termed orbital compartment syndrome. (Nguyen et al. 2017). Thrombosis of the ophthalmic or retinal artery or vein is uncommon but serious complication of orbital infections. Other ocular complications include corneal disease, retinitis, uveitis, exudative retinal detachment, optic neuropathy, endophthalmitis, and globe rupture (Gonzalez and Durairnaj 2010). Posterior extension of orbital infections may occur, with secondary intracranial complications including acute meningitis and cavernous sinus thrombosis.

## 6.3 Acute Dacryocystitis and Dacroadenitis

Acute infection or inflammation of the lacrimal sac and lacrimal duct is called acute dacryocystitis. The lacrimal sac is located inferior to the medial canthus of the orbit. Symptoms of acute infection include local discharge, epiphora, erythema, and oedema in the region of the medial epicanthus and lacrimal puncta (Asheim and Spickler 2005). The condition occurs in the very young and in older adults. Risk factors include penetrating injury, chronic sinonasal infection, and obstruction of the duct distally as it enters the inferior meatus of the nasal cavity; the latter can be secondary to tumours, dacryoliths (stones), anatomical variation, or strictures (Asheim and Spickler 2005). On CT scans, acute dacryocystitis appears as fat stranding and enhancement in the medial pre-septal periorbital tissues, and fluid may be present in the nasolacrimal duct (Fig. 45).

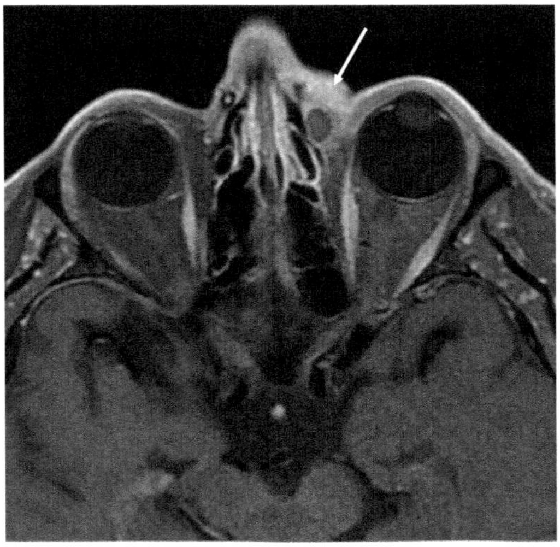

**Fig. 45** Axial fat saturated T1 weighted MRI post contrast revealing a rim enhancing fluid collection with surrounding fat stranding at the medial canthus of the left orbit (white arrow) along the upper border of the left lacrimal duct. The sinuses are largely clear

Acute dacryocystitis is treated with antibiotics to avoid abscess formation. If symptoms fail to improve, dacryocystorhinostomy may be required (Asheim and Spickler 2005). Complications of untreated infection may be identified on CECT including abscess, orbital cellulitits, periorbital cellulitis, and dacryocutaneous fistula formation.

Acute dacroadenitis is an infective or inflammatory disease of the lacrimal gland, which is most common in children and young adults. The lacrimal glands are positioned in the lateral and superior extraconal space of the orbit. Infections are usually unilateral and respond well to treatment with antibiotics (Jung et al. 2007, p. 339). On a CECT scan, involved lacrimal glands appear swollen with surrounding fat stranding in the lateral pre-septal and post-septal orbital tissues.

## 7 Acute Salivary Gland Infections

Most cases of acute infective sialadenitis of the major salivary glands are viral in aetiology, especially in children, and tend to be bilateral and self-limiting. Bacterial infection is less common, typically unilateral, and may be due to ductal obstruction by stones, strictures, or rarely by obstructing tumours. However, a large proportion of cases occur in otherwise normal salivary glands as a result of retrograde spread of microorganisms along the salivary ducts from the oral cavity, and this is more common in debilitated patients. Ultrasound or CECT may be performed initially, depending on local resources and expertise. On imaging, the affected gland is enlarged and oedematous with increased parenchymal vascularity (US) and post-contrast enhancement (CECT) (Fig. 46). Peri-glandular inflammatory changes including subcutaneous oedema and reactive lymphadenopathy are variably present. Apart from confirming the diagnosis, imaging should identify any underlying obstructive causes (Fig. 47) and acute complications including abscesses (Fig. 48) and severe cellulitis (e.g. Ludwig's angina).

## 8 Infected Congenital Cysts

Various developmental cysts in the head and neck can present acutely in children and adults as a result of infection. Other developmental anomalies such as lymphatic malformations can also become secondarily infected. With appropriate expertise, ultrasound can diagnose the majority of these and allows guided aspiration of any pus within them. In the acute setting, however, CECT may be required due to diagnostic uncertainty including concerns regarding a deep neck space collection. Branchial cysts are classified according to their embryological origin and may also have tracts extending to the skin and/or pharynx as sinuses or fistulae (Table 3). Approximately, 95% of those identified in clinical practice arise from the second branchial cleft (Harnsberger 1995). An infected branchial cyst may be diagnosed on the basis of its location (Table 3), patient age (typically children to young adults under 30 years of age), and imaging appearances. On CECT, the cyst is typically solitary and unilocular with smooth mural thickening, surrounding fat stranding and enhancement as well as adjacent

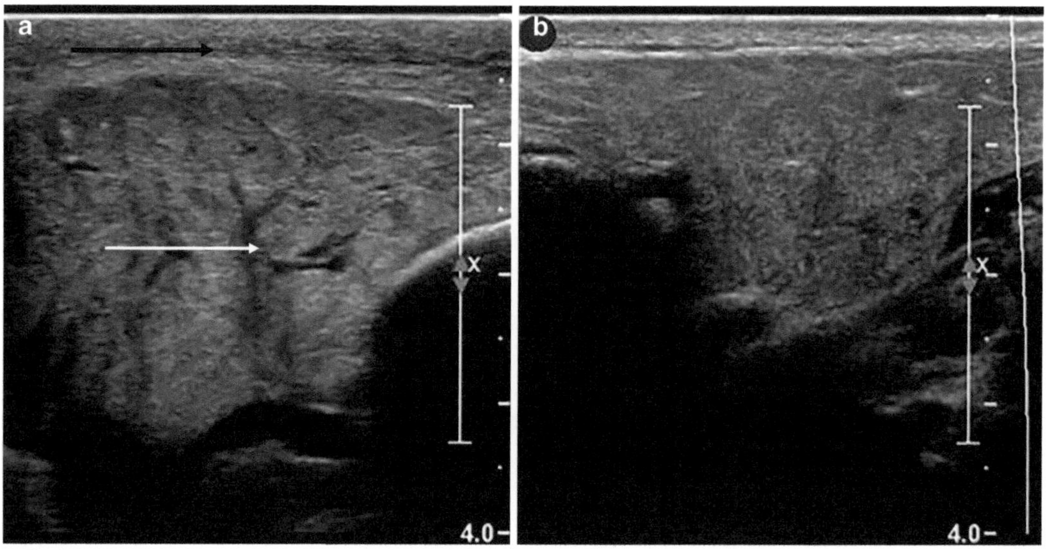


**Fig. 46** Transverse gray scale US of both parotid glands. The right parotid (**a**) is diffusely enlarged, oedematous with intraglandular duct prominence (white arrow). There is overlying subcutaneous oedema (black arrow). The left parotid (**b**) in comparison is normal

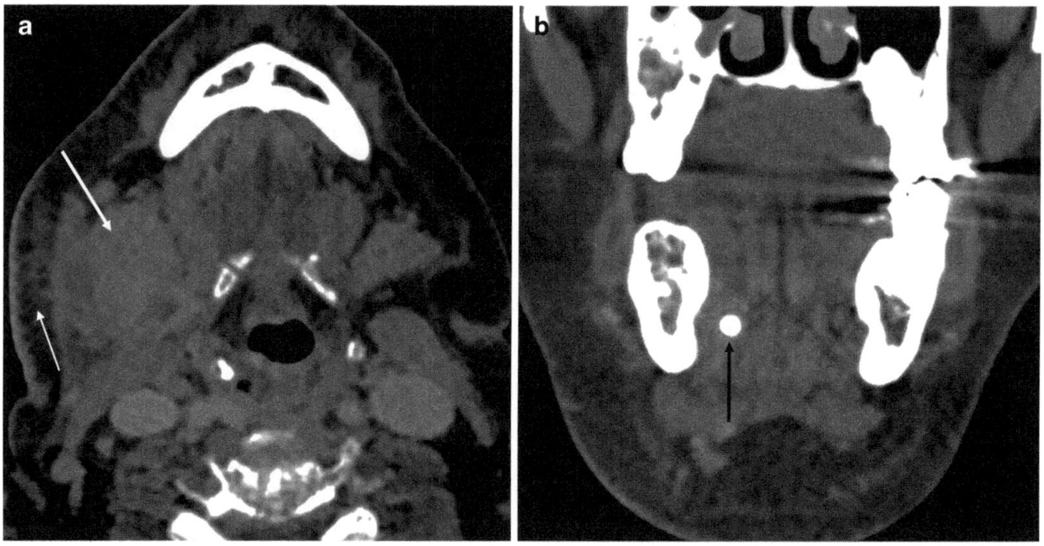


**Fig. 47** (**a**) Axial CECT showing a swollen right submandibular gland (white arrow) with associated fat stranding and phlegmon (thin white arrow). (**b**) Coronal CT showing a radiopaque calculus in the distal right submandibular duct (black arrow)

reactive lymphadenopathy (Fig. 49). In patients with a history suggestive of recurrent infections of a branchial cleft cyst, there is an increased probability of a patent communication with the pharynx, the location of which depends on the brachial cleft cyst type. Similarly, thyroid or perithyroid abscesses, which are rare in the general population, should prompt investigations to identify an underlying fourth BCC anomaly (Fig. 50).

It is worth highlighting that a cystic necrotic metastatic cervical lymph node, which is common in squamous cell carcinoma, can mimic a second or third branchial cyst on imaging, especially if complicated by superadded infection because mural thickening caused by inflammation can mask a thickened wall caused by tumour. Consequently, in adults with suspected infected second or third branchial cysts, follow-up imaging as well as fine needle or core needle biopsy of the wall is recommended to prevent potentially catastrophic misdiagnosis.

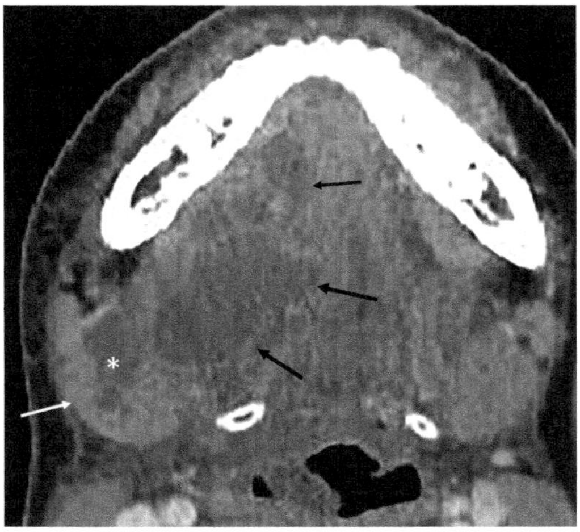

**Fig. 48** Axial CECT showing enlargement of the right submandibular gland (white arrow) with gross dilatation of the intraglandular ducts (asterisk). There is a rim enhancing abscess in the right submandibular region extending into the right floor of mouth (black arrows)

Other developmental cysts that can present acutely due to infection include dermoid cysts (often present in the midline submental or floor of mouth region) (Harnsberger 1995; Baert and Sartor 2003, p. 188), epidermoid cysts (often off-midline, typically in the sublingual space) (Sabhalok et al. 2016) (Fig. 51), and thyroglossal duct cysts. Thyroglossal duct cysts represent 70% of all congenital neck cysts and occur along the course of the embyrological tract of the thyroid gland in the midline anterior visceral space (Koeller et al. 1999). These frequently become acutely infected, causing acute swelling, pain, and tenderness in the anterior midline neck in close proximity to the hyoid bone. On US or cross-sectional imaging, thyroglossal duct cysts appear as rim enhancing, thin-walled cysts with or without internal septations. During acute infective episodes, the cyst wall becomes uniformly thickened and inflamed, the cyst contents are turbid due to inflammatory exudate, and there is a variable degree of adjacent inflammatory change.

## 9 Tuberculosis in The Head and Neck Region (Scrofula)

Tuberculosis caused by the pathogen mycobacterium tuberculosis (TB) is a global epidemic in populated areas in the developed and developing

**Table 3** Subtypes of branchial cleft cysts and their typical locations (Adapted from Bagchi et al. 2018: 599–613)

| | |
|---|---|
| **First branchial cleft cyst** | |
| Type I | Pre-auricular cyst or sinus tract adjacent to the pinna |
| Type II | Periauricular or intraparotid cyst adjacent to the facial nerve. May occur in parapharyngeal space. |
| **Second branchial cleft cyst (Bailey classification)** | |
| Type I | Deep to platysma and anterior to the sternocleidomastoid muscle (Fig. 51) |
| Type II | Lateral to the carotid sheath, anterior to the sternocleidomastoid muscle, and posterior to the submandibular gland. |
| Type III | Between the internal carotid artery and external carotid artery. May extend superiorly to the skull base. |
| Type IV | Abutting the pharyngeal wall, medial to the carotid sheath. |
| **Third branchial cleft cyst** | If in the upper neck, sited in the posterior cervical space. If in the lower neck, sited along anterior border of the sternocleidomastoid muscle. |
| **Fourth branchial cleft cyst** | Anteromedial neck mass in the lower visceral space<br>Fistula connects the pyriform sinus to the thyroid gland. Can cause episodes of suppurative thyroiditis (Fig. 50) |

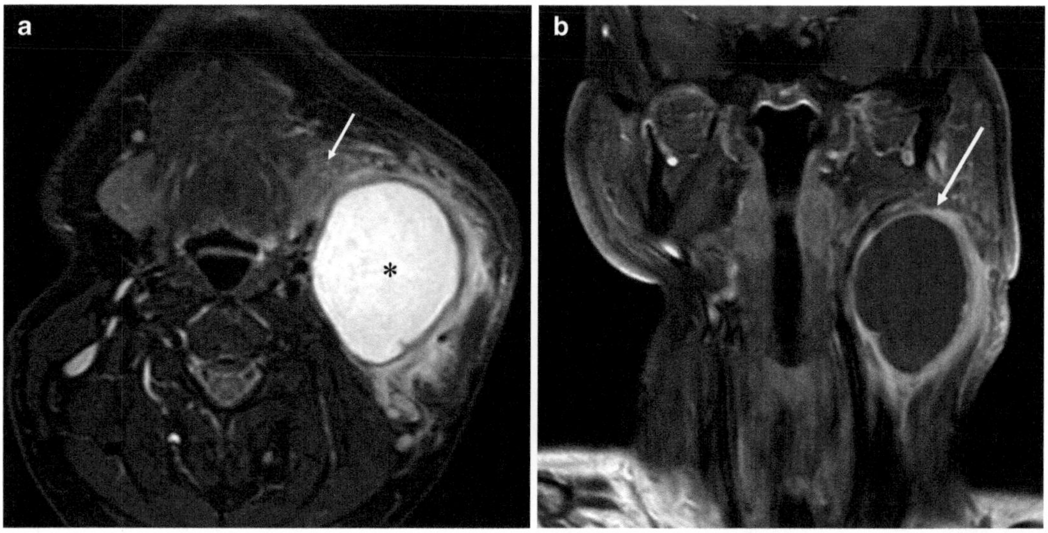


**Fig. 49** (**a**) Axial fat saturated T2 weighted MRI revealing a smooth thin-walled cyst (asterisk) in the left upper cervical region (level IIA) with surrounding fat stranding. The left submandibular gland is displaced anteriorly (white arrow). (**b**) Coronal T1 weighted fat saturated T1 weighted MRI post contrast shows enhancement of the cyst wall (white arrow)

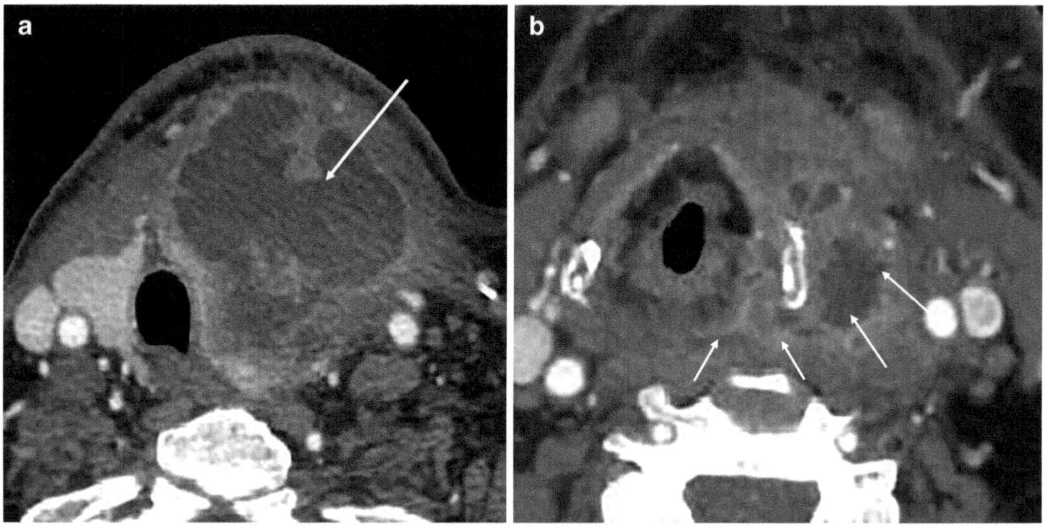


**Fig. 50** Infection of a left fourth branchial cleft anomaly (sinus) (**a**) Axial CECT demonstrating a rim enhancing abscess in the visceral space involving the left thyroid gland and tissues beyond (white arrow). (**b**) Axial CT at the level of the pyriform fossa of the hypopharynx shows a thin rim enhancing tract extending from the left pyriform fossa which communicated with the left neck collection (see white arrows)

world. Approximately ten million people were infected by TB globally in 2018 (WHO 2019). This gram-negative bacillus can infect any part of the body, although the neck is one of the most common sites. In the head and neck region, patients may present with a neck swelling secondary to lymphadenopathy or an abscess, especially in the posterior triangle or supraclavicular fossa. These masses often develop insidiously with minimal systemic or septic features, which has led to the term "cold abscess" for suppurative TB infections in the neck.

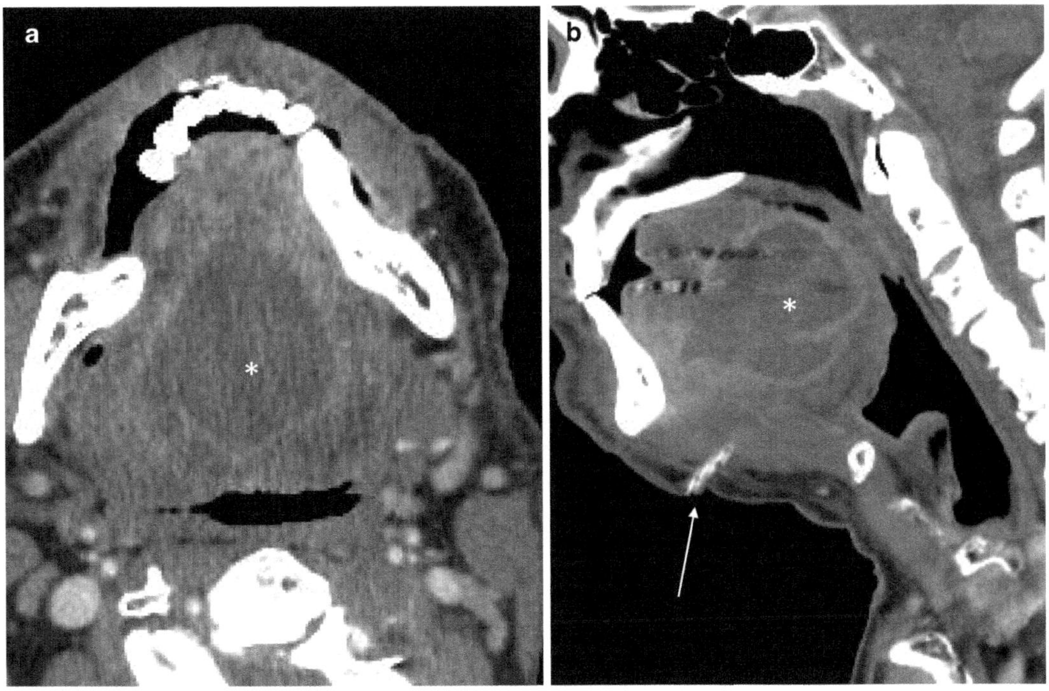


**Fig. 51** Axial (**a**) and sagittal (**b**) CECT showing a rim enhancing cystic mass in the root of the tongue (asterisk) with perilesional inflammatory changes and causing local mass effect. A corrugated drain has been inserted into it percutaneously (white arrow). Appearances were considered to be due to an abscess or infected epidermoid cyst. Pus was aspirated. The mass was subsequently excised, which confirmed an epidermoid cyst

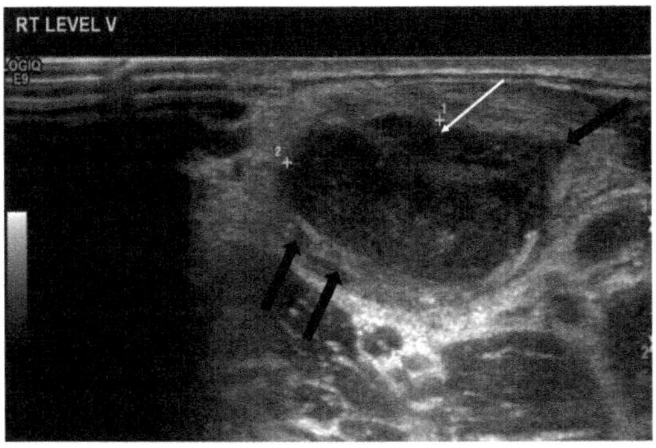


**Fig. 52** Grey scale US of the right supraclavicular fossa showing an enlarged hypoechoic lymph node (white arrow) lacking normal internal architecture with foci of surrounding perinodal oedema (black arrows)

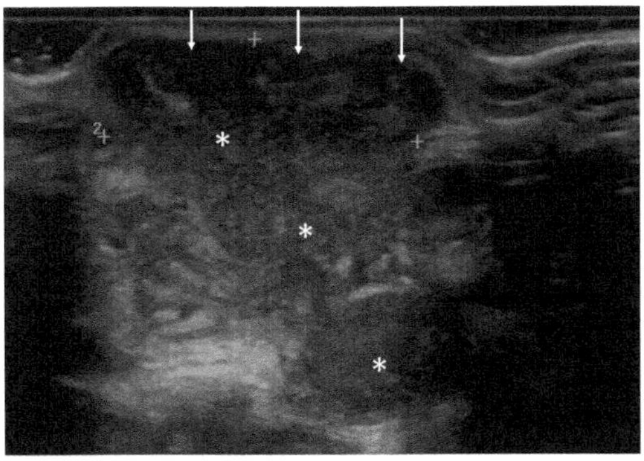

**Fig. 53** Grey scale US of the right supraclavicular fossa showing an irregular abscess (asterisk) which tracks anteriorly to just beneath the dermis (white arrows). There was minimal tenderness and no systemic features of sepsis. This is characteristic of a cold abscess from suppurative tuberculous lymphadenitis

US is widely used as the first line imaging test as it allows characterisation and image guided aspiration of pus for culture and sensitivity. On US, tuberculous nodes are enlarged, hypoechoic, and frequently display focal parenchymal abnormalities due to caseous or liquefactive necrosis. Peri-adenitis is common, resulting in nodal matting (Fig. 52). Necrotic nodes frequently coalesce and suppurate into the surrounding tissues, resulting in large irregular shaped abscesses (Fig. 53), which may even fistulate to the skin. Tuberculous abscesses may also arise in other sites including

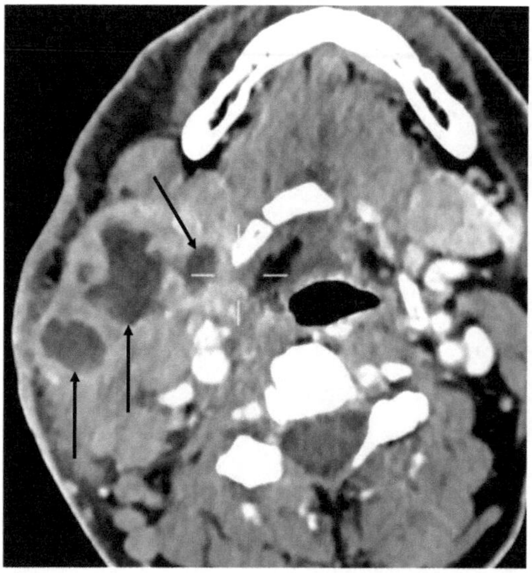

**Fig. 54** Axial CECT showing a multiloculated rim enhancing collection in the right parotid tail (black arrows)

the salivary glands, pharyngeal mucosal space, and in any deep neck space (Fig. 54).

## 10 Traumatic Infections

Traumatic head and neck infections occur in the setting of compound facial bone fractures, following penetrating assault (e.g. knives, broken glass bottles, gunshot) as well as penetrating accidents (e.g. pencils, pens, occupational, or domestic implements) (Abdelmasih et al. 2019). Patients who survive the injury and are adequately treated initially may still develop infected collections due to significant non-sterile inoculation (Fig. 55). It is important to detail the full extent of any injury on imaging as this may not be evident clinically and may require early surgical exploration and decontamination. CECT is useful for showing the extent of penetrating

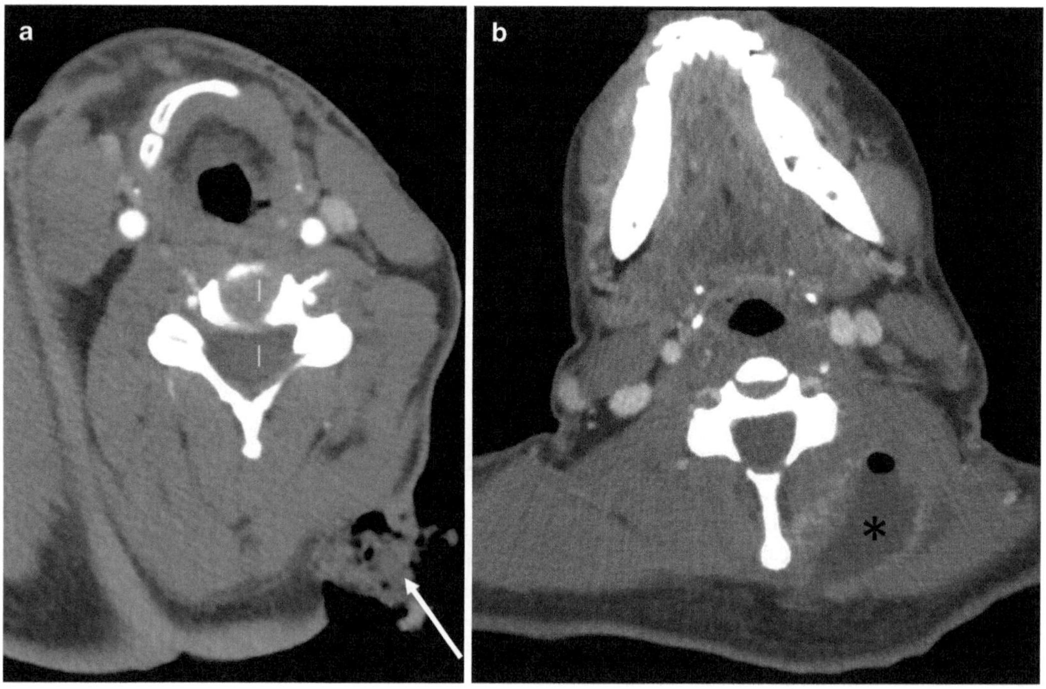


**Fig. 55** (**a**) Axial CECT performed shortly following an assault (stabbing) showing a large skin and subcutaneous defect in left posterior neck (white arrow). (**b**) Follow-up CECT 1 week later, which was performed due to localised tenderness and erythema, shows a rim enhancing air and fluid containing collection in the left posterior paravertebral muscles along the previous knife tract (asterisk)

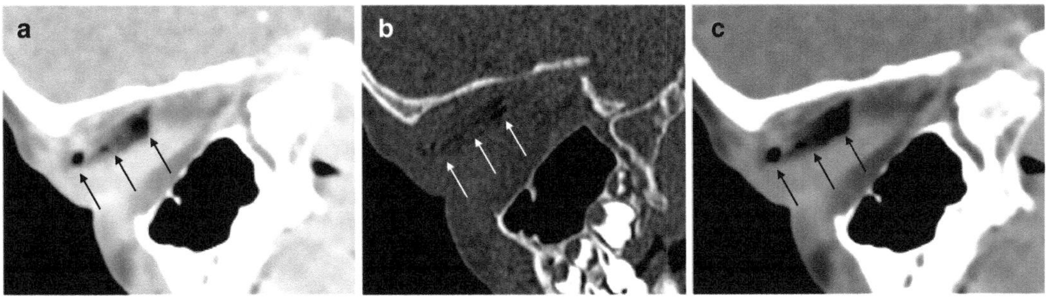


**Fig. 56** (a) Sagittal CT of the left orbit on lung window (a), bone window (b) and soft tissue window (c) settings. A geometric air containing foreign body (wood tree branch fragment) (black arrows) is lodged in the orbital fat. The fragment is inconspicuous on the bone window (white arrows), resembling surgical emphysema, whereas its shape and different density can be appreciated on the lung and soft tissue windows (black arrows)

injuries, and a portal venous phase study is especially useful to outline any haematomas and organised collections. Retained foreign bodies, particularly wood fragments and other organic material, are problematic as they are highly contaminated and act as a nidus for infection. Wood fragments are of predominantly air density and geometric in shape, which can be easily missed or mistaken for surgical emphysema if CT scans are not examined on different window settings (Fig. 56). as well as in different imaging planes. The Hounsfield unit (HU) of glass varies depending on its composition. Metal is hyperdense (>1500 HU) and associated with beam hardening artefact. Plastic is of variable density and is less irritant than organic material, thus is less likely to cause an inflammatory reaction. In bomb blast injuries, fragments of in-driven autologous or allogenic human tissue can cause infection (Offiah and Hall 2012, p. 419).

In patients with penetrating trauma, it is also important to assess the aerodigestive tract meticulously for perforating injuries, as these may be subtle or not visible directly as the lacerated mucosa may be transiently opposed, i.e. appear to be intact. The presence of tiny locules of fluid or gas in the retropharynx and parapharynx adjacent to the pharynx or oesophagus is important diagnostic clue. Initially, unrecognised perforations may result in further contamination by ingested food, resulting in severe infective complications including septicaemia, descending retropharyngitis, and mediastinitis (Offiah and Hall 2012, p. 425). Iatrogenic perforations during oesophagoduodenoscopy or intubation are also important causes.

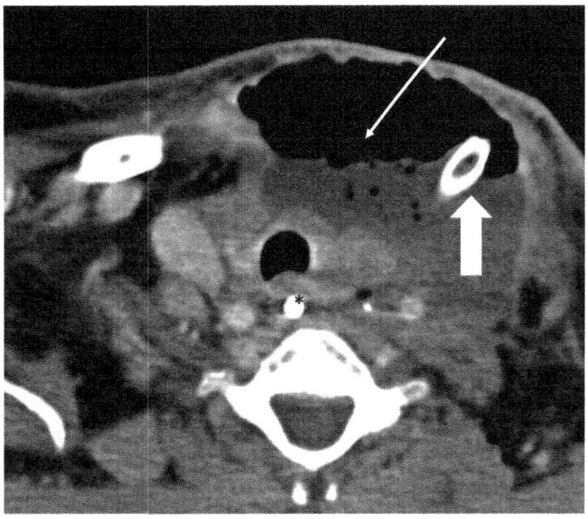

**Fig. 57** Axial CECT of the neck performed 1-week after a left partial thyroid lobectomy. There is an air and fluid density collection in the partial thyroidectomy bed (thin white arrow). A surgical drain is seen within the collection (thick white arrow). A nasogastric tube is present in the oesophagus (asterisk)

## 11 Post-Operative Infections

Imaging is often requested to exclude post-operative infective complications in head and neck surgical patients (Fig. 57). Surgical wound infections have been reported in 10–41% of head

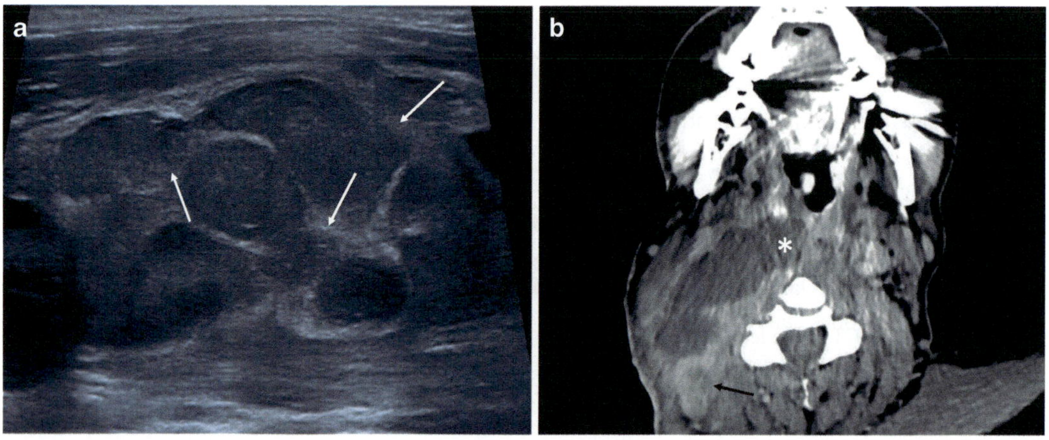


**Fig. 58** Coronal T2 weighted MRI in infective non suppurative cervical lymphadenitis (**a**) Multiple solid enlarged lymph nodes in the right anterior and posterior triangles with surrounding inflammation (white arrows). (**b**) Gray scale US demonstrating a cluster of matted, enlarged, rounded, and hypoechoic lymph nodes

and neck surgical patients, and risk factors include chemotherapy, immunosuppression, and recent prior admission to hospital (Lin et al. 2017; Ogihara et al. 2009; Penel et al. 2001). Depending on location, US or CECT can be performed. In assessing post-operative imaging, it is important to review operative notes including use of absorbable and non-absorbable packing materials, have an understanding of expected post-operative appearances as well as the spectrum of post-operative infections that may occur (e.g. abscesses, meningitis). Documenting post-operative seromas and haematomas is important as these may become secondarily infected. In addition, accidentally retained packing material such as nasal packs can cause delayed complications including toxic shock syndrome.

## 12 Acute Suppurative Lymphadenitis

Bacterial infections involving cervical lymph nodes are usually due to local infections in the head and neck. Nodes can undergo necrosis and liquefaction, termed suppurative lymphadenitis, which is more common in children. The presence of a persistent or enlarging erythematous unilateral neck mass following a recent acute pharyngitis is a common presentation, and upper cervical nodes in levels IB and II are most commonly involved. Imaging plays an important role in differentiating reactive lymphadenopathy from suppurative lymphadenitis, especially as the latter usually requires aspiration of pus or surgical drainage. Initially, non-suppurative nodes appear on US as one or more adjacent, enlarged, rounded hypoechoic nodes with increased hilar vascularity, and the perinodal fat/fascia may be inhomogeneous due to inflammation (Fig. 58). The presence of anechoic avascular parenchymal areas within a node indicates intranodal abscess. Suppurative nodes can become matted and may rupture to produce extranodal deep space collections. CECT or MRI is indicated to evaluate complex nodal masses or collections.

## 13 Other Acute Infections

### 13.1 Infections of Primary Head and Neck Tumours or Nodal Metastases

Some head and neck tumours have a tendency to become secondarily infected and/or masquerade as an acute infection both clinically and on imaging. Notable examples include squamous cell carcinomas (SCCs) of the upper aerodigestive tract such as tonsillar carcinomas mimicking acute tonsillitis, and infected Warthin tumours of the parotid glands mimicking parotid abscesses or infected sialoceles. Cystic or necrotic nodes are particularly common in head and neck cancers including SCC, papillary thyroid carcinoma, nasopharyngeal carcinoma, and high-grade nodal lymphomas (e.g. diffuse large B cell lymphoma). These metastatic nodes can resemble acute suppurative lymphadenitis on imaging, or an infected congenital cyst if solitary. Unfortunately, fine needle biopsies performed on these during an acute infective episode can be misleading in terms of showing acute inflammatory changes only. To avoid misdiagnosis, a high index of suspicion as well as careful clinical and imaging follow-up is required. Repeat FNA or a core needle biopsy of any residual abnormalities should also be considered to diagnose or exclude the presence of tumour.

## 13.2 Facial Cellulitis and Necrotising Fasciitis

Acute facial infections including those arising from skin appendages (e.g. folliculitis) are common, usually minor, self-limiting, and seldom require imaging. Occasionally, more extensive infections may occur including facial cellulitis, and imaging may be required to identify abscesses, suppurative nodes, or other secondary complications. Particular attention must be paid in terms of treating and monitoring cellulitis affecting the central face, especially an area that has been described as the "danger triangle" (extending from the corners of the mouth to the bridge of the nose), due to the risk of septic thrombophlebitis extending between the facial veins to intracranial veins including the cavernous sinuses.

Facial fillers are injected into the premaxillary soft tissues, periorbital, and perioral tissues in order to obtain a cosmetically pleasing facial contour to counteract effects of ageing, following traumatic disfigurement or in fat wasting conditions such as HIV. Some patients withhold a clinical history of facial injections or deny that the procedures have taken place. Facial fillers may be composed of transposed adipose tissue (autologous) or of biological materials or synthetics (Mundada et al. 2017). Their appearances can vary depending on composition, although on MRI, synthetic filler material typically has high T2 weighted signal. The infection rate following injection of filler material is low at 0.04% (Mundada et al. 2017). These infections can develop at any time and typically appear as localised areas of subcutaneous fat stranding, swelling, and increased enhancement, with or without abscess formation (Fig. 59a and b ).

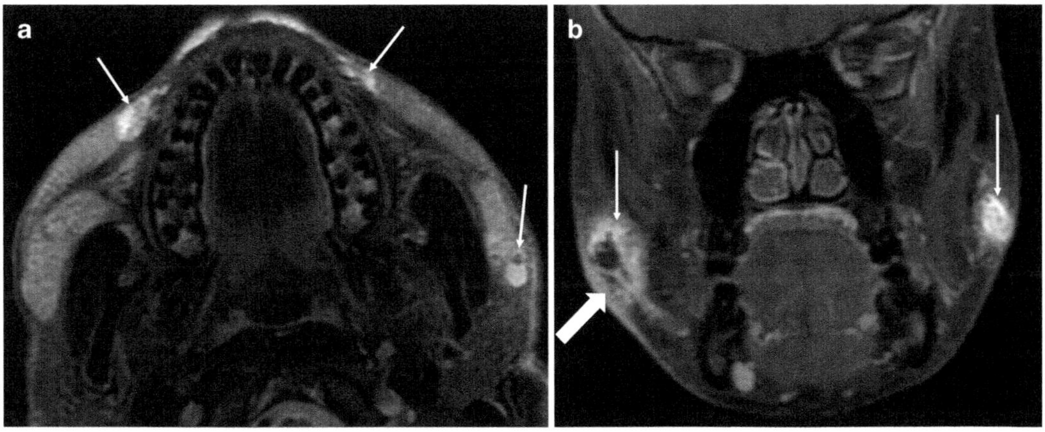


**Fig. 59** (**a**) Axial fat saturated T2 weighted MRI showing facial cosmetic filler as clusters of high signal material in the subcutaneous tissues bilaterally (white arrows). (**b**) Coronal fat saturated contrast enhanced T1 weighted MRI showing avid enhancement of the material (thin white arrows) with marked surrounding premaxillary fat stranding (thick white arrows), compatible with focal filler infection

Cervicofacial necrotising fasciitis (NF) is a rare, rapidly progressive, and life-threatening infection of the musculoaponeurotic system extending within superficial and deep fascial planes. Most are due to pharyngeal or odontogenic infections, followed by skin, post-surgical, and miscellaneous causes. Immunocompetent as well as compromised individuals may be affected, and mortality is between 10 and 20% overall but up to 30% in diabetics (Gore 2018 & Gunaratne et al. 2018). Treatment requires high dose broad-spectrum intravenous antibiotics and timely surgical debridement(s). Initial clinical findings can be subtle and overlooked, and CECT may be important in suggesting the diagnosis as well as mapping the extent (Becker et al. 1997). CECT typically shows marked inflammatory changes and fluid in the subcutaneous tissues (cellulitis) and deeper fascial planes (fasciitis), with or without muscle involvement (myositis) (Fig. 60). The presence of multiple gas locules within the involved tissues is an important feature but not essential for diagnosis and, besides, air locules are not specific as they can also occur due to surgical emphysema secondary to sinonasal injuries. Another imaging feature of NF is the presence of irregular hypoenhancing regions extending across tissue planes, which are believed to represent areas of recent necrosis (Tung-Yiu et al. 2000), and differing from abscesses, these display no or minimal rim enhancement on CECT. The mediastinum is an important review area on CECT as mediastinitis is common and associated with poorer outcomes (Becker et al. 1997).

## 14 Summary

Acute head and neck infections are varied and can be severe and life threatening. The initial assessment should include an ABCD approach as per the Advanced Trauma Life Support primary survey protocol. In particular, the risk of airway compromise must be assessed prior to imaging investigations, and early involvement of the multidisciplinary team including anaesthetists and head and neck surgeons is recommended.

Contrast enhanced CT is the best imaging modality overall, although US may be used first line for accessible soft tissue abnormalities. CECT allows rapid characterisation of organ and airway-threatening abnormalities including Ludwig's angina, parapharyngeal and retropharyngeal space abscesses, and orbital abscesses. Foreign bodies should not be missed. Deep neck space collections may be transpatial and should be described in detail to enable appropriate surgical management. The patient should be imaged from the skull base to the mediastinum if a deep neck space infection is suspected. Intracranial complications are common, and should be actively excluded in paranasal sinus, otomastoid, skull base, and severe facial infections. Several take home points for different types of infection are listed in Table 4.

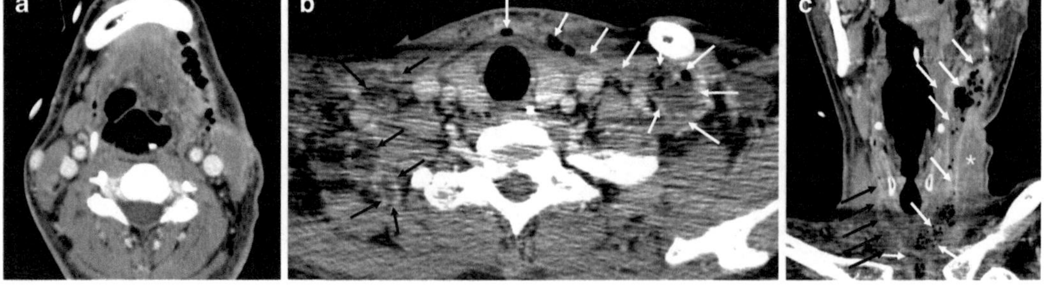


**Fig. 60** Necrotising fasciitis. Axial (**a**, **b**) and coronal (**c**) CECT showing fluid and gas within the left investing layer of deep cervical fascia (white arrows) with surrounding inflammation and myositis of the left sternocleidomastoid muscle (asterisks). This infection descended rapidly from the left submandibular space (**a**) to the supraclavicular fossa (**b**). Smaller collections are also present on the right (black arrows). Mediastinitis was present (not shown). Courtesy of Dr Julian Goh, Singapore

**Table 4** Important take home points when reviewing acute infections on head and neck CT scans

| Acute condition | Imaging tips |
|---|---|
| 1. Acute sinusitis | Incidental sinus opacification is common in the general population.<br>Sinus expansion in the presence of acute sinusitis may suggest a pyocele.<br>Exclude intracranial complications, e.g. subdural empyema, and orbital abscess.<br>Highlight the possibility of severe sinusitis including angio-invasive fungal sinusitis if there are bony erosions and inflammatory changes around the affected sinus(es).<br>Fungal sinusitis is more common in diabetic or immunocompromised patients and can be fatal due to intracranial complications including arterial thromboembolism.<br>In maxillary sinusitis, examine the upper dentition for a periapical/periodontal infective source. |
| 2. Otological and skull base infections | Coalescent otomastoiditis: mastoid opacification is associated with destruction of intramastoid osseous septations. Actively exclude extra-mastoid abscesses and intracranial complications, especially sigmoid sinus thrombosis, intracranial abscess, and petrous apicitis.<br>Petrous apicitis: suspect if clinical triad of otitis media, abducens nerve palsy, and retro-orbital pain. Patients are at risk of cavernous sinus thrombosis and meningitis.<br>Necrotising otitis externa: More common in diabetics and immunocompromised patients. Examine for cortical osseous erosions in the ear canal and mastoid process, as well as inflammatory changes around the lateral skull base. |
| 3. Dental and related infections | OPGs and plain CT may be sufficient in most cases, although CECT is required for more extensive infections associated with soft tissue complications.<br>Dental infections are a common and easily overlooked cause of other head and neck infections including facial and floor of mouth cellulitis, masticator space abscesses, sinusitis, osteomyelitis, and acute suppurative lymphadenitis. |
| 4. Pharyngeal and deep space infections | Supraglottitis, pharyngitis including tonsillitis: These can be airway emergencies. Identify complications including intramucosal abscess(es), peritonsillar abscess (medial to the constrictor muscle), extrapharyngeal abscesses (lateral to the muscle), and internal jugular vein thrombophlebitis (Lemierre's syndrome).<br>Retropharyngeal abscess: CECT coverage must extend to the upper thorax to identify mediastinal extension (mediastinitis).<br>Pitfall: Retropharyngeal inflammation/oedema can have mass effect and low CT attenuation/high T2 weighted signal, which can mimic abscesses, although only abscesses show rim enhancement.<br>Traumatic injuries: Lacerations of the pharynx/oesophagus and retained foreign bodies (fish bones) should be excluded, especially as clinical history may be unclear.<br>Parapharyngeal abscess: commonest cause is acute tonsillitis/peritonsillar abscess, although submandibular/ sublingual space and masticator space infections can also track posteriorly into this space. These can extend into the infrahyoid neck via the carotid space. These should be mapped meticulously on imaging for appropriate surgical planning. |
| 5. Orbital infections | Differentiate pre- or post-septal orbital cellulitis, especially as the latter has a high rate of serious complications. CECT is indicated to identify complications including abscesses. Document any extension of orbital infection to the orbital apex, thrombosis of ophthalmic veins, and/or cavernous sinuses.<br>Acute dacrocystitis and dacroadenitis have typical appearances on CECT. Identify acute suppurative complications including abscesses and orbital cellulitis. |
| 6. Acute salivary gland infections | Imaging should confirm the diagnosis, identify any obstructive lesions (e.g. stones, strictures, or tumours (rare)), and any acute complications including intra or extra glandular abscesses and severe facial or floor of mouth cellulitis (Ludwig's angina). |
| 7. Infected congenital cysts | Infections of branchial cleft and thyroglossal duct anomalies are most common. These may have communications (e.g. fistula or sinus) with the aerodigestive tract and skin Necrotic metastatic nodes can mimic infected second or third branchial cleft cysts on imaging, so consider imaging follow-up and fine needle aspiration of the cyst wall if presenting in adults >30 years.<br>Suppurative intra- or peri-thyroid infections (abscesses) are rare and should raise suspicion of an underlying fourth branchial cleft anomaly. |

(continued)

**Table 4** (continued)

| Acute condition | Imaging tips |
|---|---|
| 8. Traumatic infections | Document all sites of injury meticulously as they may alter treatment in terms of extent of surgical explorations and decontamination to prevent delayed sepsis. Examine wounds on different CT window settings, multiple planes, and thick sections to identify foreign bodies. Oesophageal or pharyngeal lacerations/perforations can be subtle or not directly visible; carefully inspect the adjacent neck spaces including parapharynx, retropharynx, and visceral space for locules of fluid or gas. |
| 9 Post-operative infections | Know the normal post-operative imaging appearances in order to identify abnormalities including infections. Review operative notes for any procedural complications and use of dressings/packing materials.<br>Describe any sizeable post-operative seromas or haematomas as these can become infected. |
| 10. Infected head and neck tumours or nodal metastases | Infected or inflamed head and neck tumours or metastatic nodes can mimic acute neck infections. Furthermore, needle cytology results of infected tumours can be misleading during the acute infective episode. Consequently, follow-up imaging and repeat FNA or preferably core needle biopsy should be performed after the acute episode has resolved. |
| 11. Facial infections | Infections in the central face can spread intracranially via communicating veins and may cause significant complications including septic cavernous sinus thrombosis.<br>Cosmetic facial fillers can develop acute localised infections including cellulitis and abscesses.<br>CECT has an important role in diagnosing and mapping necrotising fasciitis, especially as initial clinical signs may be mild or misleading. Diagnostic clues include extensive cellulitis and fasciitis, unexplained air locules in the soft tissues, and/or areas of poorly enhancing soft tissue (necrosis). |

## References


Abdelmasih M, Kayssi A, Roche-Nagle G (2019) Penetrating paediatric neck trauma. BMJ Case Rep 12(5):e226436

Razek AA, Huang BY (2012) Lesions of the petrous apex: classification and findings at CT and MR imaging. Radiographics 32:151–173. Published online https://doi.org/10.1148/rg.321105758

Aribandi M, McCoy V, Bazan C (2007) Imaging features of invasive and non-invasive fungal sinusitis: a review. Radiographics 27(5):1283–1296

Asheim J, Spickler E (2005) CT demonstration of dacryolithiasis complicated by dacryocystitis. AJNR 26(10):2640–2641

Baert AL, Sartor K (2003) In: King SJ, Boothroyd AE (eds) Paediatric ENT radiology. Springer, Berlin

Bagchi A, Hira P, Mittal K, Priyamvara A, Dey A et al. (2018) Branchial cleft cysts: A pictorial review. Polish Journal of Radiology 83:e204-e209. https://doi.org/10.5114/pjr.2018.76278

Becker M, Zbaren P, Hermans R (1997) Necrotizing fasciitis of the head and neck: role of CT in diagnosis and management. Radiology 202:471–476

Brook I (2003) Microbiology and management of deep facial infections and Lemierre syndrome. ORL J Otorhinolaryngol Relat Spec 65(2):117–120

Caruso P, Watkins L, Suwansaard L, Yamamoto M, Durand M, Romo L, Rincon S, Curtin H (2006) Odontogenic orbital inflammation: clinical and CT findings – initial observations. Radiology 239:187–194

Chapman MN, Rohini NN, Akman AS, Saito N, Sekiya K, Kaneda T, Sakai O (2013) Periapical lucency around the tooth: radiologic evaluation and differential diagnosis. Radiographics 33(1):E15–E32

Chengazi H, Bhatt A (2019) Pathology of the carotid space. Insights into Imaging 10(21). https://doi.org/10.1186/s13244-019-0704-z

Choi K, Park SK (2014) Petrositis with bilateral abducens nerve palsies complicated by acute otitis media. Clin Exp Otorhinolaryngol 7(1):59–62

Chul HJ, See YP, Pa-Chun W (2005) A case of tympanogenic labyrinthitis complicated by acute otitis media. Yonsei Med J 46(1):161–165

Cure J, Vattoth S, Shah R (2012) Radiopaque jaw lesions: an approach to the differential diagnosis. Radiographics 32:1909–1925

Gonzalez M, Durairnaj V (2010) Understanding paediatric bacterial preseptal and orbital cellulitis. Midd East Afr J Opth 17(2):134–137

Gore MR (2018) Odontogenic necrotizing fasciitis. A systemic review of the literature. BMC Ear Nose Throat Disord 18:14

Gunaratne DA, Tseros EA, Hasan Z (2018) Cervical necrotizing fasciitis: systemic review and analysis of

1235 reported cases from the literature. Head Neck 40:2094–2102
Hansen A, Helvik A, Nordgard S, Bugten V, Stovner L, Haberg A, Eggesbo H (2014) Incidental findings in MRI of the paranasal sinuses in adults: a population-based study. EN&T Disord 14(13). http://www.biomedcentral.com/1472-6815/14/13 Accessed online on 30 Oct 2019
Harnsberger HR (1995) Handbook of head and neck imaging, 2nd edn. Mosby, St Louis
Jung WS, Ahn KJ, Park M, Kim JY, Choi JJ, Kim B, Hahn ST (2007) The radiological spectrum of orbital pathologies that involve the lacrimal gland and the lacrimal fossa. Korean J Radiol 8(4):336–342
Koeller K, Alamo L, Adair C, Smirniotopoulos J (1999) Congenital cystic masses of the neck: radiological pathological correlation. Radiographics 19:121–146
Kool D, Blickman J (2007) Advanced Trauma life support. ABCDE from a radiological perspective. Emerg Radiology 14(3):135–141
Lin S, Melki S, Ahadizadesh E, Zender C (2017) Post-operative MRSA infections in head and neck surgery. Am J Otolaryngol 38(4):417–421
Lund V, MacKay I (1993) Staging in rhinosinusitis. Rhinology 31(4):183–184
Madani G, Beale T (2009) Sinonasal inflammatory disease. Semin Ultrasound CT MR 30:17–24
Meng Y, Zhang L, Piao Y, Lou H, Wang K, Wang C (2019) The use of magnetic resonance imaging in the differential diagnosis of allergic fungal sinusitis and eosinophilic mucin rhinosinusitis. J Thorac Dis 11(8):3569–3577
Momeni A, Roberts C, Chew F (2007) Imaging of chronic and exotic sinonasal disease: a review. AJR 189:S35–S45
Mundada R, Kohler R, Boudabbous S, Trellu L, Platon A, Becker M (2017) Injectable facial fillers: imaging features, complications, and diagnostic pitfalls at MRI and PET CT. Insights Imaging 8:557–572
Nguyen V, Singh A, Altmeyer W, Tantiwongkosi B (2017) Demystifying orbital emergencies: a pictorial review. Radiographics 37:947–962
Offiah C, Hall E (2012) Imaging assessment of penetrating injury of the neck and face. Insights Imaging 3(5):419–431
Ogihara H, Takeuchi K, Majma Y (2009) Risk factors for post-operative infections in head and neck surgery. Auris Nasus Larynx 36(4):457–460
Parikh SL, Venkatraman G, DelGaudio JM (2004) Invasive fungal sinusitis: a 15-year review from a single institution. Am J Rhinol 18(2):75–81
Penel N, Lefebvre D, Fournier C, Sarini J, Kara A, Lefebvre L (2001) Risk factors for wound infection in head and neck cancer surgery: a prospective study. Head Neck 23:447–455
Sabhalok SS, Shetty LS, Sarve PH, Setiya SV, Bharadwaj SR (2016) Epidermoid and dermoid cysts of the head and neck region. Plast Aesthet Res 3:347–350
Sahoo A, Preetam C, Samal D, Sarkar S (2017) Citelli's abscess following otitis media: a case report. Iran J Otorhinolaryngol 29(92):161–163
Scheinfeld MH, Shifteh K, Avery L, Dym H, Dym R (2012) Teeth: what the radiologist should know. Radiographics 32:1927–1944
Scrafton D, Qureishi A, Nogueira C, Mortimore S (2014) Luc's abscess as an unlucky complication of mastoiditis. Ann R Coll Surg Engl 96(5):e28–e30
Tung-Yiu W, Jehn-Shyun H, Ching-Hung C, Hung-An C (2000) Cervical necrotizing fasciitis of odontogenic origin: a report of 11 cases. J Oral Maxillofasc Surg 58:1347–1352
Warner G, Burgess A, Patel S, Martinez-Devesa P, Corbridge R (2009) Otolaryngology and head and neck surgery (oxford specialist handbooks in surgery). Oxford University Press, Oxford
Wolf G, Anderhuber W, Kuhn F (1993) Development of the paranasal sinuses in children: implications for paranasal sinus surgery. Ann Otol Rhinol Laryngol 102(9):705
World Health Organisation (2019) Global Tuberculosis Report. https://www.who.int/tb/publications/global_report/en/. accessed online 30 Oct 2019